THERAPEUTIC DRUG MONITORING

THERAPEUTIC DRUG MONITORING

Edited by

Gerald E. Schumacher, PharmD, PhD
Professor of Pharmacy
Co-Director, National Education and Research Center
for Outcome Assessment in Health Care
Northeastern University
Bouvé College of Pharmacy and Health Sciences
Boston, Massachusetts

Appleton & Lange
Norwalk, Connecticut

Copyright © 1995 by Appleton & Lange
A Simon & Schuster Company

95 96 97 98 / 10 9 8 7 6 5 4 3 2 1

Prentice Hall International (UK) Limited, *London*
Prentice Hall of Australia Pty. Limited, *Sydney*
Prentice Hall Canada, Inc., *Toronto*
Prentice Hall Hispanoamericana, S.A., *Mexico*
Prentice Hall of India Private Limited, *New Delhi*
Prentice Hall of Japan, Inc., *Tokyo*
Simon & Schuster Asia Pte. Ltd., *Singapore*
Editora Prentice Hall do Brasil Ltda., *Rio de Janeiro*
Prentice Hall, *Englewood Cliffs, New Jersey*

Therapeutic drug monitoring / edited by Gerald E. Schumacher.
     p.   cm.
   ISBN 0-8385-8946-4
   1. Drug monitoring.   I. Schumacher, Gerald E.
   [DNLM: 1. Drug Monitoring.   2. Drugs.   WB 330 T3985 1995]
RM301.9.T48 1995
615.5′8—dc20
DNLM/DLC
for Library of Congress   94-40831
                                                     CIP

Acquisitions Editor: Cheryl L. Mehalik
Production Editor: Jennifer Sinsavich
Designer: Mary Skudlarek

ISBN 0-8385-8946-4

90000

9 780838 589465

To my wife Florence,
who has always and in all ways been there.

Contributors

Judith T. Barr, ScD, MT (ASCP), CLS (NCA)
Associate Professor of Pharmacy Administration
Associate Professor of Medical Laboratory Sciences
Director, National Education and Research Center for Outcome Assessment in Health Care
Northeastern University
Bouvé College of Pharmacy and Health Sciences
Boston, Massachusetts

Joseph S. Bertino, Jr., PharmD
Assistant Director, Department of Pharmacy Services
Co-Director, Clinical Pharmacology Research Center
The Mary Imogene Basssett Hospital
Cooperstown, New York

Timothy G. Burke, PharmD
Clinical Pharmacy Specialist in Cardiology
The University of Iowa Hospitals and Clinics
Adjunct Assistant Professor of Clinical Pharmacy
The University of Iowa
College of Pharmacy
Iowa City, Iowa

Virgina E. Eaton, PharmD
Research Fellow
University of Texas
M.D. Anderson Cancer Center
Division of Pharmacy
Houston, Texas

Sharon M. Erdman, PharmD
Loyola University Medical Center
Department of Pharmacy
Maywood, Illinois

Larry Ereshefsky, PharmD, FCCP
Professor of Pharmacy
The University of Texas at Austin
Austin, Texas
Professor of Pharmacology and Psychiatry
University of Texas Health Science Center at San Antonio
San Antonio, Texas

William R. Garnett, PharmD, FCCP
Professor of Pharmacy and Pharmaceutics
Department of Pharmacy and Pharmaceutics
Medical College of Virginia
Virginia Commonwealth University
Richmond, Virginia

Thaddeus H. Grasela, Jr., PharmD
Associate Professor of Pharmacy
Director, Drug Surveillance Network
State University of New York at Buffalo
School of Pharmacy
Buffalo, New York

Terrance A. Killilea, PharmD
Director of Clinical Services
H.P.I. Health Care Services, Inc.
Albuquerque, New Mexico

Timothy Madden, PharmD
Assistant Professor
Director, Pharmaceutical Research
University of Texas
M.D. Anderson Cancer Center
Divisions of Pharmacy and Pediatrics
Houston, Texas

S. James Matthews, PharmD
Associate Professor of Clinical Pharmacy
Northeastern University
Bouvé College of Pharmacy and Health Sciences
Boston, Massachusetts

David I. Min, PharmD, MS
Assistant Professor
The University of Iowa
College of Pharmacy
Iowa City, Iowa

John E. Murphy, PharmD, FCCP, FCP
Professor and Head
Departments of Pharmacy Practice and Pharmaceutical Sciences
University of Arizona
College of Pharmacy
Tucson, Arizona

Alan H. Mutnick, PharmD
Assistant Director, Clinical Practice
The University of Iowa Hospitals and Clinics
Adjunct Associate Professor of Clinical Pharmacy
The University of Iowa
College of Pharmacy
Iowa City, Iowa

Milap C. Nahata, PharmD, FCCP
Professor of Pharmacy and Pediatrics
The Ohio State University
Colleges of Pharmacy and Medicine
Columbus, Ohio

Randy D. Pryka, PharmD
Assistant Professor of Pharmacy Practice
The University of Toledo
College of Pharmacy
Toledo, Ohio

Keith A. Rodvold, PharmD, FCCP
Associate Professor
Departments of Pharmacy Practice and Infectious Diseases
The University of Illinois at Chicago
Colleges of Pharmacy and Medicine
Chicago, Illinois

Gerald E. Schumacher, PharmD, PhD
Professor of Pharmacy
Co-Director, National Education and Research Center for Outcome Assessment in Health Care
Northeastern University
Bouvé College of Pharmacy and Health Sciences
Boston, Massachusetts

Gregory B. Toney, PharmD
Clinical Assistant Professor of Pharmacy
The University of Texas at Austin
Austin, Texas
Clinical Assistant Professor of Pharmacology
University of Texas Health Science Center at San Antonio
Clinical Pharmacologist
San Antonio State Hospital
San Antonio, Texas

Julia E. Vertrees, PharmD
Clinical Pharmacologist, Clinical Research Unit
San Antonio State Hospital
Clinical Assistant Professor of Pharmacology
University of Texas Health Science Center at San Antonio
San Antonio, Texas
Clinical Assistant Professor of Pharmacy
The University of Texas at Austin
Austin, Texas

Contents

Preface

Therapeutic drug monitoring, or TDM as it is commonly called, is about using drug serum concentrations, pharmacokinetics, and pharmacodynamics to individualize and optimize patient responses to drug therapy. It is also about understanding the merits, limitations, and applications of using serum drug concentrations in quantitative decision making.

This book evolves from my 25 years of teaching clinical pharmacokinetics and TDM to undergraduate and graduate students. The years have taught me that while it is essential to understand drug kinetics, dynamics, and therapeutics to monitor drug therapy, it is equally important to understand the ambiance that surrounds TDM: the laboratory environment that supports it, the decision analytic framework in which it is best expressed, and the assessment of outcomes resulting from applying it as an intervention.

So this is a textbook that covers in detail the drugs that are commonly monitored using serum drug concentrations as adjuncts to decision making. But it is also a reference that contains material not presently available in textbooks on TDM: how drugs are monitored, the total testing process used by the clinical laboratory to process and interpret serum drug concentrations, the test performance criteria describing the usefulness and limitations associated with using serum drug concentrations in decision analysis, and the template for characterizing outcomes of TDM from both system-related and patient-centered viewpoints.

To enhance the usefulness of this book as a learning tool for students, each chapter opens with points "To Keep in Mind," and concludes with a summary of essential concepts and the opportunity to test knowledge through questions and cases with answers.

I am grateful to the many authors who have contributed their expertise; often with eloquence. The dedication and cooperation, offered without regard to overburdened agendas, are most appreciated.

Lastly, let me hear from you; what pleases will be appreciated, the suggestions will be useful, and what displeases needs to be known.

Gerald E. Schumacher
February 1995

DRUG CONCENTRATION CONVERSIONS FOR INTERNATIONAL MARKETS

Drug	USA (Mass) Units	International (Molar) Units
Amiodarone	1.0 mg/L	1.4 μmol/L
Carbamazepine	1.0 mg/L	4.0 μmol/L
Chloramphenicol	1.0 mg/L	3.1 μmol/L
Cyclosporine	1.0 mcg/L	0.8 nmol/L
Digoxin	1.0 μg/L	1.2 nmol/L
Gentamicin	1.0 mg/L	Use USA units
Lidocaine	1.0 mg/L	4.0 μmol/L
Lithium	1.0 mEq/L	1.0 mmol/L
Phenobarbital	1.0 mg/L	4.3 μmol/L
Phenytoin	1.0 mg/L	4.0 μmol/L
Procainamide	1.0 mg/L	4.0 μmol/L
Quinidine	1.0 mg/L	3.0 μmol/L
Theophylline	1.0 mg/L	5.5 μmol/L
Tobramycin	1.0 mg/L	Use USA units
Valproic acid	1.0 mg/L	7.0 μmol/L
Vancomycin	1.0 mg/L	Use USA units

THERAPEUTIC
DRUG MONITORING

Chapter 1

Introduction to Therapeutic Drug Monitoring

Gerald E. Schumacher

Keep in Mind

- Therapeutic drug monitoring aims to promote optimum drug treatment by maintaining serum drug concentrations within a "therapeutic range," above which toxicity occurs too often and below which the drug is too often ineffective.

- Therapeutic drug monitoring is a practice applied to a small group of drugs in which there is a direct relationship between concentration and response, as well as a narrow range of concentrations that are effective and safe and for which serum drug concentrations are used in conjunction with other measures of clinical observation to assess patient status.

- Serum concentrations are used as the most practical intermediate endpoint to gauge treatment when there is no clearly observable therapeutic or toxic endpoint and other more direct, intermediate endpoints are not available for measuring response to the drug (eg, blood pressure for hypertension or prothrombin time for preventing emboli).

- The notion of a therapeutic range is more a probabilistic concept than an absolute entity. It represents a range of drug concentrations within which the probability of a desired clinical response is relatively high and the probability of unacceptable toxicity is relatively low. Some patients, however, will respond effectively below the therapeutic range, whereas others need concentrations above it. Similarly, some patients have toxic reactions within the therapeutic range.

- The most common reasons for using a serum drug level as a guide are to provide additional information to be used in conjunction with other clinical data to assist in determining patient status; to provide a basis for individualizing patient dosage regimens; and to determine if a change in drug pharmacokinetics has occurred in a patient during a course of treatment, either spontaneously or as a result of a change in physiologic state, a change in diet, or introduction of an additional drug(s) which may alter the baseline pharmacokinetics.

This book is about using drug serum concentrations, pharmacokinetics, and pharmacodynamics to individualize and optimize patient responses to drug therapy. Some call this *therapeutic drug monitoring,* as we will, but others also call it *applied pharmacokinetics* or *clinical pharmacokinetics.* By any of these names, it blends knowledge of therapeutics, pharmacology, pharmacokinetics, laboratory technology, and clinical medicine and applies it to certain drugs

1

that require determination of patient-specific dosage regimens to maximize therapeutic effectiveness while minimizing toxicity.

This book is also about adding a clinical pharmacokinetic point of view to thinking about drug therapy—how pharmacokinetics influences drug selection, the comparison of drugs, decisions about dosage regimens, and how drugs are monitored.

The early chapters focus on the environment, process, and outcome of therapeutic drug monitoring. What is the role of the clinical laboratory? How are drugs monitored? How are serum concentrations interpreted? How are these concentrations used to make decisions about treating patients? What are the strengths and limitations of therapeutic drug monitoring? How has therapeutic drug monitoring influenced patient care?

Subsequent chapters then emphasize the practice of therapeutic drug monitoring, discussing the major drugs—pharmacology, pharmacokinetics, therapeutics, monitoring parameters, and application to developing and modifying dosage regimens—along with case studies and self-assessment questions.

Stated most simply, therapeutic drug monitoring aims to promote optimum drug treatment by maintaining serum drug concentrations within a "therapeutic range," above which toxicity occurs too often and below which the drug is too often ineffective.[1] In this textbook we make a more rigorous definition by restricting the term *therapeutic drug monitoring* (and often shorten the term by using the acronym TDM) to a *small group of drugs in which there is a direct relationship between concentration and response, as well as a narrow range of concentrations that are effective and safe, and for which serum drug concentrations are used in conjunction with other measures of clinical observation to assess patient status.* This probably seems too wordy but the definition includes a number of important considerations and qualifications.

- Using a drug concentration implies that a more direct measure of patient response (blood pressure, blood coagulation time) is not readily available.
- Noting the restriction to drugs with a narrow range of effective, safe concentrations excludes the majority of drugs for which such meticulous scrutiny is unnecessary as a wide range of dosage or variation in response may be tolerated without risk.
- Evaluating patient response on the basis of a serum drug level alone is risky because this measure is only one of many factors (eg, age, severity of disease, electrolyte levels, other drugs being taken) that must be taken into account in evaluating a patient's response to a drug.

HISTORY AND EVOLUTION

Until the 1960s, drug therapy was largely a case of trial and error.[2,3] Although guidelines were generally available that provided broad ranges thought to be effective and safe, most practitioners approached dosing in an empirical manner. Dosage was usually initiated at low levels and then increased until an effect was obtained or, despite the guidelines, toxic reactions occurred. Typically, more than one half of the adverse drug reactions in a major teaching hospital in the 1960s resulted from standard dosages that were too high for the patient.[4]

Noting that some early research in the 1950s[5–8] had suggested that serum levels could be used to determine individual patient differences in pharmacokinetics and also guide responses to treatment, researchers looked to expand on this work to advance drug effectiveness and safety. For some types of drugs, serum drug concentrations were postulated to be a better index than dose to guiding treatment. Serum levels were expected to be a better indicator of drug concentrations at receptor sites, perhaps could be used to correlate drug levels and patient responses, and should be useful in determining pharmacokinetic parameters of drugs in individual patients.

So the growth in therapeutic drug monitoring was due to a combination of interacting and mutually reinforcing factors.[2] With the appreciation that standard dosage regimens led to varying patient outcomes, clinicians needed more scientific knowledge and supporting assay technology to tailor drug therapy for individual patients. These needs induced scientists to develop analytic instrumentation that could more accurately characterize the pharmacokinetic properties and therapeutic serum concentration ranges of the drugs. By the end of the 1960s, initial work on determining pharmacokinetic parameters and therapeutic serum concentration ranges for some cardiac drugs, antiepileptics, bronchodilators, and antibiotics was being published.[9-19]

Caught up in the enthusiasm for using therapeutic serum drug ranges, the 1970s and early 1980s were a period of extensive investigation and application of TDM. Physicians wanted to monitor more of their patients and this offered an excellent opportunity for pharmacists to make a contribution. Focusing on their growing knowledge of applied pharmacokinetics and clinical pharmacology, clinical pharmacists saw TDM as an opportunity for greater involvement in drug treatment. They routinely offered assistance in interpreting drug levels, calculating dosage regimens, and monitoring drugs in general. Pharmacy's enthusiasm and availability, coupled with medicine's own growing involvement and acceptance of the expanded role for pharmacists, spurred the laboratory industry to develop more rapid and accurate analytic technology, resulting in nearly a 500-fold increase in the TDM product market over the last 25 years. This led some to question the growth of TDM and wonder whether its usefulness has been overemphasized.[20-22]

RATIONALE FOR THERAPEUTIC DRUG MONITORING

Give the same dose of drug to a group of patients and responses vary. Some do not receive the desired effect, others do, and still others show adverse reactions in addition to a therapeutic effect. In those who receive a therapeutic effect without a toxic reaction, doubling the dose increases the effect without consequence for some whereas it brings on ill effects for others.

These observations lead many clinicians to the three assumptions that underlie the use of serum concentration measurements in TDM as a method for decreasing intrapatient and interpatient variability in dose versus response: (1) measuring patient drug levels provides an opportunity to adjust for variations in patient pharmacokinetics by individualizing drug dosage, because (2) the serum drug concentration is a better predictor of patient response than is dose, and (3) there is a good relationship between serum drug concentration and pharmacologic response.

In the simplest scheme, drug dose, concentration, and response are related as follows: dose $—(A)\rightarrow$ serum concentration $—(B)\rightarrow$ pharmacologic response, where A and B are referred to as the pharmacokinetic and pharmacodynamic phases of the dose–response relationship. The pharmacokinetic phase includes the processes of absorption, distribution, and clearance, which vary greatly from patient to patient. The pharmacodynamic phase, although also subject to a number of factors and patient variation, is assumed by many to be less variable than the pharmacokinetic phase and surely does bring the serum concentration closer to the end result than does the dose administered.

APPLYING CLINICAL PHARMACOKINETICS IN THERAPEUTIC DRUG MONITORING

Figure 1–1 shows the relationship between dose administered, pharmacokinetic variables, serum concentration, and pharmacologic response. The only variables that the practitioner controls in the dose-versus-response scheme are the amount of drug administered and how often it is given. These variables may be manipulated to compensate for the patient's pharmacokinetic variables, which the practitioner does not control, to achieve some designated serum concentration. If, as indicated in the scheme, a clear relationship between serum level and response has been established for a drug, then it does seem reasonable that anchoring drug therapy on serum concentration should decrease the influence of intrapatient and interpatient variation in pharmacokinetics on pharmacologic response.

Selecting a steady-state serum concentration goal is frequently referred to as using a *target concentration strategy,* a term coined by Sheiner and Tozer.[23] The target concentration falls within the range of effective and safe concentrations determined for the population at large. So the practitioner begins by assuming that the patient behaves like the average member of his or her population with respect to pharmacokinetics, serum level, and expected response, and uses average pharmacokinetic parameters to calculate the dose needed to meet the target concentra-

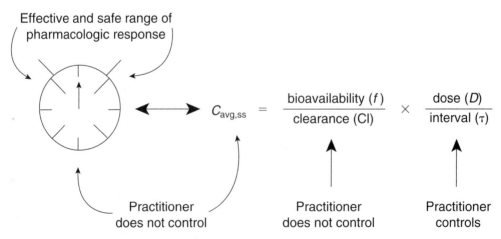

Figure 1–1. Pharmacokinetic factors influencing serum drug concentration and pharmacologic response.

tion objective. If after administering the dosage regimen until steady state is reached, the patient is responding appropriately and the measured concentration is within the therapeutic (target concentration) range, no adjustment is necessary. If, however, the starting assumption that the patient behaves similarly to the average turns out to be incorrect, because the response is subtherapeutic or toxic, due to either pharmacokinetic or pharmacodynamic behavior that is atypical for the population, then the only maneuver available to the practitioner is to manipulate the practitioner-controlled input variables, dose and frequency, to bring the pharmacologic or therapeutic response within the accepted range. Usually, but not always, an effective and safe response occurs after the dosage regimen has been adjusted to bring the serum concentration within the target concentration range. Some patients, however, will surely achieve the desired response below or above the target concentration range.

Straightforward as this process may appear, a number of factors mitigate against widespread application of therapeutic drug monitoring and restrict it to a few drugs for which the benefits of TDM outweigh the reservations:

- TDM is very costly, in terms of equipment, supplies, personnel to draw the levels and interpret the results, and investment in research to collect the necessary concentration versus response data.
- Some drugs have such a broad range of regimens that are effective and safe that using an intermediate gauge like serum concentrations is unnecessary.
- Even for some of the drugs that may potentially benefit from TDM, because they appear to have a narrow range of flexibility in dosage, the relationship between serum concentration and response is not firmly established.
- The population for which data have been obtained from studies of serum concentration versus effect (eg, males younger than 50 with congestive heart failure and normal values for renal and liver functions, thyroid, and electrolytes) may differ from the population to which the patient belongs (eg, females older than 70 with congestive heart failure, but impaired renal and/or liver function and abnormal electrolytes) for which reference data are not available.
- And for some drugs, more effective intermediate measures of response than serum level (eg, blood pressure, blood coagulation time) are available.

_____ **EXAMPLE 1–1** _____

Here is an overly simplified example of applying clinical pharmacokinetics in TDM. Refer to the scheme in Figure 1–1 and assume that theophylline is to be administered as aminophylline in a loading dose followed by a continuous intravenous infusion to a newly admitted 40-year-old male patient of average weight (~ 70 kg) who appears to have no cardiac problems, claims not to smoke, and is taking no other drugs. As the commonly accepted therapeutic range is 10 to 20 μg/mL, the clinician suggests a conservative target concentration goal of 12 μg/mL.

Start by assuming that the patient behaves like the average person in his population group. This means that the average theophylline clearance (Cl) for this patient is 0.04 L/kg/h, the volume of distribution (V) is 0.5 L/kg, and the half-life is 8 hours. As about 80% of aminophylline is theophylline, depending on the manufacturer, S is 0.8, because it denotes the fraction of the dosage form that is the active drug. Intravenous administration is fully absorbed, so f (bioavailability) is 1. The loading dose is used to bring the serum concentration up very quickly to the level that is expected to be achieved at steady state from the continuous infusion. Select the equation for the loading dose:

$$\text{loading dose} = [(C_{ss} \times V) / (S \times f)] = [(12 \text{ mg/L} \times 0.5 \text{ L/kg}) / (0.8 \times 1)]$$
$$= 7.5 \text{ mg/kg}$$

The loading dose is administered over a 15- to 30-minute period. After a 30-minute delay to permit drug distribution, many clinicians choose to determine the serum drug concentration to see if a level in the therapeutic range is achieved, as this gives some indication whether to continue using average parameters for the continuous infusion. Some practitioners would not take a level at this time, but would start a continuous infusion and settle for waiting until steady state is achieved (about 24 hours later will give an approximation). A serum concentration is obtained in this case 30 to 60 minutes after the loading dose and measures 14 µg/mL. As it is not far from the target concentration (12 µg/mL), no additional loading dose or change in the pharmacokinetic parameters assumed for the patient is considered for now.

Select the appropriate equation for continuous administration:

$$\text{dose}/\tau = [(Cl \times C_{ss}) / (S \times f)] = [(0.04 \text{ L/kg/h} \times 12 \text{ mg/L}) / (0.8 \times 1)]$$
$$\tau = 0.6 \text{ mg/kg/h}$$

One day after starting the regimen, the patient seems to be responding appropriately and without adverse reactions, and because approximately 90% of the steady-state concentration will be reached in a period of three half-lives, the time seems reasonable (24 hours after starting treatment, assuming the patient's half-life is close to the average value of 8 hours for normals) to measure the serum theophylline concentration. The level is 16 µg/mL. Because the concentration is higher than the expected target concentration of 12 µg/mL, and the only patient variable used in the equation is clearance, the patient appears to be clearing the drug more slowly than average. A patient-specific clearance may be estimated by rearranging the equation:

$$Cl = [(S \times f \times \text{dose}/\tau) / C_{inf,ss}] = [(0.8 \times 1 \times 0.6 \text{ mg/kg/h}) / 16 \text{ µg/mL}]$$
$$= 0.03 \text{ L/kg/h (a value 75% of the normal Cl of 0.04 L/kg/h)}$$

Because the patient is responding, without adversity, and the steady-state level is expected to be between 17 and 18 µg/mL (the level of 16 µg/mL obtained in the patient after three half-lives should be about 90% of steady state), the clinician recommends no change but recognizes that the serum level is on the high side of the usual therapeutic range.

Two days later when the patient is discharged, the clinician requests conversion to an oral anhydrous theophylline ($S = 1$) regimen that will produce an average steady-state concentration ($C_{avg,ss}$) during the dosage interval of 12 µg/mL. Recognizing that the equation for a continuous infusion ($C_{inf,ss}$) is the same as that for the average concentration during intermittent administration ($C_{avg,ss}$), and using the estimated patient-specific clearance,

$$\text{dose}/\tau = [(Cl \times C_{avg,ss}) / (S \times f)] = [(0.03 \text{ L/kg/h} \times 12 \text{ mg/L}) / (1 \times 1)]$$
$$= 0.36 \text{ mg/kg/h}$$
$$\sim 200 \text{ mg q8h or 300 mg q12h for a male of average weight } (\sim 70 \text{ kg})$$

THE CONCEPT OF A THERAPEUTIC RANGE

Underlying the definition of therapeutic drug monitoring at the beginning of this chapter, and the rationale for TDM just discussed, is the belief that for many drugs a specific serum concentration range can be defined that maximizes effectiveness and minimizes toxicity. Unfortunately, this concept is more complex than generally appreciated and some of the nuances of its application are commonly misunderstood:

- The notion of a therapeutic range is more a probabilistic concept than an absolute entity.[24] For any drug there are a range of serum concentrations for which the majority of patients will show an effective response with a minimum of side effects and adverse reactions. Now although the majority of patients will not show good response below this range, some patients will do so. Similarly, although most patients will show varying degrees of toxic reactions above this range, some will show no deleterious effects. Therefore, the "therapeutic range" so commonly referred to actually represents a range of drug concentrations within which the probability of a desired clinical response is relatively high and the probability of unacceptable toxicity is relatively low.
- The probabilistic concept described above refers to the likelihood of an outcome occurring within a concentration range, not to how broad the range is and, therefore, not to how much concern should be invested in it. If the effective and safe range of serum concentrations is very limited, such that reasonable intrapatient and interpatient variations in pharmacokinetics may jeopardize therapy using standard dosage guidelines, then the concept of a therapeutic range and a target concentration strategy has meaning. But if the therapeutic range for a drug covers such a wide range of serum concentrations that most patients will be effectively and safely managed within the general dosage guidelines, regardless of reasonable intrapatient and interpatient variations in pharmacokinetics, then the notion of a therapeutic range has no practical significance from a monitoring point of view.
- Drug studies characterizing serum concentration versus pharmacologic response have generally been carried out using relatively small numbers of patients and often suffer from weaknesses in study design that limit generalizations. But these data, however skimpy, have been cited repeatedly and used extensively, given the enthusiasm for TDM, so that the limitations associated with the information are often forgotten. From a statistical point of view, which is a very important consideration given the probabilistic nature of the therapeutic range, it is often difficult to make firm statements about the validity of published ranges.
- Even when properly designed studies are conducted, they may be carried out in patient populations that differ from the population in which the practitioner intends to use them. For example, a therapeutic range obtained from studies in well young volunteers may not be applicable to elderly patients. The therapeutic range for a drug obtained from patients with congestive heart failure may not apply for the drug when treating patients with arrhythmias.
- Although a patient may show an effective and safe response at a serum concentration outside the generally accepted population therapeutic range, and from the population point of view is considered an outlier, it is important to note that this likely shows that there is a patient-specific therapeutic range that should be noted and used when adjusting dosage regimens during monitoring of the patient's progress.

TABLE 1–1. THERAPEUTIC RANGE FOR COMMONLY MONITORED DRUGS

Drug	Therapeutic Range
Amikacin	20–30 µg/mL[a]
Carbamazepine	4–12 µg/mL
Digoxin	1–2 ng/mL
Gentamicin	5–10 µg/mL[b]
Lidocaine	1–5 µg/mL
Lithium	0.6–1.2 mEq/L[c]
Phenytoin	10–20 µg/mL
Procainamide	4–10 µg/mL
Quinidine	1–4 µg/mL
Theophylline	10–20 µg/mL
Tobramycin	5–10 µg/mL[b]
Valproic acid	50–100 µg/mL
Vancomycin	20–40 µg/mL[d]

[a] For peak concentration, varies with time of sampling, concentration after completion of dose; trough concentration <10 µg/mL.

[b] For peak concentration, varies with time of sampling, concentration after completion of dose; trough concentration <2 µg/mL.

[c] Morning trough concentration.

[d] For peak concentration, varies with time of sampling, concentration after completion of dose; trough concentration 5–15 µg/mL.

Given an appreciation of these caveats, the concept of a therapeutic range becomes less dogmatic than generally believed and the value of the concept is restored as a framework and anchor for therapeutic drug monitoring activities. The therapeutic ranges often cited for some of the commonly monitored drugs are shown in Table 1–1.

CHARACTERISTICS OF DRUGS APPLICABLE FOR THERAPEUTIC DRUG MONITORING

Drugs that qualify for TDM have, as a minimum, the following characteristics in common[3,21,23]:

- *Serum drug concentration is the most practical intermediate endpoint to be used when there is no clearly observable therapeutic or toxic endpoint.* Often the therapeutic endpoint is prevention of a disease, illness, or impairment. Some examples are stroke, pulmonary embolism, seizure, and renal failure. A toxic endpoint may be an arrhythmia or kidney impairment. As it is not possible to measure nonoccurrence of a condition, it is necessary to substitute some measurable response, called an *intermediate endpoint,* which has a therapeutic range that relates to prevention of the toxic condition. Examples of intermediate endpoints include blood pressure, prothrombin time, and serum drug concentration. The first two are indices more proximal to a corresponding therapeutic endpoint (blood pressure for monitoring hypertension and prothrombin time for preventing an embolus) than serum concentration. But serum levels are appropriate when a more indicative measure is not available.

- *Serum concentration is a proxy for drug concentration at the site of action.* So, for the serum concentration to be useful it should directly relate to pharmacologic effect and reflect predictable changes in response. When this is unlikely—because of either a complex relationship between concentration and effect, as seen with some drugs like the anticoagulants, or a response that may be delayed and/or outlast the decline in serum concentration, which happens for some drugs, including a few antihypertensive and psychotherapeutic agents—then serum concentration monitoring may not be useful. As proxies for response in those drugs for which a concentration-versus-response relationship has been demonstrated, drug serum levels are indicative of but not proof of outcome.
- *The range of therapeutic and safe serum concentrations is narrow.* The dose that commonly yields a subtherapeutic response is close to the dose that commonly produces toxic reactions. Another term used for characterizing the concept of the therapeutic range is the therapeutic index. The *therapeutic index* is the ratio of the top and bottom serum concentrations of the therapeutic range. Except for some antineoplastics, most drugs have a therapeutic index of 2 or more. Drugs qualifying for TDM usually have a therapeutic index of 2 to 3. For these drugs, monitoring is important because interpatient variability in pharmacokinetics results in variations in serum concentration from standard doses that may often be below or above the therapeutic range.
- *There is no predictable dose–response relationship.* A dose that produces a subtherapeutic effect in one patient may yield a toxic reaction in another. This results from a wide interpatient variability in drug absorption, distribution, and elimination. If there were little variation in patient pharmacokinetics, drug dose would be as good as serum concentration in predicting response.
- *Toxicity or lack of effectiveness puts the patient at great risk.* The notion of monitoring implies that drug therapy is important for treating or preventing the condition and that failing to produce a therapeutic result from the drug or eliciting a toxic reaction places the patient in jeopardy.
- *The pharmacologic effect observed persists for a relatively long time.* As steady-state concentrations are most reflective of pharmacologic response, acute, short, or intermittent effects are not well regulated by using serum levels.
- *A drug assay is available that is accurate, precise, and specific, requires a small sample volume, yields results quickly, and is relatively inexpensive.*

REASONS FOR MEASURING SERUM DRUG CONCENTRATIONS

Serum drug concentrations are frequently obtained as part of a pharmacokinetic analysis of the drug that contributes to determining the mean and variation in pharmacokinetic parameters in a specific population of patients or volunteers. But this is research activity intended to yield baseline data for the drug, whether or not the drug qualifies for TDM. Specific to TDM, what are the common situations in which obtaining serum concentrations from patients is necessary?[21,23,25]

- To provide additional information useful in determining patient status. Drug levels are used in conjunction with other clinical data to assist practitioners in determining how a patient is responding. Are the adverse reactions observed the result of excessive drug levels? Is the concentration of drug appropriate for the target concentration range? Is the patient's poor response due to subtherapeutic drug levels?

- To provide a basis for individualizing patient dosage regimens. A number of factors are known to modify patient pharmacokinetics and complicate the initial choice of dosage regimen.[3,25] Some of these factors include age, diet, smoking, and impairment of kidney, liver, heart, and thyroid function. A level measured early in a course of treatment provides information on how likely it is that the regimen will achieve steady-state concentrations that are in the target concentration range. A level measured during steady state determines whether the regimen achieved the desired range.
- To determine if a change in drug pharmacokinetics has occurred in a patient during a course of treatment, either spontaneously or as a result of a change in physiologic state, a change in diet, or introduction of an additional drug(s) which may alter the baseline pharmacokinetics. As noted in Figure 1–1, anything that leads to a change in pharmacokinetic parameter values may necessitate a change in dosage regimen.

Although it is common to cite patient compliance as a justification for obtaining a serum concentration, this reason is questionable. A single measurement below the therapeutic range may indicate only that a patient has missed the most recent dose, not that noncompliance is commonplace. Or, a level within or above the therapeutic range may only verify patient adherence prior to obtaining the level while it masks a general pattern of noncompliance.

TIMING OF SERUM CONCENTRATION MEASUREMENTS

When the objective is to individualize a dosage regimen, serum levels are sometimes measured early after therapy is initiated, to determine patient-specific pharmacokinetic parameters. In so doing, the dosage regimen may be tailored to the patient by using the patient-specific rather than average pharmacokinetic values for the population. But when the objective is to relate the serum level to a target concentration range, it is more common to wait to obtain a serum concentration until steady state has been achieved (three to four half-life periods after a dosage regimen has been started). This is because steady-state levels are generally used for relating to the therapeutic range. Once steady state has been reached in the patient, whether sampling time is selected to simulate the maximum, average, or minimum drug level during the dosage interval depends on what portion of the dosage interval was originally used in developing the therapeutic range now being used as a reference for the patient.

Considerations in selecting drug level sampling times are discussed more fully in Chapters 2 and 5.

INAPPROPRIATE USE OF SERUM DRUG CONCENTRATIONS

Unfortunately, serum drug levels are often obtained for reasons less justified than those cited above or are used inappropriately or even measured unneccesarily. Analyses of studies reported on serum drug level utilization conclude that as many as 50% of drug concentrations measurements may be requested unnecessarily, sampled incorrectly, or used inappropriately.[2,26] Examples include the following:

- Levels requested routinely or too often in a patient provide no new information but do incur new costs.
- Concentrations ordered for patients who appear to be responding appropriately and as expected are unnecessary. Stabilized patients do not require more serum levels unless there is reason to believe that something about the patient's status has or needs to be changed.
- Levels taken in patients who give no indication that anything has happened to modify the patient-specific drug pharmacokinetics on which the existing dosage regimen was designed are unnecessary. If the pharmacokinetics in the patient are assumed to be unchanged because status, diet, or other drugs being used have not changed, then drug levels will be as previously measured.
- Samples taken at incorrect times after administration of a dose may lead to incorrect interpretations when referenced to the therapeutic range or target concentration objective.
- Levels drawn too soon after a dosage regimen has been started or changed may provide misleading information about resulting steady-state levels. It takes a period corresponding to three to four half-lives to approximate the steady-state levels achieved after a dosage regimen has been initiated or modified.

Indiscriminant or inappropriate use of serum drug concentrations wastes much in terms of patient care, personnel time, and costs. It also compromises the value of TDM for practitioners and patients alike.

USING SERUM DRUG CONCENTRATIONS TO LINK PHARMACOKINETIC AND PHARMACODYNAMIC MODELING OF DOSAGE REGIMENS

Figure 1–1 suggests, but does not explicitly state, four things about the relationship between pharmacokinetics and pharmacodynamics in patients: (1) pharmacokinetic variability leads to the same dose rate (D/τ) producing differing serum drug concentrations in individuals because of differences in drug absorption and clearance; (2) this in turn leads to variable drug concentrations at the site of action; (3) in addition to this variation in drug concentrations at a given time during the dosage interval, the time course of serum drug concentration after dosing for many types of drugs leads to a companion time course of pharmacologic response; and (4) pharmacodynamic variability leads to the same dose rate producing differing drug responses in individuals because of differences in sensitivity or resistance to effects of the drug.

To date therapeutic drug monitoring has been practiced largely on the basis of relating the serum drug concentration to an expected response at a given time during the dosage interval, generally meaning the maximum, average, or minimum drug level during the interval at steady state, as discussed previously. In so doing, two of the considerations discussed in the preceding paragraph are not taken into account: pharmacodynamic variability and the temporal relationship of serum concentration to response. Although much success has been demonstrated in improving the number of patients with drug serum concentrations in the therapeutic range using this well-established single-point approach to TDM, and for a few drugs (principally the aminoglycoside antibiotics) a few practitioners have routinely used two measurements during the dosage interval to better monitor response, a more meaningful and useful application of serum concentration monitoring involves being able to relate the temporal course of the drug serum level to the temporal course of drug response. This is a challenging task, one that is in the very early stages of application, but the theory and progress in using serum drug concentrations to link pharmacokinetic and pharmacodynamic modeling of dosage regimens have been well reviewed.[27–30]

MOST FREQUENTLY MONITORED DRUGS

The drugs covered in this book possess the characteristics described above and are most frequently subjected to TDM:
- Antibiotics, including the aminoglycosides (amikacin, gentamicin, netilmicin, and tobramycin), vancomycin, and chloramphenicol
- Cardiac agents, including digoxin and some antiarrhythmics (amiodarone, lidocaine, procainamide, and quinidine)
- Antiepileptics, including carbamazepine, phenytoin, and valproic acid
- Psychotherapeutics, including lithium and some tricyclic antidepressants (amitriptyline, imipramine, and nortriptyline)
- Miscellaneous agents, including cyclosporine, methotrexate, and theophylline

Historically, TDM has been applied most commonly to the aminoglycosides, digoxin, phenytoin, and theophylline. This reflects not only the routine use of these drugs in therapy but also the frequency with which the drugs have been the source of investigations on TDM. Most of the other drugs, like cyclosporine, methotrexate, and the psychotherapeutic agents, are monitored in specialized clinics or circumstances. Table 1–1 summarizes the most frequently monitored drugs and commonly associated therapeutic ranges.

CLINICAL EFFECTIVENESS OF THERAPEUTIC DRUG MONITORING

Evaluation of the contribution of therapeutic drug monitoring should take therapeutic as well as economic factors into account. If TDM is of value, the practice should be reflected in increased drug effectiveness and safety but not necessarily in reduced health care costs. For it is possible that improved drug therapy could be associated with increased expense. Because the majority of studies have focused more on effectiveness and safety outcome measures than on the economic outcomes of TDM, these contributions are discussed in separate sections.

Appropriate indices of the value of TDM include direct measures of patient outcome like reduced toxicity and decreased severity or length of illness, indirect measures of outcome like a greater proportion of serum concentrations in the therapeutic range, and more prudent use and better interpretation of serum levels by practitioners. Few studies, however, have been designed with the appropriate rigor in methodology or with a sample size large enough to allow for demonstrating the value of TDM beyond question.[2,31]

But selecting the best-designed studies and combining them using the principles of meta-analysis have yielded aggregated data of sufficient sample size to permit evaluations of statistical significance. Two such investigations have demonstrated that TDM does reduce the number of patients encountering drug toxicity, which is a direct measure of outcome, and also ensures that more patients have serum drug concentrations within the appropriate therapeutic range, which is an indirect measure, when these data are compared with those for patients administered the same drugs without benefit of TDM.[32,33]

Small studies with individual drugs have also shown the benefit of TDM, depending on the specific study, through one or more of the following indices: improved effectiveness,[34–36,38,44] reduced toxicity,[33,37] decreased length of stay,[37,38] fewer hospital admissions,[39] more patients with serum levels within the appropriate therapeutic range,[32,37] and more rational use of serum concentration measurements by practitioners.[32] Some examples with commonly monitored drugs have been the aminoglycosides,[19,34,38,40–43] theophylline,[35,37,44] digoxin,[13,14,44,45] procainamide,[11] and the antiepileptics.[15,35,36,46]

On the other hand, some studies largely using the aminoglycosides have been unsuccessful in demonstrating the clinical advantages of TDM.[47–49] In these studies, one or more critical variables that would demonstrate the usefulness of TDM were not observed to differ significantly between TDM and control groups. These variables included cure rate, drug-induced rate of adverse reactions, and value of computer-assisted compared with manual or intuitive approaches to dosing.

More discussion on the usefulness and limitations of therapeutic drug monitoring is included in Chapters 5, 7, and 8.

ECONOMIC CONTRIBUTIONS OF THERAPEUTIC DRUG MONITORING

Even the demonstration of the beneficial therapeutic contributions of TDM does not guarantee that serum level monitoring justifies the resource allocation of equipment, supplies, and personnel. The practice of therapeutic drug monitoring in a facility, whether pursued casually or aggressively, consumes resources that must be justified against other expenses incurred by the facility as well as the health benefits gained for the resources expended.

Most economic evaluations of TDM have not been conducted with the rigor associated with well-accepted methods for cost-minimization, cost-effectiveness, or cost-benefit analyses.[2,50,51] Two of the better-designed studies[34,52] have demonstrated that the therapeutic or monetary benefits of TDM, or both, outweigh the costs incurred, resulting in an improved quality of care and a net benefit for society.

Nonetheless, one of the most important challenges for therapeutic drug monitoring in an era of cost containment and high expectations of therapeutic success is to show with appropriate research design and scientific rigor that TDM services enhance patient outcomes and are also cost effective.

More discussion on the economic evaluation of therapeutic drug monitoring is included in Chapter 8.

RESPONSIBILITIES OF A THERAPEUTIC DRUG MONITORING SERVICE

Therapeutic drug monitoring in a hospital or clinic may be as limited as providing consultation on one drug class such as the aminoglycosides for hospitalized patients or antiepileptics for patients in the neurology clinic, or the practice may include a number of drugs for inpatients and outpatients. In some facilities, TDM may include responsibility for assaying samples as well as interpreting the results. But in most institutions, the assay is the province of the clinical laboratory, and interpretation is the role of the pharmacy. Regardless of the scope of activities, therapeutic drug monitoring when viewed as an institutional service should meet certain expectations for responsibility.

According to recent guidelines published by the American College of Clinical Pharmacy,[53] when the pharmacy department assumes responsibility for the TDM service, but does not perform the assay, these activities include the following:

- Providing patient-specific consultations for therapeutic, toxicologic, or diagnostic management
- Developing institutional guidelines regarding appropriate use of measured drug concentrations and pharmacokinetic methodology (eg, software, dose initiation protocols, nomograms)
- Contributing to quality-assurance processes relevant to pharmacokinetics practice
- Contributing to drug usage evaluation criteria for drugs routinely monitored by drug concentration analysis
- Serving as an educational resource to professional staff and patients

This means that a TDM service should recommend guidelines for and influence the use of serum drug concentrations, advise when samples should be taken, interpret concentrations, recommend dosage regimens based on the data, communicate the information to physicians and nurses, educate practitioners through newsletters and seminars, and participate in studies collecting and analyzing patient data.

―――――― QUESTIONS ――――――

1. Define therapeutic drug monitoring.

2. The therapeutic range for digoxin is commonly cited as 1 to 2 ng/mL. What does this mean? What are the limitations in using the range?

3. A physician requests that a serum concentration be obtained for a patient taking gentamicin. This is the sixth day of treatment and the last level was obtained 3 days ago. Under what conditions is it appropriate to request the level?

4. For which specific drugs is therapeutic drug monitoring most commonly used?

5. What outcomes would you take into account to determine whether a TDM service has an effect on patient care?

BIBLIOGRAPHY

Benet LZ, Massoud N, Gambertoglio JG, eds. *Pharmacokinetic Basis for Drug Treatment.* New York: Raven Press; 1984.

Evans WE, Schentag JJ, Jusko WJ, eds. *Applied Pharmacokinetics: Principles of Therapeutic Drug Monitoring.* 3rd ed. Spokane, WA: Applied Therapeutics; 1992.

Murphy JE, ed. *Clinical Pharmacokinetics—Pocket Reference.* Bethesda, MD: American Society of Hospital Pharmacists: 1993.

Taylor WJ, Diers Caviness MH, eds. *A Textbook for the Clinical Application of Therapeutic Drug Monitoring.* Irving, TX: Abbott Laboratories; 1986.

REFERENCES

1. Richens A, Marks V, eds. *Therapeutic Drug Monitoring.* Edinburgh: Churchill Livingstone; 1981.
2. Barr JT. *The Interaction of Therapeutic Drug Monitoring and DRG Impact Levels: A Background Paper for DRG Payment and Medical Technology.* Washington, DC: Office of Technology Assessment, U.S. Congress; 1985.
3. Robinson JD, Taylor WJ. Interpretation of serum drug concentrations. In: Taylor WJ, Diers Caviness MH, eds. *A Textbook for the Clinical Application of Therapeutic Drug Monitoring.* Irving, TX: Abbott Laboratories; 1986:31–45.
4. Koch-Weser J, Sidel VW, Sweet RH, et al. Factors determining physician reporting of adverse drug reactions: Comparisons of 2000 spontaneous reports with surveillance studies at the Massachusetts General Hospital. *N Engl J Med.* 1969;280:20–29.
5. Sokolow M, Edgar AL. Blood quinidine concentrations as a guide in the treatment of cardiac arrhythmias. *Circulation.* 1950;1:576–592.
6. Talbott JH. Use of lithium salts as a substitute for sodium chloride. *Arch Intern Med.* 1950;85:1–10.
7. Geraci JE, Heilman FR, Nichols DR, et al. Some laboratory and clinical experiences with a new antibiotic, vancomycin. *Antibiot Annu.* 1956–1957;1957:90–106.
8. Buchtal F, Svensmark O, Schiller PJ. Clinical and electroencephalographic correlations with serum levels of diphenylhydantoin. *Arch Neurol.* 1960;2:624–630.
9. Smith TW, Butler VP, Haber E. Determination of therapeutic and toxic serum digoxin concentrations by radioimmunoassay. *N Engl J Med.* 1969;281:1212–1216.
10. Harrison DC, Stenson RE, Constantino RT. The relationship of blood levels, infusion rates and metabolism of lidocaine to its antiarrhythmic action. In Sandoe E, Flensted-Jensen E, Olesen K, eds. *Symposium on Cardiac Arrhythmias.* Stockholm: AB Astra; 1970:427–447.
11. Koch-Weser J, Klein SW. Procainamide dosage schedules, plasma concentrations, and clinical effects. *JAMA.* 1971;215:1454–1460.
12. Beller GA, Smith TW, Abelman WH, et al. Digitalis intoxication: A prospective clinical study with serum level correlations. *N Engl J Med.* 1971;284:989–997.
13. Olgilvie RI, Ruedy J. An educational program in digitalis therapy. *JAMA.* 1972;222:50–55.
14. Jelliffe RW, Buell J, Kalaba R. Reduction of digitalis toxicity by computer-assisted glycoside dosage regimens. *Ann Intern Med.* 1972;77:891–906.
15. Lund L. Effects of phenytoin in patients with epilepsy in relation to its concentration in plasma. In David DS, Prichard BNC, eds. *Biological Effects of Drugs in Relation to Their Concentration in Plasma.* Baltimore: University Park Press; 1972:227–239.
16. Jenne JW, Wyze E, Rood FS, et al. Pharmacokinetics of theophylline: Application to adjustment of the clinical dose of aminophylline. *Clin Pharmacol Ther.* 1972;13:349–360.
17. Mitenko PA, Olgilvie RI. Rational intravenous doses of theophylline. *N Engl J Med.* 1973; 289:600–603.
18. Koch-Weser J, Duhme LW, Greenblatt DJ. Influence of serum digoxin concentration measurements on frequency of digitoxicity. *Clin Pharmacol Ther.* 1974;16:284–287.

19. Noone P, Parson TMC, Pattison JR, et al. Experience in monitoring gentamicin therapy during treatment of serious Gram-negative sepsis. *Br Med J.* 1974;1:477–481.
20. Sjoqvist F. Interindividual differences in drug response: An overview. In Rowland M, Sheiner LB, Steimer J, eds. *Variability in Drug Therapy.* New York: Raven Press; 1985:1–10.
21. Spector R, Park GD, Johnson GF, Vesell ES. Therapeutic drug monitoring. *Clin Pharmacol Ther.* 1988;43:345–353.
22. McInnes GT. The value of therapeutic drug monitoring to the practising physician—An hypothesis in need of testing. *Br J Clin Pharmacol.* 1989;27:281–284.
23. Sheiner LB, Tozer TN. Clinical pharmacokinetics: The use of plasma concentrations of drugs. In Melmon KL, Morelli HF, eds. *Clinical Pharmacology.* New York: Macmillan; 1978:71–109.
24. Evans WE. General principles of applied pharmacokinetics. In Evans WE, Schentag JJ, Jusko WJ, eds. *Applied Pharmacokinetics: Principles of Therapeutic Drug Monitoring.* 2nd ed. Spokane, WA: Applied Therapeutics; 1986:1–8.
25. Pippenger CE, Massoud N. Therapeutic drug monitoring. In Benet LZ, Massoud N, Gambertoglio JG, eds. *Pharmacokinetic Basis for Drug Treatment.* New York: Raven Press; 1984:367–393.
26. Einarson TR, Segal HJ, Mann JL. Serum drug level utilization: A literature analysis. *Can J Hosp Pharm.* 1989;42:63–68.
27. Lalonde RL. Pharmacodynamics. In Evans WE, Schentag JJ, Jusko WJ, eds. *Applied Pharmacokinetics: Principles of Therapeutic Drug Monitoring.* 3rd ed. Spokane, WA: Applied Therapeutics; 1992:4-1–4-31.
28. Schentag JJ, Ballow CH, Paladino JA, Nix DE. Dual individualization with antibiotics: Integrated antibiotic management strategies for use in hospitals. In Evans WE, Schentag JJ, Jusko WJ, eds. *Applied Pharmacokinetics: Principles of Therapeutic Drug Monitoring.* 3rd ed. Spokane, WA: Applied Therapeutics; 1992:17-1–17-20.
29. Gibaldi M. *Biopharmaceutics and Clinical Pharmacokinetics.* 4th ed. Philadelphia: Lea & Febiger; 1991:176–186.
30. Shargel L, Yu ABC. *Applied Biopharmaceutics and Pharmacokinetics.* 3rd ed. Norwalk, CT, Appleton & Lange; 1993:465–492.
31. Reents S, Hatton RC. Influence of methods on the evaluation of therapeutic drug-monitoring services. *Am J Hosp Pharm.* 1991;48:1553–1559.
32. Ried LD, McKenna DA, Horn JR. Meta-analysis of research on the effect of clinical pharmacokinetics services on therapeutic drug monitoring. *Am J Hosp Pharm.* 1989;46:945–951.
33. Ried LD, Horn JR, McKenna DA. Therapeutic drug monitoring reduces toxic drug reactions: A meta-analysis. *Ther Drug Monit.* 1990;12:72–78.
34. Destache CJ, Meyer SK, Bittner MJ, Hermann KG. Impact of clinical pharmacokinetic services on patients treated with aminoglycosides: A cost–benefit analysis. *Ther Drug Monit.* 1990;12:419–426.
35. Mungall D, Marshall J, Penn D, et al. Individualizing theophylline therapy: The impact of clinical pharmacokinetics on patient outcomes. *Ther Drug Monit.* 1983;5:95–101.
36. Reynolds EH, Shorvon SD, Galbraith AW, et al. Phenytoin monotherapy for epilepsy: A long-term prospective study, assisted by serum level monitoring, in previously untreated patients. *Epilepsia.* 1981;22:485–488.
37. Hurley SF, Dziukas LJ, McNeil JJ, Brignell MJ. A randomized controlled clinical trial of pharmacokinetic theophylline dosing. *Am Rev Respir Dis.* 1986;134:1219–1224.
38. Crist KD, Nahata MC, Ety J. Positive impact of a therapeutic drug-monitoring program on total aminoglycoside dose and cost of hospitalization. *Ther Drug Monit.* 1987;9:306–310.
39. Wing DS, Duff HJ. The impact of a therapeutic drug monitoring program for phenytoin. *Ther Drug Monit.* 1989;11:32–37.
40. Dillon KR, Dougherty SH, Casner P, Polly S. Individualized pharmacokinetic versus standard dosing of amikacin: A comparison of therapeutic outcomes. *J Antimicrob Chemother.* 1989;24:581–589.

41. Moore RD, Smith CR, Lietman PS. Association of aminoglycoside plasma levels with therapeutic outcome in Gram negative pneumonia. *Am J Med.* 1984;77:657–663.
42. Zaske DE, Irvine P, Strand LM, et al. Wide interpatient variation in gentamicin dosage requirements for geriatric patients. *JAMA.* 1982;248:3122–3126.
43. Whipple JK, Ausman RK, Franson T, et al. Effect of individualized pharmacokinetic dosing on patient outcome. *Crit Care Med.* 1991;19:1480–1485.
44. Whiting B, Kelman AW, Bryson SM, et al. Clinical pharmacokinetics: A comprehensive system for therapeutic drug monitoring and prescribing. *Br Med J.* 1984;288:541–545.
45. Koch-Weser J, Duhme LW, Greenblatt DJ. Influence of serum digoxin concentration measurements on frequency of digitotoxicity. *Clin Pharmacol Ther.* 1974;16:284–287.
46. Sherwin AL. Clinical pharmacology of ethosuximide. In Pipenger CE, Penry JK, Kutt H, eds. *Antiepileptic Drugs: Quantitative Analysis and Interpretation.* New York: Raven Press; 1978:283–295.
47. Arroyo JC, Milligan L, Davis J, et al. Impact of aminoglycoside serum assays on clinical decisions and renal toxicity. *South Med J.* 1986;79:272–276.
48. Leehey DJ, Braun BI, Tholl DA, et al. Can pharmacokinetic dosing decrease nephrotoxicity associated with aminoglycoside therapy? *J Am Soc Nephrol.* 1993;4:81–90.
49. Kemme DJ, Daniel CI. Aminoglycoside dosing: A randomized prospective study. *South Med J.* 1993;86:46–51.
50. Vozeh S. Cost-effectiveness of therapeutic drug monitoring. *Clin Pharmacokinet.* 1987;13:131–140.
51. Gardner DM, Hardy BG. Cost-effectiveness of therapeutic drug monitoring. *Can J Hosp Pharm.* 1990;1:7–12.
52. Bootman JL, Wertheimer AI, Zaske D, Rowland C. Individualizing gentamicin dosage regimens in burn patients with Gram-negative septicemia: A cost–benefit analysis. *J Pharm Sci.* 1979;68:267–272.
53. ACCP Position Statement. Practice guidelines for the clinical pharmacokinetics consultation service. *Pharmacotherapy.* 1991;11:175–177.

Chapter 2

Pharmacokinetic Concepts in Therapeutic Drug Monitoring

Gerald E. Schumacher

Keep in Mind

- To develop a dosage regimen, the practitioner selects a steady-state serum target concentration, estimates the pharmacokinetic parameters in the patient (Cl, f, V, $t_{1/2}$), usually by using mean population parameters to start, and then adjusts dose and τ to produce the C_{ss} target. If the resulting C_{ss} is appreciably different than expected, one or more of the pharmacokinetic variables in the patient is markedly varied from the population mean. The practitioner then adapts by readjusting dose and τ to obtain the desired C_{ss}.

- Most drugs subject to TDM exhibit linear pharmacokinetic behavior wherein clearance is independent of serum concentration and a change in dose yields a proportional and predictable change in serum concentration. For these drugs, the pharmacokinetic variables used in developing dosage regimens are bioavailability (f), clearance (Cl), volume of distribution (V), and half-life ($t_{1/2}$). Clearance is the most important of these variables in determining the dosage regimen. Clearance links the bioavailable dose rate with the steady-state average serum concentration at steady state: $(Cl) (C_{avg,ss}) = (f)$ (dose rate). Overall drug clearance is the sum of each of the organs contributing to clearance and consists of two processes for each organ: blood flow to the organ (Q) and the capacity of the organ to remove the drug from circulation (extraction ratio, ER). Half-life is another important variable that determines how long it takes for a drug to accumulate to steady-state levels and how long it takes for a drug to be eliminated from the body; it is also used to determine how often to dose a drug. It is composed of two terms: $t_{1/2} = V/1.4(\text{Cl})$.

- Some TDM drugs, however, exhibit nonlinear pharmacokinetics wherein clearance is not a constant, but is variable, and a change in dose yields a nonproportional and nonpredictable change in serum concentration. For these drugs, V_{max} and K_m are used in equations and replace Cl, V, and $t_{1/2}$ used for linear pharmacokinetics.

- Accumulation is the process whereby a drug administered continuously or intermittently by a constant dosage regimen increases in serum concentration until a plateau is reached wherein, for intermittent administration, the serum concentration versus time profile is constant for each dosage interval or, for continuous administration, a plateau level is reached.

- Steady state is the condition achieved when accumulation of a dosage regimen is complete. For a drug exhibiting linear pharmacokinetic behavior, 90% of steady state is achieved in a period equal to $3.3t_{1/2}$.

- The portion of the dosage interval used to obtain the patient's serum concentration depends on what portion of the interval was associated with the pharmacologic effect used to determine the therapeutic range for the drug. When this is unknown, most practitioners use the midpoint of τ to estimate $C_{avg,ss}$ or the end of τ (before the next dose is given) to estimate $C_{min,ss}$. $C_{max,ss}$ is used infrequently, unless specifically recommended, because the timing of the value is uncertain and the necessary postabsortion, postdistribution equilibrium may not have yet been achieved.

- For renally impaired patients, normal dosage regimens may be adjusted to compensate for reduced clearance by estimating the patient's creatinine clearance (Cl_{cr}), using Cl_{cr} to estimate a patient-specific drug clearance (Cl) or half-life ($t_{1/2}$), and then using these parameters to calculate a revised dosage regimen.

Therapeutic drug monitoring requires a working knowledge of pharmacokinetic principles, background that is assumed for readers of this book. This chapter presents a cursory review of some of the clinical pharmacokinetic concepts and equations that have particular relevance to TDM. More extensive discussion of these principles is available in pharmacokinetic textbooks and publications like those cited in the bibliography at the end of the chapter.

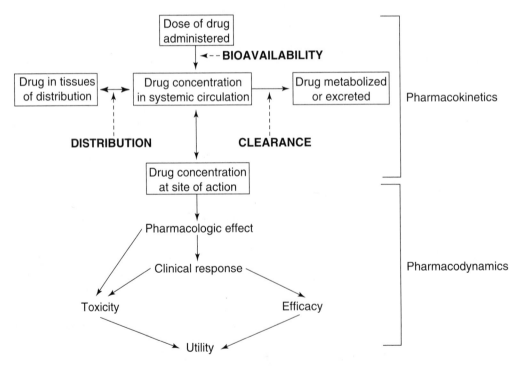

Figure 2–1. Relationship between the pharmacokinetic and pharmacodynamic phases of drug transit through the body. *(From B. G. Katzung, ed.* Basic and Clinical Pharmacology. *5th ed. Norwalk, CT: Appleton & Lange; 1992, with permission.)*

The schematic in Figure 2–1 depicts the relationship between the pharmacokinetic and pharmacodynamic phases of drug transit through the body.[1] Three pharmacokinetic variables—bioavailability, volume of distribution, and clearance—influence the temporal change in serum or plasma concentration (terms used interchangeably in this chapter). The serum concentration is assumed to have a direct relationship to the pharmacologic effect. As TDM anchors on maintaining selected drugs within a narrow range of serum concentrations, understanding the influence of the pharmacokinetic variables on concentration is essential.

Figure 2–2 shows the mathematical and dynamic relationships between dose, frequency of administration, pharmacokinetic variables, serum concentration, and pharmacologic response. This scheme shows how the practitioner-controlled variables, dose and frequency (τ), are combined with the pharmacokinetic variables contributed by the patient, bioavailability and clearance (f and Cl, respectively), to obtain a given steady-state serum concentration, in this case the average steady-state concentration ($C_{avg,ss}$) achieved during the dosage interval. To start treatment with a drug, $C_{avg,ss}$ is usually selected to be within a target concentration range that generally corresponds to a portion of the commonly accepted therapeutic range for the drug. Then average values are assumed for the pharmacokinetic variables of the drug in the patient—these are often called population values—and the dose rate (dose/τ) is calculated to obtain the desired $C_{avg,ss}$. If the resulting pharmacologic response is not as desired or adverse effects are apparent in the patient, then the practitioner manipulates the only variables under her or his control, dose and τ, to increase or decrease the serum level. This may happen because the patient's variables in the pharmacokinetic phase (dose to serum concentration) differ from the assumed average values for the population or because the patient's variables in the pharmacodynamic phase (serum concentration to pharmacologic response) differ from what is usually expected.

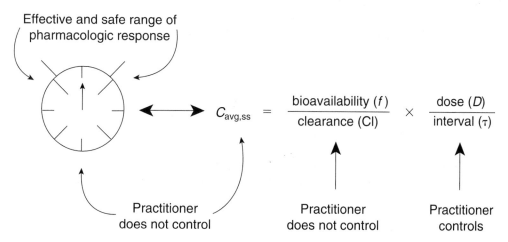

Figure 2–2. Pharmacokinetic factors influencing serum drug concentration and pharmacologic response.

PHARMACOKINETIC VARIABLES

The pharmacokinetic variables shown in Figures 2–1 and 2–2 are bioavailability, volume of distribution, and clearance. Although these variables are patient specific, individual values for a large cohort of patients are averaged to yield a mean value for each parameter. This mean value is often called the population value. As the mean represents all of the individual values, a specific patient is unlikely to have the same value as the population measure, but if this patient's value is within a standard deviation of the mean, he or she is usually termed a *normal*. Pathologic and physiologic changes, however, may further alter these normal values in the patient.

Bioavailability (f)

Bioavailability is the fraction of unchanged drug that reaches the systemic circulation after administration. As a fraction, it is a dimensionless term that is the product of two factors, absorption and presystemic extraction.[1-3] Presystemic extraction in itself comprises two types of mechanisms[3]: "first-pass" metabolism of absorbed drug via the liver before reaching the systemic circulation, and metabolism or biotransformation of absorbed drug in the gastrointestinal tract by mucosal cells or flora prior to systemic availability. The first of these mechanisms, first-pass metabolism by the liver, has been much more extensively studied than the latter and is probably the markedly dominant mechanism of presystemic extraction of drugs. Furthermore, little is known in humans about the effect of the gastrointestinal tract mechanisms of presystemic extraction. As such, the following discussion focuses on first-pass extraction by the liver alone.

$$f = \text{(fraction absorbed) (fraction not metabolized by first-pass extraction)} \qquad (2\text{–}1)$$

For intravenous administration, f is 1. For other routes of administration, f may be less than 1. For oral administration, f may be less than 1, not only because of incomplete absorption through the gut but also because of metabolism that occurs in the liver during the first pass through the portal circulation prior to reaching the systemic circulation. For oral administration of theophylline, the population value for f is nearly 1, because little first-pass metabolism occurs. For lidocaine, on the other hand, f is less than 0.2, because of extensive first-pass metabolism. An estimate of the fraction of drug that escapes first-pass metabolism is obtained from the extraction ratio, a concept discussed later under Clearance (Cl).

In the equations to be used throughout the chapter, bioavailability refers only to the *extent* of absorption, as described above. More broadly, bioavailability also includes the *rate* of drug absorption into the circulation as well as the extent of absorption. Although rate may have an influence on the intensity and duration of pharmacologic response, most use of dosage regimen equations clinically assumes that absorption occurs so much more rapidly than elimination for a drug that interpatient variation in absorption rate is not generally an important factor.

Volume of Distribution (V)

When a drug enters the systemic circulation, it distributes to varying extent to other body fluids and tissues. The volume of distribution, often expressed in units of liters or liters/kilogram, may be estimated from

$$V = \frac{\text{amount of drug in body}}{C} \qquad (2\text{--}2)$$

where C is the concentration of drug in serum. Measuring the distribution in this manner assumes that the body behaves as a homogenous system, rather than discrete tissues and fluids that accept the drug with varying avidity, so the parameter is referred to as the apparent volume of distribution. The magnitude of distribution depends on the physicochemical properties of the drug that influence diffusion through tissues as well as the extent of drug binding to proteins in fluids and tissues. A drug like digoxin has a population V of more than 7 L/kg, indicating extensive binding in some tissues, whereas a highly polar antibiotic like gentamicin is much more restricted with a value less than 0.3 L/kg. Blood and total body water constitute 0.08 and 0.6 L/kg, respectively.

When practitioners simplify the use of dosage regimen equations and monitoring, as they do whenever possible, by making the assumption that the drug distributes instantaneously into the body acting as homogenous vessel, the body is viewed as a single compartment and the drug is considered to follow one-compartment pharmacokinetic behavior or model. For a few drugs, however, this simplifying assumption is inadequate and the body must be viewed as consisting of at least two compartments, one composed of tissues perfused rapidly by the drug and the other comprising tissues perfused more slowly. This two-compartment model increases the complexity of the equations to be used and the considerations in monitoring. The various drugs affected will be discussed in subsequent chapters.

Instead of trying to attach some general physiologic meaning to various drug distribution volumes, as may be discussed for various drugs in later chapters, it is best for now simply to identify the parameter as the measure that relates the serum concentration of drug to the amount of drug in the body.

Clearance (Cl)

Clearance of a drug is the most important pharmacokinetic variable for interpreting serum concentrations and determining dosage regimens during TDM.[1,4] Physiologically, it reflects the ability of the body to eliminate a drug, as measured by the volume of serum, plasma, or blood that is cleared of the drug per unit of time, and is often expressed in milliliters/minute or liters/kilogram/hour. In pharmacokinetic terms, it is the parameter that mathematically links the bioavailable dosage rate with the average steady-state serum concentration during the dosage interval ($C_{avg,ss}$):

$$(\text{Cl})\,(C_{avg,ss}) = (f)\,(\text{dose}/\tau) \qquad (2\text{--}3)$$

Clinically, clearance is the parameter most responsible for the great interpatient variability observed in TDM. It is also the variable most subject to alteration from normal by pathologic and physiologic conditions that may occur in patients, factors such as heart, kidney, and liver disease, as well as aging in general.

Eliminating a drug from the body may involve one or more organs, principally the kidney and liver, but other organs may also contribute, so that the overall term *clearance* refers to the sum of the various organ clearances and is called the *total systemic clearance:*

$$Cl = Cl_{systemic} = Cl_{kidney} + Cl_{liver} + Cl_{other} \qquad (2\text{--}4)$$

Each of these pathways has the potential to become saturated if the dose is high enough and this is shown mathematically by an expression like the Michaelis–Menten equation in enzyme kinetics:

$$Cl = \frac{V_{max}}{K_m + C_{avg,ss}} \qquad (2\text{--}5)$$

Here V_{max} is the maximum amount of drug that may be eliminated per unit of time and K_m is the serum concentration at which the rate of elimination is 50% of V_{max}.

For most drugs encountered in TDM, $K_m \gg C_{avg,ss}$, so clearance reduces in Equation 2–5 to the expression $Cl = V_{max}/K_m$, which is a constant for a patient given stable clearance by the contributing organs. Under these conditions, clearance is independent of serum concentration and a change in dose rate yields a proportional and predictable change in serum concentration. Drugs with clearance that behaves in this manner exhibit *linear* pharmacokinetic behavior.

But for those drugs (eg, phenytoin, salicylates) with therapeutic serum concentrations similar (or greater) in magnitude to K_m, the denominator of Equation 2–5 cannot be simplified as above. As such, as noted in Equation 2–5, clearance varies with serum concentration and is not independent of serum level, and a change in dose rate yields a disproportionate and not readily predictable change in serum concentration. This is shown in Figure 2–3. At serum concentrations much less than K_m, the dose rate-versus-serum level relationship appears linear. As the serum concentration approaches and exceeds K_m, linearity is lost. Drugs with clearance that behaves in this manner exhibit *nonlinear* pharmacokinetic behavior.

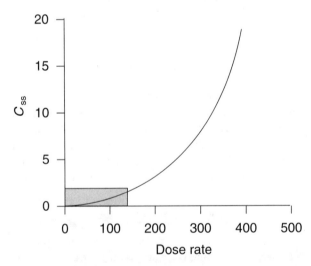

Figure 2–3. Relationship between dose rate and steady-state serum drug concentration. Drugs with linear pharmacokinetic behavior occupy the shaded area. Drugs with nonlinear pharmacokinetics encompass the entire curve. (*From B. G. Katzung, ed. Basic and Clinical Pharmacology. 5th ed. Norwalk, CT: Appleton & Lange; 1992, with permission.*)

Clearance may also be defined for a specific organ as a function of two factors, blood flow to the organ (Q) and the extraction ratio (ER), the latter being a measure of the fraction of drug entering the organ that is cleared on exit.[1] The faster the blood flow or the more pronounced the extraction ratio, the greater the clearance by the organ. With the liver as an example,

$$Cl_{liver} = (Q) (ER) \qquad (2\text{--}6)$$

Drugs with a great affinity for metabolizing enzymes in the liver show a high extraction coefficient. Therefore, clearance by metabolism is rate dependent on the rate of delivery of drug to the liver (Q). For these drugs, conditions that compromise blood flow (eg, congestive heart failure, cirrhosis, hypotension) are of importance in monitoring. Most of these drugs are not subject to TDM, however. Some examples are the ß blockers, tricyclic antidepressants, some narcotics, verapamil, and lidocaine.

Most drugs subject to TDM have a relatively low affinity for the metabolizing enzymes, so for these drugs metabolism is more dependent on enzyme capacity (ER) than on hepatic blood flow. For these drugs, greatest attention is paid to conditions that modify the production, number, and affinity of metabolizing enzymes, conditions like liver disease and enzyme inhibition or stimulation. Some examples are digoxin, phenytoin, procainamide, quinidine, salicylates, theophylline, and warfarin.

The extraction ratio also influences drug bioavailability, as noted previously in Equation 2–1. As the bioavailable fraction of drug administered reflects first-pass metabolism, which is characterized by ER, drugs with substantial extraction have a markedly reduced bioavailability. This is observed when rewriting Equation 2–1 as follows: $f = $ (fraction absorbed) $(1 - ER)$.

For drugs showing linear pharmacokinetics, clearance may be defined in terms of the volume of distribution and half-life:

$$Cl = \frac{V}{1.4t_{1/2}} \qquad (2\text{--}7)$$

This equation emphasizes that changes in V or $t_{1/2}$ can lead to modifications in clearance.

Half-Life ($t_{1/2}$)

For drugs showing linear pharmacokinetic behavior, half-life is one of the most useful pharmacokinetic variables for clinicians:

- $t_{1/2}$ determines the time it takes for a dosage regimen to reach steady-state serum levels; 50%, 75%, 88%, and 94% of steady state is achieved in one, two, three, and four half-life periods, respectively.
- $t_{1/2}$ contributes to knowing how much greater serum levels will be at steady state compared with the first dose. When the ratio of $\tau/t_{1/2}$ is 0.5, 1, and 2, the buildup of serum concentrations at steady state is 3.4, 2, and 1.3 times the corresponding levels after the first dose, respectively.
- $t_{1/2}$ determines how long it takes for the serum concentration to be reduced after a dose; 50%, 75%, 88%, and 94% of the drug is lost from the system in one, two, three, and four half-life periods, respectively.
- $t_{1/2}$ influences the choice of dosage interval. The longer the half-life, the less often the drug needs to be administered.

- $t_{1/2}$ influences the choice of sampling time for measuring serum concentrations. When the half-life is longer than τ, little fluctuation in serum level occurs during the dosage interval, so the time selected for sampling, once drug distribution equilibrium in the body is achieved, is not critical. On the other hand, when half-life is shorter than τ, sampling time is critical, because serum level fluctuation is great.

As $t_{1/2}$ is so conceptually appealing to practitioners, it is used in this chapter in preference to the elimination rate constant, k, for concepts and equations. In terms of rate constant or clearance, half-life is defined as follows, with units expressed in terms of reciprocal time (eg, h^{-1}):

$$t_{1/2} = \frac{1}{1.4k} = \frac{0.69}{k} \qquad\qquad 2\text{--}8$$

$$t_{1/2} = \frac{V}{1.4(\text{Cl})} = \frac{0.69V}{\text{Cl}} \qquad\qquad 2\text{--}9$$

Using the half-life as a guide in monitoring requires some caution. As $t_{1/2}$ is composed of two independent variables, volume of distribution (V) and clearance (Cl), changes in both may not alter the half-life. Alternately, a change in $t_{1/2}$ may not necessarily indicate a change in Cl.

Protein Binding

Most drugs are bound to some degree by proteins in plasma and tissues. Some are bound avidly, although the extent of binding is not detected by most drug level assays because the analysis usually reports the total drug concentration, which comprises both bound and unbound portions of the drug.[4,5] That attachment is reversible, so the bound and free forms are in equilibrium. But it is the unbound, free portion of the drug in plasma that is responsible for distribution through tissues, for clearance by the liver and kidney, and for interaction with the sites of action to produce pharmacologic response.

Two factors determine the extent of protein binding in plasma: the binding affinity of the drug for the proteins and the number of binding sites available. As for the other pharmacokinetic variables discussed previously, there is an average population value and normal range for plasma protein concentrations. Conditions that decrease the concentration of plasma proteins in patients, or patients with concentrations less than normal for the population, will show decreased protein binding for drugs. The resulting increase in free drug concentration provides the potential, which may or may not be realized, for increased distribution and clearance and, perhaps, a transient increase in response. Displacement of bound drug from proteins, as a result of disease or coadministration of additional drugs with high binding capacity, may lead to the same result as above. Acidic drugs like phenytoin and the salicylates are bound primarily to albumin. Basic drugs like quinidine and the tricyclic antidepressants are bound largely to globulins.

For drugs of similar composition:
- The greater the binding in plasma, given that plasma binding is not trivial compared with tissue binding, the lower the volume of distribution. Digitoxin is bound more than 90% to plasma proteins, whereas digoxin is bound less than 30%. This contributes in great measure to digitoxin having a volume of distribution more than 15 times smaller than that of digoxin.
- Increases in binding contribute to decreases in extraction ratio and clearance. Digitoxin

clearance is much lower than digoxin clearance, in part because bound drug is not cleared by the liver and kidney. So clearance must wait for the liberation of free drug molecules from bound sites over time.

- Although the reasons contributing to pharmacologic response are complex, digitoxin is less potent than digoxin, in part because it is the free form of drug molecules that reacts at receptor sites.

From a clinical viewpoint, protein binding becomes an important issue in TDM for drugs bound 80% or more. Although this threshold is arbitrary, it reflects the observation that a small displacement from protein bound sites for highly bound drugs results in a large increase in free drug. For a drug bound 95%, a 5% displacement that reduces binding to 90% leads to a twofold increase in free drug (5% to 10%). Intrapatient and interpatient variation in protein binding for highly bound drugs is always a potential explanation for unexpected alterations in drug pharmacokinetics and pharmacodynamics.

ACCUMULATION AND STEADY STATE

When a dose of drug is administered continuously, the serum concentration increases until a plateau is reached wherein the rate of drug input (dose/time) to the body equals the rate of drug output ($C_{ss} \times Cl$). The same process occurs when a dose is given intermittently (eg, q8h). As shown in Figure 2–4, this process of drug buildup is called accumulation and the plateau condition reached from continuous administration, or the constant serum concentration-versus-time

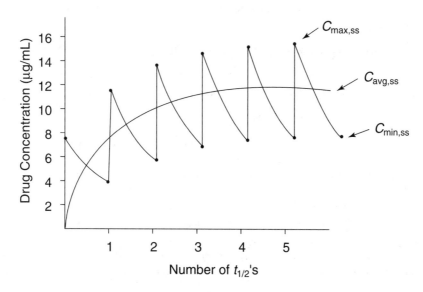

Figure 2–4. Drug accumulation during multiple dose or continuous administration showing achievement of steady state. (*From W. J. Taylor and M. H. Diers Caviness, eds., A Textbook for the Clinical Application of Therapeutic Drug Monitoring. Irving, TX: Abbott Laboratories; 1986, with permission.*)

profile during each dosage interval for intermittent administration, is called *steady state*. The relationship between drug input and output at steady state is shown in the equation:

$$(S)\,(f)\,(\text{dose}/\tau) = (C_{ss})\,(\text{Cl}) \tag{2–10}$$

where S is the fraction of the dosage form that is the active moiety, dose/τ is the amount of drug administered during each arbitrary unit of time (eg, minute, hour) within the dosage interval (τ), and C_{ss} is the steady-state serum concentration of drug. For administration of a continuous infusion, C_{ss} is more specifically designated $C_{inf,ss}$, whereas for intermittent dosing, C_{ss} becomes $C_{avg,ss}$, the average steady-state concentration during the dosage interval.

Accumulation and steady state are useful concepts for TDM:

- After initiating a dosage regimen, the time for accumulation of drug concentrations to steady-state levels is just a function of drug half-life ($t_{1/2}$). The time it takes to achieve 90% of steady state is calculated by multiplying the half-life by 3.3. So, given an estimate of $t_{1/2}$, it is easy for the practitioner to calculate a clinically useful approximation of the time or number of dosage intervals it will take to reach full therapeutic levels of the drug.
- Accumulation is a measure of how much greater drug levels are at steady state compared with the first dose. Accumulation is a function of $t_{1/2}$ and τ, and is not determined by the amount of dose administered. A useful approximation is:

$$\text{accumulation} = \frac{C_{ss,t=x}}{C_{fd,t=x}} = \frac{1}{1 - 10^{-0.3(\tau/t_{1/2})}} \tag{2–11}$$

where $C_{ss,t=x}$ and $C_{fd,t=x}$ represent steady-state and first dose concentrations, respectively, measured at the same time $(t=x)$ after the doses are administered, and the expression $1 - 10^{-0.3\,(\tau/t_{1/2})}$ represents the fraction of dose administered that is lost from the body during the dosage interval.

$$\text{fraction of drug in body lost per dosage interval} = 1 - 10^{-0.3(\tau/t_{1/2})} \tag{2–12}$$

- The ratio of a loading dose (dose$_L$) to the maintenance dose (dose), for a given dosage frequency (τ), is determined by accumulation:

$$\text{dose}_L/\text{dose} = 1 / [1 - 10^{-0.3(\tau/t_{1/2})}] \tag{2–13}$$

Using Equations 2–12 and 2–13 demonstrates the common observation that when a dosage regimen for a drug is administered at a frequency (τ) equal to the half-life ($t_{1/2}$), the fraction of drug lost during the dosage interval is 0.5 and accumulation therefore is twofold.

- Knowledge of accumulation and the time it takes to reach steady state is one of the factors that practitioners take into account in determining whether giving a loading dose is useful to initiate an intended dosage regimen. It likely is if the wait for steady state is long or accumulation will be large. But if steady state occurs quickly or accumulation will be small, then a loading dose is probably not indicated, at least on the basis of pharmacokinetics.
- Once steady state is reached, the temporal drug concentration profile is constant for each dosage interval unless something happens to alter the drug's pharmacokinetic parameters in the patient.

When to Sample After Starting or Modifying a Regimen

The therapeutic range for a drug is based on steady-state serum concentrations. Levels drawn too soon after a dosage regimen has been started or changed may provide misleading information because it takes a period corresponding to three to four half-lives to approximate steady-state levels. For example, digoxin has a $t_{1/2}$ of 1.5 to 2 days in nonelderly adults with normal clearance. After the daily regimen is established, it takes about 1 week for steady state to be achieved. During a dose given after steady state has been reached, sampling should occur only after absorption and distribution are complete, during the period of postabsorption and postdistribution equilibrium. For oral digoxin this takes 4 to 8 hours, so a level measured 8 to 24 hours after one of the daily doses (assuming a q24h regimen) given 7 or more days after starting treatment is appropriate. Changing the regimen, either because the response is inappropriate or the pharmacokinetics appear to have been altered, means waiting another period of three to four times the estimated $t_{1/2}$ before drawing a new sample.

Sampling times and the frequency of sampling are drug specific and are discussed for each drug in subsequent chapters.

RELATING SERUM CONCENTRATION TO PHARMACOLOGIC RESPONSE FOR MONITORING

In therapeutic drug monitoring, three common steady-state serum concentration measurements are used for intermittent administration, as shown in Figure 2–4: $C_{avg,ss}$, $C_{max,ss}$, and $C_{min,ss}$. For continuous administration, $C_{inf,ss}$ is equivalent to $C_{avg,ss}$. Because a fundamental premise for TDM is that serum concentration is related to pharmacologic response, and the anchor for TDM is the selection of a target serum concentration within the drug's therapeutic range, it is important to select the monitoring time during the dosage interval that corresponds to the time monitored when the reference therapeutic range was determined.

For example, does the commonly accepted therapeutic range of 10 to 20 ug/mL for theophylline mean that dosage regimens should be adjusted to ensure that $C_{max,ss}$, or $C_{avg,ss}$, or $C_{min,ss}$ should be maintained within this range? Or does the therapeutic range mean that $C_{max,ss}$ should not exceed, and $C_{min,ss}$ should not fall below, the therapeutic range? When data for setting the therapeutic range for theophylline were obtained, was the pharmacologic response observed in comparison to serum levels sampled at or near the maximum ($\sim C_{max,ss}$), the midpoint ($\sim C_{avg,ss}$), or the end ($\sim C_{min,ss}$) of the dosage interval?

Unfortunately, this question is not always resolved by practitioners when monitoring drugs. The choice of dosage regimen and the equation used to determine it depend on the target serum concentration to be achieved and the portion of the dosage interval for which this concentration is to be maintained. To illustrate, serum levels for aminoglycosides are commonly monitored for effectiveness with reference to a therapeutic range based on $C_{max,ss}$ and for toxicity with reference to $C_{min,ss}$. Lithium monitoring is referenced to $C_{min,ss}$. Digoxin, because of its long half-life, is monitored for $C_{avg,ss}$ or $C_{min,ss}$. And most practitioners seek to maintain theophylline levels within its therapeutic range ($C_{max,ss}$ and $C_{min,ss}$ are retained within the range throughout the dosage interval).

In truth, many therapeutic ranges have been developed without careful consideration of these issues so it may not be clear which portion of the dosage interval applies for sampling. In general, unless a level estimating the maximum during the dosage interval is indicated, TDM tries to use the midpoint or the end of the dosage interval to estimate $C_{avg,ss}$ or $C_{min,ss}$, respectively. These measures are preferred, when it is known or can be assumed that these measures are adequate indices of a drug's effectiveness and safety, because timing is more accurate than $C_{max,ss}$. $C_{max,ss}$ measures are uncertain with respect to timing and also are confounded by the multicompartmental pharmacokinetic behavior of drugs; sampling too early after a dose may be misleading if the drug distribution phase is still in progress and postdistribution equilibrium has not yet been achieved.

USING DOSAGE REGIMEN EQUATIONS

Using the following equations to initiate or modify a dosage regimen requires knowledge of population or patient-specific pharmacokinetic parameters. Generally, mean population values are used to initiate a regimen. When drug levels are measured after starting the regimen with the specific purpose of obtaining patient-specific pharmacokinetics, the dosage regimen may then be individualized to meet the target concentration objective. Equations 2–14 to 2–35, are summarized in Table 2–1.

TABLE 2–1. EQUATIONS COMMONLY USED IN THERAPEUTIC DRUG MONITORING

$C_{avg,ss}$: *Average Steady-State Concentration During the Dosage Interval Resulting from Intermittent Administration at a Given Dose Rate (dose/τ)*

$$2\text{–}14 \qquad C_{avg,ss} = \frac{(S)(f)(\text{dose}/\tau)}{Cl}$$

$$2\text{–}15 \qquad C_{avg,ss} = \frac{1.4(S)(f)(t_{1/2})(\text{dose}/\tau)}{V}$$

dose/τ: *Dose Rate to Achieve an Average Steady-State Concentration ($C_{avg,ss}$) During the Dosage Interval Resulting from Intermittent Administration*

$$2\text{–}16 \qquad \text{dose}/\tau = \frac{(C_{avg,ss})(Cl)}{(S)(f)}$$

$$2\text{–}17 \qquad \text{dose}/\tau = \frac{(C_{avg,ss})(V)}{1.4(S)(f)(t_{1/2})}$$

$C_{inf,ss}$: *Steady-State Concentration Resulting from Continuous Administration at a Given Dose Rate (dose/t_{inf}):*

$$2\text{–}18 \qquad C_{inf,ss} = \frac{(S)(f)(\text{dose}/t_{inf})}{Cl}$$

$$2\text{–}19 \qquad C_{inf,ss} = \frac{1.4(S)(f)(t_{1/2})(\text{dose}/t_{inf})}{V}$$

$dose/t_{inf}$: Dose Rate to Achieve a Steady-State Concentration ($C_{inf,ss}$) Resulting from Continuous Administration

$$2\text{--}20 \qquad dose/t_{inf} = \frac{(C_{inf,ss})(Cl)}{(S)(f)}$$

$$2\text{--}21 \qquad dose/t_{inf} = \frac{(C_{inf,ss})(V)}{1.4(S)(f)(t_{1/2})}$$

$C_{max,ss}$: Maximum Steady-State Concentration During the Dosage Interval Resulting from Intermittent Administration at a Given Dose Rate ($dose/\tau$)

$$2\text{--}22^a \qquad C_{max,ss} = \frac{(S)(f)(dose/V)}{1 - 10^{-0.3(\tau/t_{1/2})}}$$

$$2\text{--}23^a \qquad C_{max,ss} = \frac{(S)(f)(dose/V)}{1 - e^{-0.7(\tau/t_{1/2})}}$$

$C_{min,ss}$: Minimum Steady-State Concentration During the Dosage Interval Resulting from Intermittent Administration at a Given Dose Rate ($dose/\tau$)

$$2\text{--}24 \qquad C_{min,ss} = (C_{max,ss})\,[10^{-0.3(\tau/t_{1/2})}]$$

$$2\text{--}25 \qquad C_{min,ss} = (C_{max,ss})\,[e^{-0.7(\tau/t_{1/2})}]$$

$dose_L$: Loading Dose to Achieve an Initial Target Concentration (C_0)

$$2\text{--}26 \qquad dose_L = \frac{(C_0)(V)}{(S)(f)}$$

Nonlinear Pharmacokinetics, $C_{avg,ss}$: Average Steady-State Concentration During the Dosage Interval Resulting from Intermittent Administration at a Given Dose Rate ($dose/\tau$)

$$2\text{--}27 \qquad C_{avg,ss} = \frac{(K_m)(S)(f)(dose/\tau)}{V_{max} - (S)(f)(dose/\tau)}$$

Nonlinear Pharmacokinetics, $dose/\tau$: Dose Rate to Achieve an Average Steady-State Concentration ($C_{avg,ss}$) During the Dosage Interval Resulting from Intermittent Administration

$$2\text{--}28 \qquad dose/\tau = \frac{(V_{max})(C_{avg,ss})}{(K_m + C_{avg,ss})(S)(f)}$$

Renal Impairment for $(C_{avg,ss})_{ri} = (C_{avg,ss})_n$

$$2\text{--}30 \qquad \frac{(dose/\tau)_{ri}}{(dose/\tau)_n} = \frac{dose_{ri} \times \tau_n}{dose_n \times \tau_{ri}} = 1 - F + F\,[(Cl_{cr})_{ri}/(Cl_{cr})_n]$$

Renal Impairment for $(C_{max,ss})_{ri} = (C_{max,ss})_n$

$$2\text{--}35 \qquad dose\ per\ \tau_{ri} = (dose_L)\,[1 - 10^{-0.3(\tau_{ri}/t_{1/2ri})}]$$

$^aC_{max,ss}$ is usually overestimated because drug clearance during absorption, time of administration, or both are ignored.

Linear Pharmacokinetics

The linear pharmacokinetic parameters used are f, Cl, V, and $t_{1/2}$. The techniques for obtaining these values from patient data are described in various textbooks, two of which (Winter; Rowland and Tozer) are cited in the bibliography at the end of the chapter.

Using $C_{avg,ss}$

To estimate $C_{avg,ss}$ resulting from intermittent administration at a given dose rate (dose/τ), use the following equations, depending on the specific pharmacokinetic variables with data available:

$$C_{avg,ss} = \frac{(S)(f)(\text{dose}/\tau)}{\text{Cl}} \tag{2–14}$$

$$C_{avg,ss} = \frac{1.4(S)(f)(t_{1/2})(\text{dose}/\tau)}{V} \tag{2–15}$$

Here, dose/τ refers to the dose of drug divided by the dosage interval, called the dose rate.

Conversely, to estimate a dose rate, given a target $C_{avg,ss}$,

$$\text{dose}/\tau = \frac{(C_{avg,ss})(\text{Cl})}{(S)(f)} \tag{2–16}$$

$$\text{dose}/\tau = \frac{(C_{avg,ss})(V)}{1.4(S)(f)(t_{1/2})} \tag{2–17}$$

To estimate $C_{inf,ss}$ resulting from continuous administration at a given dose rate (dose/t_{inf}).

$$C_{inf,ss} = \frac{(S)(f)(\text{dose}/t_{inf})}{\text{Cl}} \tag{2–18}$$

$$C_{inf,ss} = \frac{1.4(S)(f)(t_{1/2})(\text{dose}/t_{inf})}{V} \tag{2–19}$$

where dose/t_{inf} refers to the dose of drug divided by the infusion time, called the dose rate.

To estimate a dose rate, given a target $C_{inf,ss}$,

$$\text{dose}/t_{inf} = \frac{(C_{inf,ss})(\text{Cl})}{(S)(f)} \tag{2–20}$$

$$\text{dose}/t_{inf} = \frac{(C_{inf,ss})(V)}{1.4(S)(f)(t_{1/2})} \tag{2–21}$$

Note in Equations 2–14 to 2–21 the similarity of $C_{inf,ss}$ to $C_{avg,ss}$. The steady-state concentration resulting from continuous administration ($C_{inf,ss}$) is the same as the average value during the dosage interval for intermittent administration ($C_{avg,ss}$). Compare Equation 2–14 with 2–18, 2–15 with 2–19, 2–16 with 2–20, and 2–17 with 2–21.

Using $C_{max,ss}$

The equations for $C_{max,ss}$ make two assumptions: (1) for oral administration, absorption rate is much faster than elimination rate so that the lag time for absorption is ignored, and (2) for intravenous administration, the time for administering the drug (t_{inf}) is relatively brief compared with $t_{1/2}$, so drug loss during administration is ignored. These assumptions simplify clinical application but the result is usually an overestimation of $C_{max,ss}$.

To estimate $C_{max,ss}$ resulting from intermittent administration at a given dose rate (dose/τ), depending on the form of the exponent used in the calculation,

$$C_{max,ss} = \frac{(S)(f)(\text{dose}/V)}{1 - 10^{-0.3(\tau/t_{1/2})}} \tag{2-22}$$

$$C_{max,ss} = \frac{(S)(f)(\text{dose}/V)}{1 - e^{-0.7(\tau/t_{1/2})}} \tag{2-23}$$

Using $C_{min,ss}$

The assumptions described above for estimating $C_{max,ss}$ will influence the estimate of $C_{min,ss}$. To estimate $C_{min,ss}$ resulting from intermittent administration at a given dose rate (dose/τ),

$$C_{min,ss} = (C_{max,ss})\,[10^{-0.3(\tau/t_{1/2})}] \tag{2-24}$$

$$C_{min,ss} = (C_{max,ss})\,[e^{-0.7(\tau/t_{1/2})}] \tag{2-25}$$

Calculating a Loading Dose

When a loading dose is indicated, either to shorten the time required to build serum levels up to steady state or to provide an initial bolus dose, Equations 2–26 and 2–13 provide reasonable estimates. Equation 2–26 may be used when estimates of V and f are available. Equation 2–13, discussed previously, calculates the loading dose in terms of a ratio to the maintenance dose and requires knowledge of the intended maintenance dose, frequency of administration, and one pharmacokinetic estimate, $t_{1/2}$. In Equation 2–26, C_0 denotes the target concentration sought:

$$\text{dose}_L = \frac{(C_0)(V)}{(S)(f)} \tag{2-26}$$

$$\text{dose}_L/\text{dose} = 1/[1 - 10^{-0.3\,(\tau/t_{1/2})}] \tag{2-13}$$

Estimating Clearance

Individualization of drug therapy is improved by obtaining a patient-specific drug clearance, in preference to using a population value, whenever possible. At steady state, Equation 2–16 may be rearranged for use in estimating clearance from intermittent administration, as dose/rate and S are known and an estimate of $C_{avg,ss}$ may be obtained in the patient. The remaining variable, f, may be estimated, or it may be ignored, as the same value would be used again when a new regimen is developed using Equation 2–16. For continuous administration, clearance may be estimated using a rearrangement of Equation 2–20.

Nonlinear Pharmacokinetics

The nonlinear pharmacokinetic parameters used are V_{max} and K_m, rather than Cl, V, and $t_{1/2}$ used for linear pharmacokinetics. The techniques for obtaining these values from patient data are described in various sources cited in the bibliography (Shargel and Yu; and Winter are particularly useful) at the end of the chapter.

Using $C_{avg,ss}$

To estimate $C_{avg,ss}$ resulting from intermittent administration at a given dose rate (dose/τ),

$$C_{avg,ss} = \frac{(K_m)(S)(f)(\text{dose}/\tau)}{V_{max} - (S)(f)(\text{dose}/\tau)} \tag{2-27}$$

$$\text{dose}/\tau = \frac{(V_{max})(C_{avg,ss})}{(K_m + C_{avg,ss})(S)(f)} \tag{2-28}$$

Using Equations 2–27 and 2–28, intended for drugs demonstrating nonlinear pharmacokinetic behavior, requires knowledge of V_{max} and K_m. These values may be obtained by various linear or bayesian graphing techniques[6,7] that require at least one set of dose-versus-steady-state $C_{avg,ss}$ values (for bayesian) or two or more sets of these values (for linear graphing).

One example of linear graphing is shown in Figure 2–5. In this approach, the dose rate (as dose/d) is plotted on the vertical axis and drug clearance (as dose/d/$C_{avg,ss}$) is plotted on the horizontal axis. The line of best fit through the data yields a slope of K_m (actually the negative value of K_m as the slope is negative) and the intercept on the vertical axis represents V_{max}. When the data are plotted as actual dose rate (as shown in Figure 2–5) the resulting V_{max} is an *apparent* value, if the actual dose rate assumes that $S = 1.0$. This apparent value is then used in Equations 2–27 and 2–28. If, as shown in Figure 2–5, the data represent the use of phenytoin capsules (for which $S = 0.92$) the apparent V_{max} of 630 mg/d is actually 8% higher than the true value.

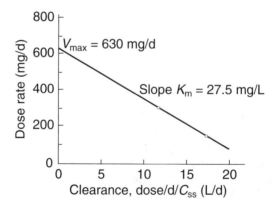

Figure 2–5. Plot of dose rate versus clearance for a drug with nonlinear pharmacokinetics. The negative slope of the line yields K_m and the intercept on the dose rate axis gives the V_{max}. (*From L. Shargel and A. B. C. Yu,* Applied Biopharmaceutics and Pharmacokinetics. *3rd ed. Norwalk, CT: Appleton & Lange; 1993, with permission.*)

EFFECT OF AGING ON PHARMACOKINETIC VARIABLES

Most pharmacokinetic data used as reference values have been obtained in 25- to 60-year-old adults; however, studies have shown that pediatric and geriatric populations do not necessarily share the population data obtained in young and middle-aged adults.[8,9] In general terms, renal drug clearance reaches full maturity by 1 year and remains stable until it begins declining in the early twenties. Drug metabolism and hepatic clearance generally reach a maximum between years 1 and 12 and then begin to decrease with age. As noted from the equations discussed above, when pharmacokinetic variables are different for the young and old compared with the usually accepted adult reference values, changes in dose rate are indicated if it can be assumed, as it often is, that a drug's therapeutic range in the reference population elicits the same effects in the young and the elderly.

In the pediatric population, renal function normalized for body surface area generally increases until adult values are reached by 1 year. Drug distribution volumes normalized for body weight decrease from a high point in neonates, reaching adult values in late childhood. Extracellular fluid volume is 50% greater at age 1 than it is as an adult. Metabolic patterns are complex but generally show increasing enzyme activity from the neonatal period through late childhood. As a result of these observations, drug dosage is often higher (mg/kg) in children than adults. Much work remains to be done, however, in evaluating pharmacodynamic and pharmacokinetic changes with age.

In the geriatric population, renal and hepatic function decline 0.5 to 2% per year after 20 years of age. The influence of aging on renal function generally appears to be more marked than on hepatic function, however. The clearance of drugs dependent primarily on the kidney for elimination declines by nearly 50%, and often the half-life nearly doubles, over a 40- to 50-year period from young adulthood; the aminoglycosides, digoxin, lithium, and vancomycin are examples. Drugs primarily metabolized do not show a consistent pattern, however. Some drugs show no significant age-related effect (eg, phenytoin, salicylates, theophylline), whereas others exhibit reduced clearance (eg, some benzodiazepines and tricyclic antidepressants). Much of the increased pharmacodynamic response for drugs attributed to aging is more likely the result of administering doses more appropriate for younger adults.

EFFECT OF DISEASE ON PHARMACOKINETIC VARIABLES

It is clear from looking at Equations 2–13 to 2–28 that factors modifying any of the pharmacokinetic variables may lead to changes in steady-state levels. As TDM depends on maintaining C_{ss} values within a target concentration range, pharmacokinetic changes may necessitate a modification in dose rate to adjust C_{ss}. Pharmacokinetic alterations influence dose adjustments in two ways: (1) dosage regimens developed using population pharmacokinetic parameters for normals may need to be changed for patients with kidney, liver, or heart disease, and (2) deteriorating physiologic status during a course of treatment may necessitate dosage adjustment.

Hepatic Impairment

The influence of liver disease on drug pharmacokinetics is complex.[10,11] Two processes contribute to hepatic clearance of a drug: blood flow rate in delivering drug to the liver and the intrinsic capacity of the liver enzymes to metabolize the drug. Drugs that are efficiently metabolized (high extraction ratio) show hepatic clearance largely dependent on hepatic blood flow (see Equation 2–6 and associated discussion). Drugs that are inefficiently metabolized (low extraction ratio) exhibit clearance that is rate limited by enzyme function.

In general terms, moderate to severe hepatic disease is expected to slow overall clearance and prolong half-life for drugs highly dependent on the liver for elimination. For drugs subject to TDM, this includes most antiarrhythmics, antiepileptics, cyclosporine, and theophylline. Studies on highly extracted drugs (eg, lidocaine among the above drugs) verify these general trends. Liver impairment often slows hepatic blood flow, resulting in decreased clearance. But for poorly extracted drugs, which includes most of the above, the studies show less consistency. Although liver disease slows clearance and increases half-life for some drugs, it has no apparent effect on others.

Most clinicians approach serious hepatic disease in patients with caution, close monitoring, and the expectation that a decrease in dose rate may be necessary. Unfortunately, in contrast to kidney disease to be discussed below, no quantitative markers relating the extent of liver disease to decreases in drug clearance are available to guide the practitioner.

Cardiac Impairment

Serious heart disease decreases hepatic and renal clearances, reduces volume of distribution, and may slow absorption for some drugs.[12] The effect of compromised perfusion is most critical for drugs that have high extraction ratios and are highly dependent on the liver for clearance. For these drugs (eg, lidocaine), hepatic blood flow is the rate-limiting step. Even drugs rate limited by enzyme capacity (eg, quinidine, theophylline) are influenced by cardiac impairment, presumably by modifying the activity of some enzymes. Like liver disease, no quantitative markers for indicating the relationship between the extent of cardiac impairment and decreases in drug clearance are available to guide clinicians.

Renal Impairment

For renal impairment there is a physiologic marker that can be used to make quantitative estimates of the influence of kidney disease on drug clearance. Many of the contributions of TDM have focused on studying and validating data and methods for modifying drug dosage regimens when renal function declines.[13–16] This condition applies not only during renal disease but also during aging for the healthy elderly. Drugs with narrow therapeutic ranges and a high dependence on the kidney for clearance require close monitoring during moderate to severe renal impairment. These drugs include the aminoglycosides, digoxin, lithium, and vancomycin.

There are two common methods for adjusting dosage regimens when kidney function declines because of either disease or aging. For most drugs, the goal is to maintain the same $C_{avg,ss}$ during renal decline as under normal conditions. For a few drugs, for example, antibiotics like the aminoglycosides and vancomycin, keeping $C_{max,ss}$ the same during kidney impairment and normal conditions is the objective. Both approaches are described below.

Using $C_{avg,ss}$ as a Target

When the pharmacokinetic objective is to maintain serum concentrations such that $C_{avg,ss}$ for a drug in the impaired patient is set equal to the $C_{avg,ss}$ sought in normals, the following equalities apply:

$$\frac{(Cl)_{ri}}{(Cl)_n} = \frac{(t_{1/2})_n}{(t_{1/2})_{ri}} = 1 - F + F\,[(Cl_{cr})_{ri}/(Cl_{cr})_n] \tag{2--29}$$

$$\frac{(dose/\tau)_{ri}}{(dose/\tau)_n} = \frac{dose_{ri} \times \tau_n}{dose_n \times \tau_{ri}} = 1 - F + F\,[(Cl_{cr})_{ri}/(Cl_{cr})_n] \tag{2--30}$$

In these equations, the subscripts ri and n denote renal impaired and normal conditions, respectively, Cl_{cr} is the creatinine clearance, and F is the fraction of drug administered that is eliminated unchanged (not metabolized). The expression $1 - F + F\,[\,(Cl_{cr})_{ri}\,/\,(Cl_{cr})_n]$ is called the *dosage reduction factor* and represents the fraction of the normal daily dose given to the impaired patient that maintains $(C_{avg,ss})_{ri} = (C_{avg,ss})_n$.

Equations 2–29 and 2–30 state that the following are all equal to the dosage reduction factor:
- Fraction of drug clearance compared with normal, for a given degree of renal impairment
- Fraction of normal half-life compared with renal impairment
- Fraction of daily dose in renal impairment compared with normal

If the objective is to estimate pharmacokinetic parameters during kidney disease, Equation 2–29 shows that when a practitioner knows the population values in normals for a drug (Cl, F, and $t_{1/2}$), and the extent of renal decline in a patient as estimated by the creatinine clearance, then an estimate of Cl or $t_{1/2}$, or both, in the patient may be calculated. Alternately, if the goal is to estimate a modified dosage regimen during renal impairment, Equation 2–30 states that knowledge of the population values in normals allows calculation of a dosage regimen.

Using the dosage reduction factor requires an estimate of $(Cl_{cr})_{ri}$ for the patient. Creatinine clearance is considered the most accurate index of renal function. Obtaining an accurate measure of Cl_{cr} is difficult, however, because it requires a 24-hour collection of urine. This is burdensome and costly. Fortunately, the concentration of creatinine in serum may be used to estimate creatinine clearance. The most commonly used and validated equation for estimating Cl_{cr} takes serum creatinine, age, weight, and gender into account, and was developed by Cockcroft and Gault[17]:

$$Cl_{cr}\,(mL/min,\ males) = \frac{(140 - age)(weight)}{(Cr_s)(72)} \tag{2--31}$$

$$Cl_{cr}\,(mL/min,\ females) = (0.85)\,(Cl_{cr}\ in\ males) \tag{2--32}$$

where age is in years, weight in kilograms, and serum creatinine (Cr_s) in milligrams/deciliter.

Using Equations 2–31 and 2–32 assumes that Cr_s is stable, not changing daily, and weight approximates normal muscle mass, as expressed by ideal (lean) body weight. When the patient's weight seems excessive, the following equations may be used to estimate the ideal weight estimate required for Equations 2–31 and 2–32:

$$\text{ideal body weight (kg, males)} = 50 + 2.3 \text{ (height} - 60) \qquad (2\text{–}33)$$

$$\text{ideal body weight (kg, females)} = 45 + 2.3 \text{ (height} - 60) \qquad (2\text{–}34)$$

Here height is in inches.

In addition to needing an estimate of Cl_{cr} to calculate the dosage reduction factor in Equations 2–29 and 2–30, a population value for F, the fraction of drug excreted unchanged, is required. The larger the value of F, the more likely that a moderate to serious decline in renal impairment will require a modification of the normal dosage regimen. Some values for TDM drugs follow:

	F
Lithium	1.0
Aminoglycosides	0.98
Vancomycin	0.95
Digoxin	0.8
Procainamide	0.5
Quinidine	0.2
Theophylline	0.1
Phenytoin	<0.1

To estimate a modified dosage regimen for a drug requires four steps:

1. Obtain the population pharmacokinetic parameters and the $C_{avg,ss}$ used in normals.
2. Determine the dosage regimen used in normals.
3. Estimate Cl_{cr} using Equation 2–31 or 2–32.
4. Use Equation 2–30 to estimate dose rate. Alternately, vary τ to calculate different doses best matched to available dosage forms and/or convenience of τ.

Using Equation 2–30 provides a variety of dosage regimens, all yielding the same daily dose (eg, 400 mg q24h, 200 mg q12h, 100 mg q6h). Each of these regimens produces the same $C_{avg,ss}$, but $C_{max,ss}$ and $C_{min,ss}$ values vary, as shown in Figure 2–6. The choice of regimens may depend on which resulting serum concentration-versus-time profile best fits the therapeutic range.

Using $C_{max,ss}$ as a Target

When the pharmacokinetic objective is to maintain serum concentrations such that $C_{max,ss}$ for a drug in the impaired patient is set equal to the $C_{max,ss}$ used in normals, the following general approach is recommended for estimating a modified dosage regimen:

1. Determine the target $C_{max,ss}$ used in normals.
2. Estimate, perhaps using Equation 2–26, the loading dose (dose$_L$) needed to achieve the target $C_{max,ss}$.

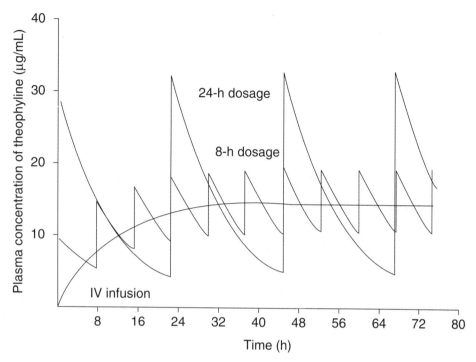

Figure 2–6. Relationship between frequency of dosing and maximum and minimum serum drug concentrations when steady state is achieved. (*From B. G. Katzung, ed.* Basic and Clinical Pharmacology. *5th ed. Norwalk, CT: Appleton & Lange; 1992, with permission.*)

3. Estimate Cl_{cr} using Equation 2–31 or 2–32.
4. Use Equation 2–29 to estimate $(t_{1/2})_{ri}$.
5. Select a desired τ_{ri} and then, using the $(t_{1/2})_{ri}$ estimated above, calculate the fraction of drug lost during the selected τ_{ri} by using Equation 2–12.
6. The maintenance dose for τ_{ri} is calculated using steps 2 and 5:

$$\text{dose per } \tau_{ri} = (\text{dose}_L)(\text{fraction of drug lost during } \tau_{ri}) \qquad (2\text{--}35)$$

7. The estimated regimen will produce the same $C_{max,ss}$ in the renally impaired patient as it does in normals. If the dose is inconvenient or otherwise not available, then steps 5 and 6 may be repeated until the best balance of dose and frequency is achieved.

Using Equations 2–29 to 2–35 assumes that renal impairment does not change pharmacokinetic parameters in the patient other than Cl and the relationship between C_{ss} and pharmacologic response. As metabolism, protein binding, absorption, or the volume of distribution may occasionally be altered as a result of kidney disease in the patient, close monitoring is always required after initiating the modified regimen.[16]

An example of estimating a modified dosage regimen for the renally impaired patient is included at the end of this chapter.

Dialysis

Hemodialysis is often used in patients with end-stage renal disease. As these patients are frequently using drugs with dosage regimens tailored to a narrow therapeutic range, TDM is concerned with determining if the period of dialysis removes enough drug to require a supplementation in dose.[14,15,18] The aminoglycosides, lithium, procainamide, and theophylline are examples of commonly monitored drugs that are cleared from the body by hemodialysis.

The half-life of a drug in a patient during the period in which no dialysis is occurring is characterized by Equation 2–9,

$$t_{1/2} = \frac{V}{1.4(Cl_{pat})}$$

where the subscript pat is added to clarify that the only clearance factors operating are those of the patient. During the period in which dialysis is occurring, the contribution of the dialysis shortens the half-life to

$$t_{1/2} = \frac{V}{1.4(Cl_{pat} + Cl_{dial})} \tag{2–36}$$

where the subscript dial refers to the contribution of dialysis. The primary question asked by the practitioner is whether the drug half-life during the period of dialysis (Equation 2–36) will be decreased significantly when compared with the baseline period of no dialysis (Equation 2–9). If so, the fraction of drug lost during the dialysis period will be substantially greater than baseline, using Equation 2–12 (where τ in this case refers to the duration of dialysis). In this situation, a supplementation of dose will be required after dialysis. If $t_{1/2}$ is not expected to be significantly different from Equations 2–9 and 2–36, then no additional dose is indicated.

A number of characteristics contribute to predicting whether dialysis will contribute significantly to drug clearance:

- *Molecular weight.* Drugs with molecular weights less than 500 do cross the dialysis membrane. This rules out common TDM drugs like digoxin and vancomycin.
- *Water solubility.* Highly polar drugs partition efficiently into the dialysis fluid. This rules out TDM drugs like phenytoin that are poorly soluble at physiologic pH.
- *Protein binding.* Highly bound drugs do not dialyze efficiently because only the unbound molecule passes through the dialysis membrane. This rules out many antiepileptics, some antiarrhythmics, and warfarin.
- *Volume of distribution.* Drugs with large distribution volumes have too little drug in blood, and too much in tissues, to be efficiently dialyzed. This rules out TDM drugs like digoxin.
- *Drug dialysis clearance (dialysance) compared with patient clearance.* As discussed above for Equation 2–36, dialysis will not make a meaningful contribution to drug loss if dialysance does not approach patient clearance in magnitude.

APPLICATION OF DOSAGE REGIMEN EQUATIONS

——————— EXAMPLE 2–1 ———————

Using $C_{avg,ss}$ to develop the regimen. The commonly accepted therapeutic range for theophylline is 10 to 20 µg/mL. What is a typical oral dosage regimen for anhydrous theophylline ($S = 1$) in an average patient? Assume that the population pharmacokinetic parameters in normals are Cl = 0.67 mL/kg/min, $V = 0.5$ L/kg, and $f = 1$.

Use Equation 2–16 for intermittent administration, set an arbitrary target concentration objective of 13 µg/mL (usually the conservative portion of the therapeutic range is used) for maintaining the average steady-state concentration ($C_{avg,ss}$) during τ, and convert the pharmacokinetic parameters to consistent units:

$$\text{dose}/\tau = \frac{(C_{avg,ss})(Cl)}{(S)(f)}$$

$$\text{dose}/\tau = \frac{(13 \text{ mg/L})(0.04 \text{ L/kg/h})}{(1)(1)} = 0.52 \text{ mg/kg/h}$$

$$= 4.16 \text{ mg/kg/8 h} = 291 \text{ mg/70 kg/8 h}$$

$$= 6.24 \text{ mg/kg/12 h} = 437 \text{ mg/70 kg/12 h}$$

The average-weight patient needs 250 to 300 mg q8h or 400 to 500 mg q12h.

——————— EXAMPLE 2–2 ———————

Using $C_{max,ss}$ and $C_{min,ss}$ to develop the regimen. A common dosage regimen for intravenous tobramycin is 1.5 mg/kg q8h (each dose administered over a 30-minute period). Most clinicians adjust regimens for severe systemic infections to achieve peak (maximum) levels of 6 to 10 µg/mL for effectiveness and trough (minimum) levels less than 2 µg/mL to reduce the risk of toxicity. Does this dosage regimen meet these target concentration objectives in normal patients? Assume that the population pharmacokinetic parameters in normals are Cl = 0.09 L/kg/h, $t_{1/2} = 2.2$ h, and $V = 0.25$ L/kg. For intravenous administration, $f = 1$, and $S = 1$ for the dosage form.

Use Equation 2–22, because $C_{max,ss}$ is the target concentration sought, divide the dose rate by the volume of distribution to convert the numerator to concentration terms (mg/L), and accept the assumption of the equation that drug loss during the 0.5-hour infusion is negligible:

$$C_{max,ss} = \frac{(S)(f)(\text{dose}/V)}{1 - 10^{-0.3(\tau/t_{1/2})}}$$

$$C_{max,ss} = \frac{(1)(1)(1.5 \text{ mg/kg}) / (0.25 \text{ L/kg})}{1 - 10^{-0.3(8 \text{ h}/2.2 \text{ h})}} = 6.5 \text{ mg/L (µg/mL)}$$

Then use Equation 2.24 to estimate $C_{min,ss}$:

$$C_{min,ss} = (C_{max,ss}) [10^{-0.3\, \tau/t_{1/2}}]$$

$$C_{min,ss} = (6.5) [10^{-0.3\, (8\, h/2.2\, h)}] = 0.5\ mg/L\ (\mu g/mL)$$

The regimen will meet the target concentration objectives in normal patients. But because the $C_{max,ss}$ of 6.5 µg/mL represents the average value for the population, a slightly higher dose will ensure that more patients achieve levels greater than 6.5 µg/mL.

_____ **EXAMPLE 2–3** _____

Effect of renal impairment. What happens when the above tobramycin regimen of 1.5 mg/kg/h is administered to a 60-year-old, 70-kg male patient with a serum creatinine (Cr_s) of 2.5 mg/dL?

As normal Cr_s is approximately 1 mg/dL, the patient has reduced renal function. Use Equation 2–31 to estimate Cl_{cr}:

$$Cl_{cr}\ (males) = \frac{(140 - age)(weight)}{(Cr_s)(72)}$$

$$Cl_{cr}\ (males) = \frac{(140 - 60\ y)(70\ kg)}{(2.5\ mg/dL)(72)} = 31\ mL/min$$

Then use Equation 2–29 to estimate $(t_{1/2})_{ri}$, assuming the population values of $F = 0.98$, $(t_{1/2})_n = 2.2$ hours, and $(Cl_{cr})_n = 120$ mL/min:

$$\frac{(t_{1/2})_n}{(t_{1/2})_{ri}} = 1 - F + F\,[(Cl_{cr})_{ri} / (Cl_{cr})_n]$$

$$\frac{(2.2\ h)}{(t_{1/2})_{ri}} = 1 - 0.98 + 0.98\,[31\,/\,120] = 0.27$$

$$(t_{1/2})_{ri} = 8.1\ h$$

Use Equation 2–22 to estimate $C_{max,ss}$:

$$C_{max,ss} = \frac{(S)(f)(dose/V)}{1 - 10^{-0.3(\tau/t_{1/2})}}$$

$$C_{max,ss} = \frac{(1)(1)(1.5\ mg/kg)\,/\,(0.25\ L/kg)}{1 - 10^{-0.3(8\ h/8.1\ h)}} = 12.1\ mg/L\ (\mu g/mL)$$

Then use Equation 2–24 to estimate $C_{min,ss}$:

$$C_{min,ss} = (C_{max,ss}) [10^{-0.3\,(\tau/t_{1/2})}]$$

$$C_{min,ss} = (12.1) [10^{-0.3\,(8\ h/8.1\ h)}] = 6.1\ mg/L\ (\mu g/mL)$$

Using the same regimen for this patient as for normals results in $C_{max,ss}$ and $C_{min,ss}$ levels that are both above the target concentration ranges and puts the patient at some risk for a toxic reaction.

——————— **EXAMPLE 2–4** ———————

Modifying the regimen during renal impairment. For the renally impaired patient in Example 2–3, what should be done to modify the typical tobramycin regimen of 1.5 mg/kg q8h used for normals in Example 2–2? From Examples 2–3 and 2–2, the estimates of $t_{1/2}$ and V in this patient are 8.1 hours and 0.25 L/kg, respectively.

To achieve the maximum target concentration range of 6 to 10 μg/mL, as noted in Example 2–2, use Equation 2–26 to calculate a loading dose, selecting an arbitrary target concentration of 7 μg/mL:

$$\text{dose}_L = \frac{(C_0)(V)}{(S)(f)}$$

$$\text{dose}_L = \frac{(7 \text{ mg/L})(0.25 \text{ L/kg})}{(1)(1)} = 1.75 \text{ mg/kg}$$

As Example 2–3 shows that a dosage interval of q8h yields potentially toxic levels, extending the interval to q12h or q24h should be considered. Trying q24h, calculate the fraction of the loading dose that is lost during τ by using Equation 2–12:

fraction of drug in body lost per dosage interval $= 1 - 10^{-0.3 \, (\tau/t_{1/2})}$

fraction of drug in body lost per dosage interval $= 1 - 10^{-0.3 \, (24 \text{ h}/8.1 \text{ h})} = 0.87$

Then use Equation 2–35 to calculate the dose to be administered q24h:

$$\text{dose per } \tau_{ri} = (\text{dose}_L)\,(\text{fraction of drug lost during } \tau_{ri})$$

$$\text{dose per } \tau_{ri} = (1.75 \text{ mg/kg})\,(0.87) = 1.5 \text{ mg/kg q24h}$$

The above regimen of 1.5 mg/kg q24h will sustain the $C_{max,ss}$ of 7 μg/mL produced by the loading dose. The final consideration is whether this regimen will also provide a $C_{min,ss}$ below the 2 μg/ml range noted in Example 2–2 for reducing the risk of toxicity. Use Equation 2–24:

$$C_{min,ss} = (C_{max,ss})\,[10^{-0.3 \, (\tau/t_{1/2})}]$$

$$C_{min,ss} = (7 \text{ μg/mL})\,[10^{-0.3 \, (24h/8.1 \, h)}] = 0.9 \text{ μg/mL}$$

A loading dose of 1.75 mg/kg followed by a regimen of 1.5 mg/kg q24h is expected to produce serum levels within the accepted ranges. For reference, a q12h regimen requires a dose of 1.1 mg/kg and yields estimated $C_{max,ss}$ and $C_{min,ss}$ levels of 7 and 2.5 μg/mL, respectively. This suggests that in the average patient with this degree of renal impairment, q12h may be less preferable than q24h. On the other hand, some clinicians would choose q12h, despite the potentially greater risk of nephrotoxicity, because therapeutic serum concentrations would be maintained for a longer portion of each day than with q24h.

_____ QUESTIONS _____

1. The commonly accepted therapeutic range for digoxin is $C_{avg,ss}$ = 0.8 to 2 ng/mL. Does the typical dosage regimen of 250 µg/day po (S = 1, f = 0.7) produce an average steady-state serum concentration during the dosage interval that is within the therapeutic range for 70-kg normals? Assume the following population pharmacokinetic parameters: V = 7 L/kg, Cl = 2 mL/kg/min, and $t_{1/2}$ = 40 hours.

2. The commonly accepted therapeutic range for vancomycin is to seek, during the steady-state dosage interval, maximum levels for therapeutic effectiveness and minimum levels to preserve effectiveness while minimizing toxicity of 20 to 40 and 5 to 15 µg/mL, respectively. Will a regimen of 1000 mg q12h intravenously (S = 1, f = 1) produce levels within the target concentration ranges for 70-kg normals? Assume the following population parameters: V = 0.7 L/kg, Cl = 1.2 mL/kg/min, and $t_{1/2}$ = 7 hours.

3. A continuous infusion of intravenous aminophylline (S = 0.8, f = 1) produced a steady-state level ($C_{inf,ss}$) of 6 µg/mL when a regimen of 36 mg/h was administered to a 60-kg patient with normal renal and hepatic function. How does this patient's clearance compare with the population value? Assume the following population parameters: V = 0.5 L/kg, Cl = 1 L/kg/d, and $t_{1/2}$ = 8.5 hours.

4. Procainamide has a commonly accepted therapeutic range of 4 to 10 µg/mL. (1) If a regimen of 500 mg q4h produces a $C_{avg,ss}$ of 8.3 µg/mL in a specific 70-kg patient, what regimen is needed to lower the $C_{avg,ss}$ to 5 µg/mL? Procainamide exhibits linear pharmacokinetic behavior. Available oral dosage forms contain 250, 375, and 500 mg of procainamide hydrochloride. (2) Assume the following population parameters: V = 2 L/kg, Cl = 0.4 L/kg/h, $t_{1/2}$ = 3.5 h, and f = 0.85. For procainamide hydrochloride dosage forms, S = 0.87. How does the clearance for this patient compare with the population value? Is this patient's steady-state level higher, lower, or about the same as expected in the average patient?

5. A nurse, medical resident, and pharmacy student disagree over the intravenous tobramycin regimen to be prescribed for a patient with pseudomonas septicemia who has the following characteristics: female, 30 years old, 60 kg, 5 ft 6 in., and a serum creatinine (Cr_s) of 3 mg/dL.

Nurse	1.5 mg/kg bolus (load)	Then 0.75 mg/kg q24h (0.5-hour infusion)
Medical resident	No bolus	1.5 mg/kg q24h (0.5-hour infusion)
Pharmacy student	No bolus	3.0 mg/kg q24h (0.5-hour infusion)

Assume in normals a mean population tobramycin $t_{1/2}$ of 2.5 hours and a creatinine clearance of 120 ml/min. Because the $t_{1/2}$ is surely long in this patient compared with the time required to first infuse the drug and then wait to sample for $C_{max,ss}$, it is reasonable to ignore drug loss in the calculations during this period as it is negligible.
    Which regimen seems most appropriate?

BIBLIOGRAPHY

Benet LZ, Massoud N. Pharmacokinetics. In Benet LZ, Massoud N, Gambertoglio JG, eds. *Pharmacokinetic Basis for Drug Treatment.* New York: Raven Press; 1984:1–28.

Benet LZ, Mitchell JR, Sheiner LB. Pharmacokinetics. In Gilman AG, Wall TW, Nies AS, Taylor P, eds. *Goodman and Gilman's the Pharmacological Basis of Therapeutics.* 8th ed. New York: Pergamon Press; 1990:1–32.

MacKichan JJ, Comstock TJ. General pharmacokinetic principles. In Taylor WJ, Diers Caviness MH, eds. *A Textbook for the Clinical Application of Therapeutic Drug Monitoring.* Irving, TX: Abbott Laboratories; 1986:pp 3–30.

Rowland M, and Tozer TN. *Clinical Pharmacokinetics: Concepts and Applications.* 2nd ed. Philadelphia: Lea & Febiger; 1989.

Shargel L, Yu ABC. *Applied Biopharmaceutics and Pharmacokinetics.* 3rd ed. Norwalk, CT: Appleton & Lange; 1993.

Winter ME. *Basic Clinical Pharmacokinetics.* 2nd ed. Spokane, WA: Applied Therapeutics; 1988.

REFERENCES

1. Benet LZ. Pharmacokinetics: Absorption, distribution, and elimination. In Katzung BG, ed. *Basic and Clinical Pharmacology.* 4th ed. Norwalk: CT, Appleton & Lange; 1989:29–40.
2. MacKichan JJ, Comstock TJ. General pharmacokinetic principles. In Taylor WJ, Diers Caviness MH- (eds): *A Textbook for the Clinical Application of Therapeutic Drug Monitoring.* Irving, TX: Abbott Laboratories; 1986:3–30.
3. Greenblatt DJ. Presystemic extraction: Mechanisms and consequences. *J Clin Pharmacol.* 1993; 33:650–656.
4. Holford NHG. Clinical interpretation of drug concentrations. In Katzung BG, ed. *Basic and Clinical Pharmacology.* 4th ed. Norwalk, CT: Appleton & Lange; 1989:802–809.
5. Winter ME. *Basic Clinical Pharmacokinetics.* 2nd ed. Spokane, WA: Applied Therapeutics; 1988:13–20.
6. Tozer TN, Winter ME. Phenytoin. In Evans WE, Schentag JJ, Jusko WJ, eds. *Applied Pharmacokinetics: Principles of Therapeutic Drug Monitoring.* 3rd ed. Spokane, WA: Applied Therapeutics; 1992:25-29–25-34.
7. Shargel L, and Yu ABC. *Applied Biopharmaceutics and Pharmacokinetics.* 3rd ed. Norwalk, CT: Appleton & Lange; 1993:387–391.
8. Green TP, Mirkin BL. Clinical pharmacokinetics: Pediatric considerations. In Benet LZ, Massoud N, Gambertoglio JG, eds. *Pharmacokinetic Basis for Drug Treatment.* New York: Raven Press; 1984: 269–282.
9. Massoud N. Pharmacokinetic considerations in geriatric patients. In Benet LZ, Massoud N, Gambertoglio JG, eds. *Pharmacokinetic Basis for Drug Treatment.* New York: Raven Press; 1984:283–310.
10. Wilkinson GR. Influence of hepatic disease on pharmacokinetics. In Evans WE, Schentag JJ, Jusko WJ, eds. *Applied Pharmacokinetics.* 2nd ed. Spokane, WA: Applied Therapeutics; 1986:116–138.
11. Williams RL. Drugs and the liver: Clinical applications. In Benet LZ, Massoud N, Gambertoglio JG, eds. *Pharmacokinetic Basis for Drug Treatment.* New York: Raven Press; 1984:63–75.
12. Benowitz NL. Effects of cardiac disease on pharmacokinetics: Pathophysiologic considerations. In Benet LZ, Massoud N, Gambertoglio JG, eds. *Pharmacokinetic Basis for Drug Treatment.* New York: Raven Press; 1984:89–104.
13. Brater DC, Chennavasin P. Effects of renal disease: Pharmacokinetic considerations. In Benet LZ,

Massoud N, Gambertoglio JG, eds. *Pharmacokinetic Basis for Drug Treatment.* New York: Raven Press; 1984:119–147.

14. Gambertoglio JG. Effects of renal disease: Altered pharmacokinetics. In Benet LZ, Massoud N, Gambertoglio JG, eds. *Pharmacokinetic Basis for Drug Treatment.* New York: Raven Press; 1984: 149–171.

15. Gibson TP. Influence of renal disease on pharmacokinetics. In Evans WE, Schentag JJ, Jusko WJ, eds. *Applied Pharmacokinetics.* 2nd ed. Spokane, WA: Applied Therapeutics; 1986:83–115.

16. Turnheim K. Pitfalls of pharmacokinetic dosage guidelines in renal insufficiency. *Eur J Clin Pharmacol.* 1991;40:87–93.

17. Cockcroft DW, Gault MH. Prediction of creatinine clearance from serum creatinine. *Nephron.* 1976;16:31–41.

18. Gibson TP, Nelson HA. Drug kinetics and artificial kidneys. *Clin Pharmacokinet.* 1977;2:403–426.

Chapter 3

The Total Testing Process Applied to Therapeutic Drug Monitoring

Judith T. Barr

Gerald E. Schumacher

Keep in Mind

- The Total Testing Process (TTP) refers to all aspects of the steps of laboratory testing beginning with a clinical question that is prompted by the patient–clinician encounter and concluding with the impact of the test result on patient care.

- TTP emphasizes that therapeutic drug monitoring must be considered a process involving a series of steps and interrelated activities and should not be viewed simply as a numerical value for a serum drug concentration.

- TTP focuses on identifying all steps of the therapeutic drug monitoring (TDM) testing process, highlighting where variations and errors can occur, interpreting drug serum concentration test results in light of the steps involved and the variations and errors that may occur, and improving the contribution of testing to achieving desired patient outcomes.

- There are four components and 11 steps in TTP. The preanalytic component consists of four steps: (1) clinical question, (2) test selected, (3) test ordered, and (4) specimen collected. The analytic component includes three steps: (5) sample prepared, (6) analysis performed, and (7) result verified. The postanalytic component comprises four steps: (8) result reported, (9) clinical answer, (10) action taken, and (11) effect on patient care. These three components are affected by the fourth component, the regulatory environment within which TDM is performed.

- TDM can intervene to improve many of the steps in TTP: providing education, drug information, and research to improve the formulation of the clinical question and interpretation of the test results; assessing the appropriateness of the TDM test order; scheduling specimen collection; developing drug dosing guidelines; and providing written and oral consultation concerning TDM results.

   Although serum drug level assays have been a part of clinical practice for more than 30 years, in many institutions therapeutic drug monitoring remains a disjointed service. Physicians or other clinicians write orders for serum drug concentrations in charts, ward secretaries transcribe these orders to laboratory forms, nurses administer the drugs, pharmacists may schedule the sample collection times, phlebotomists obtain the blood samples, clinical laboratory scientists perform the laboratory assays, and physicians or other clinicians interpret the results. When well designed and implemented, TDM can represent the best of an integrated, interdisciplinary team approach to health care, building on the knowledge and skills of each team member while requiring cooperation and communication within the unit. When TDM is poorly organized, errors can occur throughout the process, and TDM inadvertently can lead to patient harm.

The clinical pharmacokinetic service (CPKS) is one model for providing comprehensive TDM care (Parent Drug and Active Metabolites under Step 2). In this approach, clinical pharmacists assume a major portion of the responsibility for all aspects of TDM; they directly intervene in the process of TDM testing, order serum drug concentrations, schedule specimen collection, and issue interpretative reports containing recommendations for drug therapy modifications. Although there are many variations of this model (eg, some CPKSs perform drug assays as part of the service, others rely on the routine clinical laboratory for the analyses), national reports are not available concerning the number of CPKSs, the structure and function of these services, and the methods that are used to ensure quality wherever drugs are being therapeutically monitored.

Regardless of how an institution structures the process by which serum drug concentrations are obtained, the fact remains that for optimal patient care (1) each step of the process must be explicitly identified, (2) responsibility assigned, (3) quality assurance measures developed, and (4) outcomes assessed. This is especially important in TDM, where different professions may participate at various steps in the process and where errors can occur both within and between the numerous steps.

THE TOTAL TESTING PROCESS

The Total Testing Process (TTP) refers to all aspects of the steps of laboratory testing beginning with a clinical question that is prompted by the patient–clinician encounter and concluding with the impact of the test result on patient care. This broad view of laboratory testing has evolved through a series of institutes sponsored by the Centers for Disease Control (CDC).[1,2] At these invitational institutes, laboratorians, clinicians, equipment and supply manufacturers, and laboratory regulators were challenged to examine laboratory quality from a broad patient-centered perspective rather than their narrow, discipline-specific frame of reference. Multidisciplinary group discussions led participants to appreciate the complexity and interrelationship of the multiple steps required to convert a test request into a test result that could impact patient care.

The Total Testing Process has direct application to the field of therapeutic drug monitoring. TTP requires that we consider TDM as a process, not simply a numerical value for a serum drug concentration. At a minimum, we could improve the interpretation of TDM testing by identifying all steps of the TDM testing process, determining where variations and errors can occur, and interpreting TDM results in the light of these factors. But we should move beyond improved interpretation to build TDM testing systems that prevent errors from occurring in all steps of the Total Testing Process and that maximally contribute to an improved patient outcome. We use this perspective as we describe the various components of the process of therapeutic drug monitoring and suggest strategies to improve the quality of TDM testing.

First we present an overview of the major steps in the generic Total Testing Process; in the remainder of the chapter, we analyze the components of TDM using the Total Testing Process model. We chronologically describe the total TDM testing process and suggest methods by which quality can be improved in each step of the process. In aggregate, attention to quality issues in each step of the testing process should provide the foundation for a TDM total quality management program and a framework for increased communication among all involved in TDM testing.

As seen in Figure 3–1, the Total Testing Process begins and ends with patient care and consists of four major components: preanalytic, analytic, postanalytic, and the regulatory environment within which the test is performed. The *preanalytic component* begins with a clinician–patient encounter that raises a clinical question that could be answered by a test. The clinician considers what tests might be appropriate to answer the clinical question and then selects a test(s). The selection is translated into a test order either directly by the clinician placing an electronic order or indirectly by a ward secretary transferring the written order to a labo-

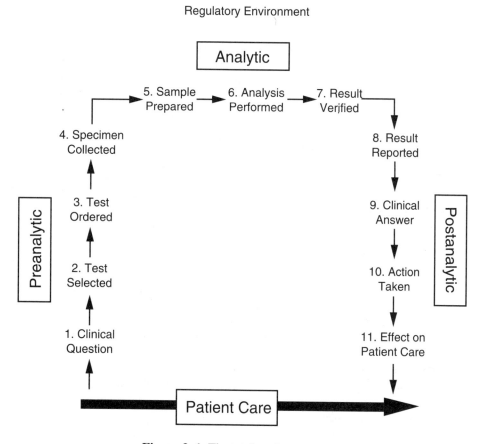

Figure 3–1. The total testing process.

ratory slip. The preanalytic component concludes with specimen collection and the transport of the specimen to clinical laboratory.

The *analytic component* involves the intralaboratory processing and testing of specimens and the verification of test results. As the ability to process and analyze the specimen accurately is dependent on the characteristics of the analytic system, considerations involving the selection of test methodology and quality-control procedures are also included in this section. The *post-analytic component* comprises the reporting of the test result, the interpretation of the result in light of the original clinical question, actions taken in response to the result, and the result of these actions on patient care and ultimate patient outcome.

All of these components are affected by the *regulatory environment* within which TDM is performed. Mandatory federal, state, and local laws as well as "voluntary" accreditation standards from the Joint Commission on the Accreditation of Healthcare Organizations (JCAHO) and the College of American Pathologists (CAP) influence the structure and process of TDM testing. In the final section of this chapter, we examine the effect of the federal regulations related to the Clinical Laboratory Improvement Amendments of 1988 (CLIA 88) and the standards of JCAHO on how a CPKS can be organized and therapeutic drug monitoring is performed.

Clinical pharmacokinetic services can intervene to improve many of the steps in the Total Testing Process: providing education, drug information, and research to improve the formulation of the clinical question and interpretation of the test results; assessing the appropriateness of the TDM test order; scheduling specimen collection; developing drug dosing guidelines; and providing written and oral consultation regarding TDM results with dosage recommendations.[3] The effectiveness of these efforts is briefly described in this chapter; a more complete examination of CPKSs is presented in Chapters 4 and 8.

Additional information about the testing of specific drugs can be found in the chapters that follow. Also, other general overviews of many of the steps in therapeutic drug monitoring[4,5]—for tricyclic antidepressants in particular[6]—are available.

PREANALYTIC COMPONENT

Step 1: Clinical Question

The goals of drug therapy are to achieve beneficial effects by curing illness, reducing symptoms, or preventing disease while producing minimal adverse effects in the patient. For certain drugs, this is not straightforward. Large interindividual variations exist in the absorption, distribution, and metabolism of the drugs so that a direct relationship does not exist between the dose of drug and its concentration at the receptor site. Not only do these drugs have wide interindividual variation, they also have a narrow range of drug concentrations within which they can exert a therapeutic effect. Above the top end of this narrow therapeutic range, the drug can be toxic, and below the low end of the range, the drug may elicit a subtherapeutic effect. The signs and symptoms of these toxic or subtherapeutic effects may be difficult to distinguish from those of the underlying disease and the therapeutic effects are sometimes difficult to measure.[6,7] Therefore, TDM was developed to assist in the optimal achievement of drug therapy by providing serum drug concentration data to assist clinicians to (1) design individual drug dosage regimens, (2) assess possible subtherapeutic and toxic conditions, and (3) monitor drug activity and patient drug-taking compliance behavior.

Therapeutic drug monitoring is based on the premise that a relationship exists between the drug concentration in a body fluid such as serum and its concentration in tissue where the drug exerts its therapeutic effect. This implies that an association exists between serum drug levels and subtherapeutic, therapeutic, and toxic effects at the drug's receptor sites. Generally, too high a drug level suggests toxicity; too low, a subtherapeutic response.

Although TDM is a testing process, the process involves a laboratory test, and as with any laboratory test, it should be performed only in response to a need to answer a specific clinical question(s). Questions arise during the clinician–patient encounter when the clinician detects certain signs or symptoms or needs additional data to guide therapy. Before tests are ordered, clinicians should not only raise the questions, but should accompany each question with a patient-specific probability assessment of how likely the patient is to have the condition or to need a dosage change. This probability estimate, taken before a test is ordered, is called a *prior probability* (also *pretest probability*). It can be based on the clinician's previous experience or use models to determine a specific patient's risk of toxicity.[7-9] Later in the TDM testing process, this prior probability is combined with the information provided by the serum drug concentration to yield a revised estimate of patient status, called the *posterior probability* (also *posttest probability*). An expanded discussion of prior and posterior probability estimates in TDM is found in Chapter 7.

Some generic questions[10,11] and associated prior probability estimates that can arise throughout the course of therapy include the following:

- After the initiation of therapy, and particularly after a loading dose, is this population dose appropriate given the patient's individual pharmacokinetics? What is the prior probability that this dose will yield a serum drug concentration that is estimated to be within the therapeutic range?
- If a therapeutic response is not achieved, is the lack of clinical response related to a subtherapeutic drug concentration? What is the prior probability that the patient will have a subtherapeutic response?
- If clinical symptoms suggest a possible toxic condition, are they related to drug toxicity? What is the prior probability that these symptoms are related to drug toxicity?
- If the patient's renal or hepatic function is changing, how is the change affecting the serum drug concentration? What is the prior probability that this changing clearance will result in a serum drug concentration outside the therapeutic range?
- Following conversion from an IV to a PO route of administration, is the resultant serum drug concentration appropriate for the patient? What is the prior probability that the dosage modification will yield a serum drug concentration within the therapeutic range?
- At admission or during follow-up visits, what is the baseline value or has the patient been compliant? What is the prior probability that the patient will be compliant?

In general, laboratory tests are overused,[12] and serum drug concentrations are no exception. In a review of 14 studies that determined appropriateness of TDM testing based on institution-specific utilization criteria, Einarson and co-workers determined that overall 34.7% of the serum drug concentrations were not clinically indicated; institution-specific rates of inappropriate utilization ranged from 10.9% to 70.4%.[13]

Overall, patients monitored by clinical pharmacokinetic services appear to undergo fewer

TDM tests as compared with patients not monitored by these services, although the effect is complex. Ried and colleagues conducted a meta-analysis of 16 articles to determine if CPKS had an effect on the number of serum drug assays ordered for drug monitoring. Aminoglycoside patients monitored by a CPKS were ordered more serum aminoglycoside concentrations than nonmonitored patients, whereas patients receiving other monitored drugs had fewer TDM tests ordered. When the CPKS also directed other aspects of the Total Testing Process, such as collection time (Step 4) and adjustment of drug dosage (Step 10), monitored patients were ordered fewer TDM tests than nonmonitored patients.[14] It is likely that appropriate dosage adjustments based on properly sampled assays led to better monitored patients and a reduced need for TDM testing.

Step 2: Test Selected

After determining that the patient's clinical condition warrants the determination of a serum drug concentration, the clinician selects the TDM test as well as other tests needed to monitor the patient's status. For example, in addition to the TDM determination, for patients receiving aminoglycosides, digoxin, and lithium, renal function should be monitored, and for patients on theophylline, hepatic function tests are indicated.

Given the nature of a patient's condition and the drug being monitored, the clinician may select special TDM testing. Two alternatives to routine testing are measuring (1) only the free (unbound) serum drug concentration and (2) the concentrations of the active metabolites as well as the parent drug. These examples are described next.

Total Drug Versus Free and Bound Drug Concentrations

Drugs in the circulation exist as two forms: those bound to protein transport molecules and those that are unbound, circulating freely, and available for diffusion into target cells. Although TDM methods routinely assay the total of bound and free forms of drugs, the free drug component is more reflective of the drug's pharmacologic activity at its receptor site. When blood proteins are decreased, there are fewer carrier molecules and more of the absorbed drug is present in the unbound or free form. For drugs that are highly protein bound, this protein decrease can lead to an increase in free drug with more drug activity at the receptor site and unexpected drug-related toxicity with serum drug concentrations within the therapeutic range.[15] For example, for a drug such as phenytoin, which is 90% protein bound, the free drug component could double if reduced protein concentrations permitted only 80% of the phenytoin to be bound. The drug's activity at the target site would be doubled, whereas the TDM assay result, based on the total serum drug concentration, would remain unchanged.

Other clinical situations exist in which the amount of free drug is lowered. During acute phase reactions associated with acute myocardial infarction, infectious disease, injury, severe burns, or shock, α_1-acid glycoprotein is elevated and increases the binding of basic drugs such as disopyramide, imipramine, lidocaine, phenytoin, propranolol, and quinidine.[16] In these situations, although the total drug concentration may appear to be in the therapeutic range, the free drug component is lowered, less drug is available for diffusion into the target tissue, and a clinical effect may not be achieved with standard dosing regimens.

The free drug concentration can be measured, but it is a more time-consuming and expensive process. After the cellular elements are removed from the sample, the protein must be precipitated to remove the bound drugs, and then the remaining free drug can be measured. Clinicians should, however, consider the selection of a free drug assay when blood proteins are decreased or when an apparent toxic reaction is associated with a therapeutic level of a drug that is highly protein bound (eg, outpatient with high probability of toxic reaction and total phenytoin level within normal range).

Parent Drug and Active Metabolites

Some drugs are biotransformed by the liver into both active and inactive forms of the parent drug. Depending on the specificity of the testing method (see Step 6), some assays will measure the parent drug and its metabolites or only the parent drug. Chromatography can separately detect all forms of a monitored drug, whereas immunoassays are dependent on the specificity of the drug's antibody to react only with the parent drug, to be less targeted and measure the combined concentration of forms of the parent drug, or to react only with its active metabolites. For example, assays are available to quantitate the levels of both procainamide and N-acetylprocainamide (NAPA), which has 50% of the activity of its parent drug, procainamide. An assay method measuring only procainamide will underestimate the amount of active drug forms present in the circulation; however, the degree of underestimation is not constant as the rate of conversion of procainamide to NAPA varies from 20% to 50% within the population.[17] Therefore, with procainamide, serum concentrations of both the parent drug and its active metabolite are useful.

At present, clinicians should determine what form(s) of the drug the laboratory is measuring and, when clinically indicated and available, request drug assays specific for the compound of interest, for example, parent drug, active metabolites, or both. Although the laboratory community recommends that drug metabolites be quantified,[18] existing methods are limited. In the future, as testing technology evolves and immunologic reagents become more selective, the test selection step will likely become more complicated. Clinicians will be able routinely to select from methods that quantitate only the parent drug, only the active components, or both the parent drug and its active metabolites. As with any laboratory test, there will be a potential for indiscriminant ordering of the various methods to evaluate drug therapy, and clinicians must base their test selection behavior on the value of the additional information provided by more comprehensive, but also more expensive, testing protocols.

Step 3: Test Ordered

In this step, the clinician's test selection is converted into a test order. This can be done by the clinician writing an order in the chart or order book that is then transcribed to an order form by a second person, usually the ward secretary. Alternatively, in computerized clinical environments, the clinician can directly place the order at the time the test is selected.

Expanded test request forms or computer-guided ordering can be used to collect important information that can improve the test ordering phase as well as earlier and later steps in the TDM testing process. Modifications of test forms have been recommended to improve ordering of laboratory tests,[12,19] and various modifications of TDM forms have been reported in the literature.[20-24] Table 3.1 identifies essential information for TDM request forms to ensure proper collection and interpretation of TDM tests.[25]

Three examples illustrate the value of an improved test order form:

1. For clinicians who are not following the steps in the Total Testing Process and are reflexively ordering TDMs without asking if they are clinically needed (eg, ordering daily therapeutic drug monitoring although the patient was doing fine), a TDM request form[26] or computer ordering package can be designed to ask the clinician to identify the clinical reason the test is being ordered from a list of appropriate indications. If the patient's condition does not meet any of the clinically appropriate reasons for ordering, the clinician may reconsider and not place the TDM test order.
2. By having the dosing history available on the test request form, the laboratory or clinical pharmacokinetic service can schedule the phlebotomist to ensure that the sample is taken at the correct time (see Step 4).
3. Complete dosing and clinical information help in the interpretation step (see Step 9).

Some laboratories have used the introduction of a revised TDM order form and an associated educational program as a method to improve the ordering of TDM tests. For example, improvement was seen in several steps of the Total Testing Process by coupling an educational program to the introduction of a redesigned TDM form requesting information on the indication for TDM, relevant disease states, concurrent drug therapy, and plasma sampling time. Appropriate indications for TDM testing rose from 62% before the new forms to 85% after their introduction, appropriate timing of TDM sampling rose from 40% to 74%, and adequate response to the TDM result rose from 53% to 72%.[26]

Although educational programs are necessary, they are not sufficient and stronger interventions are needed to improve TDM utilization.[12] When these programs are coupled with a voluntary compliance system using improved test request forms, improvements in ordering patterns will be seen, but some clinicians elect not to comply with the voluntary nature of the program. In the future, it can be anticipated that computer-based, laboratory ordering systems will require additional patient data for the TDM request to be recognized and processed. These mandatory, institutional system changes will prompt input on TDM-related patient data and help direct the appropriate frequency of TDM orders and timing of specimen collection.

Step 4: Specimen Collected

The goal of TDM is to measure, in vitro, the concentration of drug that is most representative of the concentration in the tissue where the drug is exerting its therapeutic effect. Generally that involves obtaining samples at steady state and permitting sufficient time from the last dose to achieve postdistribution equilibrium. For certain drugs, peak and trough drug concentrations are of interest. Therefore, proper timing of the collection phase is critical to ensuring a representative, in vivo drug concentration. Other considerations during the specimen collection phase include determination of the type of specimen (serum, plasma, or whole blood; fingertip or venous collection site), type of blood collection devices, and other substances that could interfere at this step in the Total Testing Process.

Proper identification of the patient and labeling of the specimen are central to specimen col-

TABLE 3–1. ESSENTIALS OF REQUEST FORMS FOR THERAPEUTIC DRUG MONITORING

Patient Specific Information

Name, address, identification number

Hospital number, outpatient/inpatient, room number

Physician, specialty service

Patient Characteristics

Age, sex, pregnancy, ethnicity

Height, weight

Primary disease process

Organ involvement, especially renal, hepatobiliary, cardiac, gastrointestinal, endocrine

Fluid balance

Laboratory studies, serum albumin, creatinine clearance

Specimen Information

Time of collection

Nature of specimen: blood, urine, other body fluids

Site of collection

Order of sample, if one of a series

Type of container, preservative

Time of receipt in laboratory

Purpose of Assay and Urgency of Request

Therapeutic confirmation

Suspected toxicity

Drug overdose

Monitoring of active metabolites

Suspected drug interactions

Comprehensive pharmacokinetic evaluation and consultation

Absence of therapeutic response

   Drug failure

   Noncompliance

   Altered clearance

Drug Information

Name of drug(s) to be assayed

Time of last dose, frequency of prescribed dose, quantity of dose, route of administration

Personnel Audit Trail

Identification of phlebotomist, nurse, clinical pharmacist, laboratory personnel

From Taylor WJ, Robinson JD, Slaughter RL. Establishing a pharmacy-based therapeutic drug monitoring service. *Drug Intell Clin Pharm.* 1985;19:821.

lection. The patient's identity must be positively established prior to obtaining the specimen, and the specimen must be completely labeled before leaving the patient. Failure in each of these processes could result in misidentification of the specimen and lead to a situation in which an analytically correct serum drug concentration could cause patient harm because action for one patient would be taken on a result for someone else.

Sampling Considerations Related to Timing of Specimen Collection

Steady State. The frequency and timing of specimen sampling protocols vary. Some recommend that the first sample after the start of a dosage regimen should not be obtained until sufficient time has elapsed for the drug to accumulate in the body and reach a steady state at the receptor site. Samples obtained prior to steady state will underestimate the steady-state drug concentration, and clinicians responding to the lower than expected serum concentrations may make inappropriate dosage changes. Generally four to five drug half-lives are required to achieve serum drug concentrations that approximate steady state.

Other clinicians, however, like to obtain serum drug concentrations prior to reaching steady state in some circumstances, mainly those related to administration of a loading dose or to determination of patient-specific pharmacokinetic values. When a loading dose is administered, most dosage regimens are initiated using average values for the patient population of interest. Under this condition, early sampling allows the clinician to see if the level is within the desired therapeutic range and, if it is, to validate the continued use of the population parameters for the subsequent maintenance regimen. Some clinical researchers also suggest that a few drug concentrations be obtained during the early dosage period to estimate the patient-specific pharmacokinetic values needed to individualize dosage regimens. But, by far, the most prudent and common use of serum drug levels occurs during the steady-state period.

Time from Last Dose Administered. Once steady state has been reached in the patient, whether the post dose sampling time is selected to simulate the maximum, average, or minimum drug level during the dosage interval depends on what portion of the dosage interval was originally used in developing the therapeutic range that is being used as a reference for monitoring the patient.

Unfortunately, some commonly accepted therapeutic ranges have been developed without careful consideration of a consistent period of sampling during the dosage interval, so it may not be clear which portion of the interval applies for sampling. In general, unless a level estimating the maximum during the dosage interval is indicated, TDM tries to use the midpoint or end of the dosage interval for monitoring to estimate the average ($C_{avg,ss}$) or trough ($C_{min,ss}$) levels during the interval, respectively. These measures are preferred when it is known or can be assumed that these measures are adequate indices of the effectiveness and safety of a drug, because timing is more accurate than estimating the maximum level ($C_{max,ss}$). $C_{max,ss}$ measures are uncertain with respect to timing and also are confounded by the multicompartmental pharmacokinetic behavior of drugs; sampling too early after a dose may be misleading if the drug distribution phase is still in progress and postdistribution equilibrium has not yet been achieved.

The ability of clinicians to interpret serum drug concentrations is severely limited when they lack information concerning the timing of the specimen in relation to the last dose. For example, is a patient's unexpectedly high serum drug concentration related to a physiologic change or to a specimen that was taken at an inappropriate time? Educational programs targeted at improving the appropriateness of serum aminoglycoside concentration collection, coupled with a revision in the test order form to require the inclusion of dosing and collection time information, were able to improve the collection time, which yielded an increase in the proportion of patients within the therapeutic range.[27] Also, standardized dosing times with dosing guidelines can reduce errors in the timing of TDM specimens.[28–30]

Combined Assessment of the Appropriateness of Specimen Collection. In a literature analysis of 25 articles to quantify the amount of inappropriate sampling, Einarson and colleagues reviewed 25 studies published between 1976 and 1986. Each study established acceptable criteria for sampling appropriateness against which it compared the sampling times of TDM samples submitted for testing. Overall, 47.1% of the combined 3855 samples were inappropriately sampled with institutional rates ranging from 2.3% to 69.2% incorrect sampling times.[13]

Given the poor quality of sampling times for TDM tests, can individual pharmacists or a CPKS improve the overall quality of sample collection? What is the impact on the quality of TDM testing if a clinical pharmacist from a centralized CPKS service or a satellite pharmacy evaluates the patient's medication administration record and schedules the TDM sampling time either in the patient record or on the laboratory request form?

Based on a meta-analysis of 11 studies with a combined population of 3543 patients, Ried and co-workers[31] determined that although more samples were properly collected in CPKS-monitored than in nonmonitored patients, the difference between the two populations improved but did not reach statistical significance. Because the authors reported a composite evaluation of collection appropriateness, results from the meta analysis do not provide information on the effect of a CPKS on the individual components of specimen collection, such as time from last dose and steady-state time. Further studies are needed to determine methods to improve sampling appropriateness and to evaluate the role of the CPKS in this step of the Total Testing Process.

Sampling Considerations Related to Type of Specimen

Serum Versus Plasma. Serum (cell-free component of *clotted* blood) from a venipuncture specimen is the traditional sample for TDM testing; however, analytic methods have been, and are being, developed to assay drug concentrations in whole blood and plasma (cell-free component of *unclotted* blood) from venipuncture, whole blood from finger punctures, and easily obtainable saliva. Plasma and whole blood offer the advantage of more rapid processing because time is not required for the blood to clot. Urine is not used to guide drug therapy; the varying fluid intake and renal functioning of each patient affect the concentration of drugs in urine.

Is there a difference between a drug's concentration in serum and in plasma? Although the answer to that question is incomplete, some results indicate that a small, but statistically significant, difference does exist between the two specimens. Ebert and colleagues found that plasma aminoglycoside concentrations were 7.8% lower than serum results in 208 samples tested using the same method. The authors indicated that they did not believe that this difference was "of significant magnitude to be of clinical significance."[32]

Venous Versus Capillary Blood. Several methods are now available to measure serum drug levels using whole blood, usually fingertip blood, obtained by capillary sampling techniques. These are designed primarily for clinic- or office-based testing, but capillary blood also is an alternative to venous blood when venipuncture is difficult. The question, however, arises: For TDM, are results from capillary blood equivalent to those from venous blood?

Although limited information is available, results from the two sample sources appear to be clinically similar when the same assay method is used. In a comparison of capillary and venous results from 18 patients, each receiving one of three classes of drugs (aminoglycosides, theophylline, or digoxin), Murphy and colleagues did detect a statistically significant difference between the two sampling methods. Although results from capillary samples were 3.76% lower than those from venous sources, the authors concluded that, for the drugs evaluated and at the drug concentrations assayed, there was not a clinically significant difference.[33] Additional studies are needed to include a larger patient sample, a broader evaluation of drug classes, and a wider range of serum drug levels.

Saliva as a Sample Source for Therapeutic Monitoring of Drugs. Saliva offers many advantages as a sample source for therapeutically monitored drugs: ease of collection, patient preference, and lack of exposure to blood for health care professionals. Methods that use saliva are particularly helpful in pediatric settings or other situations when venipuncture is difficult. Because drugs exist in saliva in the unbound, biologically active form of the drug, TDM results derived from saliva reflect a more active picture of the drug's activity at the target site.

To prevent several aspects of the Total Testing Process related to saliva-based TDM testing from getting lost in the more general discussion of blood-based testing, we combine them here. For methods using large amounts of saliva, the masticatory stimulation of saliva to produce sufficient quantity of the sample may result in a diluted drug concentration.[34] Although the lower concentration was not considered to be clinically significant, newer methods, requiring 30 to 100 μl, eliminate the need to stimulate saliva production.[35] After the sample is obtained, it should not be centrifuged; some of the drug may be lost with the debris. If the analysis cannot be immediately performed, the specimen should be placed in a sealed glass tube and frozen.[34] To improve the interpretation of saliva-based TDM results, studies are needed to determine the magnitude of the intra- and interpatient variations in the ratio of the concentration of the drug in saliva to the drug in serum.[35]

Sources of Error Related to Collection Methods

Care must be taken not to contaminate the patient's blood specimen with external sources of the drug being measured. This could lead to a falsely elevated serum drug concentration. For example, if the blood sample is correctly timed and analyzed, but the specimen is drawn from a catheter that had earlier been used to administer the drug, the serum drug concentration will be falsely elevated.[36]

For certain drugs, even the type of blood collection tube can affect the serum drug concentrations. The stoppers of the Vacutainer brand of blood collection tubes have been reported to contain tris(2-butoxyethyl)phosphate, a compound that appears to displace lidocaine, propranolol, quinidine, alprenolol, and imipramine from α_1-acid glycoprotein. In the blood collection tube, the displaced, unbound drug quickly diffuses into the red blood cells, leaving a lowered drug concentration in the serum fraction of blood. If serum is assayed to determine the drug concentration, the drug level will be spuriously low; however, the whole blood level remains unchanged. Although one company that manufactures this product (Becton-Dickinson) has removed this compound from its product,[25] check with your manufacturer to determine if tris(2-butoxyethyl)phosphate is present. And Venojet red-top tubes, supplied by Terumo Corporation, have been reported to contain a substance that causes a serious interference with phenytoin, leading to falsely elevated phenytoin levels when the drug is assayed by high-performance liquid chromatography methods.[37]

Falsely elevated drug concentrations also occurred when a finger stick was used to obtain a sample from patients who had handled the medication. Fine particles of the tablet medication remained on the fingertip, and when the finger-stick blood sample was taken, the external drug contaminated the collected specimen. Even when the finger was swabbed, sufficient digoxin residue remained on the finger to produce falsely toxic levels in volunteers who had handled tablets but were not taking digoxin. Carbamazepine tablets also left residue, but swabbing the finger reduced this source of error. Residue from paracetamol accounted for artificial concentrations of up to 500 μmol/L in volunteers not taking the drug. If, however, patients were taking paracetamol, the contamination level coupled with a therapeutic postdistribution paracetamol concentration would be likely to yield an assayed drug concentration in the toxic range and acetylcysteine might be initiated to prevent hepatotoxicity. Tablets with glossy surfaces were less likely to result in falsely elevated drug concentrations.[38]

Another example of finger contamination has been reported in children receiving oral doses of cyclosporine.[39] Children appeared to contaminate their fingers when they put them in their mouths after receiving oral cyclosporine, a drug known to accumulate in the skin.[40] Following an observation that pediatric cyclosporine levels in capillary blood ranged from 2.5 to more than 6 times higher than parallel serum levels, healthy adult volunteers were asked to place fingers from one hand in a liquid form of the drug. Sixteen hours later, although the fingertip was thoroughly disinfected and cleaned, fingertip capillary specimens from the contaminated hand yielded extremely high drug levels, whereas the control hand had nondetectable levels. These results suggest that fingertip blood from children should be avoided, and if capillary blood is the preferred specimen, ear lobe sampling should be considered.

Other Sources of Error

Fluorescein dyes used in diagnostic imaging can interfere with TDM test systems such as the Abbott TDx that use fluorescein-labeled antigens to quantitate drug concentrations. Either specimen collection should be delayed for 13 hours after a fluorescein dose, or another test method should be selected (see TDM Considerations under Step 6).[41]

ANALYTIC COMPONENT

Step 5: Specimen Prepared

For most forms of TDM testing, Step 5 involves the transportation of the specimen to the testing site, the logging in of the specimen in the laboratory and assignment of a laboratory acquisition number, the separation of the serum or plasma from cellular elements of blood, and the storage of the sample if testing is not performed immediately.

Specimen Transportation

For most TDM testing, the specimen is transported from the patient's bedside or the clinic to the central laboratory for processing. Generally, special precautions are not needed to ensure that transport of the specimen does not affect the integrity of the serum drug concentration. In a patient receiving both antipseudomonal antibiotics such as carbenicillin, ticarcillin, and piperacillin and aminoglycosides, however, the antipseudomonal antibiotics inactivate the aminoglycoside antibiotics in vitro.[42–44] To prevent this inactivation, some testing centers require that all samples for aminoglycoside testing be placed on ice immediately after collection and kept cool or frozen until the assay is performed.[45]

Laboratory Log-in and Assignment of Acquisition Number

When specimens reach the laboratory, the time of receipt is noted and the specimens are logged in. Acquisition numbers or codes are assigned, and the number for each coded sample is placed on the TDM worksheet. This phase in the TDM testing process is labor intensive, with many possibilities for transcription and other system error. Laboratory computer systems are being used to reduce the number of unit processes by having the computer generate worksheets from its centralized log-in record.

Bar codes are being used to reduce errors in this step. Some hospitals have total hospital information systems that use patient-specific bar codes, assigned at admission, that are placed on all order forms for that patient. When the TDM specimen is obtained from the patient, one of the bar codes is placed on the tube of blood and another on the laboratory request form. When the specimen is received in the laboratory, an optical scanner, linked to the laboratory's computer, reads the bar code and enters the patient's identity into the laboratory's system. The requested test is entered and the computer generates laboratory worksheets. Other computer-based systems are under development to simplify the log-in process, minimize transcription steps, and reduce the associated errors.

Blood Separation

If serum is used in the testing process, blood is generally collected in a red-top vacuum tube, some of which contain a gel that assists in separation of the serum from the cellular elements of blood. These serum separator tubes (SSTs) represent a potential source of error for TDM assays. If left in contact with serum, the gel in some brands of SSTs appears to absorb some drugs, reducing their serum drug concentration.[46–48] For example, phenytoin concentration decreased 18% in a Becton-Dickinson SST kept for 24 hours at room temperature, decreased 25% when kept for the same period at 32°C, but was not affected at 15°C,[48] whereas another study determined that the gel extracted phenytoin even with immediate separation of the serum.[49] The Monoject Corvac SST was unsuitable for lidocaine assays using all storage methods.

Given than SSTs are widely used in specimen collection, several precautions should be followed. Phenytoin should be collected in a tube without a gel separator. If SSTs are used to collect other TDM specimens, the tube should be filled to capacity.[49] If testing is delayed beyond 1 or 2 hours, the serum should be decanted from the gel to prevent falsely lower TDM results. This is particularly important for samples that are collected for testing at a remote laboratory; it would be best to remove the serum from the gel and decant into another tube prior to transit.

Step 6: Analysis Performed

TDM Assay Considerations
In selection of a TDM assay system, five major points should be considered:

1. Analytic performance, including accuracy, reliability, specificity of reaction, and concentration of drug detection
2. Practicality, including ease of performance, time of analysis, volume of sample required, equipment calibration requirements, and computer compatibility
3. Availability of laboratory equipment and supplies
4. Range of drugs that can be tested by the system
5. Economic aspects, including the initial purchase of equipment and reagent, quality control, and personnel costs

In the sections that follow, you should consider these five characteristics as we describe the common chemical and immunologic testing methodologies, the TDM instruments available for laboratory and office use, and other factors affecting the analytic process.

TDM Assay Methodologies
Immunoassay and chromatography are the two major methodologies used to assay therapeutically monitored drugs. Immunoassay methods, such as the homogenous enzyme multiplied immunotechnique (EMIT), fluorescence immunoassays, radioimmunoassay (RIA), and the apoenzyme reactivation immunoassay system (ARIS), are currently the most common assay methods. Most immunoassays have good accuracy and precision, are not technically demanding, rely on automated or semiautomated instrumentation with commercially available reagents or kit forms, and have a rapid turnaround time. Chromatography is a highly sensitive method, but the expensive equipment, longer turnaround time, and need for highly trained personnel limit its current use to drug assays that are not available from commercial manufacturers.

All immunoassay procedures involve an interaction between a specific antigen and an antibody that will react with that specific antigen. In the case of TDM immunoassays, a specific antibody is commercially produced to react with each of the monitored drugs. During the immunoassay, the drug to be measured in the patient's serum is mixed with the specific, commercially prepared antibody. In theory, the antibody will react only with the specific drug antigen; however, some cross-reactions have been reported.

Many of the immunoassay systems create a competitive antigen–antibody binding reaction by adding a second source of the drug to be measured (a commercially prepared drug, labeled to permit detection) to compete with the patient's drug for the antibody binding sites. The concentration of the commercially labeled drug is known; therefore, the proportion of it bound to the antibody is related to the concentration of the patient's drug that competes with the antibody. The various immunoassays differ primarily in the method used to quantitate directly or indirectly the amount of drug in the patient's sample that reacts with the drug antibody.

Enzyme Multiplied Immunoassay (EMIT). The EMIT system was developed by Syva Corporation in 1972. In this procedure, the patient's serum with an undetermined amount of drug is mixed with a commercially prepared standard amount of the same drug that has been bound to an enzyme. Then the mixture is added to antibodies specific for the drug. The patient's drug and the test drug coupled to the enzyme compete for reaction sites on the antibodies. How much of each binds to antibody is directly proportional to its respective concentration. When the drug–enzyme combination attaches to antibody, the antibody reduces the enzyme's catalytic activity. The degree to which the enzyme is changed can be measured and then related to the amount of drug–enzyme complex that attached to antibody. The more the enzyme is changed and unable to catalyze the indicator reaction, the more drug–enzyme complex has bound to the antibody, indicating that low levels of the drug are present in the patient's serum and competing for the antibody sites. Conversely, if there is high enzymatic activity in the indicator reaction, less of the drug–enzyme complex has been bound to the drug-specific antibody because the higher drug concentration in the patient's sample bound more of the antibody sites.

An EMIT can be performed by both manual and automated methods. Although most testing protocols use primarily serum, methods have been developed for saliva and whole blood.

Fluorescence immunoassay (FIA). Fluorescence immunoassays are used to quantitate serum drug concentrations in most clinical laboratories. They serve as the analytic method for the Syva Advance system (fluorescence detection in a homogenous enzyme immunoassay), Ames fluorogenic substrate (dye-labeled substrate producing a fluorescent detection signal), and Abbott TDx system (fluorescence polarization immunoassay).

In the fluorescence polarization immunoassay (FPIA), quantification of the patient's serum drug concentration is based on an antigen–antibody reaction detected by fluorescence polarization. The drug-specific test reagent contains a known quantity of the fluorescein-labeled drug and an antibody specific for the drug. The patient's serum, containing an unknown quantity of the drug to be measured, is mixed with a known quantity of the fluorescein-labeled drug and the antibody. The patient's drug and the fluorescein-labeled drug compete for sites on the antibody. Binding of the antibody to the labeled drug produces a large molecule that demonstrates increased fluorescence polarization, which is measured. As this is a competitive binding assay, the concentration of the labeled drug bound to the antibody and, consequently, the degree of fluorescence polarization are inversely related to the concentration of unlabeled drug in the sample.

Radioimmunoassay (RIA). Radioimmunoassay was the first of the immunoassays to be widely used in drug monitoring. The method is based on the interaction of the antigen (drug) in the patient's serum with commercially produced antibody that is simultaneously mixed with a radioactively labeled form of the same drug. After the free radioactive drug is separated from that bound to antibody, the amount of radioactive drug bound to the antibody is measured. This is inversely related to the amount of drug in the patient's serum; that is, if a large amount of radioactively labeled drug is bound to antibody, a small amount of the drug is available in the patient's serum to occupy sites on antibody.

Radioimmunoassay methods are extremely sensitive and are commonly used to detect small nanogram concentrations of digoxin; however, alternative immunoassays have been developed to replace RIA methods and avoid the analytic separation steps and the use of radioactive material.

Apoenzyme Reactivation Immunoassay System (ARIS). ARIS uses a dry-phase, immunochemical reaction to quantitate serum drug concentrations. Only 30 µl of sample is required. To initiate a multistep biochemical reaction, the sample is manually diluted and placed on a paper reagent matrix of a plastic strip containing flavin adenine dinucleotide (FAD)/drug-specific conjugate, drug-specific antibodies, and a glucose oxidase apoenzyme system. The drug in the patient's sample competes with the matrix's FAD/drug-specific complex for binding sites on the drug-specific antibody. Free FAD/drug combines with another reagent on the strip, glucose oxidase apoenzyme, to form the active enzyme, glucose oxidase, that releases peroxidase and turns an indicator system blue. Reflectance photometry is used to detect the color intensity of the indicator system which is directly related to the concentration of the drug in the patient's sample.

The Ames Seralyzer uses this system for some of its drug assays. The 90-second reaction time of the Seralyzer assay offers an advantage for physician offices or other situations where turnaround time is at a premium. In this system, saliva can be used as a test sample.[35]

Chromatography. In chromatography, compounds are separated on the basis of their differences in attraction to one of two different phases: a *mobile* phase that flows by a *stationary* phase column. In general, the compound to be assayed is in the mobile phase and is absorbed onto a stationary phase in a column. The two principal forms of chromatography, classified by the composition of the two phases, are gas–liquid and liquid chromatography.

	Mobile Phase	*Stationary Phase*
Gas–liquid chromatography (GLC)	Gas	Liquid
Liquid chromatography (LC)	Liquid	Solid

In high-pressure liquid chromatography (HPLC), the mobile liquid phase is inserted into the stationary column under high pressure.

Chromatography is used to separate different compounds based on their affinity to the substance in the column. The drugs to be identified and quantitated are injected into the mobile phase and then pass along the stationary phase. Drugs that have a strong attraction to the stationary phase are slowed as they pass through the column, whereas compounds that are weakly attracted quickly pass through and exit first. The compounds are captured as they leave the column; a detector records the time required for passage through the column and indicates the quantity of each drug as it exits the column.

Chromatography was the first method used in TDM testing. An important advantage is its ability to simultaneously detect and measure the concentration of multiple drugs within the same class as well as the metabolites of the parent drug. It is both labor and time intensive, requiring highly skilled personnel, and has largely been replaced by FPIA and EMIT testing for the most commonly monitored drugs. Chromatographic methods are frequently used for the monitoring of tricyclic antidepressants, although the interlaboratory coefficients of variation were in the range 19% to 26%, as reported from a large European quality-assurance program.[50]

TDM Testing Instrumentation

TDM concentrations can be assayed by both manual and automated methods. Automated methods may be performed either with an instrument specifically designed for TDM testing or with an analyzer, which also is used for a wide range of other types of analysis routinely performed in the clinical chemistry laboratory. In addition to the traditional clinical laboratory instrumentation, rapid assay methods have been developed for use in near-patient locations such as clinics and physician offices. Examples of these classes of TDM instruments are found in Table 3–2.

TABLE 3–2. EXAMPLES OF TDM TESTING INSTRUMENTS

Automated Instruments for TDM Testing Only (dedicated TDM systems)

Abbott TDx (Abbott Laboratories, Irving, TX)

Autocarousel (Syva Co. Inc., Palo Alto, CA)

Automated Instruments for Clinical Chemistry Including TDM (multifunctional)

DuPont ACA (Dupont, Wilmington, DE)

Cobas Fara II centrifugal analyzer (Hoffman–LaRoche, Basel, Switzerland)

Stratus (Baxter Dade Co., Miami, FL)

Vision (Abbott Laboratories, Chicago, IL)

Semiautomated Instruments for Clinical Chemistry Including TDM

Ames Seralyzer III (Ames Division, Miles Laboratories, Elkart, IN)

Instruments Designed for Physician Office Laboratory (51) and Near-Patient Testing

AccuLevel (Syntex Medical Diagnostics, Palo Alto, CA)

Vision (Abbott Laboratories, Chicago, IL)

Kodak Ektachem (Eastman Kodak, Rochester, NY)

EMIT QST (Syva Co., Inc., Palo Alto, CA)

Seralyzer ARIS (Ames Division, Miles Laboratories, Elkart, IN)

As summarized under TDM Assay Considerations, many factors must be considered in the selection of an instrument for TDM testing. It must deliver clinically useful results (acceptable accuracy, reliability, reaction specificity, drug detection levels), be appropriate for the technical skill of the test performer, provide acceptable turnaround time for test performance, offer the range of drug assays needed to support the clinical service, have adequate capacity, and be economically feasible. Cost factors should include not only the initial purchase price, but also the cost of reagents, supplies, quality control material, personnel, and any physical modifications that would be needed to accommodate the instrument. The amount of blood required for test performance should be considered, especially for populations in which blood sampling is difficult. For large laboratories, the issue of computer compatibility also should be investigated.

Many studies, too numerous to cite, have evaluated single TDM testing systems for their accuracy, reproducibility, time requirements, and other characteristics.[52–57] Others, also too numerous to cite, have conducted intermethod comparisons.[58–63] When considering instruments for possible incorporation into clinical practice, consult the single instrument evaluations and intersystem comparisons, other published literature, manufacturer's product descriptions and specifications, and individuals using the instrument for similar purposes and in similar situations.

Measurement of Method's Analytic Variation.

In selecting a method for TDM analysis or when interpreting the results produced from a selected system, clinicians should be aware of the degree of variation that is inherent in the analytic testing system. How reproducible/reliable are the test results? For example, if you analyzed the same stable sample each day for 30 consecutive days, what amount of variation would you have among those 30 results? The coefficient of variation (CV) is the unit of measurement quantitating that variation. By using the same stable sample on each of our 30 days, we have eliminated all sources of variation except those in the analytic performance step of the Total Testing Process. Because the degree of difference among the results (captured by the standard deviation statistic) would vary depending on the mean of the test result (eg, results measured in milligrams will have a smaller absolute range of values than results measured in grams), the coefficient of variation quantifies variation by relating the standard deviation of test results to their mean:

$$\frac{\text{standard deviation}}{\text{mean}} \times 100 \ = \text{coefficient of variation (\%)}$$

To reduce variation in the Total Testing Process, an analytic system with a low CV is desired. The new automated systems with improved testing methodologies have increased the reproducibility of test results and reduced the CVs. For example, the CVs of tests for the tricylic drugs fell by 38% to 46% in the mid-1980s.[50] Although variations may exist among different manufacturers' test kits and products, as a class, most TDM immunologic methods have high accuracy and CVs in the range of 5% to 10%. In a comparison of 10 immunologic and chromatographic methods measuring 15 different TDM drugs, the most consistently precise TDM method was polarization fluoroimmunoassay. Various chromatographic methods were less reliable, having CVs in the 10% to 15% range.[64]

Specificity of TDM Reactions

For the TDM immunologic testing systems, the accuracy of the test results depends on the specificity of the antigen–antibody reaction. Two examples of factors that can adversely affect the specificity are (1) interference from metabolites of parent drugs and other similar drug compounds in the patient's sample that cross-react with the drug-specific antibody and (2) interference from circulating antibodies in the patient's sample that cross-react with the enzyme or other substances used in the detection system.

Reactions with Metabolites and Other Drugs. Many of the drugs that are therapeutically monitored have active and inactive metabolites that may or may not react with the immunoassay reagents depending on the specificity of the immunologic testing reagents. If a nonspecific drug antibody reacts with the parent drug compound and both its active and inactive metabolites, the resultant drug concentration will overestimate the drug's activity at the receptor site. For example, digoxin immunoassay reagents are known to lack specificity and cross-react with digoxin metabolites and digoxin-like immunoreactive substances.[65,66] Thus, when a nonspecific immunoassay yields a digoxin concentration of 2.5 ng/mL, the clinician does not know if all the digoxin is in a metabolically active form or if a substantial part of immunologically reactive drug is in a metabolically inactive form because of the large interpatient variation in the rate and extent of digoxin metabolism. Soldin suggests that the nonspecificity of the assay reaction is probably responsible for the lack of consensus as to the correlation between serum digoxin concentration and either its therapeutic or toxic effects.[66]

The measurement of cyclosporine poses particular problems. Although chromatography can isolate and quantitate the active cyclosporine compounds, early immunoassay methods used nonspecific, polyclonal antibodies that reacted with all cyclosporine-like substances.[67] Although manufacturers have improved the specificity of the antibody in their detection systems, they have achieved differential results with the specificity of their new, more specific, "monoclonal" products. In one study, the monoclonal antibody of a fluorescence polarization immunoassay yielded cyclosporine results that were 12.5% higher than those yielded by the monoclonal antibody used in a radioimmunoassay method, which in turn were 5.9% higher than those detected by the monoclonal antibody used in an automated EMIT method.[68] The differences in cyclosporine quantification have created problems in following individual patients whose tests have been performed at different laboratories that used different methods, as well as in interpreting clinical results from multicenter trials and in establishing serum drug levels associated with improved clinical effectiveness.

Not only inactive metabolites, but also other drugs can interfere with TDM testing. Spironolactone and its metabolites cross-react with some immunoassay reagents used in the detection of digoxin. For example, one study found that patients taking spironolactone, but not digoxin, had a digoxin level of 0.4 ng/ml. This would lead to falsely elevated digoxin concentrations in those patients who were taking digoxin and spironolactone.[69]

Non-Drug Related Reactions with Commercial Test Reagents. Patients may have antibodies that cross-react with reagents in the testing systems. For example, it has been reported that the serum of some patients contains antibodies that cross-react with the bacterial enzyme used to label aminoglycosides in the Stratus system's competitive binding method. The reagent drug, labeled with alkaline phosphatase derived from *Escherichia coli,* competes with the drug present in the patient's serum for the aminoglycoside antibody. If, however, the patient has endogenous antibodies against the bacterial enzyme as a result of *E. coli* septicemia or other severe infection, the patient's antibody will modify the bacterially derived alkaline phosphatase label. Both falsely elevated and falsely depressed aminoglycoside levels have been reported.[70] Good clinician–laboratorian communication is required to select appropriate testing methodologies to prevent this source of interference in patients with severe *E. coli* infections.

Quality Control
As applied in the clinical laboratory, quality control is a structured system to monitor the precision of analytic measurement and ensure the medical usefulness of testing results. Based on performance standards, the general laboratory equipment, supplies, reagents, and test analyzers are monitored to ensure they are operating properly, are not outdated, and can generate accurate and reproducible results.

Specifically related to therapeutic drug monitoring, the quality of the analytic component of TDM testing is monitored daily with the use of quality-control (QC) specimens. QC specimens are samples of known concentration that are analyzed along with patient samples in every test batch. Generally, two QC specimens are used: one of high and one of low concentration. Within the test run, they are placed before the patient samples; some systems recommend that QC specimens also be placed at intervals throughout the test run or at the end of a long run of patient specimens. This would detect any drift (a gradual shift to higher or lower values) in the analytic system from the beginning to the end of the test run.

At the completion of a test run, the QC specimens are checked to ensure that they are within plus or minus two standard deviations of their known concentrations. If they are outside that range, the QC specimens are run through again, and if then found to be within range, the results are released. Repeat quality-control results still outside the acceptable range point to a systematic error in the test system. No results are released until the test system is corrected and the QC specimens are within range.

Examples of other aspects of a quality-control system include daily temperature checks of refrigerators and water baths, calibration of the centrifugal speed used for blood sample separation, and implementation of other preventive measures to reduce errors and variability in the testing systems.

Testing Location

Although TDM testing has traditionally been performed in the clinical laboratory, miniaturization and simplification of testing technology now provide the opportunity to perform TDM in CPKS laboratories and near-patient locations such as clinics and physician offices. In the latter locations, near-patient testing can significantly reduce the patient's waiting time. In one study of patients in an epilepsy clinic, waiting time for TDM results was reduced from 112 to 16 minutes with the use of a system designed for near-patient testing. Although near-patient testing and reagent costs were higher than traditional laboratory testing costs due to confirmation of the clinic results, overall there was a savings of 20% related to reduced medical and nursing staff time and an increase of 23% in patient throughput.[71] These investigators caution that only trained technical staff should perform the testing because they are experienced in preventing and detecting errors in the testing system.

Acculevel, Seralyzer, and Vision systems are three near-patient TDM testing devices, marketed for their ability to provide answers within several minutes. All use monoclonal antibody technology; however, Vision is an automated system; Seralyzer, a partially automated system; and Acculevel, a noninstrumented system. The Vision and Acculevel systems can use whole blood, thus removing the potential sources of error in the blood separation step and conserving processing time. Coefficients of variation for each of the three systems are less than 10%, and the total testing time is under 30 minutes, with the Vision system producing results in under 20 minutes. In a 1988 cost analysis, depending on test volume, the average cost per sample assayed with the Vision system ranged from $14 to $24; with the Seralyzer, $5 to $9; and with the Acculevel system, $15 (one unit cost independent of test volume).[60]

Step 7: Results Verified

Within the laboratory, results are verified prior to their release to patient care areas. First, the quality-control specimens that are run in parallel with the patient samples are checked to ensure that they are within plus or minus two standard deviations of their known concentrations as described earlier. Next, samples yielding extremely high or low values, exceeding a predetermined level for each analyte, generally are repeated. All test systems are subject to occasional random error; this step is a method to separate these random errors from valid patient results and prevent erroneous results from leaving the laboratory. A random error is unlikely to recur, whereas an abnormally high or low patient result will remain abnormal.

Additionally, some laboratories have the capability to perform a "delta check" on patient samples. A *delta check* is defined as a procedure to measure the difference between the present and most recent test results. After the quality-control results have been verified, a delta check is performed; if the difference between the two values exceeds a preestablished level, the patient's sample is rerun. This check is designed to separate a true change in the patient's results from a false change related to random errors in the analytic testing process. If the present test is repeated and the result still exceeds the delta check, there is a high likelihood that the patient experienced a true physiologic change. Specimens that return to earlier levels probably were affected by random errors. Computerized laboratory systems can be programmed to perform a delta check for each test result and to identify results that are beyond the normal delta check limits.

POSTANALYTIC COMPONENT

Step 8: Result Reported

For routine test results, the TDM result is transferred from the laboratory worksheet onto the laboratory request form and returned to the floor where it is entered in the patient's chart. Values exceeding predetermined limits are considered of critical importance to patient care, and the floor or clinician is directly notified. For institutions with integrated computer systems, the transcription steps can be eliminated and potential sources of error reduced by having test results entered directly into the computerized patient record.

Several models have been developed for cooperative reporting systems between the laboratory and the clinical pharmacokinetic service. Some institutions have a direct computerized laboratory–CPKS linkage and results are reported to both the patient floor and the CPKS. Others rely on the clinical pharmacist reviewing all TDM results and identifying results that merit CPKS follow-up.

Both hard-copy and computerized TDM results frequently are accompanied by the "therapeutic range" for the drug that was assayed. The *therapeutic range* is a range of serum concentrations within which a drug is likely to produce a therapeutic effect. This implies that above the top of the range, a patient is likely to manifest toxic effects related to the drug, whereas below the range, a patient is likely not to receive a therapeutic effect.

Many of these ranges were developed in the 1970s when TDM was first developed; however, recent studies have indicated that there is a great deal of overlap in serum drug concentrations that are therapeutic, toxic, or subtherapeutic among different patients. Given the wide interindividual variation associated with different patterns of metabolism, elimination, age, plasma protein binding, presence of other drugs, and type and severity of disease, the predetermined therapeutic range is often irrelevant.[72,73] For many drugs, a TDM result above the therapeutic range is not highly predictive that the drug is toxic. And conversely, a result in the therapeutic range could be associated with a toxic or subtherapeutic effect.[74–76]

The information content of a TDM report could be improved if each test result were accompanied by the range likelihood ratio associated with a narrow range of results containing the specific patient's serum drug concentration. This measure, described more fully in Chapter 8, is the ratio of the prevalence of a toxic (or subtherapeutic) response in a specific range to the prevalence of a therapeutic response in that same range. The range likelihood ratio can be combined with the clinician's estimate of the patient's prior probability of clinical status (therapeutic, subtherapeutic, toxic) to yield a posterior probability of clinical status that serves as an individualized interpretation of the patient's drug concentration.

Step 9: Clinical Answer

Clinicians use the TDM results to answer the clinical question(s) they raised at the beginning of the Total Testing Process. But correct interpretations of TDM results depend not only on the test value, but also on information about the quality of all preceding steps as well as characteristics of individual patients. That is not a simple matter. As Friedman and Greenblatt[77] indicate:

> The simple act of ordering a serum drug level does not ensure that the information will be meaningful or useful. The interpretation of serum concentrations can be profoundly influenced by such factors as timing of sample, the patient's clinical state, the drug's pharmacokinetics and metabolism, and the tube type and analytic methodology. The likelihood of obtaining clinically meaningful and useful results can be maximized when these factors are taken into account.

We describe five methods to obtain more information to improve the interpretation of TDM results: (1) include information provided on the comprehensive laboratory request form accompanying the TDM request, (2) adjust for intrapatient TDM variation, (3) adjust pretest probabilities of therapeutic, subtherapeutic, or toxic conditions based on the test performance characteristics, (4) use dosage adjustment aids such as bayesian computer packages, and (5) involve individuals who can make dosage decisions based on clinical pharmacokinetic information.

TDM Test Request Forms
Clinicians should consult the TDM test request forms for information that could assist in the interpretation of TDM results. As described under Step 3, a comprehensive and properly completed laboratory request form should provide information concerning the patient's clinical condition, dosing regimen, time of last dose, suspected drug interactions, specimen collection time, and type of specimen. In interpreting the TDM result, clinicians should be able to obtain from the laboratory request form answers to such questions as: Was the patient receiving medication that could interfere with TDM testing? What was the reason for ordering the test? What was the patient's probability of a toxic or subtherapeutic response? Are other conditions indicated that could affect TDM levels? When was the first dose? When was the last dose? When was the sample collected? Answers to these questions provide some of the information needed to modify a dosing regimen or derive a posttest probability of a toxic or subtherapeutic response.

Posttest Probability of Patient's Status
The interpretation of a serum drug concentration should incorporate as much information as possible about both the specific patient and the test performance characteristics of the specific TDM test methodology. One approach to combining patient and test information involves Bayes' theorem and the determination of a patient-specific, posttest probability estimate.[78] Bayes' theorem is most useful when the clinician is trying to answer either of two clinical questions that arise in the first step of the Total Testing Process: (1) What is the probability that this patient's condition is associated with a *subtherapeutic response?* (2) What is the probability that this patient's condition is associated with *drug-related toxicity?* Although Chapter 7 presents a more complete discussion of Bayes' theorem and its application to the calculation of posttest (posterior) probabilities, a summary is presented at this point in the description of the Total Testing Process.

The interpretation of a TDM result should be made in the light of the clinical question raised in the first step of the Total Testing Process. When a toxic or subtherapeutic response is suspected, the clinican should estimate a pretest probability of the condition in the patient. This pretest probability is based on the patient's symptoms, other information about the patient, and the clinical experience of the clinician. Then, when the test result is received, the clinician uses Bayes' theorem to modify the patient's pretest probability based on the TDM test results and the test's ability to differentiate between toxic and therapeutic or subtherapeutic and therapeutic responses at that serum drug concentration using information contained in the range likelihood ratio. Thus, rather than interpreting the TDM result on the basis of whether it is "in" or "out" of the "therapeutic range," this approach yields a patient-specific interpretation of the TDM test result based on the patient's clinical symptoms and the sensitivity and specificity of the TDM testing system.

Additional clinical research can improve this interpretative step in the Total Testing Process. As mentioned under Step 8, TDM "therapeutic ranges" need to be reexamined. Clinical epidemiology can be used to better describe the relationships among drug dosages, serum drug levels, and subtherapeutic, therapeutic, and toxic responses. On the basis of these epidemiologic data, computer programs can be developed, using bayesian logic, to integrate the patient's prior probability, patient-specific pharmacokinetic and dosing information, the sensitivity and specificity of the TDM method, and the test result to yield the revised, patient-specific probability needed to answer the original clinical question. Area-under-the-curve monitoring, rather than peak or trough levels, also needs to be further explored and may be more informative, especially for cyclosporine.[79–81]

Effect of Intrapatient Variation

Clinicians should consider intrapatient variation when TDM results are used to guide drug dosage regimens. For example, Dobbs and co-workers[82] found that one third of digoxin doses that seemed to be optimal, based on one TDM result, produced serum drug concentrations outside the "therapeutic range" when repeated: 21% were too high and 13% too low. When two levels were used to guide dosing, only 3% of the resultant serum drug concentrations were outside the "therapeutic range." Based on this study designed to reduce exogenous sources of variation (eg, patients were compliant, blood collection was properly timed and at steady state), the authors suggested that the variation from expected levels was not related to collection or testing effects, but rather to a high within-patient variation (TDM within-patient CV, 25%; creatinine clearance CV, 12%). To guide dosing regimens appropriately, they cautioned that "when prescribing seemed optimal as judged by the measurement of the digoxin concentration in a single sample, the chance of any single repeat measurement falling outside the conventional therapeutic range would be one in three. . . . A striking improvement in prediction can be made by basing prescription on the digoxin concentrations in samples taken on two or more occasions."

Aids to Improve Drug Dosing in Response to TDM Results

Given the complexity of multicompartments, nonlinear dosage responses, and saturation kinetics as well as the individual differences that exist in drug metabolism and elimination, many opportunities exist for errors to occur in the interpretation of TDM results and their application to drug dosing. For example, after four follow-up serum drug concentrations in patients followed at two epileptic clinics, 90% of patients receiving carbamazepine were within the therapeutic range as compared with only 59% of patients receiving the more pharmacokinetically complex drug, phenytoin.[83]

Nomograms, graphic methods, programmable hand-held calculators, least-squares regression models, and bayesian computer forecasting models are among the tools that have been developed to aid clinicians in modifying dosing regimens based on TDM results.[84-86]

Contribution of Clinical Pharmacists

Methods exist for improving the interpretation of TDM results. Clinical pharmacists, practicing either as part of a structured clinical pharmacokinetic service or independently, can provide an interpretation of serum drug concentrations and make recommendations in the chart to optimize patient dosages. Several studies have been published reporting the success of the CPKS in improving the last three steps of the Total Testing Process: (9) interpretation of serum drug levels, (10) actions taken by physicians, and (11) outcomes of patients. For example, using a one-compartment, computerized, bayesian model for pharmacokinetic interpretation of serum levels, a CPKS placed notes in patient charts indicating interpretations of aminoglycoside concentrations and dosage recommendations. As compared with patients whose physicians incompletely followed all CPKS recommendations, patients whose physicians did follow all recommendations had a 34% shorter febrile period resulting in a 54% shorter length of stay with a 64% reduction in mean direct hospital costs.[87] When all CPKS recommendations were followed, patients also did better than patients receiving no input from the service.[88] This suggests that a CPKS can improve the interpretation of serum blood concentrations, and if appropriate actions are taken, patient care can be improved.

TDM interpretation can also be improved by explicitly recognizing the magnitude of variation that is inherent in the Total Testing Process. If the patient's serum drug concentration has changed, clinicians need to be able to distinguish changes related to analytic and patient variability from changes related to a real physiologic difference between this result and previous TDM determinations.

Step 10: Action Taken

The clinical pharmacist interprets TDM results, recommends dosage changes, and increasingly initiates dosage modifications. Historically, however, it has been the physician who decides whether to take action as a result of a TDM value. Studies indicate that in some cases they may not be taking appropriate action. One report even suggests that for a significant number of their patients, the decision to act or not act is made without information; 60% of patients were discharged before the TDM results were entered into charts.[89]

In a literature analysis of 24 studies that evaluated the quality of physicians' use of TDM results, Einarson and co-workers reported that overall, 40% of the TDM results were inappropriately used; that is, 40% of the time, physicians either took action when not indicated or did not take action when indicated (study range: 10.9% to 86.1% inappropriate use of TDM results).[13] While acknowledging that serious problems exist in physicians' actions related to TDM interpretation and that improvement is definitely needed in this step, one should view these results with caution. Each study defined its own guidelines for appropriate use of TDM results, usually indicating that (1) no action was needed if results were within the therapeutic range, and

(2) action was needed if the results were outside the therapeutic range, or if pharmacokinetic projections indicated that unless the current dosage was modified, future TDM results would be too high or too low. None, however, qualified the degree to which inappropriate action deviated from indicated action (eg, what percentage of TDM results not acted on were only slightly versus significantly above the therapeutic range?), and few acknowledged those patients with results outside the therapeutic range who were being treated safely and effectively. By judging the appropriateness of actions primarily on the basis of the therapeutic range, these studies inflated the rate of inappropriate response to TDM results by not examining which of these errors were clinically significant.

Although we do not know the magnitude of inappropriate TDM use that is clinically significant, most acknowledge that problems do exist in this step. Can clinical pharmacokinetic services improve the use of TDM results? Ried et al identified seven studies that measured the impact of a CPKS on the quality of TDM actions. Studies were limited to those that included either a control population that did not receive CPKS input or a baseline period during which CPKS services were not provided. Five of the studies showed significant improvements, ranging from 27.3% to 81.1% increase in appropriate use, whereas two studies did not detect any change. A meta-analysis based on these seven studies detected a trend toward improvement related to CPKS input; however, a statistically significant improvement was not measured, possibly because of the small number of studies that included a control population or baseline period and substantial variation in the effect size among the studies.[31]

But there is an assumption that underlies all of these studies: adjusting the patient drug concentration to within the therapeutic range is the correct course of action, and not responding to a TDM result in the subtherapeutic or toxic range is an inappropriate clinical response. Although further work is needed in this area, clinicians are cautioned that treating the patient and the associated clinical signs is much more important than treating the serum drug concentration.[90]

Step 11: Effect on Patient Care

In this section we examine the effect of TDM on patient care. This effect can be captured indirectly by measuring the degree to which therapeutic guidelines were achieved (eg, percentage of patients with results within the therapeutic range) or directly by determining the effect of TDM on patient outcome (eg, resolution of breathing problems or infection). Both indirect and direct effects of TDM on patient care are discussed more thoroughly in Chapter 8.

Effect on Indirect Measures of Patient Care

In a meta-analysis of 27 articles, Ried and co-workers[31] evaluated the ability of clinical pharmacokinetic services to increase the number of patients with therapeutic peak and trough serum drug concentrations, reduce the number of patients with inappropriate peak and trough concentrations, and increase the number of patients with concentrations in the appropriate therapeutic range. As displayed in Table 3–3, when all 41 individual studies from the 27 articles were combined, patients followed by a CKPS did better overall than 77% of the patients who were not monitored. Because fewer studies examined the effect of each of the five variables, a statistically significant positive effect was shown for only two of the five individual variables: more patients with results within the therapeutic range and fewer patients with toxic trough concentrations. The confidence intervals for the remaining three comparisons included zero, indicating that although

TABLE 3–3. EFFECT OF CLINICAL PHARMACOKINETIC SERVICES ON APPROPRIATENESS OF SERUM DRUG CONCENTRATIONS

Variable	Number of Studies	% CPKS-Monitored Patients Better than Nonmonitored	95% Confidence Interval
Overall appropriateness	41	77	0.34 to 1.16
Within therapeutic range	12	82	0.19 to 1.63
Toxic troughs	7	83	0.12 to 1.82
Toxic peaks	7	52	−0.53 to 0.65
Therapeutic troughs	6	87	−0.37 to 2.68
Therapeutic peaks	9	69	−0.34 to 1.36
Assays used appropriately	7	Not given	−0.46 to 2.88

more CPKS patients had appropriate serum levels, at the 95% confidence level, there was a statistical possibility that there was no difference between the CPKS-monitored and nonmonitored patients.

This meta-analysis also examined if assay results were used appropriately. Although it would seem logical that the improved overall appropriateness of serum concentrations reported above should be related to an improved use of assay results, only one of the nine appropriate use studies also examined the appropriateness of serum concentrations. The lack of parallel studies, coupled with the limited number of studies that examined the appropriate use of assay results ($n = 9$), may have prevented the detection of a statistically significant difference in appropriate assay use between CPKS-monitored and unmonitored patients. Improved use of assay results was detected in CPKS-monitored patients, but the difference between monitored and unmonitored populations did not reach statistical significance.

Although the variables examined by Ried and co-workers were generally accepted measures of quality, they are only indirect indicators of patient outcome. The various investigators defined *appropriateness* to be that all patients should be within the therapeutic range for clinical effectiveness to be achieved, but few asked the question more directly related to patient outcomes: Of patients whose TDM results were outside the therapeutic range and who did not have their doses adjusted, what percentage *clinically* needed dosage adjustments because of toxic or subtherapeutic symptoms? This is the more valid question. Rather than assuming that TDM results outside the therapeutic range are associated with poor patient care if dosage changes are not made, examining the clinical status of those patients in whom the decision was made not to modify the dosage regimen must be examined.

Effect on Patient Outcome

What effect has therapeutic drug monitoring and clinical pharmacokinetic services had, not on indirect measures of effect such as proportion of serum drug concentrations within the therapeutic range or sampled at an appropriate times from last dose, but on outcomes that more directly measure the impact on the course of a patient's clinical outcome? Although Chapter 8 will examine this question more thoroughly, key studies assessing the clinical impact of therapeutic monitoring of aminoglycosides and antiepileptic agents are summarized in this section.

Several studies used patient survival as an outcome measure to assess the contribution of drug monitoring to patient care. Bootman[91] and Zaske[92] and their co-workers have reported that in a series of burn patients with bacteremia, individualized aminoglycoside monitoring and associated dosage adjustments increased survival in patients. Moore and colleagues demonstrated that, in both Gram-negative bacteremia and pneumonia, early peak concentrations of aminoglycosides (gentamicin or tobramycin > 5 mg/L or amikacin > 20 mg/L) were associated with significantly higher survival.[93,94] But in a randomized study, while individualized aminoglycoside dosing did result in more patients being within the target ranges, the small sample size prevented the detection of a significant difference in patient survival.[95]

Another study examined survival, hospital length of stay, time for resolution of infection, and incidence of decreased renal function in patients with pneumonia or bacteremia randomized to be followed by a clinical pharmacokinetic service or by routine hospital care. Although there was no difference in the number of deaths between the two groups, vital signs of the CPKS-monitored patients return to normal 45% faster and these patients spent 32% fewer hours in the hospital.[96] Within the CPKS-monitored patients, some of the physicians followed 100% of the CPKS dosing recommendations and some did not. When the physicians did follow the recommendations, patients had a 34% reduction in febrile period, 54% reduction in hospital stay, and 64% reduction in direct costs as compared with patients who had appropriate TDM testing but whose physicians elected not to follow the CPKS recommendations.[87] This study implies that a CPKS can contribute to an improvement in important patient outcomes, and that improvement can be maximized when physicians follow the recommendations of the CPKS.

Therapeutic drug monitoring has been an important part of antiepileptic care since early TDM testing. In 1982, however, Beardsley reported that the availability of rapid TDM testing for antiepileptic agents was not sufficient to ensure that the results would be used properly to modify dosing regimens.[97] When clinicians made inappropriate responses to the TDM results, only 2% of the patients had an improvement in their seizure control; when they appropriately used the results, 51% of the patients experienced improvement in their seizure control. In a later study, when the availability of rapid TDM was combined with CPKS dosing advice, patients in an outpatient epilepsy clinic had an increase not only in the percentage of phenytoin levels within the therapeutic range, but also in important patient care outcomes—significant improvements in seizure control and reductions (but not reaching statistical significance) and in the incidence of adverse reactions, emergency room visits, and hospital admissions.[98]

Not all studies have shown either a direct or indirect effect of TDM on patient care. In determining optimal therapeutic response to theophylline, some investigators have indicated that pulmonary function tests should be used to guide therapy in patients with chronic obstructive pulmonary disease rather than theophylline drug concentration monitoring. In a majority of the patient population, pulmonary function tests reached their maximum when theophylline was at subtherapeutic concentrations, and even decreased when the theophylline level increased. Large interpatient variation in therapeutic effect resulted in a wide range of theophylline concentrations at which pulmonary function tests were optimal. In this population, TDM did not contribute to improved patient care. If clinicians had dogmatically forced theophylline levels within the therapeutic range, pulmonary function may have been compromised.[99]

More and better outcome studies are needed to assess the clinical effectiveness of therapeutic drug monitoring and the relevance of therapeutic ranges. These topics are further discussed in Chapter 8.

REGULATORY ENVIRONMENT

The Total Testing Process is performed within an environment that is regulated by federal, state, and local governmental laws and by voluntary standards from such organizations as the Joint Commission for the Accreditation of Healthcare Organizations (JCAHO) and the National Committee for Clinical Laboratory Standards (NCCLS). Of course, policies and procedures of individual institutions and departments also influence the environment within which tests are performed.

Clinical Laboratory Improvement Amendments of 1988

The Congress of the United States passed the Clinical Laboratory Improvement Amendments (CLIAs) in 1988 to improve the quality of clinical laboratory testing. All locations that perform testing on human specimens for health assessment or for the diagnosis, prevention, or treatment of disease must adhere to the comprehensive CLIA. According to the CDC summary of the Amendments:

> Each laboratory must establish and follow written policies and procedures for a comprehensive quality assurance (QA) program designed to monitor and evaluate the ongoing and overall quality of the total testing process. The regulations list specific requirements for assessing patient test management, quality control, proficiency testing personnel; comparing test results when a laboratory or institution performs the same test by more than one method or at more than one site; correlating test results with patient information; rectifying communication breakdowns; investigating complaints; reviewing QA assessments with staff; and maintaining QA records.[100]

Some specific regulations are related to TDM testing: (1) Quality-control requirements specify that instruments must be calibrated every 6 months and two levels of controls are performed daily. (2) Proficiency testing requirements specify that each year the laboratory must participate in a proficiency testing program that provides at least three shipments of five samples for each analyte or test. (3) Personnel requirements for individuals performing the tests are linked to the moderate or high complexity of the test methodology. (4) Patient test management regulations specify requirements for specimen submission and handling, test requisitions, specimen handling, and test records and reports.

For further CLIA 1988 information consult the CDC summary of the regulations,[100] the CLIA 1988 regulations as published in the *Federal Register* (FR), and the clinical laboratory in your institution.

Joint Commission for the Accreditation of Healthcare Organizations (JCAHO)

Although the Pathology and Clinical Laboratory Services and Pharmaceutical Services chapters of the JCAHO's *Accreditation Manual for Hospitals, 1993* include standards related to some aspects of TDM testing, it is the Quality Assessment and Improvement chapter that is most relevant for fostering the elements of the Total Testing Process.[101] The standards of the chapter are based on principles, several of which are quoted here:

- A hospital can improve patient care quality—that is, increase the probability of desired patient outcomes—by assessing and improving those governance, managerial, clinical, and support processes that most affect patient outcomes.

- Whether carried out by one or more groups, the processes must be coordinated and integrated. . . .
- Opportunities to improve the processes—and, thus, improve patient outcomes—arise much more frequently than mistakes or errors. Consequently, the hospital's principal goal should be to help everyone improve the processes in which he/she is involved.

It is clear that the principles of the Total Testing Process and the JCAHO's Quality Assessment and Improvement standards are mutually reinforcing. In the JCAHO chapter, the standards encourage hospitals to expand their assessment and improvement activities. Examine how closely the Total Testing Process matches five JCAHO-identified areas of importance:

1. *The full series of interrelated governance, managerial, support, and clinical processes that affect patient outcomes.* The TTP recognizes that not only the laboratory is involved in a TDM test. Rather there is a complex interaction among the patient, physician, nurse, pharmacist, laboratorians, and various clerical and support staff throughout the Total Testing Process. The process occurs within, and is bounded by, the governance and managerial organization of the institution. For change and improvements to occur, the coordinated efforts of all parties are necessary.

2. *Organizing quality assessment and improvement activities around the flow of patient care, in which interrelated processes are often cross-disciplinary and cross-departmental.* As we have described, the 11 steps of the Total Testing Process are built on the flow of patient care. Each step can be further teased apart to identify additional factors that influence the quality of TDM testing and its impact on patient care. Once all steps and potential problems are identified, quality assessment measures can be designed to monitor the frequency and severity of the problems. Then, problem areas can be targeted for improvement.

3. *Focusing on how well the processes in which individuals participate are performed, how well the processes are coordinated and integrated, and how the processes can be improved.* This is part of the quality assessment program referred to above. As described in this chapter, therapeutic monitoring of drugs can be improved by targeting specific areas where it has been documented that errors occur and by better coordinating the different departments and individuals who contribute throughout TDM testing.

4. *Trying to find better ways to carry out processes, as well as initiating action when a problem is identified.* Given the interdisciplinary nature of TDM testing, isolated changes in several individual departments will not likely have the same effect of an interdisciplinary effort designed to improve communications, strengthen the health care team, and lead to improvements in TDM testing and, ultimately, better patient care. Cooperation and collaboration are necessary to solve many of the problems in TDM testing. Once the group suggests and implements changes, it must monitor its efforts and determine its effectiveness.

5. *Integrating efforts to improve patient outcomes with efforts to improve efficiency, that is, improving value.* Throughout the process of TDM testing, investing in methods to improve TDM testing has the potential to lead to better patient care. Also,

doing something right the first time is likely to save money in the long run. For example, better timing of specimen collection offers the opportunity to improve patient care and reduce costs. Samples taken at appropriate postdistribution times more accurately reflect tissue concentrations and, thus, provide clinicians with clinically correct TDM results, increasing the probability of optimal patient care. Improved patient care reduces the need for additional TDM testing and the potential for inappropriate clinical action based on unrepresentative TDM results. Doing it right the first time improves patient care and saves money.

SUMMARY

Therapeutic drug monitoring is a multistep process, beginning and ending with the needs of the patient. Identification of the steps in the Total Testing Process helps us better understand the complexity of TDM testing, the problems that can arise during testing, and the nature of the interdisciplinary team needed to improve the process and offer optimal patient care. Communications among departments and the development of interdepartment guidelines are necessary to improve the utilization, sampling, performance, and interpretation of TDM tests. A commitment to the continuous improvement of TDM testing requires the participation of pharmacists, nurses, physicians, laboratorians, clerical staff, equipment and supply manufacturers, computer programmers, and administrators. Many of the problems are commonly known. Now it is time for every institution performing therapeutic drug monitoring to bring individuals together, collectively identify solutions, implement an improvement plan, and then evaluate the effectiveness of their efforts using outcome measures that both directly and indirectly relate to improved patient care. Doing it right the first time will both benefit the patient and conserve our limited health care dollars.

QUESTIONS

1. Briefly describe what is meant by the *Total Testing Process*.

2. What are the three analytic components of the Total Testing Process? Which steps are included in each component?

3. Which steps most involve the pharmacist?

4. What pharmacy-based activities will improve the specimen collection step in the Total Testing Process?

5. What specific types of problems can occur during the Total Testing Process?

REFERENCES

1. Inhorn SL, Addison BV, eds. *Proceedings of the 1986 Institute on Critical Issues in Health Practices: Managing the Quality of Laboratory Test Results in a Changing Health Care Environment.* Wilmington, DE: DuPont; 1987.

2. Martin ML, Addison BV, Eagner WM, Essien JDK. *Proceedings of the 1989 Institute on Critical Issues in Health Laboratory Practice: Improving the Quality of Health Management through Clinician and Laboratorian Teamwork.* Wilmington, DE: DuPont; 1991.

3. Ambrose PJ, Smith WE, Palarea ER. A decade of experience with a clinical pharmacokinetic service. *Am J Hosp Pharm.* 1988;45:1879–1886.

4. Dobbs RJ, Dobbs SM. Problems with the use of drug blood levels in patient management. In Lasanga L, ed. *Controversies in Therapeutics.* Philadelphia: WB Saunders; 1980:106–117.

5. Cox S, Walson PD. Providing effective therapeutic drug monitoring services. *Ther Drug Monit.* 1989;11:310–322.

6. Orsulak PJ, Gerson B. Therapeutic monitoring of tricyclic antidepressants: Quality control considerations. *Ther Drug Monit.* 1980;2:233–242.

7. Garrison MW, Rotschafer JC. Clinical assessment of a published model to predict aminoglycoside-induced nephrotoxicity. *Ther Drug Monit.* 1989;11:171–175.

8. Sawyers CL, Moore RD, Lerner SA, Smith CR. A model for predicting nephrotoxicity in patients treated with aminoglycosides. *J Infect Dis.* 1986;153:1062–1068.

9. Slaughter RL. Probability assessment approach to therapeutic drug monitoring: Tobramycin. *Drug Intell Clin Pharm.* 1989;23:240–244.

10. Aronson JK. Indications for the measurement of plasma digoxin concentrations. *Drugs.* 1983; 26:230–242.

11. Friedman H, Greenblatt DJ. Rational therapeutic drug monitoring. *JAMA.* 1986;256:2227–2233.

12. Barr JT. Improved laboratory utilization and information production: The administrator's new role. *J Med Technol.* 1986;3:511–521.

13. Einarson TR, Segal HJ, Mann JL. Serum drug level utilization: A literature analysis. *Can J Hosp Pharm.* 1989;42:63–68.

14. Ried LD, McKenna DA, Horn JR. Effect of therapeutic drug monitoring services on the number of serum drug assays ordered for patients: A meta-analysis. *Ther Drug Monit.* 1989;11:253–263.

15. Greenblatt DJ, Sellers EM, Koch-Weser J. Importance of protein binding for the interpretation of serum or plasma drug concentrations. *J Clin Pharmacol.* 1982;22:259–263.

16. Piafsky KM. Disease-induced changes in the plasma binding of basic drugs. *Clin Pharmacokinet.* 1980;5:246–262.

17. Connolly SJ, Kates RE. Clinical pharmacokinetics of *N*-acetylprocainamide. *Clin Pharmacokinet.* 1982;7:206–220.

18. Pippenger CE. Commentary: Therapeutic drug monitoring in the 1990s. *Clin Chem.* 1989;35:1348–1351.

19. Wong ET, McCarron MM, Shaw ST. Ordering of laboratory tests in a teaching hospital: Can it be improved? *JAMA.* 1983;249:3076–3080.

20. Ives TJ, Parry JL, Gwyther RE. Serum drug level utilization review in a family medicine residency program. *J Fam Pract.* 1984;19:507–512.

21. Job ML, Ward ES, Murphy JE. Seven years of experience with a pharmacokinetic service. *Hosp Pharm.* 1989;24:512–519.

22. Pitterle ME, Sorkness CA, Wiederholt JB. Use of serum drug concentrations in outpatient clinics. *Am J Hosp Pharm.* 1985;42:1547–1552.

23. Wallace SM, Gesy K, Gorecki DKJ. Establishing a clinical pharmacokinetic service for gentamicin in a community hospital. *Can J Hosp Pharm.* 1984;37:10–14.

24. Whiting B, Kelman AW, Bryson SM, et al. Clinical pharmacokinetics: A comprehensive system for therapeutic drug monitoring and prescribing. *Br Med J.* 1984;288:541–545

25. Taylor WJ, Robinson JD, Slaughter RL. Establishing a pharmacy-based therapeutic drug monitoring service. *Drug Intell Clin Pharm.* 1985;19:821.

26. Pearce GA, Day RO. Compliance with criteria necessary for effective drug concentration monitoring. *Ther Drug Monit.* 1990;12:250–257.

27. Carroll DJ. Effect of education on the appropriateness of serum drug concentration determinations. *Ther Drug Monit.* 1992;14:81–84.

28. Greenlaw CW, Henrietta GC, Stolley SN. Standardized heparin dosage schedule using pharmacokinetic principles. *Am J Hosp Pharm.* 1979;36:920–923.

29. Lynch TJ, Possidente CJ, Cioffi WG, Hebert JC. Multidisciplinary protocol for determining aminoglycoside dosage. *Am J Hosp Pharm.* 1992;49:109–115.

30. Matzuk MM, Shlomchik M, Shaw LM. Making digoxin therapeutic drug monitoring more effective. *Ther Drug Monit.* 1991;13:215–219.

31. Ried LD, McKenna DA, Horn JR. Meta-analysis of research on the effect of clinical pharmacokinetics services on therapeutic drug monitoring. *Am J Hosp Pharm.* 1989;46:945–951.

32. Ebert SC, Leroy M, Darcey B. Comparison of aminoglycoside concentrations measured in plasma versus serum. *Ther Drug Monit.* 1989;11:44–46.

33. Murphy JE, Peltier T, Anderson D, Ward ES. A comparison of venous versus capillary measurements of drug concentration. *Ther Drug Monit.* 1990;12:264–267.

34. Mucklow JC. The use of saliva in therapeutic drug monitoring. *Ther Drug Monit.* 1981;3:151–157.

35. Miles MV, Tennison MB, Greenwood RS, et al. Evaluation of the Ames Seralyzer for the determination of carbamazepine, phenobarbital, and phenytoin conentration in saliva. *Ther Drug Monit.* 1990;12:501–510.

36. Longley JM, Murphy JE. Falsely elevated digoxin levels: Another look. *Ther Drug Monit.* 1989;11:572–573.

37. Leslie J, Busby M, Khazan E. Interference from a red top Venojet tube in high-performance liquid chromatographic analyses. *Ther Drug Monit.* 1989;11:724–727.

38. Roberts GW, Aldis JJE. Falsely high serum drug concentrations caused by blood samples from contaminated fingers. *Ther Drug Monit.* 1990;12:559–561.

39. Lindholm A, Elinder CG, Ekqvist B. Falsely high-trough cyclosporine levels in capillary samples due to topical contamination. *Ther Drug Monit.* 1990;12:211–213.

40. Niederberger W, Lemaine M, Maurer G, et al. Distribution and binding of cyclosporine in blood and tissues. *Transplant Proc.* 1983;15:203–205.

41. Toler SM, Porter WH, Chandler MHH. Evaluation of precision and accuracy of a fluorescence polarization immunoassay system after dilution of serum samples containing fluorescein dye. *Ther Drug Monit.* 1990;12:300–302.

42. Ambrose PJ, Borchardt C, Henke R, Evans S. Spurious aminoglycoside results using the Stratus immunoassay. *Ther Drug Monit.* 1988;10:116.

43. Pickering LK, Gearhart P. Effect of time and concentration upon interaction between gentamicin, tobramycin, netilmicin, or amikacin and carbenicillin or ticarcillin. *Antimicrob Agents Chemother.* 1979;15:592–596.

44. O'Bey KA, Jim LK, Gee JP, et al. Temperature dependence of the stability of tobramycin mixed with penicillins in human serum. *Am J Hosp Pharm.* 1982;39:1005–1008.

45. Ebert SC, Jorgensen JH, Drutz DJ, Clementi WA. Comparative assessment of in vitro inactivation of gentamicin in the presence of carbenicillin by three different gentamicin assay methods. *J Clin Microbiol.* 1984;20:701–705.

46. Bailey DN, Coffee JJ, Briggs JR. Stability of drug concentrations in plasma stored in serum separator blood collection tubes. *Ther Drug Monit.* 1988;10:352–354.

47. Levy AB, Walters M, Stern SL. Reduced serum tricyclic levels due to gel separators. *J Clin Psychopharmacol.* 1987;7:423–424.
48. Parish RC, Alexander T. Stability of phenytoin in blood collected in vacuum blood collection tubes. *Ther Drug Monit.* 1990;12:85–89.
49. Koch TR, Platoff G. Suitability of collection tubes with separator gels for therapeutic drug monitoring. *Ther Drug Monit.* 1990;12:277–280.
50. Wilson JF, Tsanaclis LM, Williams J, et al. External quality assurance of tricyclic antidepressant measurements in serum: Eight years of progress? *Ther Drug Monit.* 1989;11:196–199.
51. Oles KS. Therapeutic drug monitoring analysis systems for the physician office laboratory: A review of the literature. *Drug Intell Clin Pharm.* 1990;24:1070–1077.
52. Chan KM, Walton KG, Koenig J. Evaluation of the theophylline procedure on the Abbott Vision analyzer. *Clin Chem.* 1986;32:1051. Abstract
53. Monaco F, Gianelli, Dimancio U, Mutani R. A simple and disposable visual measuring device to assay antiepileptic drugs from whole blood samples. *Ther Drug Monit.* 1990;12:359–361.
54. Oeltgen PR, Shank WA, Blouin RA. Clinical evaluation of the Abbott TDx fluorescence polarization immunoassay analyzer. *Ther Drug Monit.* 1984;6:360–367.
55. St. Louis PJ, MacDonald, Giesbrecht E, Soldin SJ. An evaluation of the Kodak Ektachem clinical chemistry slide for theophylline. *Ther Drug Monit.* 1989;11:93–96.
56. Vaughan LM, Weinberger MW, Milavetz A. Evaluation of the Ames Seralyzer for therapeutic drug monitoring of theophylline. *Drug Intell Clin Pharm.* 1986;20:118–121.
57. Zaninotto M, Secchiero S, Paleari CD, Burlina A. Performance of a fluorescence polarization immunoassay system evaluated by therapeutic monitoring of four drugs. *Ther Drug Monit.* 1992;14:301–305.
58. Boyce EG, Lawson LA, Gibson GA, Nachamkin I. Comparison of gentamicin immunoassays using univariate and multivariate analyses. *Ther Drug Monit.* 1989;11:97–104.
59. Busch RP, Virji MA. Serum theophylline assay by Ames Seralyzer compared with Abbott TDx in pediatric care. *Clin Chem.* 1985;31:1247–1248.
60. Clifton GD, West ME, Hunt BA, Burki NK. Accuracy and time requirements for use of three rapid theophylline assay methods. *Clin Pharm.* 1988;7:462–466.
61. Leppik IE, Oles KS, Sheehan ML, et al. Phenytoin and phenobarbital concentrations in serum: A comparison of Ames Seralyzer with GLC, TDx, and EMIT. *Ther Drug Monit.* 1989;11:73–78.
62. Lindholm A, Henricsson S. Comparative analyses of cyclosporine in blood and plasma by radioimmunoassay, fluorescence polarization immunoassay, and high-performance liquid chromatography. *Ther Drug Monit.* 1990;12:344–352.
63. Wilson JF, Tsanalis LM, Williams J, et al. Comparison of nonisotopic and radioimmunoassay techniques for digoxin: A study based on external quality assurance measurements. *Ther Drug Monit.* 1989;11:477–479.
64. Wilson JF, Tsanaclis LM, Perrett JE, et al. Performance of techniques of therapeutic drugs in serum. A comparison based on external quality assurance data. *Ther Drug Monit.* 1992;14:98–106.
65. Iosefsohn M, Soldin SJ, Hicks JM. A dry-strip immunometric assay for digoxin on the Ames Seralyzer. *Ther Drug Monit.* 1990;12:201–205.
66. Soldin SJ. Digoxin—Issues and controversies. *Clin Chem.* 1986;32:5–12.
67. Shaw LM. Advances in cyclosporine pharmacology, measurement, and therapeutic monitoring. *Clin Chem.* 1989;35:1299–1308.
68. Morris RG, Saccoia NC, Ryall RG, et al. Specific enzyme-multiplied immunoassay and fluorescence polarization immunoassay for cyclosporin compared with Cyclotrac [125I] radioimmunoassay. *Ther Drug Monit.* 1992;14:226–233.
69. Foukaridis GN. Influence of spironolactone and its metabolite canrenone on serum digoxin assays. *Ther Drug Monit.* 1990;12:82–84.

70. Ambrose PJ, Borchardt C, Henke R, Evans S. Spurious aminoglycoside results using the Stratus immunoassay. *Ther Drug Monit.* 1988;10:116.
71. Elliot K, Watson ID, Tsintis P, et al. The impact of near-patient testing on the organization and costs of an anticonvulsant clinic. *Ther Drug Monit.* 1990;12:434–437.
72. Hasegawa GR. Antiarrhythmic monitoring: Misplaced emphasis. *Clin Pharm.* 1991;10:211–212.
73. Spector R, Park GD, Johnson GF, Vesell ES. Therapeutic drug monitoring. *Clin Pharmacol Ther.* 1988;43:345–353.
74. Schumacher GE, Barr JT. Applying decision analysis in therapeutic drug monitoring: Using decision trees to interpret serum theophylline concentrations. *Clin Pharm.* 1986;5:325–333.
75. Schumacher GE, Barr JT. Making serum drug levels more meaningful. *Ther Drug Monit.* 1989;11:580–584.
76. Schumacher GE, Barr JT. Using population-based serum drug concentration cut-off values to predict toxicity: Test performance and limitations compared with bayesian interpretation. *Clin Pharm.* 1990;9:88–96.
77. Friedman H, Greenblatt DJ. Rational therapeutic drug monitoring. *JAMA.* 1986;256:2227–2233.
78. Weinstein M, Fineberg HV. *Clinical Decision Making.* St. Louis, MO: Mosby; 1980.
79. Grevel J, Welsh MS, Kahan BD. Cyclosporine monitoring in renal transplantation: Area under the curve monitoring is superior to through-level monitoring. *Ther Drug Monit.* 1989;11:246–248.
80. Grevel J, Napoli KL, Gibbons S, Kahan BD. Area-under-the-curve monitoring of cyclosporine therapy: Performance of different assay methods and their target concentrations. *Ther Drug Monit.* 1990;12:8–15.
81. Lindholm A, Napoli K, Rutzky L, Kahan BD. Specific monoclonal radioimmunoassay and fluorescence polarization immunoassay for trough concentration and area-under-the curve monitoring of cyclosporine in renal transplantation. *Ther Drug Monit.* 1992;14:297–300.
82. Dobbs RJ, Nicholson PW, Denham MJ, et al. Therapeutic drug monitoring of digoxin—Help or hindrance? *Eur J Clin Pharmacol.* 1986;31:491–495.
83. Privitera MD. Dosing accuracy of antiepileptic drug regimens as determined by serum concentrations in outpatient epilepsy clinic patients. *Ther Drug Monit.* 1989;11:647–651.
84. Godley PJ, Ludden TM, Clementi WA, et al. Evaluation of a bayesian regression program for nonsteady-state phenytoin pharmacokinetics. *Clin Pharm.* 1987;6:634–639.
85. Privitera MD, Homan RW, Ludden TM, et al. Clinical utility of a bayesian dosing program for phenytoin. *Ther Drug Monit.* 1989;11:285–294.
86. Vozeh S, Uematsu T, Ritz R, et al. Computer-assisted individualized lidocaine dosage: Clinical evaluation and comparison with physician performance. *Am Heart J.* 1987;113:928–933.
87. Destache CJ, Meyer SK, Rowley KM. Does accepting pharmacokinetic recommendations impact hospitalization? A cost–benefit analysis. *Ther Drug Monit.* 1990;12:427–433.
88. Destache CJ, Meyer SK, Bittner MJ, Hermann KG. Impact of a clinical pharmacokinetic service on patients treated with aminoglycosides: A cost–benefit analysis. *Ther Drug Monit.* 1990;12:419–426.
89. Kumana CR, Chan YM, Kou M. Audit exposes flawed blood sampling for "digoxin levels." *Ther Drug Monit.* 1992;14:155–158.
90. Chadwick DW. Overuse of monitoring of blood concentrations of antiepileptic drugs. *Br J Med.* 1987;294:723–724.
91. Bootman JL, Wertheimer AL, Zaske DE, et al. Individualized gentamicin dosage regimens in burn patients with Gram-negative septicemia: A cost–benefit analysis. *J Pharm Sci.* 1979;68:267–272.
92. Zaske DE, Bootman JL, Solem LB, et al. Increased burn patient survival with individualized dosages of gentamicin. *Surgery.* 1982;91:142–149.
93. Moore RD, Smith CR, Lietman PS. The association of aminoglycoside plasma levels with mortality in patients with Gram-negative bacteremia. *J Infect Dis.* 1984;194:443–448.
94. Moore RD, Lietman PS, Smith CR. Clinical response to aminoglycoside therapy: Importance of the ratio of peak concentration to minimal inhibitory concentration. *J Infect Dis.* 1987;155:93–99.

95. Begg EJ, Atkinson HC, Jeffrey GM, Taylor NW. Individualized aminoglycoside dosage based on pharmacokinetic analysis is superior to dosage based on physician intuition at achieving target drug concentrations. *Br J Clin Pharmacol.* 1989;28:137–141.

96. Destache CJ, Meyer SK, Padomek MT, Ortmeier BG. Impact of a clinical pharmacokinetic service on patients treated with aminoglycosides for Gram-negative infections. *Drug Intell Clin Pharm.* 1989;23:33–38.

97. Beardsley RS, Freeman JM, Appel FA. Anticonvulsant serum levels are useful only if the physician appropriately uses them: An assessment of the impact of providing serum level data to physicians. *Epilepsia.* 1983;24:330–335.

98. Ionnides-Demos, Horne MK, Tong N, et al. Impact of pharmacokinetics consultation service on clinical outcomes in an ambulatory-care epilepsy clinic. *Am J Hosp Pharm.* 1988;45:1549–1551.

99. Ashutosh K, Bajaj R, Cho C, Sangani G. Use of theophylline level as a guide to optimum therapy in patients with chronic obstructive lung disease. *J Clin Pharmacol.* 1990;30:324–329.

100. Centers for Disease Control. Regulations for implementing the Clinical Laboratory Improvement Amendments of 1988: A summary. *MMWR.* 1992;41:1–17 No.RR-2.

101. Joint Commission for the Accreditation of Healthcare Organizations. Quality assessment and improvement. In *Accreditation Manual for Hospitals, 1993.* Chicago: American Hospital Association, 1993:139–144.

Chapter 4

Developing and Operating a Therapeutic Drug Monitoring Service

John E. Murphy
Terrance A. Killilea

Keep in Mind

- Between 1978 and 1988 the proportion of surveyed hospitals that reported providing clinical pharmacokinetic services on a daily basis rose more than fivefold from 6.2 to 38%. This growth is continuing.

- Many early services were justified based on improving poor utilization and reporting of drug concentration measurements. This justification remains today in many health systems.

- Developing a therapeutic drug monitoring service requires many steps. A well-thought-out plan and consistent follow-through will increase the likelihood of success.

- There are three extremely important considerations in promoting and expanding a therapeutic drug monitoring service. These are the three V's: visibility, visibility, and visibility.

> A journey of a thousand miles begins with a single step.
> A Chinese proverb.

Establishment and operation of therapeutic drug monitoring (TDM) or clinical pharmacokinetic monitoring services (CPKS) (terminology to be used interchangeably for this chapter), or both, and their impact on hospital costs and patient care have received much attention in the last 15 years. Research and writing have focused on establishing the service,[1-21] describing the impact of the service,[22-38] determining the utility of drug concentration measurements for TDM[39-44] and the cost–benefit/effectiveness of provided services,[45-58] ensuring the quality of services provided,[59-63] and documenting the incidence of provision of such services.[64-70] Services provided outside of the traditional hospital setting have been depicted,[71-74] and methods for obtaining reimbursement for pharmacokinetic and other clinical services have been described.[2,4,8,9,75-80] Many of these articles addressed more than one of the issues listed above.

The term *pharmacokinetics* was introduced by F. H. Dost in 1953 and many of the equations frequently used in characterizing the pharmacokinetics of drugs in humans were described from the 1930s through the 1970s.[81] With the development of specific and sensitive assay methods for the high-performance liquid chromatography (HPLC) and other somewhat complicated techniques (in terms of technical skill required), application of pharmacokinetic principles to patient care began to develop in the United States. It was, however, the development of easy-to-use assay instruments for accurate immunoassay methods (eg, EMIT by Syva and TDX by Abbott) and the advances in hand-held calculator and computer technology that provided the tools necessary for the rapid evolution of pharmacokinetic monitoring in the clinical setting.

Two national surveys conducted 10 years apart indicated that the provision of CPKSs on a daily basis in hospitals had increased from 6.2% of the surveyed respondents to 35% between 1978 and 1988.[64,65] Two other surveys by a group of authors found that 27 institutions provided CPKSs in 1979 compared with 63 institutions by 1983.[66,67] A 1990 national survey found that 42.1% of responding hospitals reported provision of CPKSs and that 82.5% of recommendations by members of the CPKSs were accepted.[68] Researchers in a 1987 regional study found that 40% of responding hospitals in the area reported provision of CPKSs, that the mean (± SD) number of patients monitored per day was 25 ± 82 (though the median number was only 4), and that the median pharmacist time spent per patient per day was 32 minutes.[69] In the 1983 survey, CPKSs employed a mean (± 1 SD) of 1.25 ± 1.2 FTE pharmacists in their programs.[67] An earlier survey of members of a pharmacokinetics special interest group indicated similar results in terms of number of consultations. The mean (± 1 SD) number of monthly consultations was 35.1 ± 33.8 (range: 1–95).[12] The 1983 survey found CPKSs averaging 102.4 ± 180.7 consultations per month.[67] The provision of CPKSs has also been found to vary by hospital size and type and by region of the country.[68]

A 1990 statewide survey in Georgia found that aminoglycoside monitoring made up the bulk of consultations in the majority of institutions reporting CPKS provision.[70] This same study showed that almost half of the institutions with CPKSs provided consultation on 20 or fewer patients monthly and that only 38% charged for the service. In addition, though only 23.3% of the respondents indicated providing a CPKS in this survey, 47% of those without a CPKS had plans to initiate one in the future.

These surveys provide interesting information and raise important questions relative to CPKSs and TDM. First, the provision of these services is increasing fairly rapidly across the United States and there appears to be strong interest in providing the service in hospitals not currently doing so. This trend is occurring despite limited charging for service provision. Second, the scope of service provided is limited and does not impact on all patients who might benefit from these services, particularly outside of aminoglycoside TDM. Two questions demand answers: Why have CPKSs not expanded to include many drugs for TDM? Why is charging for service not more widespread if it is accomplished in a substantial number of institutions. One reason for the limited growth of charging for service may be the growth of capitated payment systems. In systems where reimbursement for an inpatient admission is fixed, charging for services will not amount to reimbursement. On the other hand, billing the patient or third party in conjunction with or in a similar fashion as a physician can lead to actual reimbursement for services. Other important questions concern who will be providing pharmacokinetic service and how can different professionals best interact to ensure optimal patient outcome through collaborative efforts in the use of TDM.

The establishment and operation of a CPKS or TDM service remains of great importance and should be of considerable interest to the 60% or more institutions nationwide that do not currently provide these services. TDM will be an integral part of the provision of pharmaceutical care to patients, thus ensuring continuation of such monitoring for many years to come. The structure of these services may change as the majority of pharmacists (who have traditionally provided the bulk of CPKS monitoring) begin to practice pharmaceutical care and issues such as differences between "clinical" and "staff" pharmacist positions and job duties begin to blur. In addition, TDM will be conducted in many settings outside of the traditional institutions, further enhancing the potential for pharmacists and other health care professionals to provide pharmaceutical care.

The remainder of this chapter deals with traditional and nontraditional methods used to date to establish and maintain TDM or pharmacokinetic services.

JUSTIFYING THE NEED FOR A PHARMACOKINETIC SERVICE

Many early services were established based on documentation of problems with the utilization of drug concentration measurements (DCMs) and demonstration that scheduling and control of DCMs by TDM services improved usage.[1,5,16,17,25,46] The potential for improving patient care was also often discussed with hospital administrators and others making decisions on the service; however, because of the difficulty of performing the studies necessary to prove patient outcome benefits internally, and the economic advantages of DCM scheduling noted and easily demonstrated at any hospital, this aspect of the service was considered an added, though unproven, benefit when proposing new service establishment.

A recent meta-analysis of research on the effect of CPKSs on TDM demonstrated that patients monitored by CPKSs were more likely to have DCMs within acceptable ranges than those not monitored.[36] CPKS-monitored patients also had more DCMs collected and used appropriately. This meta-analysis illustrates why the approach of documenting the potential benefit of CPKSs through improvement of DCM utilization has remained effective through the years.

As experience with CPKSs grew, studies were initiated and reported focusing on ensuring the quality of the consultations provided by members of CPKSs along with some discussion of influence on patient outcome.[54–63] Finally, the impact of CPKS provision on patient outcome began to play a more dominant role in the literature.[26,28,31,33,37,45,48,55,56] This time line was not absolute and certain of the papers written discussed DCM usage, quality, and outcome in early and late periods.

Effective justification of the need for a pharmacokinetic service should now be a matter of gathering a representative sample of the literature, developing a proposal, gathering support, and selling administration. Requests by administrators to document the need for a CPKS in each individual hospital should be discouraged if at all possible, as this documentation consumes much time and effort that might be better spent in staff development and service organization. Utilization of the wide variety of studies available along with the presentation of a well-formed plan should replace the need to document potential benefit in every institution. As hospital pharmacy leader Herbert Carlin stated, "Administration and medical staff . . . must show enough faith to allow a truly comprehensive program to grow and develop and eventually demonstrate its value."[82]

When it is necessary to document the need for a CPKS, several standards, both process and outcome oriented, can be used (Table 4–1). An effective manner to demonstrate achievable benefit is to examine retrospective records of previous DCMs and illustrate (1) that the CPKS (in

TABLE 4–1. DEMONSTRATING A NEED: STANDARDS

Standard	Orientation
Frequency of inappropriate drug concentration measurements (DCMs)	Process
Frequency of dose modification in response to inappropriate DCMs	Process
Time to achieve therapeutic range (particularly useful—heparin/warfarin)	Outcome
Occurrence of adverse drug reaction with subsequent elevated DCM	Outcome

some cases using pharmacokinetic software) could have predicted the nonoptimal DCM, and (2) the CPKS could have avoided the nonoptimal DCM by using pharmacokinetic analysis. Selecting an appropriate forum for presentation of the data to a large group of key prescribers and administrators can enhance the utility of the data gathered. Occasionally, this "show and tell" method of presenting institution-specific information will be a pharmacy's first opportunity to demonstrate the potential benefit of a CPKS to a large group of physicians or administrators (as opposed to prolonged, labor-intensive development with individual physicians).

In discussing the beneficial effects of TDM, appropriate use of pharmacoeconomic terms can enhance credibility. Discussions can range from noneconomic improvement in patient outcome/survival to frank financial savings. Cost–benefit analysis places all achieved improvements in monetary terms. Cost–effectiveness analysis uses improved outcome as measurement of end effect. These concepts can be blended by placing economic value on beneficial therapeutic outcome. This approach can focus on economic benefit to the hospital (shown via decreased length of stay or costs) or to society in general (via lower health care costs or improved productivity).

The benefits of TDM services have been summarized in four areas[54]:

1. *Achievement of therapeutic concentrations is associated with increased efficacy and reduced frequency of side effects.* This effect has been demonstrated in patients receiving valproic acid,[39] theophylline,[40] tricyclic antidepressants,[41] and methotrexate.[42]

2. *Without TDM a large proportion of patients will have serum concentrations outside the therapeutic range.* Aminoglycosides have demonstrated wide interpatient variability.[83] Empiric, non-patient–specific dosing lacks precision in aminoglycoside therapy.

3. *Making drug assays without a TDM service available to physicians does not improve the quality of treatment.* Serum drug concentrations alone do not improve patient outcome.[43,44] Inappropriate drawing of samples and noninformed action on receipt of DCMs impair the ability to improve and can, in fact, impair the quality of patient care.

4. *Dose adjustment based on appropriate interpretation of DCMs reduces the proportion of patients with serum concentrations outside the therapeutic range.* There is convincing evidence that TDM is effective when interpretation of results is appropriate. This has been demonstrated for aminoglycosides,[84] theophylline,[40] and lidocaine.[85] The introduction of a broad-based pharmacokinetic service has been shown to be effective in increasing the proportion of samples of digoxin, theophylline, and phenytoin within the therapeutic range.[7]

It should be noted that placing a definitive economic value on the benefits of a service is very difficult. With the current emphasis on quality improvement, cost–effectiveness analysis can be blended with cost–benefit analysis to demonstrate the true value of a TDM service to administrators and other health care professionals.

The beneficial effects of TDM have been broken down into direct and indirect effects.[54] The direct benefits include improvement in survival, reduction in length of treatment, improvement in recuperation, reduction in treatment costs due to side effects, and improvement in patient symptoms (disease status). The indirect benefits include physician education, patient compliance, and site-specific pharmacokinetic data.

Of particular interest are the improved opportunities for physician education. The benefits of physician education can be exhibited in several areas.

1. *Improved utilization/empiric dosing.* As the TDM program matures, physicians may begin to select empiric dosing regimens that require less intense pharmacokinetic monitoring. This is a result of the feedback physician groups receive regarding the dosing strategies of a successful TDM service.

2. *Confidence in traditional, cost-effective agents.* A good example of this potential benefit is the antibiotic gentamicin. With increased confidence in safe, effective dosing of gentamicin, use of this valuable, cost-effective antibiotic will continue. The potential cost–benefit of sustained gentamicin use is extensive.

3. *Increased professional interaction between medical staff and pharmacy staff.* This benefit can be long-lasting and beneficial to patients and the institution. Pharmacokinetic consultation is a distinguished area through which a pharmacy can demonstrate its ability to excel in therapeutic challenges. If positioned correctly, a strong TDM service can demonstrate that the members of the pharmacy department are partners in pharmacotherapy and not dispensatory policeman. This level of interaction can lead to the next two developments.

4. *Pharmacy review of the entire pharmacotherapeutic regimen.* With the demonstration of valuable insight, additional pharmacy input into therapeutic options may become viable. The next logical step after evaluation of the dosing of an agent that is monitored with serum concentrations is evaluation of all medications that should have dosing modifications in patients with impaired renal function. Antibiotic selection, either empiric or after culture and sensitivity results are available, is another area of therapeutics that can be investigated in conjunction with a TDM service.

5. *Dosing protocol development.* If areas requiring pharmacokinetic modification are identified, this approach can prospectively address the avoidance of nonoptimum initial therapy. In addition, this precedent can lead to broader areas of influence as described above.

DEVELOPING THE SERVICE

Table 4–2 lists steps in the development of a CPKS. These are not necessarily in the order in which they should be accomplished; considerable overlap in timing is likely.

TABLE 4–2. STEPS IN THE DEVELOPMENT OF A CLINICAL PHARMACOKINETIC SERVICE

    I. Instill desire (if necessary) in individuals who will work in and with the service.

   II. Formulate a proposal and plan.

      A. Identify potential problems in patient care and resource utilization that might be alleviated by a clinical pharmacokinetic service (CPKS). Review the literature on the benefits of CPKSs and provide any in-house data.

      B. Determine the scope of the service.

         1. Hours of operation

         2. Number of drugs for which consultation will be provided

         3. Limitations on availability

         4. Quality assurance

      C. Evaluate the personnel available and those needed.

      D. Determine the necessity for additional training.

      E. Evaluate the equipment available and that needed.

      F. Assess the cost of the service.

      G. Develop a reimbursement plan.

  III. Recruit support for the service among other health care professionals.

  IV. Approach decision makers (administration, pharmacy and therapeutics committee, etc.) with the proposal.

   V. Develop policies and procedures for the service.

  VI. Develop a promotion campaign to announce the service.

 VII. Educate ancillary personnel.

VIII. Initiate the service.

  IX. Maintain a high level of visibility and promote the service.

   X. Document the benefits of the service to justify its continuation.

  XI. Expand the service into other areas of patient care demonstrating a need.

Instilling Desire in Service Personnel

Though most schools and colleges of pharmacy have focused some course work on the area of pharmacokinetics in the last two decades, many practicing pharmacists have had little training in pharmacokinetics. Thus, initiating a CPKS may be a source of substantial stress for those who have had little or no training and for the many pharmacists who have not kept up with the discipline. If the service is to function with these individuals, extensive training and staff development are necessary. To use pharmacists or other health professionals with limited training effectively, their support must be gained as much of the educational efforts will fall on them as individuals. Rewriting job descriptions, establishing reward systems for extra effort (including career ladders for participation), and setting reasonable expectations may prove useful in gaining support from staff.

    For some institutions, hiring a pharmacist(s) with extensive skill in clinical pharmacokinetics may be essential. In others, the development of appropriate training programs and a strong desire by the staff may suffice.[20,21] Regardless, safe and efficacious dosing is the responsibility of each pharmacist dispensing medications.

Formulating a Proposal and Plan for the Service

Potential Problems in Patient Care and Resource Utilization
The following procedure and decision-making problems might be avoided with the institution of a CPKS or TDM service.

Inappropriate Timing of DCMs. DCMs are notoriously mismanaged in terms of utilization without some method of close monitoring of scheduling relative to dose administration. Two studies demonstrated very poor utilization of DCMs. In the first, only 49% of DCMs were considered usable.[24] Only 54% of samples in the second were obtained at the appropriate time.[27] DCMs should be drawn at suitable times relative to dose administration to be clinically useful, and the time of dosing and sample collection should be readily available (preferably on the final permanent report of the DCM). This is particularly important for drugs with a short half-life and somewhat less important for drugs with a long half-life relative to dosage interval. The positive impact of CPKS monitoring of and education relative to DCM scheduling and collection procedures has been documented in numerous reports.[5,13,22,32,34,35]

Inappropriate Use of DCMs. DCMs reported without timing information or those drawn at inappropriate times can lead to incorrect decisions about future therapy. CPKSs have also led to better decision making by physicians using DCMs[30] and to better use of DCMs for therapeutic decisions.[5,30,37]

Suboptimum Dosing Patterns and Therapeutic Range/Outcome Achievement for a Certain Drug or Drugs. Studies have frequently documented poor achievement of the therapeutic range prior to CPKS involvement and improvement after initiation of the service.[1,7,31] Therapeutic outcome of patients has been improved by CPKS monitoring and rapid achievement of targeted drug concentrations.[26,28,31,33,48,55] One author has suggested that direct and indirect benefits are associated with TDM.[54] Direct benefits can include improvement in survival, reduction of the length of treatment, improvement in recuperation, reduction in treatment costs due to side effects, and improvement in patient symptoms. Potential indirect benefits include physician education, patient compliance enhancement, and gathering of pharmacokinetic data. Appropriate utilization of TDM by CPKS members can increase the likelihood of these benefits being manifested.[86]

Development of Adverse Effects from Dosing (Dose-Related Toxicity). Studies have documented reduced toxicity associated with TDM and CPKSs.[28] Effective TDM can prevent the development of toxicity; however, it should be considered that more aggressive dosing for therapeutic response could potentially lead to a slightly greater incidence of minor toxic effects.

Scope of the Service
Numerous options on the scope of service that can be provided occur and appear to be in place.[11] In the surveys of CPKS provision discussed earlier, it is obvious that a wide range of coverage exists. The minimum TDM service might include a part-time practitioner, available by request only and only at certain times of the day or week, who monitors only one drug class (eg, aminoglycosides) solely in a limited segment of the institution (eg, ICU or pediatrics), who may only

provide verbal suggestions without documentation of activities in the patient's chart, and who does not monitor the scheduling of DCM measurements.

The maximum service would be staffed by a number of pharmacokineticists backing up general practitioners who are providing pharmaceutical care to all patients throughout the institution, would be available 24 hours per day and 7 days per week, would interact on all drugs for which TDM is possible, would also comment on other drug therapy during patient assessment, would document all interactions as permanent records in patient charts, and would be considered an indispensable member of the patient care team in the institution. Somewhere between these minimum and maximum approaches for CPKSs fit the majority of services in existence today.

In determining the scope of service, it is useful to consider the possible activities of personnel involved. Both the American Society of Hospital Pharmacists and the American College of Clinical Pharmacy have put forth guidelines for pharmacokinetic services.[14,18] At a minimum, both indicate that professionals providing these services should provide patient-specific consultations that enhance drug efficacy, reduce toxicity, and/or provide diagnosis; communicate with, collaborate with, and educate professional staff; conduct quality-assurance and drug usage evaluation studies; develop protocols and guidelines to enhance TDM in the institution; and conduct pharmacokinetic research to advance the discipline. Table 4–3 lists some of the functions of a CPKS that might be considered.

Hours of Operation. Determination of the hours of operation depends on the integration of the service expected and the availability of staff. Continuous availability provides for rapid institution of patient-specific TDM but is expensive in terms of staffing. In addition, patient care may only be moderately affected with reduced hours, particularly if dose initiation protocols are in place and widely used. Providing a partial service is better than no service at all, as other health care providers can learn from the service team.[22,23,38] A recent study found that 93% of physicians responding to a questionnaire on an aminoglycoside CPKS felt that the CPKS had improved their ability to select an appropriate aminoglycoside dosing regimen.[38]

Number of Drugs for Which Consultation Will Be Provided. Determining the number of drugs for which consultation can be provided by the CPKS depends largely on the experience and knowledge of the CPKS team. Several approaches have been used to generate consultations.

TABLE 4–3. PHARMACOKINETIC SERVICE FUNCTIONS

I. Ensure correct timing, drawing, and reporting of drug concentration measurements (DCMs).

II. Cancel unnecessary DCMs.

III. Design individualized dosage regimens and monitoring.

    A. Attain therapeutic range rapidly through loading doses.

    B. Determine initial maintenance dose based on population pharmacokinetic estimates and determine initial monitoring required.

    C. Calculate patient's pharmacokinetic parameters based on DCM results and knowledge of dosing history.

    D. Adjust dosage regimens in response to DCM results and patient response.

    E. Continue to monitor patient response and design individualized monitoring program.

The traditional method, in which the consultation is requested by a physician, has the distinct advantage that the clinician requesting the consultation wishes information to be provided to him or her. A second, fairly traditional approach has been to have all patients receiving a targeted drug for which a DCM is ordered receive a consultation from the CPKS. The disadvantage of this approach is that the clinician may not have an interest in having another group of clinicians comment on her or his drug therapy. The down side of the requested consultation approach is that many patients who could benefit from pharmacokinetic consultation on a given drug will not be affected by a CPKS. This deficiency conversely becomes the positive side of the approach of having all patients receiving a target drug with DCM ordered receive a consultation from the CPKS. In a third approach, the CPKS is given full dose adjustment authority on a given drug or drugs that may be monitored by TDM. This may occur more often in a specific unit that generally has a finite number of physicians practicing.

Another approach is to have the CPKS comment on any DCM that falls outside of a specified range, either subtherapeutic or toxic. An offshoot of this type of monitoring would be a service that examines elevated laboratory tests such as serum creatinine to adjust doses of renally excreted drugs. Another similar example would be the monitoring of culture and sensitivity reports for appropriate antibiotic therapy.

Two types of therapeutic agents have been identified that require TDM. The first group of agents exhibits an erratic or unpredictable dose–response relationship, for example, phenytoin. The second group of agents comprises those that have a narrow therapeutic to toxic range; the aminoglycosides and theophylline are useful examples of this group.

Limitations on Availability of the Service. A pharmacokinetic service would ideally be available 24 hours a day, 7 days a week. There are numerous times when patients would require the benefits of the service in late evening, when traditional pharmacy services may not be available; however, the number of times that such availability is required will tend to be limited unless the hospital is very large. It is important to remember that patients can be initiated with protocol management and the ordering of appropriately timed DCMs that will allow the CPKS to interact quickly with the patient on any given morning. Also, as pointed out earlier, physicians tend to learn from consultations with a CPKS and therapy initiation may not be hampered if availability is not around the clock. Though a traditional 40-hour week may be satisfactory in most cases, it seems likely that availability of the service 7 days per week is the most desirable. A challenging situation, often found in community nonteaching hospitals, is that of providing adequate therapeutic drug monitoring with limited personnel. Although it may not have the ability to provide a pharmacokinetic consult for every patient in the institution, a department can screen readily available data to focus limited resources on those patients who might benefit the most (Table 4–4).

Quality Assurance. Quality assurance involves the correct timing, drawing, and reporting of DCMs; consultations among team members; and patient outcome.

Correct Timing, Drawing, and Reporting of DCMs. As discussed above, many early pharmacokinetic services justified their existence on the basis of improving the quality of DCM utilization and the resulting cost avoidance. The three main criteria for evaluation of DCMs have tended to be (1) appropriateness of indication for ordering a DCM, (2) accuracy and completeness of infor-

TABLE 4–4. MAXIMIZING BENEFIT WITH LIMITED PERSONNEL

1. Screen list from lab; respond to drug concentration measurements less or greater than an established threshold for a given drug.
2. Focus interventions on ICU patients only.
3. Focus interventions on elderly patients receiving renally cleared drugs.
4. Implement optimal sampling strategies, such as a decision tree for aminoglycoside serum sampling.
5. Use single-point estimations via non-steady-state Bayesian modeling (available in some commercial pharmacokinetics software).

mation provided, and (3) appropriateness of action taken on DCM results. The appropriateness of indication and action taken on DCMs can be influenced by usage evaluation, educational efforts, and restriction of use.

To improve the scheduling, drawing, and reporting of DCMs, a reporting mechanism may be instituted that records (1) the drug concentration measured, (2) the time the last dose was administered, and (3) the time the blood sample was taken from the patient. It is recommended that periodic audits be conducted for each of these aspects of appropriate documentation of DCM results.

Consultations. Ensuring the consistency of the consultations among members of the CPKS team according to appropriate criteria is important for documenting the quality of the service. A number of authors have addressed this need.[23,59–62] Quality-assurance programs should evaluate the internal consistency of consultation among the practitioners of the CPKS. Target concentrations for various disease states, monitoring parameters that should be evaluated, frequency of evaluation, length of therapy, and actions to take in case of poor outcome should all be evaluated by the service.

Patient Outcome. Quality-assurance and therapeutic outcome evaluation of patients treated by the service can provide useful information for JCAHO accreditation and for evaluation of need for more extensive involvement in patient care. When these data can be compared with those for patients not evaluated by the service, even more useful information can be obtained. It may also be helpful to use such data to compare outcome for various members of a CPKS team. Careful attention to development of equivalency of comparison groups will enhance the utility of the gathered information.

Availability of Personnel

The majority of costs associated with a CPKS will be in personnel. A 1983 survey of 63 CPKSs found that the average annual salary costs were ~$30,000 compared with only $500 in equipment.[67] Thus, as pointed out by one group of authors, "The availability of appropriate personnel and the budget to recruit these personnel are therefore major rate-limiting steps in determining the scope of the service."[11] Integration of CPKS duties with routine pharmacist activity may minimize the necessity to increase the personnel budget.

Necessity for Additional Training

The amount of training necessary for members of a CPKS is directly tied to the scope of services to be offered. The number of drugs for which consultation will be provided, the number of patients who receive these drugs, the willingness of physicians to request consultation assistance, other activities that the service provides, and the previous training of the staff providing CPKSs all affect educational needs. Obviously, individuals previously experienced with the running of a pharmacokinetics service and who have experience with a wide variety of drugs for consultation will be a strong asset for the service. Individuals who have little background in pharmacokinetics will need training in both basic pharmacokinetic principles and in the application of pharmacokinetics to patient care. Many potential practitioners concerned with integrating TDM into an overall practice of pharmaceutical care may also require extensive background training in therapeutic aspects of treatment.

A number of textbooks and self-guided training manuals are available for pharmacokinetics teaching. In addition, software programs have been developed to aid in training of individuals wishing to enhance their skills in basic pharmacokinetic principles. The formation of study groups for improving pharmacokinetic skills may be useful in developing the service. It may also be advantageous to perform practice consultations on patients and scrutinize recommendations of all individuals who review the same patient for internal consistency. This practice evaluation/consultation of patients can help build the confidence of pharmacists who may have had limited experience in providing such consultation in the past.[20]

Availability of Equipment

This section addresses the equipment that might be necessary to run the pharmacokinetics service. Some departments may already have computer systems that are tied in to the main hospital computer system. Such mainframe computers can provide accessibility to the software that is desired by members of the pharmacokinetics service who are spread throughout the institution. On the other hand, personal and laptop computers may be sufficient if ready accessibility is ensured.

Software programs that provide for advanced pharmacokinetic consultations and data collection may be very useful. These also allow for the fulfillment of one of the recommendations of both ACCP and ASHP regarding the conduct of pharmacokinetic research by the consultation service.

Two recent articles provide useful information on selecting clinical pharmacokinetic software.[87,88] Each article covers the features of a large number of the currently available software programs and discusses issues of importance for the buyer and user.

Although many useful computer-based pharmacokinetic programs are available, one of the most difficult challenges is convincing the medical staff that the "black box" used is based on science. The practitioner establishing a CPKS should be prepared to present the medical, pharmacologic, and mathematic basis of the methods and programs employed. The opportunity to educate physicians in various areas of pharmacology can increase interest and allow for greater physician–pharmacist interaction. However, as stated by Vozeh, "physicians' acceptance is one of the most important reasons why dosage algorithms with a high level of sophistication are often overlooked while simple methods with inferior performance receive great interest."[54]

Cost of the Service

The cost of the service is directly related to the scope of the services to be provided. How well the CPKS activities of staff pharmacists can be integrated into daily routines can have a significant effect on the added expense of providing a CPKS. If a hospital has instituted satellite pharmacy services, daily routines can include analysis of pharmacokinetic dosing in specific care areas. This allows the pharmacist to become proficient in dosing of medications in particular patients (eg, oncology, neurology, trauma).

Where pharmacists are not positioned in the patient care area, implementing the strategies outlined in Table 4–4 will maximize benefit and impact. Instituting methods to improve efficiency of pharmacy operations (eg, unit dose, increased technician responsibilities) may be all that is required to provide the additional time for pharmacists to provide baseline pharmacokinetic service. These strategies can be used to commence a CPKS program without additional personnel costs. In a larger institution, a pharmacist position dedicated partially (such as a clinical coordinator) or completely to CPKS functions (including quality assurance) may be necessary. In such an institution, the large number of patients on agents requiring pharmacokinetic monitoring is conducive to cost justification using cost–benefit and cost–efficiency methods described earlier.

If a large-scale CPKS is planned, acquiring a proprietary pharmacokinetic software package may be of great benefit. Contrary to the early 1980s, pharmacokinetic packages that assist dosing of many (>10) agents, provide contemporary state-of-the-art algorithms for pharmacokinetic analysis, and are quite user friendly are available for under $500.[87,88] Pharmacokinetic packages that require quarterly updates or other long-term contracts can be cost-inefficient in the long term. The functional requirements for a useful pharmacokinetic software package are to:

1. Provide dependable, accurate projections of future dose/serum concentrations (a refereed, published evaluation is optimal)
2. Be simple enough to allow all pharmacists to use the program with a reasonable amount of training
3. Be able to process steady-state as well as non-steady-state data
4. Be able to provide steady-state as well as non-steady-state projections of serum concentrations
5. Have the ability to print a summary of dose/serum predictions as well as a graphic representation of estimations

Obviously, compatibility with existing computer hardware is helpful. With coordination of hardware operation, purchase of an additional computer system may not be necessary. If purchasing an additional computer is necessary, the expense can be justified (in addition to benefits from the CPKS) by improving clinical information exchange among pharmacists via institution of an electronic mail system or database-derived tracking program. The consistent decrease in the cost of computers has made this expense less of a factor than in the 1980s.

Reimbursement Plan

Reimbursement for pharmacist's cognitive services is an issue of great importance today. Several task forces are working on assessment of this issue. Previous articles have reported on the current status of reimbursement for such cognitive pharmacy services.[76–80] Reimbursement for CPKSs has been discussed and several methods have been used. Current methods seem to revolve around direct billing of third-party payors or patients for the service, billing through another provider (eg, a physician), adding a fee to the drug products dispensed by the institutional pharmacy to pay for the CPKS (or other clinical pharmacy services), or adding a fee to the charge for DCMs. Working with financial reimbursement specialists in the institution may help to identify the most appropriate method or methods for a CPKS.

Recruiting Support for the Service Among Other Health Care Professionals

The value of a CPKS can be demonstrated to other members of the patient care team via convincing data as well as the general concept of patient outcome management. When the true potential benefit to the patient is demonstrated to nurses and physicians, few will argue that a CPKS does not improve the quality of patient care. The challenge in building alliances with other health care professionals is to demonstrate the potential benefit without infringing on their perceived area of practice (or influence) or placing additional burdens on their busy schedule. Proper prospective planning and marketing can avoid conflicts.

Nursing Staff

The nursing staff often have quality of patient care as their utmost concern. Discussion of the ability of a CPKS to improve the quality of care can successfully enlist nursing support for CPKS. Two primary issues are often integral in encouraging nursing staff participation in a successful CPKS: (1) the DCMs that they have been drawing for years will now truly be contributing to improved quality of care, and (2) better utilization of DCMs will require less frequent drawing of blood levels and therefore less demand on nursing staff. Needless to say, including nursing management input on the design of a coordinated CPKS from the beginning will serve to avoid future conflict in implementing the program.

Laboratory Services

The laboratory services of a hospital can be enlisted as an ally in developing a strong CPKS. Although the sole responsibility for processing and interpreting DCMs lies with the laboratory in some institutions, more often the pharmacy (or no department at all) is responsible for CPKS functions. Where the laboratory is the sole site of pharmacokinetic consultations, the clinical expertise of a well-trained pharmacist can be offered to improve interpretation proficiency. Thorough guidelines for the integration of pharmacy and laboratory services in providing CPKSs have been published.[89] This approach is useful when the analytical laboratory has an existing service or desires to become involved in providing CPKSs.

Where the analytical laboratory has not instituted interpretive services for DCMs, the implementation of a pharmacy-based CPKS can be positioned to augment existing laboratory procedures. As stated by the College of American Pathologists, the responsibilities of an analytical chemistry lab are to (1) provide precise, accurate results, and (2) notify physicians of "critical" values.[90] As previously discussed, interpreting serum levels as just numbers, without regard to sampling times and dosing patterns, can lead to inappropriate response. Assisting the laboratory in enhancing physician practice patterns and improving patient care is a strong marketing tool to encourage cooperation of the analytical laboratory.

Medical Staff

One of the greatest challenges faced in instituting a CPKS is garnering physician support. It is important to focus discussions of benefits from CPKSs on improvement of patient outcome. The potential benefit to patients can be shown in (1) results from a retrospective drug usage evaluation (DUE) demonstrating opportunities to improve and (2) concurrent "show-and-tell" on selected patients.

The DUE should be performed to minimize perceptions of pharmacy as a big brother watching over outcome. Recent publications in prestigious medical journals have discussed the need for rational therapeutic drug monitoring.[91] Discussion of programs at other hospitals, either nationally or locally prominent, may lend credence to the discussion. If acceptable, implementing pharmacokinetic methods in retrospective analysis can show that nonoptimal DCMs or patient outcomes can be avoided. These data should be presented in a positive fashion ("this is what the service could have done for you and your patients") as opposed to a negative fashion ("this is what you did wrong and here is how the service could have done better").

More concurrent is the method of active "show-and-tell." This approach involves offering pharmacokinetic dosing advice on selected patients to demonstrate prospectively the benefits of pharmacokinetic analysis. Three caveats should hold: (1) Only qualified individuals should be offering advice. (2) Services should be focused on patients who can be accurately analyzed with available pharmacokinetic resources. (3) Only physicians who are known to be open to input regarding pharmacotherapy should be enrolled. Once 10 to 20 patients have been successfully managed via the CPKS, a summary of data should be presented to the physicians involved as well as to the pharmacy and therapeutics committee. Data obtained using DUE can also be presented at this time. A problem that may occur after such presentations is strong physician demand, which can dramatically increase CPKS utilization and responsibilities, thereby stressing a fledgling service. This is the time that strong managerial leadership and coordination of services are essential to ensure that timely, accurate, and physician-solicited consultations are provided. This is also the time to begin to approach the hospital administration regarding increased resources to provide service to the medical staff.

It is essential that routine pharmacy services do not suffer as the CPKS begins to grow. It is also essential that the pharmacy staff be instructed not to (1) overstep boundaries of responsibilities, leading to physician staff intimidation and alienation; (2) shun routine duties, thus placing higher stress on other members of the pharmacy staff; and (3) go beyond existing protocols or enrolled physicians to expand the service independently. In the early stages of developing a CPKS, the best approach may be one that is conservative and organized, adhering strictly to protocol and building a collegial relationship with the medical staff. Once members of the medical staff have confidence in the abilities of the CPKS, and responsibilities and protocols are delineated, organized growth that builds on the initial success can lead to a CPKS that is viewed as professional and essential to optimal patient care.

Approaching Decision Makers with the Proposal

After demonstration of achievable benefits from a CPKS, a formal proposal should be made to the hospital administration. The key administrators who should be included in the discussion include assistant administrators of all areas that will be affected by the service, the medical administrator of the hospital, members of the medical and administration staff who are responsible for quality assurance (including risk management), supporting physicians who have had a positive experience with the program, and the chair of the pharmacy and therapeutics committee. Previously discussed benefits of the program (eg, improved patient outcome, achievable cost savings, avoidance of unnecessary toxic effects) should be emphasized. In the presentation of the proposal to hospital administrators, comparison with hospitals of similar size or nature can be valuable. Statistics describing the provision of pharmacokinetic services in hospitals of various sizes and alignments have been published.[92]

Incorporating the CPKS into the current movement of outcome management and continuous quality improvement will serve to position the service as an essential benefit. Development of indicators, standards, and thresholds of performance will allow for objective analysis of the performance of the system. It may be advisable to avoid discussions that are overly scientific. It may also be wise to focus on the broad issues that are well understood by nonmedical administrators. Although not essential, approval of a formal program can lead to firm funding of necessary personnel and equipment and advancement of the CPKS as an institution of good pharmacotherapeutic practice in a hospital.

Developing Policies and Procedures for the Service

Policies and procedures for the CPKS can help to ensure quality, guide members of the team, and develop an understanding of service goals. Several articles have discussed quality-assurance standards which can be used to develop CPKS policies.[59–63]

Developing a Promotion Campaign to Announce the Service

In business and home sales it is often said that there are only three important considerations and they all begin with the letter L: location, location, and location. Pharmaceutical care and clinical pharmacy services benefit from the three V's. In terms of advancing services and utilization of the cognitive expertise of the pharmacist, these are visibility, visibility, and visibility. Pharmacists who are physically in patient care areas participating in pharmaceutical care of patients have a much greater likelihood of having their expertise requested than pharmacists sequestered "in the basement."

A promotion campaign might include announcements in the pharmacy newsletter describing the CPKS and how to receive consultation advice, lectures to the various constituencies who will be affected by the service, notes on charts offering advice, wall charts, stickers for telephones, and other marketing devices. The marketing possibilities are beyond the scope of this chapter; however, as many institutions have personnel skilled in public relations, utilization of these skills might well enhance the usage of the CPKS.

Educating Ancillary Personnel

Phlebotomists, ward clerks, laboratory technicians and secretaries, IV administration nurses, medication nurses, and many other health care professionals may be affected by the CPKS. As their cooperation may be vital in securing useful DCM and dosing information and results, it is extremely important that they understand their importance in patient care related to TDM. If a DCM is drawn at a time different from that scheduled, if a nurse gives a dose late and does not inform the CPKS when DCMs are scheduled around the dose, or if a laboratory technician does not inform the CPKS of assay problems, the potential for error increases dramatically. These individuals play a critical role in ensuring that the information obtained is accurate and useful and their importance should be accorded the time it deserves.

Initiating a Formal Pharmacokinetic Service

Several procedures should be delineated prior to initiating a formal CPKS. These include establishing the privilege of pharmacists to take verbal orders from physicians for medication as well as laboratory orders, establishing the pharmacist's privilege to write notes directly in the patient's chart to document the pharmacist's input in patient care and to enhance reimbursement potential, coordinating the laboratory and nursing staff to delineate DCM sampling times and procedures, establishing administration times for many of the drugs commonly analyzed by a CPKS, and coordinating methods for obtaining DCM results. This last procedure may be difficult if a hospital-based computer system is not in place. A report of results generated by the laboratory to be obtained by the pharmacy at a given time may allow for efficient flow of information.

In the early stages of implementing CPKSs, limiting the service to specific practice groups, such as internal medicine, can provide several benefits. These include the ability to assess the personnel requirements of the established CPKS, to focus analysis on whether established protocols are performing well in a controlled group, to ensure good quality control that will impress members of other medical specialty groups, and to allow for the practitioners involved in the early implementation of the program to serve as educators and role models for subsequent participants in the service.

Maintaining a High Level of Visibility and Promoting the Service

Visibility will lead to continuing promotion of the service. Speaking with nurses and physicians to remind them of the availability of the CPKS can enhance opportunities to participate in patient care. Writing articles for newsletters related to pharmacokinetics, giving lectures on pharmacokinetic topics, and participating on hospital committees as a member of the CPKS team all lead to greater visibility for the CPKS. Again, working with the institution's public relations personnel can help to promote the service and give publicity to positive aspects of the CPKS.

Documenting the Benefits of the Service to Justify Continuation

A successful CPKS can justify continuation or expansion by several methods. The previously discussed concepts of cost–benefit and cost–effectiveness analysis are vital to demonstrating benefit to patients and the hospital. Focusing on avoidance of inappropriately drawn DCMs and improved interpretation can yield significant cost–benefit data.[23] If possible, comparing service data with prospectively collected, preservice data will increase validity.[93]

Cost-efficiency may be more difficult to demonstrate adequately. Some analyses of CPKSs have shown a positive effect on quality-of-care issues such as length of hospital stay and febrile periods,[56] whereas others have not demonstrated such an effect.[30] To maximize credibility, comparing similar patients groups (with respect to age, severity of illness, concomitant diseases) is important. Although this may limit the size of the study, it focuses on results that maintain credibility.[57]

Expanding the Service to New Areas Demonstrating Need

Once the pharmacokinetic service has established itself as a vital aspect of quality patient care, expansion of the service into other areas and to other agents should not be as difficult as the initiation of the service. Building on the successes of previous programs should be much easier. Methods similar to those used to initiate the service can be used. In addition, once the physician groups are accustomed to collegial input from members of the pharmacy staff, disease-based DUEs may discover additional areas of pharmaceutical use that could benefit from CPKS involvement.

───────── QUESTIONS ───

1. Discuss four areas in which the benefits of TDM services have been realized.

2. Describe five direct benefits of pharmacokinetic services.

3. Describe methods of ensuring the training of individuals who will participate in the TDM service and the types of training resources available.

4. Describe the steps in development of a TDM service.

REFERENCES

1. Taylor JW, McLean AJ, Leonard RG, et al. Initial experience of clinical pharmacology and clinical pharmacy interactions in a clinical pharmacokinetics consultation service. *J Clin Pharmacol.* 1979;19:1–7.
2. Moore TD, Schneider PJ, Nold EG. Developing reimbursable clinical pharmacy programs: Pharmacokinetic dosing service. *Am J Hosp Pharm.* 1979;36:1523–1529.
3. Hoffman DS, Kerr RA. Responsibility charting in a consultative pharmacy service. *Contemp Pharm Pract.* 1980;3(2):68–74.
4. Maddox RR, Vanderveen TW, Jones EM, et al. Collaborative clinical pharmacokinetic services. *Am J Hosp Pharm.* 1981;38:524–529.
5. Bollish SH, Kelly WN, Miller DE, et al. Establishing an aminoglycoside pharmacokinetic monitoring service in a community hospital. *Am J Hosp Pharm.* 1981;38:73–76.
6. Maddox RR, Lampasona V. Administrative aspects of clinical pharmacokinetic services. *Top Hosp Manage.* 1982;May:61–73.
7. Whiting B, Kelman AW, Bryson SM, et al. Clinical pharmacokinetics: A comprehensive system for therapeutic drug monitoring and prescribing. *Br Med J.* 1984;288:541–545.
8. Moore RA, Tonnies RD. Aminoglycoside dosing service provided by baccalaureate-level pharmacists. *Am J Hosp Pharm.* 1984;41:98–105.
9. Rietscha WJ, Heissler JF, Paulson JF, et al. Collaborative clinical pharmacokinetics service in a community hospital. *Am J Hosp Pharm.* 1984;41:473–477.

10. Maddox RR. *Clinical Pharmacokinetic Monitoring: Administrative Considerations.* Indianapolis, IN: Dista Products Co, 1984.

11. Taylor WJ, Robinson JD, Slaughter RL. Establishing a pharmacy-based therapeutic drug monitoring service. *Drug Intell Clin Pharm.* 1985;19:818–824.

12. Pieper JA. ASHP clinical pharmacokinetics practice SIG membership questionnaire. 1987, Fall. American Society of Hospital Pharmacists SIG Membership Communique.

13. Job ML, Ward ES Jr, Murphy JE. Seven years of experience with a pharmacokinetic service. *Hosp Pharm.* 1989;24:512–526.

14. American Society of Hospital Pharmacists. ASHP statement on the pharmacist's role in clinical pharmacokinetic services. *Am J Hosp Pharm.* 1989;46:804–805.

15. Burkle WS. Development and implementation of clinical pharmacokinetic services. *Am J Hosp Pharm.* 1990;47:391–394.

16. Murphy JE, Ward ES, Job ML. Implementing and maintaining a private pharmacokinetics practice. *Am J Hosp Pharm.* 1990;47:591–597.

17. Murphy JE. Management consultation. *Am J Hosp Pharm.* 1990;47: 2213–2218.

18. ACCP Position Statement. Practice guidelines for the clinical pharmacokinetics consultation service. *Pharmacotherapy.* 1991;11(2):175–177.

19. Jorgenson JA, Rewers RF. Justification and evaluation of an aminoglycoside pharmacokinetic dosing service. *Hosp Pharm.* 1991;26:605–615.

20. Walker DG, Washington GS. Jump starting the pharmacy department on the road to comprehensive pharmaceutical care—First stop: A pharmacokinetic service. In: *Proceedings of the American Society of Hospital Pharmacists' 48th Annual Meeting; June 1991; San Diego, CA.*

21. Prevost RR. Therapeutic drug monitoring by staff pharmacists in a newborn center. In: *Proceedings of the American College of Clinical Pharmacy's 2nd Annual Winter Forum;* February 1992; Phoenix, AZ.

22. Carroll DJ, Austin GE, Stajich GV, et al. Effect of education on the appropriateness of serum drug concentration determination. *Ther Drug Monit.* 1992;14:81–84.

23. D'Angio RG, Stevenson JG, Lively BT, et al. Therapeutic drug monitoring: Improved performance through educational intervention. *Ther Drug Monit.* 1990;12:173–181.

24. Flynn TW, Pevonka MP, Yost RL, et al. Use of serum gentamicin levels in hospitalized patients. *Am J Hosp Pharm.* 1978;35:806–808.

25. Elenbaas RM, Payne WW, Bauman JL. Influence of clinical pharmacist consultations on the use of drug blood level tests. *Am J Hosp Pharm.* 1980;37:61–64.

26. Mungall D, Marshall J, Penn D, et al. Individualizing theophylline therapy: The impact of clinical pharmacokinetics on patient outcomes. *Ther Drug Monit.* 1983;5:95–101.

27. Mason GD, Winter ME. Appropriateness of sampling times for therapeutic monitoring. *Am J Hosp Pharm.* 1984;41:1796–1801.

28. Sveska KJ, Roffe BD, Solomon DK, et al. Outcome of patients treated by an aminoglycoside pharmacokinetic dosing service. *Am J Hosp Pharm.* 1985;42:2472–2478.

29. Cahill RJ, Myers RM, Bauer LA, et al. Impact of an aminoglycoside kinetic service on aminoglycoside use in a community hospital. *Hosp Pharm.* 1986;21:734–737.

30. Winter ME, Herfindal ET, Bernstein LR. Impact of decentralized pharmacokinetics consultation service. *Am J Hosp Pharm.* 1986;43:2178–2184.

31. Smith M, Murphy JE, Job ML, et al. Aminoglycoside monitoring: Use of a pharmacokinetic service versus physician recommendations. *Hosp Formul.* 1987;22:92–102.

32. Ambrose PJ, Nitake M. Kildoo CW. Impact of pharmacist scheduling of blood-sampling times for therapeutic drug monitoring. *Am J Hosp Pharm.* 1988;45:380–382.

33. Destache CJ, Meyer SK, Padomek MT, et al. Impact of clinical pharmacokinetic service on patients treated with aminoglycosides for Gram-negative infections. *Drug Intell Clin Pharm: Ann Pharmacother.* 1989;23:33–37.

34. Ambrose PJ, Smith WE, Palarea ER. A decade of experience with a clinical pharmacokinetics service. *Am J Hosp Pharm.* 1988;45:1879–1886.
35. Klamerus KJ Munger MA. Effect of clinical pharmacy services on appropriateness of serum digoxin concentration monitoring. *Am J Hosp Pharm.* 1988;45:1887–1893.
36. Ried LD, McKenna DA, Horn JR. Meta-analysis of research on the effect of clinical pharmacokinetic services on therapeutic drug monitoring. *Am J Hosp Pharm.* 1989;46:945–951.
37. Wing DS, Duff HJ. Impact of a therapeutic drug monitoring program for phenytoin. *Ther Drug Monit.* 1989;11:32–37.
38. Lackner TE, Manchester R. Physicians' perceptions of the effect of a pharmacokinetic service on their ability to independently function. *Hosp Pharm.* 1991;26:618–632.
39. Gram L, Flachs H, Wurtz-Jorgensen A, et al. Sodium valproate, serum level and clinical effect in epilepsy: A controlled study. *Epilepsia.* 1979;20:303–312.
40. Vozeh S, Kewitz G, Perruchoud A, et al. Theophylline serum concentration and therapeutic effect in severe acute bronchial obstruction: The optimal use of intravenously administered aminophylline. *Am Rev Respir Dis.* 1982;125:181–184.
41. Kragh-Sorensen P, Hansen CE, Baastrup PC, et al. Self-inhibiting action of nortriptyline's antidepressive effect at high plasma levels. *Psychopharmacology (Berl).* 1976;45:305–312.
42. Evans WE, Crom WR, Abromowitch M, et al. Clinical pharmacodynamics of high-dose methotrexate in acute lymphocytic leukemia. *N Engl J Med.* 1986;314:471–476.
43. Froscher W, Eichelbaum M, Gugler R, et al. A prospective randomized trial on the effect of monitoring plasma anticonvulsant levels in epilepsy. *J Neurol.* 1981;224:193–201.
44. Bussey HI, Hoffman EW. A prospective evaluation of therapeutic drug monitoring. *Ther Drug Monit.* 1983;5:245–248.
45. Bootman JL, Wertheimer AI, Zaske D, Rowland C. Individualizing gentamicin dosage regimens in burn patients with Gram-negative septicemia: A cost–benefit analysis. *J Pharm Sci.* 1979;68:267–272.
46. Greenlaw CW, Blough SS, Haugen RK. Aminoglycoside serum assays restricted through a pharmacy program. *Am J Hosp Pharm.* 1979;26:1080–1083.
47. Bootman JL, Zaske DE, Wertheimer AI, et al. Cost of individualizing aminoglycoside dosage regimens. *Am J Hosp Pharm.* 1979;36:368–370.
48. Lehmann CR, Leonard CR. Effect of theophylline pharmacokinetic monitoring service on cost and quality of care. *Am J Hosp Pharm.* 1982;39:1656–1661.
49. Sesin GP, Baptista RJ. Utilizing the clinical pharmacist to modify tobramycin dosage regimens: Accuracy of prediction and potential cost-effectiveness. *Hosp Pharm.* 1984;19:806–810.
50. Schloemer JH, Zagozen JJ. Cost-analysis of an aminoglycoside pharmacokinetic dosing program. *Am J Hosp Pharm.* 1984;41:2347–2351.
51. Meisel S. Cost–benefit analysis of clinical pharmacy services in a community hospital. *Hosp Pharm.* 1985;20:904–906.
52. Holt RJ. Cost savings from kinetic services. *Am J Hosp Pharm.* 1985;42:786–787.
53. Kimelblatt BJ, Bradbury K, Chodoff L, et al. Cost–benefit analysis of an aminoglycoside monitoring service. *Am J Hosp Pharm.* 1986;43:1205–1209.
54. Vozeh S. Cost-effectiveness of therapeutic drug monitoring. *Clin Pharm.* 1987;13:131–140.
55. Destache CJ, Myer SK, Bittner MI, et al. Impact of a clinical pharmacokinetic service on patients treated with aminoglycosides: A cost–benefit analysis. *Ther Drug Monit.* 1990;12:419–426.
56. Destache CJ, Meyer SK, Rowley KM. Does accepting pharmacokinetic recommendations impact hospitalization: A cost–benefit analysis. *Ther Drug Monit.* 1990;12:427–433.
57. Pippenger CE. The cost-effectiveness of therapeutic drug monitoring. *Ther Drug Monit.* 1990;12:418.
58. Krinsky D, Trent D, Beck D. Financial impact of clinical interventions by a pharmacokinetic dosing service. In: *Proceedings of the American College of Clinical Pharmacy's 2nd Annual Winter Forum; February 1992; Phoenix, AZ.*

59. Burkle WS, Matzke GR, Lucarotti RL. Development of competency standards for quality assurance in clinical pharmacokinetics. *Hosp Pharm.* 1980;15:494–496.
60. Lawson LA, Blouin RA, Parker PF, et al. Quality assurance program for a clinical pharmacokinetic service. *Am J Hosp Pharm.* 1982;39:607–609.
61. Walker DJ, Smith SR. Assuring the quality of a clinical pharmacokinetics service. *Am J Hosp Pharm.* 1986;43:2184–2188.
62. Miller DA, Stankiewicz RF, Zarowitz BJ, et al. Developing and implementing standards of practice for clinical pharmacy services. *Hosp Pharm.* 1987;22:772–783.
63. Beck DE, Bradley EL, Farringer JA. Predicting need for pharmacokinetic consultation follow-up using discriminant analysis. *Clin Pharm.* 1988;7:681–688.
64. Deiner CH, ed. *Lilly Hospital Pharmacy Survey 1979.* Indianapolis, IN: Eli Lilly and Co; 1979.
65. Flohrs WJ, ed. *Lilly Hospital Pharmacy Survey 1989.* Indianapolis, IN: Eli Lilly and Co; 1989.
66. Rich DS, Gallina JH, Jeffrey LP. National survey of pharmacokinetic consultation services. *Am J Hosp Pharm.* 1981;38:551–552.
67. Rich DS, Jeffrey LP. Pharmacokinetic consultation services: 1979 versus 1983. *Am J Hosp Pharm.* 1984;41:56.
68. Crawford SY. ASHP national survey of hospital-based pharmacy services—1990. *Am J Hosp Pharm.* 1990;47:2665–2695.
69. Raehl CL, Bond CA, Pitterle ME. Hospital pharmacy services in the Great Lakes region. *Am J Hosp Pharm.* 1990;47:1283–1303.
70. Murphy JE, Capers CC, Carroll DJ, et al. A statewide survey of pharmacokinetic service provision in Georgia. *Hosp Pharm.* 1991;26:711–716.
71. Frakes ME, Pepin S, Godes T, et al. Reimbursable pharmacokinetic dosing services in long-term care facilities. Presented at the American Society of Consultant Pharmacists' 13th Annual Meeting; November 1982.
72. Robinson JD, Lopez LM, Stewart WL. How to establish a pharmacokinetic consulting service for ambulatory patients. *Am J Hosp Pharm.* 1984;41:2048–2056.
73. Einarson TR, Bootman JL, McGhan WF, et al. Establishment and evaluation of a serum cholesterol monitoring service in a community pharmacy. *Drug Intell Clin Pharm.* 1988;22:45–48.
74. Sawada JM. Development and implementation of a home-care pharmacokinetic service. *Pharmaguide.* 1991;4(4):1–3.
75. Crisp CB, Lane Jr, Murray W. Audit of serum drug concentration analysis for patients in the surgical intensive care unit. *Crit Care Med.* 1990;18:734–737.
76. Petersen SD, Patterson LE. Reimbursement for pharmacokinetic consultation in a community hospital. *Am J Hosp Pharm.* 1980;37:1466.
77. ASHP Reports. ASHP guidelines for implementing and obtaining reimbursement for clinical pharmaceutical services. *Am J Hosp Pharm.* 1981;38:386.
78. Kelly WN, Gibson GA, Miller DE. Obtaining reimbursement for clinical pharmacokinetic monitoring. *Am J Hosp Pharm.* 1982;39:1662–1665.
79. Nahata MC. Financial support for clinical pharmacy services. *Drug Intell Clin Pharm.* 1986; 20:988–989.
80. Hutchinson RA, Vogel DP, Witte KW. A model for inpatient clinical pharmacy practice and reimbursement. *Drug Intell Clin Pharm.* 1986;20:989–992.
81. Wagner JG. The history of pharmacokinetics. *Drug Intell Clin Pharm.* 1977;11:747–748.
82. Carlin HS. Patient accountability—Pharmacist's future. *Am J Hosp Pharm.* 1978;35:263–267.
83. Vozeh S, Steiner J. Feedback control methods for drug dosage optimization. *Clin Pharmacokinet.* 1985;10:457–476.
84. Zaske DE, Irvine P, Strand LM, et al. Wide interpatient variations in gentamicin dose requirements for geriatric patients. *JAMA.* 1982;248:3122–3126.

85. Burton ME, Brater C, Chen PS, et al. A bayesian feedback method of aminoglycoside dosing. *Clin Pharmacol Ther.* 1985;37:349–357.
86. Vozeh S, Uematsu T, Schmidlin O, et al. Computer-assisted individualized lidocaine dosage: Clinical evaluation and comparison with physician performance. *Am Heart J.* 1987;113:928–933.
87. Buffington DE, Lampasona V, Chandler MHH. Computers in pharmacokinetics: Choosing software for clinical decision making. *Clin Pharmacokinet.* 1993;25:205–216.
88. Poirier TI, Giudici RA. Survey of clinical pharmacokinetic software for microcomputers. *Hosp Pharm.* 1992;27:971–972, 975–977.
89. Cox S, Walson PD. Providing effective therapeutic drug monitoring services. *Ther Drug Monit.* 1989;11:310–322.
90. *Inspection Checklist, Toxicology/Therapeutic Drug Monitoring.* Skokie, IL: College of American Pathologists, Commission on Laboratory Accreditation. 1987:2–7.
91. Friedman H, Greenblatt DJ. Rational therapeutic drug monitoring. *JAMA.* 1986;256:2227–2233.
92. Raehl CL, Bond CA, Pitterle ME. Pharmaceutical Services in U.S. hospitals in 1989. *Am J Hosp Pharm.* 1992;49:323–346.
93. Makela EH, Davis SK, Piveral K, et al. Effect of data collection method on the results of serum digoxin concentration audit. *Am J Hosp Pharm.* 1988;45:126–130.

Chapter 5

Monitoring Drug Therapy

John E. Murphy

Keep in Mind

- For every drug a patient receives, there should be a therapeutic goal and a plan to avoid complications.
- There are four fundamental cornerstones of monitoring drug therapy:
    1. Understand the desired therapeutic outcome of drug therapy and a reasonable length of therapy for the individual patient.
    2. Assess the potential efficacy of the drug versus other possible therapies for the specific patient.
    3. Determine monitoring parameters (laboratory tests, symptom relief, etc) that will indicate optimal therapeutic outcome.
    4. Determine monitoring parameters that will indicate toxic or adverse reactions caused by the drug.
- There must be a correlation between drug concentration and therapeutic outcome for useful therapeutic drug monitoring.
- Drug concentrations are often measured in excess. Increasing efficiency and utility should be a goal for all who use drug concentrations to guide therapy.
- Many factors affect an individual's therapeutic range for a given drug.
- Though a number of exceptions exist, many clinicians recommend drawing almost all drug concentration measurements at steady state to best relate response and concentration.
- For many drugs for which therapeutic drug monitoring is used, the timing of the sample relative to dose administration is critical for appropriate assessment of the resulting concentration compared with patient response.
- Those who use therapeutic drug monitoring in practice must be detectives, ensuring that all aspects of the process are sound.

Drugs are monitored to evaluate their effects and to prevent toxic reactions in individual patients. As not all patients respond equally to a certain dose or schedule or to a certain drug concentration in serum or plasma, monitoring response and toxicity is necessary to enhance the potential for optimal patient outcome. This monitoring, however, is often haphazard and not provided for each patient. Donald E. Francke once said that "Today's drugs may be likened to ballistic missiles with atomic warheads, while we prescribe, dispense, and administer them as if they were bows and arrows."[1] Hepler wondered how pharmacists could provide "a drug, a poison, to a patient without knowing what effect the drug should produce?"[2] He further questioned how pharmacists could know if a drug was working or not if the therapeutic goal is unknown.[2]

For every drug a patient receives there should be a purpose, that is, an anticipated outcome (or therapeutic goal), and a plan to avoid complications from the drug. Appropriate monitoring of drug therapy can enhance the potential for successful outcome and reduce the potential for adverse effects in patients.

Drug therapy monitoring can be accomplished in a variety of ways. The traditional approach has been to determine a patient's problem, select a drug with known or suspected potential to affect the problem, determine an initial empiric dose and schedule (often based on "standard doses"), and begin therapy. Next, a determination is made of whether the patient is responding adequately and without toxicity. For those patients not responding well, the dose may be increased or another drug or therapy added or substituted. For those who respond well and exhibit no toxic effects, the dose can remain as initially prescribed. For those who respond but exhibit toxic effects, the dose may be reduced. For those patients whose therapy is adjusted, the same cycle is repeated at the next patient contact. One major problem associated with this method is the potential adverse effect that patient noncompliance can have on decision making.

Therapeutic drug monitoring (TDM) is the application of drug concentration measurements (DCMs) to the preceding general plan. For drugs with a correlation between concentration and outcome (positive or negative), the use of DCMs to guide therapy can allow for quicker achievement of target concentrations, assessment of toxic reactions despite the usual doses, assessment of subtherapeutic outcome despite the usual doses, and evaluation of a patient's compliance. Unfortunately, DCMs are not universally useful and often demonstrate poor correlation with therapeutic outcome. Thus, other methods of monitoring drugs are necessary. For drugs with a large therapeutic index (ie, substantial difference in concentrations producing efficacy and toxic reactions), the need to use DCMs to guide therapy is limited or nonexistent.

There are four cornerstones to the monitoring of therapy with any drug.

1. Understand the desired therapeutic outcome of drug therapy and a reasonable length of therapy for the individual patient.
2. Assess the potential efficacy of the drug versus other possible therapies for the specific patient.
3. Determine monitoring parameters (laboratory tests, symptom relief, etc) that will indicate optimal therapeutic outcome.
4. Determine monitoring parameters that will indicate toxic or adverse reactions caused by the drug.

Drug therapy should be designed to "improve the patient's quality of life through (1) cure of a disease, (2) elimination or reduction of symptoms, (3) arrest or slowing of a disease process, or (4) prevention of a disease or symptoms."[3] Careful monitoring using the four cornerstones or what Strand and colleagues call the "pharmacists' work-up of drug therapy"[4] can facilitate optimum outcome of the drug therapy.

This chapter focuses on the application of TDM. A review of the general aspects of TDM is beyond the scope of the chapter and the reader is urged to study outcome monitoring for specific drugs in pharmacotherapy texts or reviews.

MONITORING DRUGS

Necessary Relationships: Drug Concentration and Response/Toxic Reaction

The therapeutic value of using DCMs to guide decision making with respect to drug use should be determined before the assays are made routinely available to clinicians as part of regular patient care. There must be a correlation between drug concentration and therapeutic outcome, or the feedback provided by a DCM may lead to inappropriate decisions regarding current or future treatment. It has been suggested that TDM may, in fact, be justified for only a small number of drugs.[5]

Researchers have demonstrated that commonly accepted therapeutic ranges are less a gold standard and more frequently only a rough guide to outcome with a drug.[6,7] It is fairly clear that better research should be conducted to establish desirable therapeutic ranges for individual drugs. It is also likely that each patient has his or her own therapeutic range for a particular drug and those conducting TDM should keep this in mind. Figure 5–1 demonstrates the principle of therapeutic effectiveness and how it changes with concentration, but also illustrates that not all patients will be affected by either efficacy or toxicity as concentration changes.

Many authors have documented problems with utilization of DCMs leading to resource waste and potentially unsuitable decisions regarding therapy.[8–10] Other authors suggest that entire groups of patients may do just as well without the "benefit" of TDM,[11–13] thus indicating the need for routine utilization review of DCM, use similar to that conducted for drug use in all hospitals.[14] Several reviews have discussed issues associated with TDM and the authors provided suggestions for ideal use.[15–17] Finally, others call for routine procedures for the evaluation of TDM.[5,18,19]

If the value of TDM for a drug is demonstrated in research environments, application to routine patient care is still fraught with many difficulties. If accurate information (Table 5–1) is not provided to clinicians, trust will not be engendered for using TDM to guide therapy, even for appropriate situations. Information regarding DCMs should be readily retrievable and preferably documented on the final DCM report. Unfortunately, many DCMs may still be routinely ordered even when clinicians do not trust the accuracy of the system, if not to guide therapy, then to avoid potential medicolegal problems. Difficulties associated with interpretation of DCMs are discussed later.

Frequency of Sampling

The frequency of DCM sampling is governed by patient stability in terms of factors that could change absorption, distribution, and elimination of the drug. Stable patients on long-term therapy may not need evaluation more frequently than once a year. Unstable patients with rapidly changing renal or other organ function, hydration status, therapeutic response, and so on may need DCM measurements more than once a day.

Number of Samples Necessary

The number of samples necessary to adequately describe a patient's pharmacokinetic parameters to guide therapy varies. For drugs with a long half-life that are at steady state, a single DCM

THERAPEUTIC RESPONSE AND TOXICITY

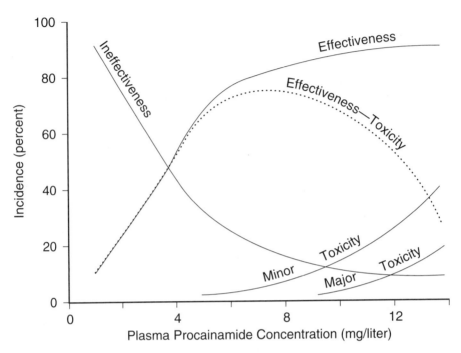

Figure 5–1. Schematic representation of the frequency of ineffective therapy, effective therapy, minor side effects, serious side toxicity, and "therapeutic effectiveness" with plasma concentration of procainamide in patients receiving this drug for the treatment of arrhythmias. Therapeutic effectiveness is defined arbitrarily as the difference in the frequency between effective therapy and toxic effects; the therapeutic effectiveness (•••) of procainamide reaches a peak at 8 mg/L. (One mg/L = 4.3 micromolar.) (From Rowland M, Tozer TN. *Clinical Pharmacokinetics: Concepts and Applications,* 2nd ed. Malvern PA; Lea & Febiger: 1989:55.)

taken at almost any time in the dosing interval may be satisfactory to estimate clearance. For drugs with a short half-life where peak and trough concentrations are important, the number of samples can range from as few as two to a "panel" of DCMs. Use of the panel (ie, three or more DCMs) reduces the effect of assay error and collection errors on estimates. Conversely, the price of monitoring increases with each additional DCM. To establish multicompartment pharmacokinetic parameters for an individual patient, several DCMs are necessary. This approach is not routinely taken for most drugs.

Drug concentration measurements are often ordered in excess. Ordering a DCM to be done daily in a patient with elevated concentrations (eg, overdose) to determine when her or his drug concentrations return to the normal therapeutic range should be discouraged. Efficient use of two or three samples can allow prediction of the time necessary to reach desired concentrations for drugs that demonstrate first-order elimination, unless patient status is rapidly changing.

TABLE 5–1. WHAT MUST BE KNOWN FOR DRUG CONCENTRATION MEASUREMENTS TO BE OF MAXIMUM VALUE

Factor	Who Is Responsible
Time last dose was given/taken	Nurse or patient
Duration of infusion (if given IV)	Nurse or patient (?)
Time sample was drawn	Phlebotomist
Relative compliance with regimen	Patient/clinician
Assay quality	Technologists

Therapeutic Range, Target Concentrations, and Patient Response

As discussed earlier, the therapeutic range, or that range between the mean minimum concentration for efficacy and the mean minimum concentration for toxicity, should be best described as an area with differing shades of gray. The therapeutic range does not tend to occur in an on–off scenario, though it may for an individual patient (eg, seizure activity to no seizures). Rather, more patients tend to respond to therapy as concentration increases across a population (eg, degree of pain control). Similarly, as concentration increases further, the incidence of toxic reactions will increase.

The concept of target concentration relates to setting an a priori desired concentration of drug for a patient (peak, trough, or average concentration) to treat some problem. Next, an initial regimen is chosen based on population average pharmacokinetic parameters. As each patient likely has his or her own therapeutic range, the target based on a population therapeutic range may not lead to maximum success even if it is achieved, but may well serve as an improvement over shooting blindly at an unknown target. The patient may more rapidly achieve a concentration that will be beneficial and future therapy can be guided by DCM results and outcome.

Factors Affecting the Therapeutic Range

Numerous factors may affect the desired target concentration. Alterations in protein binding that result in more or less unbound drug can affect response to a DCM if the concentration reported reflects both bound and unbound drug. As this is the case for most assays, the traditional "therapeutic ranges" may need to be altered based on changes in binding.[20,21]

Certain disease states and aging may also affect the desired concentration. Drug interactions that affect the pharmacodynamics of a drug can lead to changes in desired concentrations, as can the use of more than one drug to control a disease or symptoms (eg, carbamazepine monotherapy versus polytherapy for seizures).

Assay sensitivity and specificity can have an effect on the desired therapeutic range. Early quinidine assays were not very specific, measuring both metabolite and parent compound.[22] Newer quinidine assays measure parent compound, thus reducing the therapeutic range relative to early studies with nonspecific assays. The therapeutic effect of warfarin is monitored using prothrombin time. The potency of the thromboplastin used can affect the desired prothrombin ratio.[23] The effect of assay error on pharmacokinetic parameter determinations may lead to less than optimal changes in therapy. The effect of such errors has been simulated.[24]

A variety of factors can alter assay results and, indirectly, interpretation of therapeutic effect or therapeutic range. It is well known that in a number of diseases and conditions, an interfering substance is produced that mimics digoxin in many commercially available assays.[25] This has been termed *endogenous digoxin-like immunoreactive substance* (DLIS) and has led some to question previously established therapeutic ranges for the drug.[26] This phenomenon occurs in neonates and in patients with liver and renal disease.[26,27] Also well known is the degradation that occurs when aminoglycosides are mixed with various penicillins. This interaction occurs when IV solutions of the drugs are mixed prior to administration. It has also been observed to occur in unrefrigerated blood samples containing both drug types and in patients with renal failure in whom contact with both drugs is prolonged. DCM results are then artifactually low, leading to the potential for inappropriate or unnecessary dosage adjustment.

The presence of active metabolites can confound assessment of therapeutic range and therapeutic outcome based on any measurement of parent drug compound alone. Procainamide is a classic example. For procainamide, most clinicians now also measure the concentration of *N*-acetylprocainamide (NAPA) when assessing therapy with this drug. Another example is the use of theophylline in neonates. Caffeine, which has activity in the treatment of neonatal apnea, is a significant theophylline metabolite only in this age group. Some clinicians routinely measure both theophylline and caffeine concentrations to guide therapy with theophylline in neonates.

Computers, Calculators, and Nomograms in Therapeutic Drug Monitoring

Because of the mathematical nature of pharmacokinetic evaluation, computers and calculators are used extensively as adjuncts to TDM. Computers rapidly provide calculations that take excessive amounts of time by hand and can also incorporate sophisticated analyses that would be virtually impossible using only a calculator. Computer analysis also speeds the calculations necessary to evaluate non-steady-state DCMs. Bayesian analysis has been developed with the use of computers and shown to be accurate and to reduce the need for multiple DCMs.[28] Nonlinear mixed-effect modeling (NONMEM) allows analysis of routinely collected DCMs that are not rigorously scheduled.[29] Computers also allow for more complicated modeling of drug disposition and elimination (eg, use of a multiple-compartment model for vancomycin). Other benefits are storage of hospital/clinic patient pharmacokinetic data or information on special patient types to develop institution-specific population values. Two recent articles provide useful evaluations of currently available clinical pharmacokinetic software and the important considerations for choosing software.[30,31]

Population average values of clearance, volume of distribution, and half-life allow clinicians to use more sophisticated empiric approaches to initiating therapy than just "standard" doses. Unfortunately, this approach frequently falls short of providing sufficient predictability to allow for the elimination of DCMs, leading many researchers studying predictability to recommend the use of DCMs to facilitate therapy.

INTERPRETING DRUG CONCENTRATION MEASUREMENTS

Effect of Steady State

Drug concentration measurements drawn prior to steady state on an initial dosing plan can be useful aids when attempting to determine a final dose and schedule to produce desired target concentrations. They are not as useful, however, in determining the potential efficacy or toxicity of the current or a future regimen. Depending on whether the final concentration will be more (insufficient or no loading dose, after dose increase) or less (eg, after a loading dose that produces concentrations higher than the maintenance dose at steady state or after dose decrease), the pharmacodynamic response to the steady-state concentration may be quite different from that observed with the non-steady-state DCMs. Thus, many clinicians recommend drawing almost all DCMs at steady state. Obvious exceptions would be when the patient exhibits signs and symptoms of drug toxicity prior to steady state and when compliance is in question.

Effect of Sample Timing

For many drugs for which TDM is used, the timing of the sample relative to dose administration is critical for appropriate assessment of the resulting concentration compared with patient response. Drugs that may be exceptions to this rule are those with very long half-lives compared with the dosing interval that do not exhibit marked multiple-compartment distribution (eg, phenobarbital). Those with marked multicompartment distribution but long half-lives may often be sampled at almost any time during the dosing interval without major change in concentration once the initial distribution phase is complete (eg, digoxin). However, it is still recommended that any sampling of such drugs would benefit from measurements conducted at roughly the same time after dosing to enable easy assessment of results.[32]

When drugs exhibit significant multicompartment distribution, it is imperative that this be accounted for in sample timing. For certain drugs such as vancomycin, multicompartment analysis of pharmacokinetic parameters is used by some clinicians and DCMs may be collected during the initial distribution phase. For other drugs such as digoxin, where efficacy is not correlated to the initial distribution, DCMs may be "falsely elevated" if drawn during the distribution phase.[33]

For drugs that undergo large fluctuations in concentration during the dosing interval, knowledge of both the time of dose administration and the time the DCM was drawn is required. For example, the DCM for an aminoglycoside antibiotic with a half-life of 2 hours in a patient would decrease by 29% in just 1 hour. Lack of knowledge of the time of sample relative to dose could dramatically influence decisions on the maintenance dose necessary to achieve desired target concentrations if the DCM is collected only 1 hour from when expected.

Effect of Compliance and Noncompliance

Obviously critical to collection of necessary information such as time of dose and time of sample collection are medication administration nurses, patients, and phlebotomists. Each of these people can help or hinder the process of data collection. Nurses must accurately chart dose administration time and report this information to the laboratory so all critical information can be printed on the DCM result. In certain cases such as administration of short infusions of drugs with a short half-life (eg, aminoglycosides in patients with normal renal function), the time the infusion ends may also be crucial for accurate calculation of pharmacokinetic parameters. If so, these data should also be documented. It is unfortunate for those involved with TDM that hospital policies often give nurses the prerogative to give doses 1 hour before or after the scheduled time without requiring them to chart the actual time of administration. This practice can cause many problems when peak or trough concentrations, or both, are ordered within one-half hour of a dose. It is also obligatory that any doses not given are clearly indicated as such on the medication administration record. Additionally, nurses (and patients) should be instructed to inform clinicians who have ordered a DCM for a patient whenever doses have been recently missed.

Another problem relates to unusual dosing intervals.[34] If odd schedules (eg, every 16 or 18 hours, every 2 or 3 days) are employed, it is essential that clinicians in institutions check medication administration records for accuracy and that those in outpatient settings adequately explain when to take the medicine to their ambulatory patients. For outpatients, a medication calendar may help them take medications correctly.

Patients may be the providers of information on the time of last dose and relative compliance in many cases. They must be educated as to the importance of taking medications correctly and that they are partners in the decision to adjust or not adjust current doses. Decisions to change the dose or schedule should not be made based on DCMs and lack of positive therapeutic outcome from noncompliant patients. Compliance enhancement should be initiated first followed by reassessment of DCM.[35]

When scheduling DCMs for ambulatory outpatients, the patients should be instructed on when to take their medication and when to come in for blood drawing. A patient who takes his or her digoxin tablet 1 hour before sampling will have a falsely elevated concentration, which will be difficult to evaluate. Sampling at the same time relative to dose when doses are adjusted in outpatients will make determination of stability or lack of stability of clearance easier.

It is mandatory for many drugs that the time of phlebotomy be accurately recorded. Educating those who draw blood as to the importance of this information can help ensure it is noted and reported. Setting up systems that require documentation of time of collection may also be necessary.

One documented method of increasing the quality, and therefore utility, of DCMs is development of a DCM scheduling service.[14,32] Such services can coordinate the appropriate timing of samples relative to dose for the phlebotomists, interface with medication administration nurses to help guarantee that the doses are given on time, and generally serve as intermediaries between laboratory, nursing, phlebotomy, and clinicians.

Effect of Predistribution Collection

Predistribution collection was referred to earlier. For digoxin, sampling before initial distribution is complete will relate poorly to patient outcome and concentrations may be very high compared with the traditional therapeutic range.[33] For drugs whose efficacy is based on distribution in the central compartment, early DCMs would relate best to efficacy. In general, it seems that many involved with TDM prefer to collect DCMs postdistribution because a smaller number of concentrations need to be measured to provide useful information.

Effect of Infusion Apparatus and Technique

Many researchers have demonstrated effects of infusion apparatus or infusion techniques (eg, duration of infusion, site of drug administration) on the DCMs achieved and subsequent pharmacokinetic parameter estimation.[36-44] Clinicians providing TDM should be very aware of the effects that these apparatus and techniques can have on DCM results and set up administration protocols to prevent problems from occurring.

Effect of Blood Sampling Through Lines for Drug Administration

Artifactually high DCMs have resulted from sampling blood through catheters used to administer the drug.[45-47] This effect can be minimized by flushing the catheter after the dose is given and by discarding a sample of blood and fluid from the catheter prior to withdrawing the final blood for sampling. Either of these two techniques used alone may be insufficient to prevent artifactual elevations of the actual drug concentration in serum.[47]

Effect of Blood Sampling from Different Sites

It is theoretically possible that sampling from different body sites might affect the DCM reported. Obvious opportunities for error exist when sampling "downstream" from an IV that is delivering the drug to be measured. One study showed minimal effect of capillary versus venous sampling in neonates.[48]

Effect of Intrapatient Variation

People change. Some do it more rapidly than others as it relates to the pharmacokinetic handling of a given drug. For some patients, after an initial assessment period to determine their ability to absorb, distribute, and eliminate the drug, they may be monitored very infrequently. DCMs will change only slightly in relatively healthy patients *unless* the patient is noncompliant. Conversely, patients in the intensive care unit with acute illness or injury may have significant alterations in absorption, distribution, and elimination, in very short periods. Clinicians should anticipate rapid changes in pharmacokinetic parameters in these seriously ill patients and look for changes by monitoring DCMs and other assessment parameters.

Clinical Intuition: Clinical Pearls

The clinician using DCMs as a guide in TDM must wear several hats. These include educator (to nurses, patients, phlebotomists, technicians), collaborator (with other health professionals and the patient), negotiator (to get things done appropriately in times of reduced resources), and, primarily, detective. Many studies have documented problems with at least half of all DCMs in institutions where some type of service is not available to coordinate the collection and measurement of drug concentrations. Thus, many of the nation's hospitals are operating with systems in which flipping a coin would provide almost as much information as the DCM. This requires practitioners of TDM to become DCM detectives.

Whenever a DCM does not appear to make sense, the detective role becomes important. It is also likely that the TDM practitioner should take on this role when DCMs appear "appropriate." Searching medication administration records and questioning patients, nurses, pharmacists, phlebotomists, and technicians may be required to sort out the potential accuracy or inaccuracy of a DCM. Discussed below are but a few of the many mysteries that have actually been observed with DCMs. The examples are followed by suggested potential "diagnoses" of these problems.

Peak Less than Trough

A patient receiving vancomycin 1 g every 12 hours as 1-hour infusions has a "trough" level ordered before an 8 PM dose and a "peak" level ordered 2 hours after the 8 PM dose. The "trough" DCM drawn at 7:30 PM is reported as 11.1 mg/L and the "peak" DCM drawn at 10 PM is reported as 9.5 mg/L.

Primary Diagnosis. The dose was not given at 8 PM and both concentrations are in the elimination phase. Check the medication administration record, and question the nurse, the pharmacy (ie, was there a stop order on the antibiotic), and the patient. It is also possible that the dose was given at a different time altogether (eg, at 4 PM), or that the "peak" and "trough" levels were drawn from two different patients, and so on.

Peak About Same as Trough

This situation is more difficult to evaluate as it approaches a circumstance where a very large volume of distribution might account for the small difference. Consider the same scenario above except that the "peak" is reported as 15.5 mg/L (assume that the clinician's pharmacokinetic estimation of peak is 20.4 mg/L).

Primary Diagnoses. The dose was started late or the infusion that was scheduled for 1 hour was actually given as a very long infusion (eg, 6 hours) and the "peak" represents only partial infusion of the dose. DCMs could also have been drawn from different patients. Use evaluation methods similar to those described above.

Grossly Elevated Digoxin DCM

A patient has a digoxin DCM scheduled for 6 hours after the last IV dose. It is reported as 10 µg/L. The patient is sitting up in bed reading.

Primary Diagnoses. The digoxin dose was given within the hour before the blood was actually collected and, therefore, the DCM was drawn prior to completion of the distribution phase. Several explanations are possible: The nurse charted medication administration at the appropriate time, forgot to give it, and finally administered the dose 1 hour before collection. Or the phlebotomist, who was up on the ward, knew she would have to collect blood on the patient for the digoxin DCM later in the day and decided to go ahead and draw the blood early, and did not document the actual collection time. As always, collection from another patient is possible.

Nonexistent Peak

A neonate is started on IV gentamicin every 12 hours. The first-dose "peak" DCM drawn 1 hour after dose infusion is started is reported as 0.2 mg/L. The first-dose "trough" DCM is drawn 30 minutes before the next scheduled dose and is reported as 1.1 mg/L.

Primary Diagnoses. The dose was not started on time or the dose was placed in the infusion apparatus too far from the neonate; the slow infusion rate prevented the drug from getting to baby in time to make the peak level accurate. The dose does appear to have been given as the trough level is near what would be expected.

Wrong Dose Given

First-dose gentamicin DCMs are drawn on a neonate. The "peak" is reported as 18.6 mg/L and the "trough" as 5.9 mg/L. The DCMs were collected 10.5 hours apart.

Primary Diagnosis. This dilemma is solved by evaluating the pharmacokinetic parameters and checking the medication drawer. The calculated volume of distribution is one-fourth that antici-pated from usual population values, while the half-life is consistent with expectations. Knowing that gentamicin is available as 40 mg/ml dosage strength for adults and 10 mg/m! for children, a check of the medication drawer might reveal that a vial of adult strength was used. If so, this would indicate that the nurse used the standard administration volume, thus giving the neonate four times the dose actually desired.

There are other reasons for erroneous assessment: The wrong drug may have been given. The wrong DCM (eg, digitoxin for digoxin) may have been ordered. The patient may not be on the drug for which the DCM is ordered. A different dosage form (regular-release product for sustained-release, or vice versa) may have been administered. A sustained-release product may have been crushed for administration down a feeding tube. The IV may have infiltrated, thus pre-venting administration of the dose. As always, noncompliance with the regimen by patients or medication administration nurses is possible.

A major caveat must always be held in evaluation of DCMs. DCMs close to those antici-pated on the basis of the dose administered and population pharmacokinetic predictions do not signify that inaccuracies have not occurred. Clinicians should always be on the lookout for potential problems that may affect the DCM result.

Taking Action on Unusual Results

The action to be taken depends on whether the erroneous DCMs can be at all useful. For exam-ple, if peak and trough concentrations are measured and only one is determined to be subject to some error, only the erroneous DCM may need to be repeated. Stage of therapy (eg, 9th day of a 10-day course of aminoglycoside) should also be considered. If, as in the example in which the adult dose of an aminoglycoside was administered to a neonate, the half-life and volume of dis-tribution can be accurately determined from the DCMs, there may not be a need to repeat DCMs beyond what usual follow-up monitoring would be if the initial dose had been correct.

─────── **QUESTIONS** ───────────────────────────

1. What are the four cornerstones of monitoring drug therapy?

2. Name five important process considerations that must be known for drug concentra-tion measurements to be of maximum value.

3. Name five factors that can affect the desired therapeutic range for an individual.

4. Discuss reasons for the recommendation to draw most DCMs at steady state.

5. Discuss reasons for drawing DCMs prior to steady state.

REFERENCES

1. *The Role of the Pharmacist in Comprehensive Medication Use Management.* APhA White Paper. Washington, DC: American Pharmaceutical Association; 1992.
2. Hepler CD. The pharmacist's job is to provide total pharmaceutical care. *US Pharmacist* 1991(Nov): 61–64,68.
3. Hepler CD, Strand LM. Opportunities and responsibilities in pharmaceutical care. *Am J Hosp Pharm* 1990;47:533–543.
4. Strand LM, Cipolle RJ, Morley PC. Documenting the clinical pharmacists's activities: Back to basics. *Drug Intell Clin Pharm.* 1988;22:63–67.
5. Hvidberg EF. Monitoring drug plasma levels in clinical practice? A procedure for evaluation is needed. *Eur J Clin Pharmacol.* 1980;17:317–319.
6. McCormack JP, Jewesson PJ. A critical reevaluation of the "therapeutic range" of aminoglycosides. *Clin Infect Dis.* 1992;14:320–339.
7. Schumacher GE, Barr JT. Applying decision analysis in therapeutic drug monitoring: Using decision trees to interpret serum theophylline concentrations. *Clin Pharm.* 1986;5:325–333.
8. Guernsey BG, Hokanson JA, Ingrim NB, et al. A utilization review of digoxin assays: Sampling patterns and use. *Hosp Pharm.* 1984;19:187–200.
9. Greenlaw CW, Blough SS, Haugen RK. Aminoglycoside serum assays restricted through a pharmacy program. *Am J Hosp Pharm.* 1979;36:1080–1083.
10. Flynn TW, Pevonka PM, Yost RL, et al. Use of serum gentamicin levels in hospitalized patients. *Am J Hosp Pharm.* 1978;35:806–808.
11. Buchanan N. Aminoglycoside monitoring in neonates—A re-appraisal. *Aust NZ J Med.* 1985; 15:457–459.
12. Massey KL, Hendeles L, Neims A. Identification of children for whom routine monitoring of aminoglycoside serum concentrations is not cost effective. *J Pediatr.* 1986;109:897–901.
13. Averbuch M, Weintraub M, Nolte F. Gentamicin blood levels: Ordered too soon and too often. *Hosp Formul.* 1989;24:598–612.
14. Job ML, Ward ES Jr, Murphy JE. Seven years of experience with a pharmacokinetic service. *Hosp Pharm.* 1989;24:512–526.
15. Gal P. Therapeutic drug monitoring in neonates: Problems and issues. *Drug Intell Clin Pharm.* 1988;22:317–323.
16. Walson PD, Edwards R, Cox S. Neonatal therapeutic drug monitoring—Its clinical relevance. *Ther Drug Monit.* 1989;11:425–430.
17. Pellock JM, Willmore LJ. A rational guide to routine blood monitoring in patients receiving antiepileptic drugs. *Neurology.* 1991;41:961–964.
18. Vozeh S. Cost-effectiveness of therapeutic drug monitoring. *Clin Pharmacokinet.* 1987;13:131–140.
19. Reynolds EH. Serum levels of anticonvulsant drugs: Interpretation and clinical value. *Pharmacol Ther.* 1980;8:217–235.

20. Winter ME, Tozer TN. Phenytoin. In: Evans WE, Schentag JJ, Jusko WJ, eds. *Applied Pharmacokinetics: Principles of Therapeutic Drug Monitoring.* Spokane, WA: Applied Therapeutics, Inc; 1986.

21. Tuten MB, Murphy JE, Tuten AT. Alteration in phenytoin protein binding at varying degrees of renal function and albumin concentration. *Georgia J Hosp Pharm.* 1991;5:21–25.

22. Ueda CT. Quinidine. In: Evans WE, Schentag JJ, Jusko WJ, eds. *Applied Pharmacokinetics: Principles of Therapeutic Drug Monitoring.* Spokane, WA: Applied Therapeutics, Inc; 1986.

23. Poller L, Taberner DA. Dosage and control of oral anticoagulants: An international collaborative survey. *Br J Haematol.* 1982;51:479–485.

24. Boyce EG, Pugh CB. Simulated effect of gentamicin assay errors on calculated pharmacokinetic parameters. *Clin Pharm.* 1988;7:307–313.

25. Pudek MR, Seccombe DW, Jacobson BE, et al. Seven different digoxin immunoassay kits compared with respect to interference by a digoxin-like immunoreactive substance in serum from premature and full-term infants. *Clin Chem.* 1983;29:1972–1974.

26. Hyneck ML. How reliable are serum digoxin assays? *Clin Pharm.* 1985;4:81–82.

27. Rosenkranz B, Frolich J. Falsely elevated digoxin concentrations in patients with liver disease. *Ther Drug Monit.* 1985;7:202–206.

28. Burton ME, Chow MSS, Platt DR, et al. Accuracy of bayesian and Sawchuk–Zaske dosing methods for gentamicin. *Clin Pharm.* 1986;5:143–149.

29. Jensen PD, Edgren BE, Brundage RC. Population pharmacokinetics of gentamicin in neonates using a nonlinear, mixed-effects model. *Pharmacotherapy.* 1992;12:178–182.

30. Poirier TI, Giudici RA. Survey of clinical pharmacokinetic software for microcomputers. *Hosp Pharm.* 1992;27:971–972, 975–977.

31. Buffington DE, Lampasona V, Chandler MHH. Computers in pharmacokinetics: Choosing software for clinical decision making. *Clin Pharmacokinet.* 1993;25:205–216.

32. Murphy JE, Winter ME. Timing drug-level determinations. *Fam Pract Recert.* 1989;11:81–94.

33. Murphy JE, Ward ES, Job ML. Avoiding erroneous serum digoxin concentrations. *Am J Hosp Pharm.* 1985;42:2418–2420.

34. Murphy JE, Job ML, Ward ES. Rectifying incorrect dosage schedules. *Am J Hosp Pharm.* 1990;47:2235–2236.

35. Ambrose PJ, Nitake M, Kildoo CW. Impact of pharmacist scheduling of blood-sampling times for therapeutic drug monitoring. *Am J Hosp Pharm.* 1988;45:380–382.

36. Boyce EG, Pugh CB. Computer-simulated effect of errors in infusion duration and blood sampling times on pharmacokinetic calculations for gentamicin. *Clin Pharm.* 1989;8:48–53.

37. Quebbeman EJ, Franson TR, Whipple JE, et al. A quality control analysis of aminoglycoside management. *Arch Surg.* 1985;120:1069–1071.

38. Nahata MC, Powell DA, Durrell DE, et al. Effect of infusion methods on tobramycin serum concentrations in newborn infants. *J Pediatr.* 1986;104:136–138.

39. Pleasants RA, Sawyer WT, Williams DM, et al. Accuracy of tobramycin delivery by four i.v. infusion methods. *Clin Pharm.* 1988;7:367–373.

40. Pleasants RA, Sawyer WT, Williams DM, et al. Effect of four intravenous infusion methods on tobramycin pharmacokinetics. *Clin Pharm.* 1988;7:374–379.

41. Cacek AT, Moore JE, Bishop TS. Effect of various infusion pump administration techniques and rates on tobramycin delivery. *Am J Hosp Pharm.* 1988;45:2381–2383.

42. Bosch DE, Williams DN. Comparison of aminoglycoside concentrations produced by two infusion methods. *Clin Pharm.* 1990;9:777–780.

43. Armistead JA, Nahata MC. Effect of variables associated with intermittent gentamicin infusions on pharmacokinetic predictions. *Clin Pharm.* 1983;2:153–156.

44. Munoz DM, Green ER, Chrymko MM, et al. Delivery of gentamicin by controlled-release infusion system versus a minibag system. *Clin Pharm.* 1988;7:303–307.

45. Longley JM, Murphy JE. Falsely elevated digoxin levels: Another look. *Ther Drug Monit.* 1989;11:572–573.
46. Murphy JE, Ward ES. Elevated phenytoin concentration caused by sampling through the drug-administration catheter. *Pharmacotherapy.* 1991;11(4):348–350.
47. Wanwimolruk S, Murphy JE. Effect of monitoring drug concentrations through lines used to administer the drugs: An in-vitro study. *Ther Drug Monit.* 1991;13:443–447.
48. Murphy JE, Peltier T, Anderson D, Ward ES. A comparison of venous versus capillary measurements of drug concentration. *Ther Drug Monit.* 1990;12:264–267.

Chapter 6

Population Approaches to Pharmacokinetics and Risk Management

Thaddeus H. Grasela, Jr.

Keep in Mind

- The increasing availability of computerized databases, the development of statistical tools for the analysis of observational data, and the growing recognition of the need for continual monitoring of patient outcome have improved our ability to identify the determinants of drug response in patient populations.

- Mixed-effect modeling provides a method for estimating pharmacokinetic parameters from data collected during the process of providing pharmacokinetic consultations.

- The three types of population pharmacokinetic parameters—the mean value, the magnitude of interindividual variability, and the magnitude of residual variability—provide important, and different, information regarding the disposition of a drug in a patient population.

- Bayesian forecasting techniques can be used to interpret drug concentrations by balancing the information content of a measured concentration(s) against the prior knowledge provided by the population pharmacokinetic parameters.

- A complete pharmacokinetic and statistical model for a population analysis requires four components:
    1. A pharmacokinetic structured model
    2. Regression models for pharmacokinetic parameters
    3. Statistical model for interindividual variability
    4. Statistical model for residual variability

- Population pharmacokinetic analysis and pharmacoepidemiology research methods provide a mechanism to gain insight into patient and drug-associated factors that can influence response to therapy.

Clinical pharmacokinetics has been one of the major activities defining the practice of clinical pharmacy. Clinical pharmacy practitioners have received extensive training in the interpretation of drug concentrations and the development of individualized patient dosing regimens based on measured drug concentrations and the patient's drug dosing history. The nature of this activity has grown in complexity and the range of responsibilities of clinical pharmacists have expanded. In large part this is due to changes in the mandates of the Joint Commission for the Accreditation of Healthcare Organizations (JCAHO).[1] Over the last several years JCAHO regulations have undergone a number of remarkable revisions, resulting in the current emphasis on monitoring patient outcomes to identify risk factors for poor outcomes and, conversely, prognostic factors associated with good outcomes. Although these regulations are aimed primarily at the pharmacy and therapeutics committee within a hospital, the responsibility for implementing drug-oriented quality-assurance programs has generally fallen to the pharmacy department.

One consequence of these regulations has been the development of outcome-oriented drug utilization evaluation programs in which clinical pharmacists concurrently assess patient outcome and determine whether adjustments in the treatment plan are warranted, including making recommendations for patient monitoring activities and the selection of drug therapy alternatives. The information collected during this prospective process is then analyzed to identify corrective measures that might be implemented to improve the overall quality of patient care. This increased emphasis on quality assurance within the hospital has important implications for all aspects of clinical pharmacy practice, including clinical pharmacokinetics.

Pharmacokinetic consults have traditionally involved the determination of the individual's pharmacokinetic parameters and the use of these parameters to design dosing regimens that would maintain the patient's drug concentrations in an appropriate therapeutic range. In the early history of clinical pharmacokinetics, simplified approaches to determining individual pharmacokinetic parameters via a test dose strategy[2] were commonly employed to facilitate the interpretation of drug concentrations and the development of dosing recommendations. In large part, these methods represented an early attempt to come to grips with the complexity of bringing together the pharmacokinetic, statistical, and data processing tools necessary for performing the task of estimating an individual's pharmacokinetic parameters from the fragmentary and sometimes unreliable data available from the patient care environment.

During this process, the focus of the pharmacokinetic consult service was the patient, and the goal of the consult was to individualize drug therapy for each patient. Unfortunately, this approach can lead to fragmented care because the prior experiences of the pharmacokineticist in the interpretation of drug concentrations are generally not formally incorporated into the consultation process. The consultations for individual patients may have been accumulated in the department files, but there were few attempts to bring this information together in a scientific manner to improve the quality of subsequent consults. Although the clinician may have noticed that a certain patient population was notoriously difficult to dose because of patient-to-patient or day-to-day variability, or that standard dosing recommendations for certain patient populations tended to systematically result in either underdosing or overdosing, it was difficult to deal with these problems in a formal way. Given the current emphasis on continued monitoring and improvement of quality of care, the case-by-case approach to pharmacokinetic consultations must be replaced with a more comprehensive and sophisticated approach. This includes not only the interpretation of drug concentrations in a patient, but also the overall assessment of the patient's likelihood of obtaining a satisfactory response to drug therapy.

Over the last several years, a number of data analysis tools have become available that greatly facilitate the analysis of patient outcome data and have the potential to alter radically the role of clinical pharmacy in the health care setting. These tools include methods for obtaining accurate estimates of population pharmacokinetic parameters from drug concentrations obtained during patient care,[3] the interpretation of drug concentrations using bayesian forecasting methods,[4] and multivariate statistical techniques, such as logistic regression, for identifying patient risk factors associated with clinical outcomes.[5] Each of these tools is discussed in the context of an integrated program to manage the risk of drug therapy in a patient population.

In 1972, Sheiner and colleagues published a paradigm for the interpretation of drug concentrations that incorporated prior knowledge about the distribution of pharmacokinetic parameters in a patient population into a mathematical and statistical framework for interpreting drug concentrations measured in a patient.[6] This approach, using a combination of bayesian forecasting and mixed-effect modeling, has become increasingly popular over the past decade for several reasons. First, clinicians have come to recognize the value of systematically examining patient outcome to drug therapy, second, the statistical tools for appropriately analyzing this type of data have become available and accessible, and third, the increasing availability of computers in the health care setting is facilitating the collection and analysis of patient data.

Although clinical pharmacists are familiar with the theory and practice of pharmacokinetics, they are much less familiar with the statistical aspects of analyzing observational pharmacokinetic data. In addition, there has been a paucity of efforts to use pharmacokinetic data in conjunction with other patient characteristics such as age, gender, and presence of concurrent illnesses, to maximize the benefit and minimize the risk of drug therapy. The first objective of this chapter is to present an overview of mixed-effect modeling as a method for the analysis of pharmacokinetic data that routinely arise during the process of providing pharmacokinetic consultations. The second objective is to discuss the incorporation of population pharmacokinetic analysis into a multivariable analysis of patient outcome data and the value of integrating these elements into an effective risk management program in the hospital setting.

DEFINITIONS OF POPULATION PHARMACOKINETIC PARAMETERS

Before discussing the methodology of mixed-effect modeling as applied to the estimation of population pharmacokinetic parameters, it is important to understand the nature of the parameters we seek to estimate and the reasons why they are of interest. In the previous section, the notion of using prior knowledge of drug pharmacokinetics to interpret the drug concentrations measured in a specific patient was introduced. The first question one must ask is, What constitutes adequate knowledge of drug pharmacokinetics for the interpretation of drug concentrations?

Three types of parameters can be used to characterize the pharmacokinetic disposition of a drug in a patient population. The first type of parameter is the typical value of the pharmacokinetic parameters in the population, such as the mean clearance and mean volume of distribution for a drug. These parameters are designated by the Greek symbol Θ. The second type of parameter is the magnitude of variability in the pharmacokinetic parameters across the individuals in the population, designated by ω^2. The third type of parameter is the magnitude of variability in drug concentrations within an individual over time, designated by σ^2. Each of these parameters provides important, and different, information regarding the pharmacokinetic properties of a drug in a patient population. Each of the parameters can be used for providing pharmacokinetic consultation and risk management in the hospital setting. Let us consider each of these parameters in greater detail and discuss how they might be used in patient care.

The first type of parameter of interest is the mean, or typical value of a pharmacokinetic parameter in a patient population. These parameters include the mean clearance in a population as a function of body weight, or the mean proportionality constant relating renal function to drug clearance. In mixed-effect modeling, these parameters are referred to as fixed-effect parameters because they describe the relationship between measurable patient characteristics, such as weight and creatinine clearance, and alterations in pharmacokinetic parameters according to a specified regression model. An example of a regression model for clearance is given by

$$\tilde{Cl}_j = \Theta_1 + \Theta_2 \cdot Cl_{cr, j} \tag{6–1}$$

where Cl_j is the typical value for drug clearance predicted in a patient given information regarding renal function, as provided by the estimated creatinine clearance, $Cl_{cr,j}$, and values of the fixed effect parameters Θ_1 and Θ_2; Θ_1 represents the nonrenal clearance of a drug; and Θ_2 is the proportionality constant relating creatinine clearance to the extent of renal elimination of the unchanged drug.

If relevant, information regarding the effects of age, renal impairment, various concomitant medications, and concurrent illnesses can be incorporated into the regression formulas to obtain the typical values for pharmacokinetic parameters in a patient population. The values of these parameters can then be used to develop initial dosing recommendations for patients based on their observable characteristics and a target drug concentration strategy.[7]

In the regression model for clearance given in Equation 6–1, the typical clearance values for all patients with a given creatinine clearance would be identical; however, the values of pharmacokinetic parameters in specific individuals with a given creatinine clearance in the population will not necessarily be equal to the typical value. Individuals are different in terms of their genetic makeup; diet; personal habits, such as smoking and alcohol consumption; organ function; use of concomitant medications; and severity of illness. Thus, we would anticipate differences in the efficiency of drug elimination across a patient population and this would translate into variability in drug clearance even among individuals with identical values of creatinine clearance.

The magnitude of variability in the distribution of a pharmacokinetic parameter across the population is the second population pharmacokinetic parameter of interest. The variance (ω^2) provides a measure of the variability in the distribution of parameter values, such as clearance, around the typical value given by the regression equation. Thus, ω^2 gives a measure of the variability that is not explained by the regression model. Consequently, as explanatory variables, such as age and gender, are added to the regression model, the magnitude of ω^2 would be expected to decrease.

The magnitude of interindividual variability is important to the clinician because the larger the magnitude of unexplained interindividual variability, the greater is the range of pharmacokinetic parameter values that are likely to be observed in the population. In the case of a normal distribution for clearance, 67% of patients in a population will have a clearance value within one standard deviation of the mean clearance. Thus, the larger the standard deviation, the broader the range of clearance values likely to be observed in a patient population. In fact, this is one of the clinical foundations for therapeutic drug monitoring. If there is a large amount of unexplained interindividual variability in pharmacokinetic parameters, patients prescribed a standard regimen will be expected to show a wide range in drug concentrations. If there is also an association between drug concentrations and the probability of drug safety or efficacy, the use of drug concentrations to individualize dosing regimens may be warranted to improve patient outcome.

The third type of population pharmacokinetic parameter, referred to as residual variability (σ^2), measures the magnitude of variability in drug concentrations observed over time within an individual. If a patient were receiving a constant drug dosing regimen and serial trough concentrations were obtained under steady-state conditions, one would expect the drug concentrations to vary over time. The variance of the distribution of these drug concentrations around the mean value quantifies the uncertainty in measured drug concentrations resulting from a number of sources including drug assay error; day-to-day fluctuations in the efficiency of organs of elimination; pharmacokinetic model misspecification, for example, use of a one-compartment model when a two-compartment model would be more appropriate; errors in data collection; and variable patient compliance. This parameter is important to clinicians because it provides a mechanism for evaluating a measured drug concentration and deciding whether a dosing adjustment is necessary. For example, a large degree of residual variability suggests that if a measured drug concentration is slightly below the therapeutic range on a given day, there is a good chance that the next time the concentration is measured it will be within the therapeutic range. Thus, it may not be necessary to act on a low drug concentration unless it is consistently low and associated with evidence of subtherapeutic response.

Both ω^2 and σ^2 are referred to as random effect parameters because they quantify the magnitude of variability that is assumed to be random for the purposes of the statistical models described below. It is important to understand the distinction between interindividual variability and residual variability. Any factor that results in consistent differences in pharmacokinetic parameters from one patient to another will increase the magnitude of interindividual variability. A factor that results in variability across time within an individual patient will increase the magnitude of residual variability. Thus, product formulation problems might affect both interindividual and residual variability. If there are consistent differences in bioavailability across individuals, interindividual variability will be affected. If, however, the formulation results in erratic absorption over multiple administrations within a patient, residual variability will increase.

NEED FOR ACCURATE ESTIMATES OF POPULATION PHARMACOKINETIC PARAMETERS

The value of accurate information regarding all three of the population pharmacokinetic parameters in patient care becomes apparent if one employs a bayesian approach to therapeutic drug monitoring.[4] In using this approach, one explicitly recognizes the value of prior information about pharmacokinetic parameters to more appropriately interpret drug concentrations measured in a particular patient. The bayesian objective function used to obtain estimates of an individual's pharmacokinetic parameters for a simple one-compartment model, given measured drug concentrations, the dosing history, and prior knowledge of population pharmacokinetic parameters is specified in the equation

$$\text{OBJ}_{\text{BAYES}} = \frac{(\text{Cl}_j - \tilde{\text{Cl}}_j)^2}{\omega_{\text{Cl}}^2} + \frac{(V_j - \tilde{V}_j)^2}{\omega_V^2} + \sum_{i=1}^{m} \frac{(C_{\text{P},i} - \tilde{C}_{\text{P},i})^2}{\sigma_i^2} \qquad (6\text{--}2)$$

where $\tilde{\text{Cl}}_j$ and $\tilde{V}_j$ are the typical values for the pharmacokinetic parameters in a population; ω_{Cl}^2

and ω_V^2 are the variances for interindividual variability; $C_{P,i}$ are the measured drug concentrations obtained in a specific patient; $\tilde{C}_{P,i}$ are the corresponding predicted concentrations given the pharmacokinetic model, the current estimates of pharmacokinetic parameters (i.e., Cl_j and V_j), and the drug dosing history; and σ_i^2 is the magnitude of residual variability.

The goal is to find values for Cl_j and V_j that minimize the right-hand side of Equation 6–2. Using a bayesian approach to interpret drug concentrations, the information content of a measured drug concentration is balanced against prior knowledge of population pharmacokinetic parameters, adjusting for the uncertainty in both sources of information, via the estimates of ω_{Cl}^2, ω_V^2, and σ^2.

For example, suppose that we are interested in obtaining a bayesian estimate of clearance and volume of distribution for a patient, and based on previous data the interindividual variability in the volume of distribution (ω_v^2) is very small, but the variability in clearance (ω_{Cl}^2) is very large. Further, suppose that we obtain a drug concentration immediately after a rapidly administered intravenous dose of drug and the measured drug concentration is spuriously elevated because of an error; either the sample was inappropriately obtained from the vein immediately distal to the infusion site or there was a drug assay problem. An experienced clinician might intuitively question the measured drug concentration and disregard or deemphasize the data. This is exactly the process employed in bayesian forecasting. During the process of minimizing the bayesian objective function given by Equation 6–2, different values for Cl_j and V_j are evaluated according to the minimization algorithm employed, and the difference between the measured drug concentration and the corresponding predicted concentration obtained from the values for the pharmacokinetic parameters and the pharmacokinetic model is calculated.

In ordinary least squares (see below) the values of the pharmacokinetic parameters that minimize the difference between the measured and predicted values are taken to be the estimates of the individual's parameters, but one does explicitly recognize that the measured drug concentration may be spurious. In a bayesian approach, however, we are penalized when the selected values for Cl_j and V_j deviate from the typical values $\tilde{Cl}_j$ and $\tilde{V}_j$, respectively, weighted by the magnitude of ω_V^2 and ω_{Cl}^2. When ω_{Cl}^2 is large, the denominator is large and deviations from the typical value will not add much to the overall objective function. Because ω_V^2 is small in our example, however, minor differences between $V_{d,j}$ and $\tilde{V}_{d,j}$ will be magnified by the small ω_V^2 in the denominator. This will result in a compromise between the current information from the patient, that is, the spuriously measured high drug concentration, and prior knowledge suggesting that it is unlikely for the volume of distribution of the drug to be small enough to produce the observed drug concentration.

If one accepts the philosophy of bayesian forecasting, important considerations are the source and accuracy of the estimates of population pharmacokinetic parameters employed in the analysis of drug concentrations from patients. During the new drug development process pharmacokinetic studies are frequently performed using select groups of patients with mild disease who have few other concurrent illnesses. As a result the population pharmacokinetic parameters, and hence the dosing recommendations, available at the time of marketing may be biased in that they do not represent the typical parameters for sicker patients who will be prescribed the drug in the postmarketing period.

Because of the logistical complexity, cost, and ethical considerations associated with traditional approaches to pharmacokinetic research it is often difficult to obtain estimates of pharmacokinetic parameters in all patient subgroups potentially of interest to clinicians.

Pharmacokinetic studies during drug development generally focus on studying the anticipated major effects in selected patient populations. Pharmacokinetic information is often not available for important patient groups such as the elderly, the very young, or critically ill patients. These patient populations are historically at the greatest risk of therapeutic failure and information about changes in pharmacokinetics within these groups would be extremely valuable in developing a priori dosing recommendations and performing bayesian forecasting. Thus, it would be advantageous if drug concentrations obtained in the course of patient care could be used to provide information about the population pharmacokinetic parameters in these patients.

Drug concentrations obtained for patient care are called nonexperimental or observational data because little or no effort is made to influence the frequency or timing of the drug concentrations. Prior to the development of mixed-effect modeling techniques, these data represented a dilemma for the pharmacokineticist. The choice was either to ignore drug concentrations obtained during patient care because of the problems associated with their analysis or to attempt to use traditional data analysis methods recognizing the risk of obtaining inaccurate and imprecise estimates of population pharmacokinetic parameters. Mixed-effect modeling provides a mechanism for explicitly dealing with the problems arising in the analysis of nonexperimental data and expands the sources of information that can be used to develop accurate and representative estimates of pharmacokinetic parameters in all patient populations of interest.

NEED FOR MIXED-EFFECT MODELING WHEN ANALYZING NONEXPERIMENTAL DATA

The problems encountered in obtaining accurate and precise estimates of population pharmacokinetic parameters can best be illustrated by an example. Consider the design and analysis of a study to estimate the clearance of a drug in a patient population. The experimental paradigm consists of maintaining subjects on a continuous, constant-rate, intravenous infusion of the drug until steady-state conditions are achieved. Each patient then has three blood samples obtained for the determination of drug concentration. Representative concentration–time curves for three patients are shown in Figure 6–1. Note that patient 1 is at steady state during the time the drug concentrations are obtained, patient 2 is not yet at steady state when the concentrations are obtained, and the blood samples in patient 3 are obtained during a time when there was a brief, but unrecognized, interruption in the infusion of the drug.

To obtain an estimate of the population mean clearance based on our assumption of steady state, one could use the following equation to estimate clearance for each of the observed drug concentrations in each subject:

$$\frac{\text{rate of infusion}}{C_{P,ss}} = \text{clearance} \qquad (6\text{–}3)$$

The average of the three estimates of clearance available for each subject would then serve as the individual's estimate of clearance. The mean and variance of the individual estimates would serve as the population mean clearance and measure of the magnitude of interindividual variability in the population, respectively. This approach has been referred to as the two-stage approach; estimates of each subject's pharmacokinetic parameters are obtained in stage 1, and in

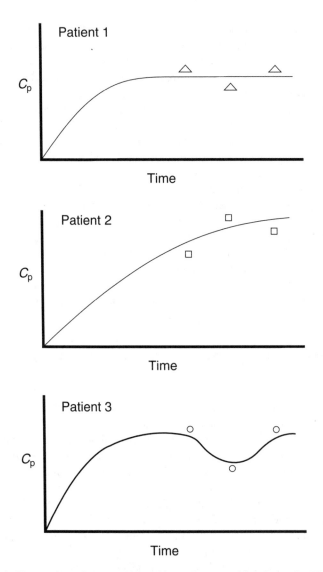

Figure 6–1. Illustration of data collected in a pharmacokinetic study. The solid line represents the individual's true concentration–time course of drug and the symbols indicate the measured values. Note that some patients violate the assumption of steady state used in the analysis.

stage 2 the population mean and variance are computed from the individual estimates. Although the two-stage approach is commonly used to analyze experimental data, significant problems are encountered when this approach is used to estimate population pharmacokinetic parameters from nonexperimental data.

The experimental paradigm used in traditional pharmacokinetic studies is designed to yield the maximum amount of data about the pharmacokinetic parameters in each subject so that accurate estimates of each individual's pharmacokinetic parameters can be obtained. The efforts made to collect a large amount of high-quality data for each subject in the experimental setting translates into a relatively straightforward data analysis. Nonexperimental data, on the other hand, are obtained during patient care with little or no effort to collect data in a systematic way. There are several consequences of the lack of structure in data collection. First, insufficient data may be available from each subject to allow the estimation of the individual's pharmacokinetic parameters. Alternatively, the quality and quantity of data available from each subject might be poor so that reliable estimates of the pharmacokinetic parameters in each patient cannot be obtained. This can result in biased estimates of the mean population parameters and the estimates of the magnitude of interindividual variability will be inflated. Second, the data obtained from different patients may vary in quality. As noted above, some of the patients violate the assumptions of the experiment; for example, they may not be at steady state when the drug concentrations are measured, or there may be problems with drug administration. In the above example, high-quality data are indiscriminately analyzed along with poor-quality data with potentially deleterious consequences.

In the experiment described above there were sufficient data available from each patient to allow the estimation of clearance in each subject using the simplified pharmacokinetic model. As frequently happens in the clinic or hospital setting, minimal numbers of measured drug concentrations may be available from each patient, and in some cases, estimates of pharmacokinetic parameters for each patient cannot be obtained from the available data. Sheiner and colleagues recognized that these drug concentrations contained information regarding drug disposition, but that the data were inadequate to meet the requirements for traditional data analysis methods. This led to the development of an innovative approach to data analysis using statistical techniques to explicitly deal with the shortcomings of nonexperimental data.[3] This approach is referred to as mixed-effect modeling because it mixes fixed and random effects in the model used for data analysis, and has been implemented in the computer program NONMEM, an acronym which stands for nonlinear mixed-effect modeling.[8]

The essence of this approach lies in the fact that although patients are different in terms of their pharmacokinetic parameters, they are also similar in other respects and with appropriate statistical methods one can explicitly recognize the similarities and adjust for the differences. Thus, even when only limited numbers of samples are available for each patient and individual estimates of pharmacokinetic parameters cannot be obtained, the population pharmacokinetic parameters can still be estimated.

To obtain these estimates, however, it is necessary to shift the focus of the data analysis from the individual to the population and develop a pharmacokinetic and statistical model that will allow us to pool the data while at the same time explicitly recognizing the correlation of drug concentrations obtained within the same individual. The population perspective for the data from Figure 6–1 is illustrated in Figure 6–2. Note that each patient has a central tendency denoted by the dotted lines and the patients' central tendencies are distributed about the population mean value, Θ_{Cl}. The distance from Θ_{Cl} to each of the individual's central tendencies is denoted by the η's and the variance of the distribution of the η's, ω_{Cl}^2, is a measure of the magnitude of interindividual variability in clearance in the population. Furthermore, within each patient there was variability in the measured drug concentrations over time and, thus, variability in the individual's estimated clearance over time. The distance between the central tendency for clearance in a

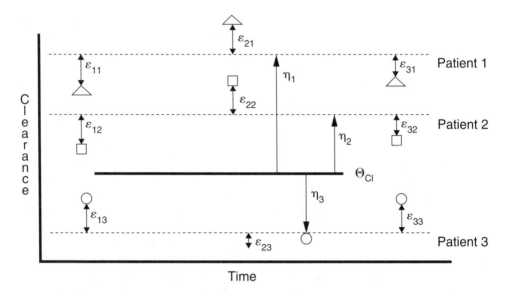

Figure 6–2. Population perspective for pharmacokinetic data. Dashed lines represent the true (unknown) values for clearance in three patients. The ϵ's represent the discrepancies between clearance values observed at different times. The η's represent the discrepancies between the time values and the population mean value, Θ_{Cl}.

patient and each of the estimates of clearance within a subject is denoted by ϵ_{ij}, where the subscript indicates the ith estimate of clearance in the jth person. The variance of the distribution of ϵ_{ij} across the entire data set, σ^2, is a measure of the magnitude of residual variability in the population.

In the usual approach to fitting pharmacokinetic data in an individual, nonlinear regression analysis using the least-squares criterion would be used to obtain estimates of the pharmacokinetic parameters for each patient. When this approach is used, there are three implicit assumptions regarding the data points to be fitted to the model: each of the data points is assumed to be independent and not correlated with one another, the errors between the measured and predicted drug concentrations have the same typical value, and the error is additive. These assumptions imply that if many replicate measurements were made for each time point the variance of the distribution of the measured values would be the same for each time point. When these conditions hold true, the ordinary least-squares objective function, given by

$$OF_{OLS} = \Sigma(C_{P,i} - \hat{C}_{P,i})^2 \qquad (6\text{–}4)$$

can be used to fit the pharmacokinetic model to the data and obtain estimates of the pharmacokinetic parameters.

Using the ordinary least-squares approach the pharmacokinetic parameters that minimize the difference between the measured drug concentrations obtained in an individual ($C_{P,i}$) and the predicted values ($\hat{C}_{P,i}$) are sought.

In practice we often find that the magnitude of assay variability increases with the measured concentration. This violation of the assumption of homoscedasticity, or constant variance, is commonly handled by using the weighted least-squares criterion as given by

$$OF_{WLS} = \Sigma \frac{(C_{P,i} - \hat{C}_{P,i})^2}{\sigma_i^2} \tag{6-5}$$

where σ_i^2 is the variance of the ith measured drug concentration. Because we do not usually have an estimate of σ_i^2, when using the weighted least-squares criterion we generally assume that the variance σ_i^2 is proportional to C_P or C_P^2.

In the case of a population pharmacokinetic analysis the problems associated with violations of the assumptions listed above become more critical and the problem of selecting a weighting scheme becomes difficult. From a population perspective the errors are now correlated, because some drug concentrations are obtained from one patient whereas others are obtained in other patients. Also, data can be collected under different clinical conditions and with varying quality with respect to determining the time of sampling and determining the measured drug concentration so that a simplistic weighting scheme is inappropriate. In the example above, for example, we may have a subset of patients, for example, patients in the intensive care unit, who for various reasons experience problems with maintaining a constant infusion rate. An explicit pharmacokinetic and statistical model must be specified to account for these problems.

In this setting, a more sophisticated and flexible weighting method must be used to analyze the data. Such a method has been developed by Sheiner and Beal and is known as extended least squares.[3] The objective function used to obtain these estimates is given by

$$OF_{ELS} = \Sigma \left[\frac{(C_{P,i} - \hat{C}_{P,i})^2}{\sigma(\Theta, \xi, x_i)^2} + \ln[\sigma(\Theta, \xi, x_i)^2] \right] \tag{6-6}$$

In this approach the variance σ^2 is modeled as a function of the data (x_i), the fixed-effect parameter (Θ), and the random-effect parameter (ξ). With this function, one can make the weighting scheme a function of the data; for example, intensive care unit patients may have more residual variability than nonintensive care unit patients, and this can be explicitly incorporated in the objective function. When using extended least squares, however, a penalty term must be added to prevent the variance function from becoming very large and resulting in a meaningless solution. This penalty is provided by the natural logarithm of $\sigma (\Theta, \xi, x_i)^2$ on the right-hand side of Equation 6–6. This objective function is extremely flexible, but its use requires considerable effort to define and interpret the statistical model, which is usually taken for granted in ordinary or weighted least-squares analysis.

PHARMACOSTATISTICAL MODELING

Unlike the two-stage approach, a mixed-effect model analysis requires an explicit statement of the complete pharmacokinetic and pharmacostatistical model, including a formal statement of fixed- and random-effect models. This model must include four components:

1. Pharmacokinetic structural model
2. Regression formulas for the typical values of pharmacokinetic parameters

3. Statistical model for interindividual variability
4. Statistical model for residual variability

A complete discussion of these four components and the implications of selecting a specific statistical model is beyond the scope of this chapter; however, the interested reader is referred to the NONMEM program documentation,[9] in particular, Part VI of the NONMEM user's guide,[10] for a complete discussion. The following is a brief overview of each component of the pharmacostatistical model.

Pharmacokinetic Structural Models

When a model is fit to data using nonlinear regression, it is necessary to specify the pharmacokinetic model to be used in generating predictions for comparison to the measured values. One example is a simple one-compartment open model with intravenous bolus administration given by

$$\hat{C}_{P,i} = \frac{D}{V} e^{[-(Cl/V)t_i]} \tag{6-7}$$

If this model were to be used in conjunction with Equation 6–4, predicted drug concentrations, $\hat{C}_{P,i}$, would be generated at times, t_i, corresponding to the times of measured drug concentrations obtained following the dose, D. Different values for the pharmacokinetic parameters Cl and V would be selected by the fitting program to find the values that minimize the objective function, such as the one given by Equation 6–4 if ordinary least squares is to be used. In an experimental setting the specification of a pharmacokinetic model is relatively straightforward because drug administration and sampling times are usually standardized for each subject.

Data collection in the clinical setting, however, is generally more complicated. The times of drug administration are usually not standardized and blood samples may be drawn at different times over multiple dosing intervals. The patient's dosing regimen may change over time; patients may switch from intravenous to oral dosing, patients may miss doses, or supplemental doses might be administered. Thus, the process of specifying the pharmacokinetic structural model becomes more difficult. In the case of mixed-effect modeling this process is even more difficult because of the need to model the influence of the random effects. This was one of the major obstacles to the use of earlier versions of the NONMEM program. Fortunately, the current version of NONMEM provides a library of subroutines, referred to as PREDPP, that facilitate the specification of a pharmacokinetic model. The available models range from a one-compartment linear model to multicompartmental disposition with nonlinear elimination. Any combination of oral or intravenous administration can be handled. These subroutines allow complete flexibility in specifying dosing events and times of drug concentration sampling so that even the most complicated dosing history can be accurately described.

Regression Models for Pharmacokinetic Parameters (Θ)

One of the primary objectives of a population analysis is the identification of observable patient features that are associated with alterations in drug pharmacokinetics. These factors are identified through the evaluation of regression formulas that allow one to explore the ability of patient covariates to explain differences in drug pharmacokinetics. For example, the following Equation is a simple regression model that states that the typical value for clearance, $\hat{C}l_j$, is equal to a constant and is unrelated to any observable patient data:

$$\tilde{C}l_j = \Theta_1 \tag{6-8}$$

We can expand this model by adding information about creatinine clearance and obtain the regression model

$$\tilde{C}l_j = \Theta_1 + \Theta_2 \cdot Cl_{cr,j} \tag{6-9}$$

which states that the typical value for drug clearance is a function of the measured creatinine clearance. This equation is identical to Equation 6–1 discussed previously and is reproduced here for ease of exposition.

In formulating the regression models for the pharmacokinetic parameters, one must consider the nature of the patient variable, that is, whether it is a continuous variable such as creatinine clearance or categorical such as gender, and whether the effect is linear or nonlinear. Examples of various types of regression models and implementation in the NONMEM program can be found in the program documentation.[10]

It is important to remember that the discovery of an association does not imply a cause–effect relationship, but it may point the way for further investigation. Thus, the finding that clearance decreases with age does not provide an explanation for the underlying mechanism for the change. Further investigation would be needed to determine what specific drug metabolizing process varies with age to produce the observed reduction in clearance.

Statistical Model for Interindividual Variability (ω^2)

The regression formula given by Equation 6–9 predicts the same typical value for clearance for all patients with the same creatinine clearance. If we were to measure the clearance of a renally excreted drug in a population and plot the values against estimated creatinine clearance we might observe something similar to the data in Figure 6–3. Note that the measured values for drug clearance are not identical to the typical values and that the variability in the measured values about the typical value increases with increasing typical values. Because of interindividual variability in the values for Θ_1 and Θ_2, there will be persistent differences between the typical value for clearance given by the regression formula and an individual's measured value. As discussed above, this persistent difference is denoted by η and a frequency distribution of the η's will have a mean of zero and a variance denoted by ω_{Cl}^2. This variance, ω_{Cl}^2, measures the amount of spread of the measured values for clearance around the typical value and quantifies the magnitude of interindividual variability.

In mixed-effect modeling, it is necessary to state a statistical model for the relationship between the typical value and the error, η. In Figure 6–3, for example, the typical size of the error increases with increasing $\tilde{C}l_j$ so that a proportional statistical model for interindividual variability as given by the following equation may be appropriate.

$$Cl_j = \tilde{C}l_j + \tilde{C}l_j \cdot \eta_j^{Cl} \tag{6-10}$$

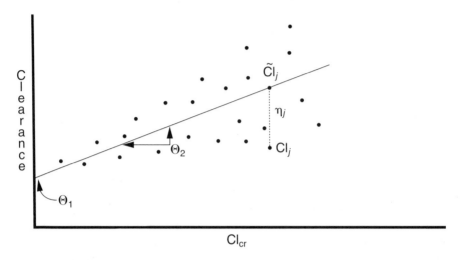

Figure 6–3. Relationship between drug clearance and renal function. Each dot represents a measured clearance value plotted at the patient's observed creatinine clearance. The typical value for clearance as a function of creatinine clearance is given by Equation 6–9. η represents the persistent difference between an individual's measured clearance and the typical value. The variance of the distribution of the η's is a measure of the magnitude of interindividual variability.

Statistical Model for Residual Variability (σ^2)

Mixed-effect model analysis also requires a statistical model for the persistent differences between the measured concentrations and the predicted concentrations obtained from the typical values of pharmacokinetic parameters and the pharmacokinetic structural models described above. This persistent difference is illustrated in Figure 6–4. The model for residual variability must have the potential to account for differences in the nature of the variability caused by different data collection schemes at different hospitals, differences in variability in different patient populations, and differences in the precision of drug concentration assays at multiple institutions. Although this model can become complex, a simple, but useful, model for residual variability is shown in the equation

$$C_{P,ij} = \hat{C}_{P,ij} + \hat{C}_{P,ij} \cdot \epsilon_{ij} \qquad (6\text{--}11)$$

The form of this model is similar to Equation 6–10 in which we state that the typical size of the error increases with increasing predicted drug concentration. The variance of the ϵ_{ij}, σ^2, measures the magnitude of residual variability.

Selection of Statistical Models

The selection of the statistical models for interindividual variability and residual variability is based on a examination of the data and the goals of the analysis. It may be of interest, for example, to determine if the interindividual or residual variability is greater in a population of inten-

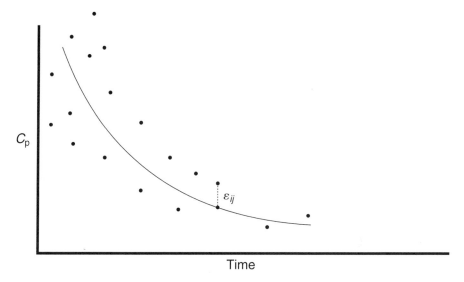

Figure 6–4. Fitting a pharmacokinetic model to individual concentration–time data. The solid curve represents an individual's true (unknown) concentration–time course of drug. The dots indicate measured values and ϵ's indicate the persistent difference between the measured and predicted values.

sive care unit patients as compared with patients in an ambulatory care setting. Statistical models can be developed to allow for such differences, but this is beyond the scope of this chapter.[10]

First-Order Approximation Used in NONMEM Program

The goal of a mixed-effect modeling analysis is to obtain accurate and precise estimates of the three types of population pharmacokinetic parameters: Θ, ω^2, and σ^2. Within the computer program NONMEM this is accomplished by using maximum likelihood estimation, in conjunction with the extended least-squares objective function from Equation 6–6. Maximum likelihood estimation was originally developed in the early 1920s by R. A. Fisher.[11] This general method allows the estimation of parameters of a statistical model given certain assumptions about the distribution of random terms in the model. In using maximum likelihood estimation one chooses the values of the parameters of the model so as to maximize the probability of obtaining the observed data. Least-squares estimation of a regression model with normally distributed errors, in which the parameters of a model are chosen to minimize the difference between observed and predicted values, is equivalent to maximum likelihood estimation.

When maximum likelihood estimation is used, a likelihood function giving the joint probability distribution of the observed data must be specified. In fitting pharmacokinetic models this requires an expression for the mean and variance of each measured drug concentration. In addition, an assumption about the distribution of the random error terms, η_j and ϵ_{ij}, must be stated. For a number of reasons, a normal distribution or at least a symmetric distribution is usually chosen.

Because even the simplest pharmacokinetic model is statistically nonlinear, not to be confused with nonlinear pharmacokinetics, the process of finding the maximum likelihood estimates is more difficult. The random effects enter into the model nonlinearly, that is, they appear in the exponent, and there can be cross-products between the different types of random variables, that is, the η's and ϵ's. The statistical models for interindividual variability (Equation 6–10) and residual variability (Equation 6–11) have been incorporated into the structural pharmacokinetic model (Equation 6–7) for a simple one-compartment model with bolus administration to illustrate the complexity of the combined model:

$$C_{P,ij} = \frac{D_j}{\tilde{V}(1 + \eta_j^V)} \, exp\left[\frac{\tilde{Cl}(1 + \eta_j^{Cl})}{\tilde{V}(1 + \eta_j^V)} \cdot t_{ij} \right] \cdot [1 + \epsilon_{ij}] \qquad (6\text{–}12)$$

Because of the way these random effects enter into the model some simplification is necessary. The partial derivatives of the η_j and the ϵ_{ij} with respect to $C_{P,ij}$ are used to approximate the nonlinear influence of the η's and the ϵ's on the predicted concentration. The η's and the ϵ's are then set to their expected values, that is, zero. In this way the random effects enter into the model in a linear way and the distribution of the predicted concentrations will be normal. The mean and variance of the concentration can then be computed and maximum likelihood estimates of Θ, ω^2, and σ^2 are obtained. Sheiner et al provide a more detailed description of this process.[3]

There has been considerable interest regarding the problem of obtaining population pharmacokinetic parameter estimates from observational data. A number of different approaches have been proposed as a way of dealing with the statistical problems that arise in dealing with this type of data.[12] Each of these approaches requires certain simplifications and assumptions which undoubtedly result in advantages and limitations in dealing with different types of data. The mixed-effect model approach used in the NONMEM program has become one of the more popular methods for population analysis. There has been considerable effort on the part of the NONMEM project group to support this method and extensive documentation for the program is available. In addition, a considerable number of reports have been published describing analyses of clinical data and a number of simulation studies have been performed to investigate the performance characteristics of the program. As additional experience with alternative methods is gained we will be better able to judge the merits of the various approaches and select the best method for a particular problem.

POPULATION PHARMACOKINETICS AND PHARMACOEPIDEMIOLOGY

In the previous sections a method was described for dealing with drug concentrations obtained during the routine clinical care of patients and identifying patient characteristics associated with altered drug disposition. We now turn our attention to the problem of evaluating patient outcomes and identifying patient or drug therapy characteristics associated with adverse, or beneficial, events. In the final section we bring together these two processes and show how they can be integrated into an overall risk management program.

In general, randomized, double-blind, placebo-controlled clinical trials represent the preferred method for demonstrating the safety and efficacy of new drugs. The results of these trials serve as the foundation for seeking marketing approval from the Food and Drug Administration, and they are also used to develop criteria for identifying the patient populations who will have the greatest likelihood of achieving a therapeutic response to a drug. Although controlled clinical trials are a powerful tool for answering important clinical questions, problems can arise when one attempts to extrapolate the study results to clinical practice. The application of strict inclusion and exclusion criteria may create a study population that does not resemble the patients who are likely to use the drug during routine clinical practice. This is completely analogous to the situation described above regarding population pharmacokinetic parameters. As with pharmacokinetics, there has been increased interest in the use of observational data to continue to study drug efficacy and safety in the postmarketing period.[13]

Pharmacoepidemiology is a relatively new area of research that combines epidemiology research methods,[14] such as the case–control study or a prospective cohort study, with biostatistics and principles of clinical pharmacology to determine the risk of adverse events or therapeutic failure in patient populations and identify patient characteristics associated with a higher probability of these events.

In a cohort study, the incidence of an adverse event in a group of patients exposed to a drug is compared with the incidence in a group of patients who are not exposed to the drug. A cohort study is similar to the design of a clinical trial with the important exception that the enrollment of patients into the various treatment or exposure groups is not randomized. Both groups are initially free of the outcome of interest and are monitored to determine the number of adverse events that occur over a specified period. The incidence of the adverse event in the exposed group is computed as the number of new cases of the adverse event detected in the exposed group divided by the total number of patients in the exposed group. A similar calculation is performed for the comparison group and the ratio of the incidence of the adverse event in the exposed group versus the incidence of the adverse event in the nonexposed group, known as the relative risk (RR), is used as the measure of association between the exposure and the outcome. The magnitude of the relative risk gives the likelihood of experiencing the outcome based on exposure status. A relative risk of 3.0, for example, means that the risk of developing the adverse event is three times more likely in the exposed versus comparison group. Conversely, a relative risk less than 1.0 suggests that the exposed group is at a reduced risk of developing the event.

In a case–control study, patients with the disease of interest (cases) and patients without the disease (controls) are identified and differences in exposures between the two groups are compared. Because incidence cannot be computed in a case–control study, the odds ratio is used to assess the probability of the outcome given the exposure. The odds ratio is computed as the ratio of the proportion of cases exposed to the factor of interest to the proportion of controls exposed. It has been shown that the odds ratio provides an approximation of the relative risk when the incidence of disease is small.

Both the cohort and case–control study methodologies can serve as a scientific framework for studying patient outcome to drug therapy, and would be well used as the basis for performing outcome-oriented drug utilization evaluations. The wealth of experience with these approaches in other settings can serve to help in the design, analysis, and interpretation of studies of adverse events in the hospital or managed care setting. Moreover, when blood sampling for the determination of drug concentrations has been performed, population pharmacokinetic analysis provides a mechanism for using this information in a risk factor analysis. Thus, there is an intimate relationship between the tools of population pharmacokinetic analysis and pharmacoepidemiology research methods. By using these tools in the context of a comprehensive pharmacokinetic and patient outcome monitoring program it is possible to evaluate the role of drug concentrations, in conjunction with patient characteristics, such as age and gender, as an independent risk factor for adverse events.

Multivariate Analysis of Patient Risk Factors

The overall relative risk obtained from a cohort study provides an average measure of a patient's risk of developing an event given exposure to a drug. It is frequently of interest to determine the risk for specific patient subgroups within the study population. Thus, we might compare the incidence of adverse events in elderly versus young patients, in men versus women, and so forth. The goal of this type of analysis is to identify the patient subgroups with the highest risk of adverse events so that efforts to reduce the risk might be implemented.

The type of analysis described above can be helpful, but it does not help in examining the influence of multiple risk factors acting simultaneously. In addition, because patients are generally not prescribed drugs in a randomized way, the role of confounding in producing the observed results must be considered. A confounding variable is a variable that is associated with both the exposure and the outcome and that independently affects the risk of developing the outcome. Thus, the observed association between the exposure and outcome may be due to differences between the exposed and nonexposed groups that have little to do with the exposure. Uncontrolled confounding is one of the major issues in assessing the validity of study results. It can result in over- or underestimates of the relative risk for an exposure and can even change the direction of the effect.

A number of multivariable data analysis techniques are available to investigate the association between multiple patient factors and outcome while simultaneously controlling for confounding factors. The specific type of multivariate analysis to be used is dependent on the nature of the outcome under study. If the outcome is a continuous variable and the error terms are normally distributed, multiple linear regression would be used. An example might be an analysis of the association between measured diastolic blood pressure, a continuous outcome variable, and age, gender, and treatment with antihypertensive medication.

The patient outcome of interest in many pharmacoepidemiology studies is often dichotomous and not continuous; that is, an adverse event occurs or it does not, the patient has a successful therapeutic outcome or he does not. In this setting, logistic regression analysis represents an appropriate method for estimating the magnitude of the association between drug exposure and the outcome while adjusting for the effects of other patient characteristics that may represent confounding factors.

In logistic regression analysis, the risk of developing the outcome of interest is expressed as a function of independent predictor variables. By defining the dependent variable to be the natural logarithm (ln) of the odds of the outcome, the independent variables can be represented by a linear function. Using notation, $P(y)$ is the probability of the outcome, and $P(y)/[1 - P(y)]$ represents the "odds" of the outcome. In logistic regression the log odds is the dependent variable and is expressed as a linear function of the independent predictor variables:

$$\ln\left[\frac{P(y)}{1 - P(y)}\right] = \beta_0 + \beta_1 x_1 + \ldots + \beta_m x_m \qquad (6\text{--}13)$$

This equation can be rewritten to give the probability of developing the outcome:

$$P(y) = \frac{1}{1 + \exp^{-(\beta_0 + \beta_1 x_1 + \ldots + \beta_m x_m)}} \tag{6-14}$$

In Equation 6–14, $P(y)$ is the probability of developing the outcome, for example, an adverse event or therapeutic failure, and the β's are coefficients of the model relating predictor variables to the probability of the event. The predictor variables can be either continuous, such as age, weight, and drug concentration, or categorical, such as gender and the presence of another concurrent illness. The coefficients can be converted to odds ratios that provide an estimate of the relative risk when the incidence of the outcome is low. When the independent variable is categorical, the exponential of the coefficient gives the odds ratio. When the independent variable is continuous, such as is the case with drug concentrations, the exponential of the corresponding β gives the magnitude of the increase or decrease in the log odds produced by a unit change in the independent variable, for example, drug concentrations, when all other factors are held constant.

For the purposes of an example, suppose that a logistic regression analysis revealed a relationship between the probability of an adverse event and the independent variables gender and magnitude of drug exposure. The results of this analysis are given by

$$P(y) = \frac{1}{1 + \exp^{-(-6 + 0.1 \times C_p + 0.725 \times \text{SEX})}} \tag{6-15}$$

where the probability of the outcome, $P(y)$, is a function of the measured drug concentration, C_p, and gender, denoted by the indicator variable SEX, where SEX has a value of 1 if the patient is a female and 0 if the patient is a male. The coefficients in Equation 6–15 were arbitrarily selected for the purposes of illustration.

The probability of the event as a function of the measured drug concentration and stratified for gender is shown in Figure 6–5.

Population Approaches to Risk Management

Other chapters in this book deal with the relationship between drug concentrations and drug efficacy and safety. Relatively little is known, however, about the role of other patient characteristics that can mitigate patient response to drug therapy. For example, is the therapeutic range of a drug different for elderly versus young patients? There have been relatively few examples where this type of analysis has been performed. This is probably the result of the independent evolution of clinical pharmacokinetics and clinical epidemiology and there have been relatively few individuals who have tried to bridge this gap. With the current interest in outcome-oriented drug utilization evaluations, however, new opportunities for individuals with knowledge at the interface between these two disciplines become apparent.

One of the goals of pharmacoepidemiology research is to determine the relative risk for an adverse event and identify patient factors that might be associated with either an increased or decreased risk of the event. A frequent component of the analysis of risk factors for adverse events is to evaluate a dose–response relationship. This can be difficult to evaluate in the context of an observational study because variability in pharmacokinetics across the population creates

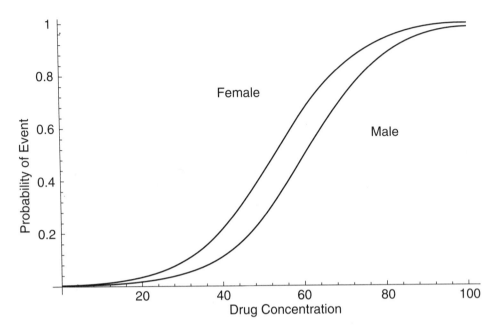

Figure 6–5. Probability of an event modeled using logistic regression. The curves were generated using Equation 6–15 to predict the probability of the event of interest for various drug concentrations stratified by the gender of the patient.

overlap in the concentrations achieved for any given dose. The ability to integrate population pharmacokinetic data as a predictive variable into pharmacoepidemiologic studies represents an important advance in our ability to study risk factors for adverse events. This enhances our ability to evaluate the relationship between drug exposure, quantified by the average steady-state drug concentration or total area under the curve, and total daily dose. By accounting for more of the variability between patients we can improve our ability to predict the factors associated with an adverse event. Although there have been a few attempts to relate drug concentrations to adverse events, these studies are limited by the relatively simplistic approach taken with respect to the drug concentrations.

An example where drug concentrations have been used as covariate of a multivariable analysis of an epidemiologic investigation was performed by Sawyers et al,[15] who identified risk factors for nephrotoxicity using data collected from 338 patients receiving aminoglycosides. In this analysis, age, sex, initial calculated rate of creatinine clearance, presence of diabetes, shock, liver disease, bacteremia, initial serum level of aminoglycoside 1 hour after administration, trough level of aminoglycoside, total dose of aminoglycoside, and duration of therapy were explored as possible risk factors for nephrotoxicity. In this study, nephrotoxicity was defined as a greater than 50% fall in the calculated rate of creatinine clearance. The results of the stepwise multivariate logistic regression analysis identified several statistically significant risk factors for nephrotoxicity. Based on these results, the probability of a patient developing nephrotoxicity (P(NT)] during a course of aminoglycoside therapy can be computed from

$$P(\text{NT}) = \frac{1}{1 + \exp^{-(-8.96 + \text{DURATION} \times 0.098 + C_{\text{P}} \times 0.234 + \text{LIVER} \times 1.49 + \text{AGE} \times 0.051 + \text{Cl}_{\text{cr}} \times 0.02 + \text{SEX} \times 0.725)}}$$

(6–16)

In Equation 6–16, duration is the duration of the aminoglycoside therapy in days, C_{p} is the initial 1-hour postdose aminoglycoside level (µg/mL), LIVER is an indicator variable that indicates the presence of liver disease (LIVER = 1) or absence (LIVER = 0), AGE is the patient's age in years, Cl_{cr} is the patient's initial rate of creatinine clearance (mL/min), and SEX is an indicator variable with a value of 1 if the patient is a female or 0 otherwise.

One clinically relevant application of this equation is to provide a mechanism to target individuals at high risk of developing nephrotoxicity for more intensive monitoring or use of non-aminoglycoside antibiotics, such as third-generation cephalosporins, to minimize the occurrence of nephrotoxicity.

From a pharmacokinetic perspective there is an important limitation to this study because the only pharmacokinetic information used as a risk factor was an initial aminoglycoside level. Drug dosages may change over time and patient pharmacokinetic parameters may change over time, resulting in marked variability in the actual magnitude of exposure over the duration of therapy. By obtaining drug concentrations over the course of patient therapy and performing a bayesian analysis to estimate the patient's pharmacokinetic parameters, some of these sources of variability, and thus the magnitude of drug exposure, could be identified and a more precise measure of drug exposure could be developed.

Risk Management in the Hospital Setting

The tools discussed in this chapter, including population pharmacokinetic analysis, bayesian analysis, and pharmacoepidemiology research methods, provide an important mechanism for clinicians to gain insight into patient factors that influence the response to drug therapy. Over time, drug concentrations measured in patients receiving drug therapy can be pooled and analyzed using a population model to obtain estimates of the population pharmacokinetic parameters. This pharmacokinetic database can then be used in the evaluation of subsequent patients. The drug dosing history and measured drug concentrations in a patient receiving a drug of interest can be collected and bayesian estimates of the individuals pharmacokinetic parameters can be obtained. These estimates can then be used to revise the dosing regimen as appropriate in a target drug concentration strategy. The initial population pharmacokinetic database can also be used to develop a priori dosing recommendations for subsequent patients admitted to the hospital. In addition, the estimates of the individual pharmacokinetic parameters can be used to compute individualized measures of drug exposure that more precisely describe drug exposure than simply total dose or total daily dose. For example, the average steady-state drug concentration, or the average daily area under the concentration–time curve, or the total area under the curve can be computed depending on the drug, clinical setting, and patient outcome under investigation.

These measures of drug exposure can then be incorporated into a pharmacoepidemiologic analysis to identify other patient-specific covariates predictive of patient outcome. In the course of performing outcome-oriented drug utilization evaluations, age, sex, concomitant medications, and concurrent illnesses are generally recorded. This information, in addition to the drug exposure information, can be incorporated into a multiple logistic regression analysis similar to that described above to identify patients at greatest risk for developing the adverse event. A similar process could be pursued to identify prognostic factors for beneficial therapeutic outcomes.

In this ongoing process, subsequent patients admitted to the hospital who exhibit characteristics associated with the high probability of therapeutic failure would then be the target of more intensive monitoring. For example, lower dosages might be employed, more frequent drug concentrations may be obtained, or alternative therapies might be selected if risk cannot be minimized to an acceptable level using patient intervention strategies.

As hospitals grow increasingly computerized the possibility of automatically flagging patients meeting certain characteristics becomes more likely, so that on admission, or during the course of hospitalization as patient status changes, a series of events might be initiated based on the specific details of each patient's clinical case. Although these strategies do not serve as a replacement for good clinical decision making on the part of physicians and pharmacists, they can serve as tools to assist in decision making and at least provide objective information on which more informed decisions might be made.

Glossary of Terms

Θ Typical value of a pharmacokinetic parameter in a population
η The difference between an individual's value of pharmacokinetics parameter and the population mean value
ω^2 The variance of η, the magnitude of unexplained variability in the distribution of pharmacokinetic parameter across the population
ϵ The difference between measured and predicted drug concentrations within an individual
σ^2 The variance of ϵ, the magnitude of residual variability in drug concentrations observed over time within an individual

——————— QUESTIONS ———————

1. Describe the difference between residual variability and interindividual variability in pharmacokinetic parameters.

2. What would be the effect of selecting the wrong pharmacokinetic structural model on the estimates of residual variability? For example, suppose that a drug exhibits a two-compartment disposition but a one-compartment model is used to analyze the data.

3. What is the critical distinction between a least-squares approach to the interpretation of a measured drug concentration and bayesian estimation procedures?

4. Using Equation 6–16, compute the probability of developing nephrotoxicity in a 65-year-old male patient with an initial creatinine clearance of 40 mL/min, receiving aminoglycosides for 10 days with an initial creatinine level of 10.0 mg/mL. Assume no evidence for liver disease.

REFERENCES

1. *Committed to Quality: An Introduction to the Joint Commission on Accreditation of Healthcare Organizations.* 4th ed. Oakbrook Terrace, IL: Joint Commission of Accreditation of Healthcare Organizations; 1990.
2. Slattery JT, Gibaldi M, Koup JR. Prediction of maintenance dose required to attain a desired drug concentration at steady-state from a single determination of concentration after an initial dose. *Clin Pharmacokinet.* 1980;5:377–385.
3. Sheiner LB, Rosenberg B, Marathe VV. Estimation of population characteristics of pharmacokinetic parameters from routine clinical data. *J Pharmacokinet Biopharm.* 1977;5(5):445–479.
4. Peck CC, Rodman JH. Analysis of clinical pharmacokinetic data for individualizing drug dosage regimens. In Evans WE, Schentag JJ, Jusko WJ, eds: *Applied Pharmacokinetics: Principles of Therapeutic Drug Monitoring.* Spokane, WA: Applied Therapeutics. 1986:55–82.
5. Hosmer DW, Lemeshow S. *Applied Logistic Regression.* New York: John Wiley & Sons; 1989.
6. Sheiner LB, Rosenberg B, Melmon KL. Modeling of individual pharmacokinetics for computer-aided drug dosage. *Comput Biomed Res.* 1972;5:441–459.
7. Gilman AG, Rall TW, Nies AS, Taylor P. *The Pharmacological Basis of Therapeutics.* 8th ed. New York: Pergamon Press; 1990:28–32.
8. Beal SL, Sheiner LB. The NONMEM system. *Am Statistican.* 1980;34:118–119.
9. Beal SL, Sheiner LB. *NONMEM Users Guide.* Regents of the University of California; 1989.
10. *Part VI of NONMEM User's Guide. Introductory Guide.* Regents of the University of California; 1989.
11. Freund JE, Walpole RE. *Mathematical Statistics.* 4th ed. Englewood Cliffs, NJ: Prentice-Hall; 1987:350–354.
12. Rowland M, Aarons L. European cooperation in the field of scientific and technical research. Presented at a conference held in Manchester, UK; September 21–23, 1991.
13. Strom BL. *Pharmacoepidemiology.* New York: Churchill-Livingstone; 1989.
14. Hennekens CH, Buring JE. *Epidemiology in Medicine.* Boston: Little, Brown; 1987.
15. Sawyers CL, Moore RD, Lerner SA, Smith CR. A model for predicting nephrotoxicity in patients treated with aminoglycosides. *J Infect Dis.* 1986;153:1062.

Chapter 7

Decision Analysis Applied to Therapeutic Drug Monitoring

Gerald E. Schumacher

Judith T. Barr

Keep in Mind

- Decision analysis has the following steps: identify the decision alternatives, structure a decision tree, assign probabilities to the chance nodes, assign a value or worth to each outcome, and calculate the expected value for each of the decision alternatives. The alternative with the greatest expected value is the preferred option.

- A bayesian approach to test interpretation involves the following sequence: the practitioner estimates the probability of the condition being present before a test is ordered (the pretest probability), then new information is obtained by a diagnostic test, and this results in a revised, posttest probability of the condition.

- In TDM, the serum drug concentration functions like a diagnostic test in which a cutoff value is used to separate either toxic from therapeutic or therapeutic from subtherapeutic populations. When test results are dichotomized in this manner, a number of test performance indices are used to characterize the quality of test information: true-positive rate (sensitivity) is the probability of observing a drug level greater than the test cutoff in patients with the condition that is being tested for; false-positive rate is the probability of seeing a drug level greater than the cutoff in patients without the condition; true-negative rate (specificity) is the probability of noting a drug level less than the cutoff in patients without the condition being tested for; false-negative rate is the probability of finding a drug level less than the cutoff in patients with the condition; and likelihood ratio (+) for a positive test result represents true-positive rate/false-positive rate. For the practitioner, two additional important characteristics are the positive and negative predictive values of a diagnostic test: positive predictive value is the probability that a patient with a drug level greater than the cutoff truly has the condition and negative predictive value is the probability that a patient with a drug level less than the cutoff truly does not have the condition. Predictive values vary with the prevalence of the condition in the population being tested, but test sensitivity and specificity do not.

- A threshold probability is the posttest probability of the condition being present that functions as a decision threshold for separating the selection of one decision alternative from another.

- A drug level should be ordered only if the test result can lead to revising the pretest probability of a condition such that the posttest probability may cause the practitioner to change the decision about the best course of action for managing the patient.

In the interpretation of serum drug levels for therapeutic drug monitoring, there is a need to decide among several available options. When a patient has signs indicating a possible drug-induced toxicity, and the serum level is above the therapeutic range, do you conclude that the patient is toxic? When a patient has suspected drug toxicity but continues to need treatment, is the best decision to discontinue the drug, lower the dosage, or continue the present regimen? When a patient does not seem to be responding appropriately to a drug, is the best course of action to increase the dosage or change to another drug? When a patient appears to be making progress with a drug but the serum level is above the therapeutic range, is the best decision to maintain the regimen as is or to lower the dosage? Each of these situations produces a number of decision options, each option leads to its own set of consequences, but the likelihood of each consequence occurring is uncertain, and therefore the best decision to make is unclear.

Decision analysis is a systematic approach to making choices under conditions of uncertainty. A clinical decision rarely involves only one possible course of action with absolute certainty of its outcome; rather, clinicians are challenged constantly with situations involving a range of diagnostic and treatment options with uncertain outcome. As few decisions are accompanied with absolute certainty of the consequences of the associated outcomes, decision analysis can be used to assist the decision maker to identify the available options, predict the consequences and outcomes of each option, assess the likelihood or probability of each result occurring, determine the value of each outcome, and select the decision option that will provide the best payoff. Decision analysis not only forces an explicit, orderly, and careful consideration of a variety of important issues; it also provides insight into the process of decision making.

Decision analysis is explicit—it forces one to structure the decision as well as identify the consequences of the possible outcomes. It is quantitative—it forces one to assign numbers to probability estimates and outcome valuations. It is prescriptive—the analysis identifies the decision route to take to maximize the expected value of the decision.

The origins of decision analysis, as well as many of the techniques presented in this chapter, can be traced to the British during World War II when principles of game theory, systems analysis, and operations research were applied to decisions involving the allocation of scarce resources. By the 1950s, these techniques were combined in the business world into the evolving field of decision analysis. The late 1950s saw the beginning of medical applications,[1] and the approach reached the medical literature in the early 1970s.[2-4] By the late 1980s, more than 200 publications had demonstrated the application of decision analysis to medical problems,[5] including economic evaluations like cost-minimization, cost-effectiveness, and cost–benefit analyses.[5-7] Two textbooks are commonly used as references for health care personnel.[6,7]

Decision analysis has seen increasing application in drug therapy,[8-23] although its use in therapeutic drug monitoring (TDM) is in the early stages.[16-23] As a limitation of use in drug therapy involves acquisition of the necessary data for applying decision analysis, this chapter is intended not only to demonstrate the concepts, principles, and techniques of decision analysis as applied to TDM, but also to stimulate interest in collecting and evaluating the data necessary for successful application of the technology.

USING SERUM DRUG LEVELS IN EXPECTED VALUE DECISION MAKING

Steps in the Decision Analytic Process

The six steps in performing a decision analysis are described below and summarized in Table 7–1. Each step is then discussed further with examples.

1. Determine who is making the decision (eg, practitioner, patient); identify the decision alternatives (eg, continue drug regimen, discontinue drug regimen); and select the time frame over which the decision is to be evaluated (eg, duration of hospital stay, a year of drug therapy for chronic illness).

2. Structure the decision process over the time frame selected. Include for each decision alternative the range of outcomes that may result (eg, in choosing drug A, the patient may respond appropriately or may be nonresponsive) and subsequent decision alternatives that may arise from an outcome (eg, nonresponse needs a subsequent decision about alternative drugs).

3. Assess the probability of each outcome occurring. Each outcome has a certain likelihood of occurring (eg, on average, 75% of patients respond appropriately to drug A and 25% do not).

4. Assign a value to each outcome pathway. The outcomes that may result from a decision have varying merit or consequence. Values may be measured in different units (eg, cost, quality of life), and each outcome should be assigned a value.

5. Select the decision alternative with the highest expected value. The sum of the product of probability multiplied by the value for each of the outcomes associated with a decision alternative represents the expected value for the decision alternative. The alternative with the highest expected value is favored.

6. Do a sensitivity analysis. Does the rank order of expected values for the decision alternatives change (and therefore the choice of favored alternative) if the probability estimates or outcome values are varied?

These six steps characterize the general use of decision analysis for situations when it is uncertain which of various alternatives is the best choice. Applied to therapeutic drug monitor-

TABLE 7–1. STEPS IN APPLYING DECISION ANALYSIS

1. Determine the decision alternatives to be studied, who is making the decision, and the time frame over which the decision process is to be evaluated.

2. Structure the decision process, including the consequences resulting from each decision alternative, over time.

3. Assess the probability that each consequence will occur.

4. Determine the value of each outcome (eg, in dollars, quality-adjusted life years saved, utilities).

5. Select the decision alternative with the highest expected value.

6. Do a sensitivity analysis, varying the more questionable outcome probabilities and values, to see if the decision changes.

ing, the serum drug concentration makes its specific contribution in Step 3 by contributing probabilistic information about the status of the patient. The six steps summarized in Table 7–1 are now discussed in detail.

Step 1: Identifying the Decision Process

One of the most common applications of serum drug levels is to provide information that assists in reassessing the probability of patient status. A typical, uncomplicated decision tree for this application is shown in general form in Figure 7–1. Let us apply the tree specifically to an example of a patient taking theophylline. The patient has experienced a side effect or adverse reaction which may be a consequence of taking the drug. The decision maker is assumed to be the physician or some other practitioner who will advise the physician, the decision alternatives are to continue the theophylline regimen unchanged or discontinue the drug, and the time frame extends from emergence of toxic symptoms to shortly after the selected decision alternative is acted on.

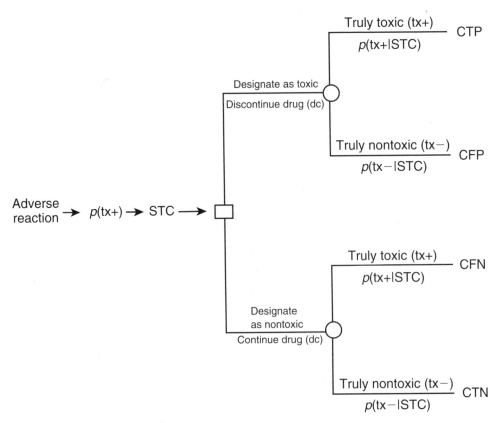

Figure 7–1. Decision tree for continuing or discontinuing drug. Theophylline is used as an example, with STC denoting the serum theophylline concentration and $p(\text{tx+}|\text{STC})$ and $p(\text{tx-}|\text{STC})$ representing the positive predictive value of toxicity and negative predictive value of no toxicity, respectively, resulting from the pretest probability of toxicity, $p(\text{tx+})$, and the STC.

Step 2: Structuring the Decision Tree

The decision noted in Figure 7–1 is structured as follows: The practitioner first makes an assessment of the pretest (sometimes called prior) probability, p(tx+), that the toxicity is induced by theophylline. *Pretest probability* is the term used to describe the likelihood of a clinical condition occurring (toxic reaction in this example) based on the available information prior to seeking additional tests or data. After the pretest probability has been set, the practitioner orders a test, in this case the serum theophylline concentration (STC). As a result of the additional information provided by the STC, the practitioner in this example has two alternatives: to designate the patient as toxic (tx+) and discontinue the drug or nontoxic (tx−) and continue the drug.

In the decision tree of Figure 7–1, the square preceding the two decision alternatives is called a choice node, meaning that the next action is determined by the decision maker and not left to chance. The clinician will choose to call the patient toxic or nontoxic based on the clinical symptoms, STC, and probability of toxicity or nontoxicity provided by the STC as a test; the latter information is commonly referred to as the test performance characteristics of the test. Regardless of which decision alternative is selected by the practitioner, the true status of the patient is unknown, because the STC cannot cleanly separate patient populations into those that are toxic and those that are nontoxic. If the patient is called toxic by the practitioner, the true status may be tx+ or tx−, and the same uncertainty applies if the patient is called nontoxic. Therefore, as tx+ and tx− are the only two true states the patient may be in, these two outcomes are noted in the tree for both decision alternatives that may be selected by the practitioner, designating the patient as toxic or nontoxic.

This uncertainty as to whether the patient is tx+ or tx− is denoted by the circle (○), called a chance node, after each of the decision alternatives, meaning that the outcomes resulting from the decision are not under the control of the practitioner. It is important to note that a number of side effects and/or adverse reactions (generically termed *toxicity* in this chapter) may be induced by theophylline and a separate tree should formally be drawn for each manifestation of toxicity because the decision may change depending on the severity of the toxicity. In practice, however, when more than one toxic effect is observed, the decision process can usually be analyzed by drawing a single tree that describes the most serious of the toxic effects. The probability notation in Figure 7–1 that is associated with each outcome (eg, p[tx+| STC]) is discussed below under Step 3 and the valuation of each of these decision pathways noted at the right of each outcome is described under Step 4.

Step 3: Assessing Probabilities of Outcomes

Step 3 in the decision process involves assigning a probability estimate for each event resulting from a chance node (○) in the decision tree, making sure that the sum of the probabilities for all of the events arising from a chance node add to 1.0 (eg, the probabilities of tx+ and tx− outcomes resulting from the chance node at the end of the "designate as tx+" decision alternative in Figure 7–1 must sum to 1.0).

The tree in Figure 7–1 describes a bayesian approach to using serum drug levels in which the additional probabilistic information gained from the serum level test is used to revise the pretest probability to estimate a posttest probability. A bayesian approach to interpreting diagnostic test information involves the following sequence: The practitioner estimates the probability of the condition being present before a test is ordered, the pretest probability, p(tx+); the test is ordered, new information is obtained from the test result, and that information is combined with the pretest probability to yield a revised probability, the posttest probability, $p(\text{tx}+|\text{STC})$. In Figure 7–1, $p(\text{tx}+|\text{STC})$, is assigned to the truly tx+ outcome pathway, and the companion probability, $p(\text{tx}-|\text{STC})$, is assigned to the truly tx– pathway. These posttest probabilities are termed *conditional probabilities,* denoting the probabilities of toxicity and nontoxicity, respectively, given the patient's STC. A conditional probability characterizes the likelihood of an event occurring given some existing condition. For example, the conditional probabilities noted above, $p(\text{tx}+|\text{STC})$ and $p(\text{tx}-|\text{STC})$, are read: "The probability of toxicity in the patient, given the STC measurement" and "the probability of nontoxicity, given the STC," respectively. These two outcome probabilities, resulting from both chance nodes in Figure 7–1, must add to 1.0 for each of the two chance nodes.

To discuss probability assessment, we introduce in Table 7–2 the retrospective analysis we performed of published data reporting drug levels and concomitant verification of toxic or nontoxic status for 280 hospitalized adults patients administered theophylline parenterally as aminophylline.[18] The distribution of serum theophylline concentrations and patient status are recorded in Table 7–2.

Bayes' formula is used to link the practitioner's pretest assessment of probability, the test performance characteristics of the test result (STC represents the test here), and the revised posttest probability, as

$$\text{posttest probability} = \frac{p(\text{tx}+)(\text{true-positive range rate})}{p(\text{tx}+)(\text{true-positive range rate}) + (1 - p(\text{tx}+))(\text{false-positive range rate})}$$
$$(7\text{–}1)$$

where $p(\text{tx}+)$ is the pretest probability of toxicity, $1 - p(\text{tx}+)$ is the pretest probability of no toxicity, true-positive range rate is the fraction of the total number of toxic patients that have a STC within a narrow range of STC values that contains the patient's measured STC, and false-positive range rate is the fraction of nontoxic patients within the same STC range. Referring to Table 7–2 for illustration, the fraction of toxic patients with a STC within the range 19 to 20.9 µg/mL is 3/39, so the true-positive range rate is 0.077. The fraction of nontoxic patients within the range is 11/241, so the false-positive range rate is 0.046.

The assessment of pretest probability, which is important to set with care, may be objective or subjective. Objective assessments may come from population-based literature data or from estimates gained at the specific hospital or clinic site. The prevalence of the condition may also be used as a population-based pretest probability. Subjective, more patient-specific estimates may reflect expert opinions of colleagues or the practitioner's own "hunch" concerning the individual patient's condition. A combination of literature awareness blended with practitioner experience is the most likely basis for estimating an individualized pretest probability.

Some find it easier to appreciate the link between pretest probability, serum drug concentration test characteristics, and posttest probability by casting Bayes' formula in its odds ratio form. Continuing with the theophylline toxicity example, the odds ratio format is shown in Equation 7–2; the formula is converted to the more common probability notation

$$\text{posttest odds of toxicity} = \text{pretest odds of toxicity} \times \text{test likelihood ratio} \qquad (7\text{–}2)$$

$$\frac{p(\text{tx}+|\text{STC})}{p(\text{tx}-|\text{STC})} = \frac{p(\text{tx}+)}{p(\text{tx}-)} \times \frac{p(\text{STC}|\text{tx}+)}{p(\text{STC}|\text{tx}-)} \qquad (7\text{–}3)$$

TABLE 7–2. DISTRIBUTION OF SERUM THEOPHYLLINE CONCENTRATIONS (STCs) FOR PATIENTS WITH VERIFIED TOXICITY STATUS[a]

STC (μg/mL)	Toxic (tx+)	Nontoxic (tx−)	Range Likelihood Ratio (+)[b]
>31	10	3	20.6
29–30.9	2	1	12.4
27–28.9	2	2	6.2
25–26.9	2	3	4.1
23–24.9	4	7	3.5
21–22.9	4	9	2.7
19–20.9	3	11	1.7
17–18.9	3	18	1.0
15–16.9	3	26	0.7
13–14.9	4	28	0.9
11–12.9	2	40	0.3
9–10.9	0	40	0
<9	0	53	0
Total	39	241	

[a]Prevalence of toxicity is 14% (39/280).

[b]True-positive range rate/false-positive range rate; p(STC range |tx+)/p(STC range |tx−).

From Schumacher GE, Barr JT. Applying decision analysis in therapeutic drug monitoring: Using decision trees to interpret serum theophylline concentrations. Clin Pharm. *1986;5:325–333, with permission.*

In these equations, test likelihood ratio refers to the range likelihood ratio associated with the serum drug level. There are two types of likelihood ratios, one resulting from a positive test result and one from a negative test. The range likelihood ratio (+) for a positive test result (patient's drug level above the test cutoff level) is the ratio of true-positive range rate, p(STC|tx+), to false-positive range rate, p(STC|tx−), within the most narrow concentration range practical, given the available data. The range likelihood ratio (−) for a negative test result (patient's drug level below the test cutoff level) is the ratio of false-negative range rate to true-negative range rate. Equation 7–3 refers to just the posttest revision due to a positive test result because the test likelihood ratio shown is the ratio of the true-positive to false-positive range rates. Another way to view the concept of the likelihood ratio is to note, on rearranging Equation 7–2, that it represents the ratio of the posttest odds to the pretest odds.

The use of odds in Equations 7–2 and 7–3 is an alternative form of expressing probability. Probability is a number between 0 and 1 that characterizes the likelihood of an event occurring. Odds represents the ratio of the likelihood of an event occurring divided by the likelihood of the event not occurring. The interconversion of odds and probability is expressed as

$$\text{probability} = \text{odds}/(1 + \text{odds}) \tag{7–4}$$

$$\text{odds} = p/(1 - p) \tag{7–5}$$

_____ **EXAMPLE 7–1** _____

A practitioner estimates that there is one chance in four that the observed adverse reaction in a patient is due to theophylline. A serum theophylline level is ordered and measures 22 μg/mL, which as noted in Table 7–2 is associated with a range likelihood ratio of 2.7. The likelihood ratio may be referred to as positive (LR+), although this designation is not necessary to determine the posttest probability, as the top of the commonly accepted therapeutic range for theophylline is 20 μg/mL and the patient's test result is therefore positive. What is the posttest probability of theophylline-induced toxicity in this patient?

The statement "one chance in four" means a pretest odds of 1/3 (one chance of a drug reaction divided by three chances of no drug reaction). After the theophylline level is obtained, Equation 7–2 is used to calculate the revised, posttest odds:

$$\text{posttest odds} = (1/3) \times 2.7 = 0.9/1$$

To convert this to probability form, use Equation 7–4:

$$\text{posttest probability} = (0.93/1) / (0.93/1 + 1) = 0.48$$

The probabilistic information contributed to the evaluation by the serum level revises the pretest odds of toxicity from 1/3 to posttest odds of almost 1/1. In probability terms, the pretest of 0.25 has been nearly doubled to a posttest of 0.47. As all outcomes resulting from a chance node must sum to 1.0, the posttest probability for the nontoxic outcome in Figure 7–1 is 0.53.

Assume that instead of the patient's level measuring 22 μg/mL, it reads 12 μg/mL. In this case, the range likelihood ratio associated with this level using the data in Table 7–2 is 0.3. The likelihood ratio may be referred to as negative as the patient's level is below the cutoff of 20 μg/mL and is therefore a negative test result. This converts the pretest odds of 1/3 to 1/10:

$$\text{posttest odds} = (1/3) \times 0.3 = 1/10$$

The two situations described in the preceding example illustrate the bayesian approach to probability revision, wherein the practitioner's individualized assessment of the patient's status has been combined with the patient's test result to provide a revised patient-specific odds or probability of toxicity. The likelihood ratio associated with the drug level results in a posttest assessment that is greater than the pretest when the likelihood ratio is greater than one. When the likelihood ratio is less than one, the posttest probability is less than the pretest. The process of converting pretest to posttest probabilities occurs each time new information is sought. Should the practitioner in the above situation decide to obtain additional information that may modify the probability of toxicity, the posttest probability of 0.48 (using the case of the theophylline level measuring 22 μg/mL) then becomes the pretest probability for the new sequence of bayesian revision.

_____ **EXAMPLE 7–2** _____

Equation 7–1 may be used as the more traditional form of Bayes' formula to determine the posttest probability in Example 7–1. The pretest odds of 1/3 are converted, using Equation 7–4, to a pretest probability, p(tx+), of 0.25. The true-positive and false-positive range rates for a serum concentration of 22 µg/mL are calculated from the data in Table 7–2:

$$\text{posttest probability} = \frac{p(\text{tx+}) \ (\text{true-positive range rate})}{p(\text{tx+})(\text{true-positive range rate}) + (1 - p(\text{tx+}))(\text{false-positive range rate})}$$

$$\text{posttest probability} = \frac{(0.25)(4/39)}{(0.25)(4/39) + (0.75)(9/241)} = 0.48$$

To reduce the effort in making these calculations for every case, a family of conditional probability curves may be constructed, as shown for theophylline in Figure 7–2. We used the data in Table 7–2, in conjunction with Equation 7–1, to construct the curves relating pretest (called prior in the figure) probability, p(tx+), to posttest (called posterior in the figure) probability, p(tx+|STC).[18] We formed each curve by using various values for the pretest probability, multiplied by the range likelihood ratio (+) for the concentration range, to calculate the various associated posttest probabilities.

The conditional probability curves in Figure 7–2 are graphic depictions of bayesian probability revision that eliminate the need to make calculations for individual patients. These curves represent the posttest probability of toxicity conditioned on the measured serum theophylline concentration. The pretest probability is located on the horizontal axis; a line is extended vertically until it intersects with the range containing the theophylline level and then is extended horizontally until it intersects the associated posttest probability on the vertical axis.

_____ **EXAMPLE 7–3** _____

Assume that Practitioner A estimates a patient's pretest probability of theophylline-induced toxicity as 0.25, obtains a STC of 20 µg/mL, and uses Figure 7–2 to estimate a revised posttest probability of 0.36. On the other hand, Practitioner B estimates the same patient's pretest probability as 0.50, which converts, using the same STC of 20 µg/mL, to a posttest probability of 0.62. This example illustrates in quantitative terms the subjective nature of probability assessment that underlies the notion of a "second opinion." Because bayesian probability blends the human perception of patient-specific risk with the population probability data contained in the patient's drug level, varying perceptions of pretest risk will lead to varying posttest probability, even with the same test (drug level) result. Practitioner A sees less risk of toxicity than does Practitioner B. The patient's drug level revises both risk levels upward but it is still lower for Practitioner A than B. If the patient is involved in the decision, or if a third practitioner must make the decision based on the input from A and B, the posttest probability to be used in the decision tree is likely to come from the practitioner viewed to be most accurate in estimating pretest probability.

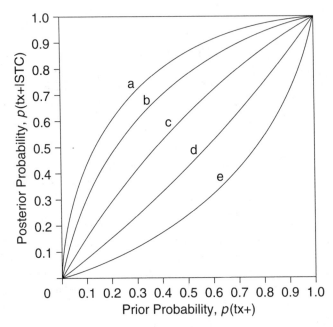

Figure 7–2. Conditional probability curves relating prior probability of toxicity, $p(\text{tx}+)$, and serum theophylline concentration (STC) to posterior probability of toxicity, $p(\text{tx}+|\text{STC})$. STC ranges and likelihood ratios (LRs) corresponding to curves a–e are as follows: (a) STC = 27–28.9 μg/mL, LR = 6.38; (b) STC = 23–24.9 μg/mL, LR = 3.55; (c) STC = 19–20.9 μg/mL, LR = 1.67; (d) STC = 15–16.9 μg/mL, LR = 0.71; (e) STC = 11–12.9 μg/mL, LR = 0.31. (*From Schumacher GE, Barr JT. Applying decision analysis in therapeutic drug monitoring: Using decision trees to interpret serum theophylline concentrations. Clin Pharm. 1986;5:325–333, with permission.*)

Step 4: Assigning Values for Outcome Pathways

Each step in the decision process leads to an outcome. Decision makers place different values or consequences on the various ways that things can turn out; some of the outcomes are valued highly, whereas others are considered inferior. The purpose of Step 4 is to quantitate the value or worth of these outcomes so that they may be compared with each other.

The tree in Figure 7–1 includes notation for the value term (sometimes called consequence) assigned to each outcome in this decision analysis. The acronyms CTP, CFP, CFN, and CTN refer to the consequences (C) associated with true-positive, false-positive, false-negative, and true-negative outcomes, respectively. These four possible outcomes are described as:

- *True-positive:* a truly toxic patient corrrectly presumed by the practitioner to be toxic.
- *False-positive:* a truly nontoxic patient falsely presumed by the practitioner to be toxic.

- *False-negative:* a truly toxic patient falsely presumed by the practitioner to be nontoxic.
- *True-negative:* a truly nontoxic patient correctly presumed by the practitioner to be nontoxic.

Using the decision tree in Figure 7–1, all would agree that a true-negative outcome is much preferable to a false-negative outcome. In the former case drug treatment is appropriately continued in a nontoxic patient but in the latter case it is continued inappropriately in a toxic patient. Alternatively stated, a false-negative action is considered to be of much greater consequence than a true-negative action, although the magnitude of the difference in value varies with the perception of the individual decision maker. Similarly, a true-positive outcome is much more desirable than a false-positive one. Less clear, however, is the relative weighting of the two types of errors, false-positive and false-negative. For a given situation, is it more of a consequence to take action based on calling a truly nontoxic patient toxic (a false-positive) or calling a truly toxic patient nontoxic (a false-negative)?

Valuing outcomes may take many forms depending on the type of decision and the data available. In some cases like the situation depicted by the decision tree in Figure 7–1, outcomes may be measured in dollars—as measured in days of hospital stay, resources consumed, and consultations sought—for each of the four outcomes. In other cases (eg, comparing two alternative antihypertensive drug regimens), nonmonetary measures may be used, such as length of hospital stay, number of sick days away from the job per year, quality of life, and, for decisions applying to a group, number of life years extended. When a specific measure is not readily apparent or is inconvenient for the analysis, or a number of factors contribute to defining a value for the outcome, a term called *utility* is used. Although different measures may be used for valuing outcomes, depending on the intent or the data available, for a given analysis, a uniform measure (eg, quality of life, dollars, utility) should be used for rank ordering each of the outcomes in a specific decision tree.

Although valuing outcomes in dollars, life years, and so on represents an objective assessment, utility is a subjective measure that reflects a decision maker's degree of preference among possible outcomes. Utility is a dimensionless number ranging from 0 to 1. For a given set of outcomes in a decision tree (eg, the four outcomes in Figure 7–1), the most desirable outcome is generally assigned a utility of 1, the least desirable is assigned 0, and the other outcomes are given intermediate values within this range. As the assignment of the intermediate utilities is subjective, and is often done intuitively, a variety of techniques (eg, standard reference gamble, time trade-off) are nonetheless available for assisting the decision maker in assigning values.* Often, when these latter techniques are used, 1 is assigned to perfect health and 0 is assigned to death. When utility values are used for valuing outcomes, the values become specific for a given decision maker in a specific decision analysis. The values for a specific outcome may vary (1) with different decision makers valuing outcomes in the same decision tree or (2) with the value of a specific outcome in one decision tree being assigned a different value when applied to a different decision tree.

---

*References 6 (pp 252–254), 7 (pp 208–220), 24.

_____ **EXAMPLE 7–4** _____

Two physicians, A and B, discuss the situation described in Figure 7–1. Although they concur on the utility values assigned to the true-negative and false-negative outcomes, they do not
agree on the relative consequences of the true-positive and false-positive results:

	Utility Value	
Outcome	A	B
True-negative (c,tx−)	1.0	1.0
True-positive (dc,tx+)	0.8	0.9
False-positive (dc,tx−)	0.7	0.6
False-negative (c,tx+)	0	0

The designations c and dc in Figure 7–1 and above denote decisions to continue and discontinue, respectively. Both physicians agree that being able to continue theophylline in a truly
nontoxic (c,tx−) patient is the best possible outcome and that inappropriately continuing
theophylline in the truly toxic patient (c,tx+) is the worst possible outcome. Toxic reactions
to theophylline are of varying severity, so for simplicity the toxicity observed is considered to
be very serious, with both physicians agreeing that it merits a utility assignment of 0. The
physicians do not agree on the relative weighting of the other outcomes, however. Physician
A considers a true-positive outcome (dc,tx+) to be more highly valued (of less consequence)
than a false-positive (dc,tx−) one. Physician B agrees with the ranking but not the weighting
and places the relative weighting of a true-positive and a false-positive outcome as more and
less, respectively, than Physician A. Both physicians perceive that discontinuing treatment,
whether the patient is toxic or not, represents a much better outcome (utility values of 0.6–0.9
assigned) than continuing in the toxic patient. Both physicians also concur in considering a
false-positive error (utility value of 0.8 or 0.9) in this situation to be highly preferable to a
false-negative error (utility value of 0).

This subjectivity in assigning utilities is one of the strengths of decision analysis. Each decision maker selects a personalized set of outcome weights which is then used to determine the
best course of action based on the unique set of preferences.

Note that for the set of four outcomes in the decision analysis of Example 7–4, a false negative was considered the worst possible outcome and was assigned a value of 0; however, for a
different decision tree including a false-negative outcome, perhaps one that also involves death
as an outcome, death would be assigned a value of 0, and a false-negative result would surely be
valued greater than 0.

Step 5: Calculating and Using Expected Values
When choosing among alternative courses of action, the alternative with the greatest expected
value (EV) should be selected because it reflects the best weighted average value for the various
outcomes resulting from the decision alternatives. This procedure of obtaining the EV for each
decision alternative is often described as "averaging out and folding back the tree," which refers
to the process of solving the tree by working from the tips of the branches at the right backward

to the root of the tree containing the choice node for the decision alternatives at the left. To do this, working from right to left, each outcome is "averaged out" by obtaining the sum of all outcomes weighted by the probability of each outcome, as shown in

$$EV = V_1 p(O_1) + V_2 p(O_2) \ldots + V_n p(O_n) \tag{7–6}$$

$$EV = \sum_{(i=1)}^{n} V_i p(O_i) \tag{7–7}$$

where V denotes the value assigned for an outcome and $p(O)$ represents the probability of the outcome (O) occurring.

In simple trees, like the decision analysis depicted in Figure 7–1, when there is only one chance node in the pathway for each decision alternative, there is only one "averaging out" to be performed for each alternative, so the alternative with the greatest EV, as calculated using Equation 7–6, is the preferred option. More complex trees, however, contain intermediate chance nodes along the pathway stemming from each decision alternative, so the EV for each chance node is calculated, working from right to left, and then the pathway is "folded back," calculating EV for each additional chance node encountered, until EV for the decision alternative is obtained.

Using the simple tree in Figure 7–1 for illustration, for each of the two courses of action there are only two possible outcomes (tx+ and tx−). Making the general form of Equation 7–6 specific for this situation leads to Equations 7–8 and 7–9 for decisions to discontinue (presume toxic) and continue (presume nontoxic), respectively:

$$EV_{dc} = V_{dc,tx+}\, p(tx+|STC) + V_{dc,tx-}\, p(tx-|STC) \tag{7–8}$$

$$EV_{c} = V_{c,tx+}\, p(tx+|STC) + V_{c,tx-}\, p(tx-|STC) \tag{7–9}$$

The decision alternative with the greatest EV in Figure 7–1 is the best decision, given the set of outcome values assigned and the probabilities of occurrence of the four outcomes.

——————— **EXAMPLE 7–5** ———————————————————————————

Using the posttest probability of toxicity for the patient in Example 7–2 and the utility values assigned to outcomes by Physician A in Example 7–4, and applying the data to the decision tree depicted in Figure 7–1, is the best decision to continue or discontinue theophylline in the patient? Using Equations 7–8 and 7–9,

$$EV_{dc} = (0.48)(0.8) + (0.52)(0.7) = 0.75$$

$$EV_{c} = (0.48)(0) + (0.52)(1.0) = 0.52$$

The decision alternative to discontinue has the greatest expected value and is therefore the preferred course of action.

Step 6: Conducting a Sensitivity Analysis

The data used to calculate expected values come from the assessment of outcome probabilities in Step 3 and the assignment of outcome values in Step 4. If some of these data are subjective, does varying the data alter the EV for the decision alternatives to the extent that the preferred course of action obtained in Step 5 is changed? For example, would realistic variations of either the utility values or the posttest probabilities used in Example 7–5 lead to changes in EV for the decision alternatives such that continuing theophylline would become the preferred alternative?

Of the data that can be manipulated, assignment of subjective values such as utility assessments for the outcomes represents the most likely candidate. If valuing outcomes is relatively objective (eg, dollars), however, there may be little flexibility in altering the outcome values except for deciding to omit or add certain categories of costs. When the probabilities associated with the outcomes are subjectively assessed, they may be altered, but when data are extensive enough to be considered objective representations, the probabilities are most likely fixed.

If large changes in variables do not alter the rank order of the EV for the decision alternatives, then the preferred decision determined in Step 5 is robust. But if small changes in variables alter the choice of decision alternative, then the result of Step 5 must be considered with some caution.

Using Serum Theophylline Concentrations to Illustrate Decision Analysis

The six steps of decision analysis outlined in Table 7–1 are now applied to the situation depicted in Figure 7–3. This is a more complex and realistic situation than shown previously in Figure 7–1. In this case, the practitioner must decide whether to continue the theophylline regimen unchanged, lower the regimen, or discontinue the drug, based on observing an adverse event which may or may not be the result of taking theophylline. Similar to the decision tree shown in Figure 7–1, the status of the patient, regardless of the decision alternative selected, is either toxic or nontoxic. This results in a tree containing three decision alternatives and six possible outcomes.

To conduct the decision analysis we again used the data discussed previously from our retrospective analysis of reported drug levels and concomitant verification of toxic or nontoxic status for 280 hospitalized adults patients administered theophylline parenterally as aminophylline.[18] We used the family of conditional probability curves shown previously in Figure 7–2 to convert pretest to posttest probabilities. The utilities we assigned for the six possible outcomes are shown in Table 7–3.[18] The utility range was set at 0.2 to 1.0; 0.2 represents the least desirable outcome of continuing the regimen unchanged in a patient who is truly toxic, and 1.0 represents the most desirable outcome of continuing the dosage regimen unchanged in a patient who is truly nontoxic.

Contrary to the tree in Figure 7–1, in which the lowest utility value of 0 was assigned for continuing the regimen unchanged in the toxic patient, we did not do this for the same outcome in the decision analysis described in Figure 7–3. In reality, some of the utility values assigned for the various outcomes would change depending on the severity of the adverse effect (eg, headache, nausea, arrhythmia, seizure) that precipitated the decision problem. Continuing treatment with a theophylline-induced headache, for example, would most likely be valued higher than continuing in the face of a drug-induced arrhythmia. As this decision analysis assumes that the patient presents with one toxic effect, yet the specific adverse effect has not been defined, the resulting tree in Figure 7–3 is a generic depiction, and the range of toxic effects have been pooled

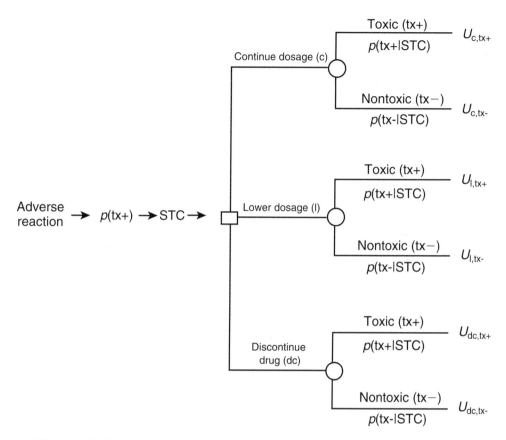

Figure 7–3. Decision tree for continuing, lowering, or discontinuing drug dosage. Theophylline is used as an example, with STC denoting the serum theophylline concentration; p(tx+|STC) and p(tx−|STC) representing the positive predictive value of toxicity and negative predictive value of no toxicity, respectively, resulting from the pretest probability of toxicity, p(tx+), and the STC; and U representing the utility value assigned to each outcome.

to assign an average utility of 0.2 for the outcome of continuing dosage unchanged in a truly toxic patient.

A utility score for an outcome reflects the overall assessment of the positive and negative aspects of the outcome. High and low utility scores represent favorable and unfavorable trade-offs of factors contributing to an outcome, respectively. As noted above, an outcome of continuing a needed drug in a patient with a side effect like nausea would generally receive a higher utility score than continuing the drug in a patient with an adverse effect like an arrhythmia. An outcome of continuing a drug in a patient with the side effect of persistent headache would likely be assigned a lower utility score if the drug has a good substitute than if it is the drug of choice with no suitable alternative.

TABLE 7–3. UTILITY VALUES ASSIGNED TO THE POSSIBLE OUTCOMES FOR THE THEOPHYLLINE DOSAGE REGIMEN DECISION PROCESS[a]

Outcome	Designation	Utility[b]
Continue same dosage in patient who is not in toxic condition	$U_{c,tx-}$	1.0
Discontinue drug in patient who is in toxic condition	$U_{dc,tx+}$	0.95
Lower dosage in patient who is in toxic condition	$U_{l,tx+}$	0.8
Lower dosage in patient who is not in toxic condition	$U_{l,tx-}$	0.6
Discontinue drug in patient who is not in toxic condition	$U_{dc,tx-}$	0.4
Continue same dosage in patient who is in toxic condition	$U_{c,tx+}$	0.2[c]

[a]Based on the situation depicted by the decision tree in Figure 7–3.
[b]The relative value of each outcome resulting from a set of decisions in which the best and worst possible outcomes are assigned utility values of 1 and 0, respectively.
[c]See text for explanation.

_____ **EXAMPLE 7–6** _____

A practitioner estimates a pretest probability of 0.25 (odds of 1/3) of a patient having a toxic effect as a result of a theophylline regimen. A STC is ordered and measures 20 µg/mL. Using the decision tree in Figure 7–3 for this case, in which the pretest probability of toxicity is modest and the drug level is at the top of the commonly accepted therapeutic range, is the best decision to continue the regimen unchanged, lower the regimen, or discontinue the theophylline? Assume that the practitioner agrees with the utility values for the outcomes shown in Table 7–3.

The posttest probability of toxicity may be estimated from inspection of the 19.0 to 20.9 µg/mL conditional probability curve in Figure 7–2. Alternately, it may be calculated using data in Table 7–2 and Equation 7–1 or Equations 7–2 and 7–4. From either approach, the posttest probability of toxicity is estimated in the patient as 0.36.

Then using the utility values in Table 7–3 and Equations 7–8 and 7–9 to calculate the expected values for decisions to discontinue and continue, respectively, and a similar equation for the decision to lower :

$$EV_{dc} = (0.36)(0.95) + (0.64)(0.4) = 0.60$$

$$EV_c = (0.36)(0.2) + (0.64)(1.0) = 0.71$$

$$EV_l = (0.36)(0.8) + (0.64)(0.6) = 0.67$$

For this set of outcome utility values, a pretest probability of 0.25 followed by a STC of 20 µg/mL and a resulting posttest probability of 0.36 leads to the greatest expected value for the decision alternative of continuing the regimen unchanged.

Table 7–4 presents eight prototypical cases for theophylline with varying pretest probability and STC values. For all cases, however, the set of utility values in Table 7–3 is constant. The cases are arranged in order of increasing posttest probability of toxicity. As the posttest proba-

TABLE 7–4. POSTTEST PROBABILITY AND GREATEST EXPECTED UTILITY FOR THEOPHYLLINE DECISION ALTERNATIVES IN VARIOUS PROTOTYPE CASES[a]

Case	Pretest Probability of Toxicity, p(tx+)	STC (μg/mL)	Posttest Probability of Toxicity, p(tx+|STC)	Decision With Greatest Expected Utility
1	0.33	16	0.26	Continue
2	0.25	20	0.36	Continue
3	0.67	12	0.39	Continue
4	0.5	16	0.42	Lower
5	0.25	22	0.47	Lower
6	0.67	16	0.59	Discontinue
7	0.5	20	0.63	Discontinue
8	0.33	24	0.64	Discontinue

[a] Based on the situation depicted by the decision tree in Figure 7–3.

bility increases, the decision changes from continue to lower to discontinue. Observe how the interplay of pretest probability and STC produces varying posttest probabilities, resulting in differing decision alternatives with the greatest EV.

Using Threshold Probabilities

Calculations of this sort are cumbersome. It would be more expeditious to have some quantitative benchmark, a decision threshold, that separates the selection of one decision alternative from another. In other words, what range of posttest probabilities of toxicity leads to favoring the decision to discontinue over the decision to continue the dosage unchanged in Figure 7–1? What posttest probability separates the decision of discontinuing from the decision of lowering or separates the decision of lowering from that of continuing in Figure 7–3? The threshold probability approach to decision making, as developed by Pauker and Kassirer,[25,26] provides a method for determining these values.

This approach, as it applies specifically to the type of decision analyses illustrated in Figures 7–1 and 7–3, states that for any given set of utility values assigned to the various outcomes resulting from two alternative courses of action (eg, continue or discontinue, continue or lower, lower or discontinue), there is a threshold probability (T) that yields identical expected values for the two alternatives. When the posttest probability in a patient is equal to T, the decision maker has no preference for the alternatives and the decision is considered a "tossup." But when the posttest probability is greater than T, the more aggressive decision alternative is favored: discontinue versus continue favors discontinue, discontinue versus lower favors discontinue, and lower vs continue favors lower. Conversely, when the posttest probability is less than T, the opposite decision alternative from above is favored.

This concept is shown in Figure 7–4 for the two decision alternatives depicted in Figure 7–1. When the posttest probability is less than T_{dc}, the probability of toxicity is not great enough to warrant discontinuing the drug. But when the posttest probability increases above T_{dc}, the probability is high enough to warrant discontinuing treatment. Figure 7–5 depicts the situation

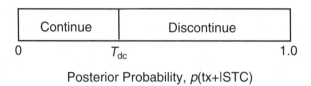

Figure 7–4. Threshold probability of toxicity for decision to continue or discontinue.

for the three decision alternatives described in Figure 7–3. When the posttest probability is less than T_1, continuing is favored over lowering the dosage. As the probability of toxicity increases above T_{dc}, however, discontinuing drug becomes preferable to lowering the dosage.

This approach has been generalized by Pauker and Kassirer[25] as the cost–benefit method of determining the threshold probability. It classifies each outcome resulting from two decision alternatives as either a benefit or cost in the decision process, defining these indices in terms of utility. The benefit of treatment applies to the outcomes of patients with the target disorder. The cost of treatment refers to the outcomes of patients without the target disorder. In general terms the target disorder may be considered a disease or illness. In the specific examples common to TDM, as shown in Figures 7–1 and 7–3, the target disorder is drug-induced toxicity.

In the example illustrated by Figure 7–1, two strategies are possible for the patient with an adverse reaction that may be drug induced: discontinuing or continuing the drug. Benefit (B) in this decision situation is defined as the net effect of dealing with the toxic patient (the target disorder). Net benefit, therefore, is the difference in utility between discontinuing and continuing in a toxic patient:

$$B_{dc} = U_{dc,tx+} - U_{c,tx+} \qquad (7\text{–}10)$$

Cost (C) in this situation is defined as the net effect of dealing with the nontoxic patient. Net cost, therefore, is the difference in utility between continuing and discontinuing in a nontoxic patient:

$$C_{dc} = U_{c,tx-} - U_{dc,tx-} \qquad (7\text{–}11)$$

The threshold probability (T) is generally defined for any two alternative decisions:

$$T = \frac{C}{C + B} \qquad (7\text{–}12)$$

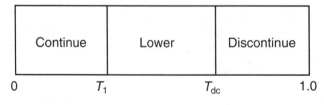

Figure 7–5. Threshold probability of toxicity for decision to continue, lower, or discontinue.

Specifically for the discontinue versus continue decision in Figure 7–1,

$$T_{dc} = \frac{C_{dc}}{C_{dc} + B_{dc}} = \frac{U_{c,tx-} - U_{dc,tx-}}{(U_{c,tx-} - U_{dc,tx-}) + (U_{dc,tx+} - U_{c,tx+})} \qquad (7\text{--}13)$$

Note in Equation 7–13 that the threshold probability depends only on the selection of utilities for the various outcomes in the decision process. Once the net benefit and cost of a decision process are determined, T_{dc} is a constant.

As the net benefit-to-cost ratio (B/C) ratio for choosing between these two decision alternatives increases, Equation 7–13 shows that the T_{dc} decreases. This is because increasing benefit (the net effect of discontinuing drug in the toxic patient) urges the decision maker to be less cautious in taking action. If two practitioners have different utilities for outcomes in the same decision analysis situation, the practitioner with the higher B/C ratio will cross the threshold for selecting discontinuing versus continuing at a lower posttest probability of toxicity.

_____   **EXAMPLE 7–7**   _____

Using the decision process described by Figure 7–1, two practitioners assign the following utilities to the four outcomes resulting from the decision process to continue or discontinue theophylline in a patient with a serious toxic effect that may be induced by the drug:

Outcome	Practitioner A	Practitioner B
$U_{c,tx-}$	1.0	1.0
$U_{dc,tx+}$	0.9	0.95
$U_{dc,tx-}$	0.7	0.6
$U_{c,tx+}$	0	0

Using Equation 7–13,

$$T_{dc} = \frac{U_{c,tx-} - U_{dc,tx-}}{(U_{c,tx-} - U_{dc,tx-}) + (U_{dc,tx+} - U_{c,tx+})}$$

$$T_{dc} \text{ for Practitioner A} = \frac{1.0 - 0.7}{(1.0 - 0.7) + (0.9 - 0)} = 0.25 \quad (B/C = 3)$$

$$T_{dc} \text{ for Practitioner B} = \frac{1.0 - 0.6}{(1.0 - 0.6) + (0.95 - 0)} = 0.3 \quad (B/C = 2.2)$$

Practitioner A reaches the threshold for converting from the continuing to discontinuing alternative at a lower posttest probability of toxicity than does Practitioner B. As the net B/C ratio of utilities is greater for A than B (3 compared with 2.2), the perceived benefit of taking action is higher for A than B. As a result, A is less cautious than B in discontinuing the drug; A discontinues at a lower posttest probability of toxicity than does B.

For the three alternative decisions depicted in Figure 7–3, two threshold probabilities exist, T_1 for the continuing versus lowering alternative and T_{dc} for the lowering versus discontinuing option. The action steps in the former and latter alternatives are lowering and discontinuing, respectively. Let us summarize the relationship between the posttest probability of toxicity and these two threshold probabilities, as noted in Figure 7–5:

- When $p(tx+|STC) < T_1$, choose the decision to continue.
- When $T_1 < p(tx+|STC) < T_{dc}$, choose the decision to lower.
- When $p(tx+|STC) > T_{dc}$, choose the decision to discontinue.

The threshold probability for the decision to continue versus lower is calculated for a given set of outcome utility values by using the equation

$$T_1 = \frac{U_{c,tx-} - U_{1,tx-}}{(U_{c,tx-} - U_{1,tx-}) + (U_{1,tx+} - U_{c,tx+})} \tag{7–14}$$

Similarly, for the decision to lower versus discontinue, we use

$$T_{dc} = \frac{U_{1,tx-} - U_{dc,tx-}}{(U_{1,tx-} - U_{dc,tx-}) + (U_{dc,tx+} - U_{1,tx+})} \tag{7–15}$$

where $U_{c,tx-} - U_{1,tx-}$ and $U_{1,tx-} - U_{dc,tx-}$ represent the net cost in Equations 7–14 and 7–15, respectively, and $U_{1,tx+} - U_{c,tx+}$ and $U_{dc,tx+} - U_{1,tx+}$ denote the net benefit in the respective equations.

In Equations 7–10, 7–11, and 7–13 to 7–15, U refers to the utility value for an outcome. Should measures other than utility be used to calculate outcome values (eg, dollars, lives saved), these measures may be substituted for utility in the equations.

_____ EXAMPLE 7–8 _____

Using the utility values shown in Table 7–3, what posttest probability of toxicity represents the threshold probability for the decision to continue versus lower the theophylline regimen for the situation depicted in Figure 7–3? What posttest probability of toxicity represents the threshold probability for the decision to discontinue versus lower the regimen?

Using Equation 7–14,

$$T_1 = \frac{1.0 - 0.6}{(1.0 - 0.6) + (0.8 - 0.2)} = 0.40$$

Using Equation 7–15,

$$T_{dc} = \frac{0.6 - 0.4}{(0.6 - 0.4) + (0.95 - 0.8)} = 0.57$$

When the posttest probability of toxicity is less than 0.40, the best decision is to continue. When the posttest probability is greater than 0.57, discontinuing the regimen is the best decision.

Table 7–5 records the threshold probabilities for the three decision alternatives shown in the tree of Figure 7–3, using the utility values shown in Table 7–3. The preferred decision is to continue the theophylline unchanged, lower the regimen, or discontinue the drug when the posttest probability of toxicity is less than 0.40, greater than 0.40 up to 0.57, or greater than 0.57, respectively. Once threshold probabilities are established for a given drug toxicity in a decision tree, it becomes unnecessary to calculate EV for each decision alternative when a decision analysis for a patient is encountered, assuming that the set of outcome utility values used to calculate T_l and T_{dc} are not changed. These threshold probabilities will not apply for other toxic effects induced by the drug, however, if the outcome utility values vary with the differing toxic effects.

The calculation of threshold probabilities in Table 7–5 provides a basis for conducting a sensitivity analysis of the theophylline decision process. Variations in pretest probability of toxicity, theophylline drug level, and/or performance characteristics of the drug level as a test will change the expected values for the decision alternatives and may result in a change in the preferred alternative. Variations in the set of outcome utilities used for calculating the threshold probabilities will, using Equations 7–14 and 7–15, lead to changes in T_l and T_{dc}, and this may change the preferred alternative for a given decision analysis.

USING SERUM DRUG LEVELS AS DIAGNOSTIC TESTS: APPLYING TEST PERFORMANCE CHARACTERISTICS

Another common application of serum drug levels is in interpreting patient status. A typical decision tree for this application is shown in Figure 7–6. The patient has experienced an adverse reaction which may be a consequence of taking the drug. The practitioner orders a serum level and uses the measurement in conjunction with other data and impressions to classify the patient as drug-induced toxic or nontoxic.

In therapeutic drug monitoring, serum drug concentrations are frequently measured for drugs with narrow ranges of therapeutic concentrations because experience suggests that there are target concentration ranges that may improve patient response and decrease toxicity. The reason for the tree depicted in Figure 7–6, however, is that serum levels are not infallible measures of patient status. It is inevitable that some patients develop drug toxicity in the therapeutic range, whereas others show a nontoxic, therapeutic response in the toxic range. As a result, the target concentration range for various drugs cannot completely separate the toxic from the nontoxic populations (or, for that matter, the therapeutic from the subtherapeutic populations).

TABLE 7–5. THRESHOLD PROBABILITIES FOR THEOPHYLLINE DECISION ALTERNATIVES

Threshold Probability,[a] p(tx+|STC)	Best Decision
< 0.40	Continue
> 0.40—0.57	Lower
> 0.57	Discontinue

[a]Based on the situation depicted by the decision tree in Figure 7–3 and the utilities assigned in Table 7–3.

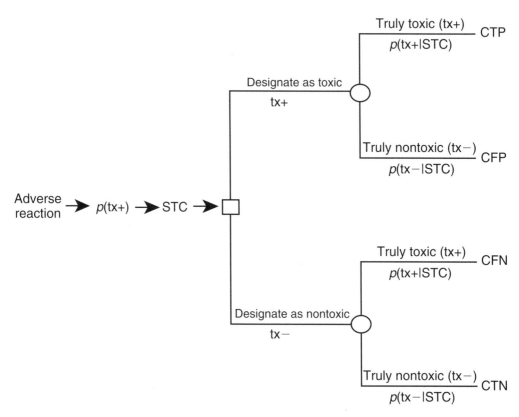

Figure 7–6. Decision tree for ruling in or ruling out drug-induced toxicity. Theophylline is used as an example, with STC denoting the serum theophylline concentration and $p(tx+|STC)$ and $p(tx-|STC)$ representing the positive predictive value of toxicity and negative predictive value of no toxicity, respectively, resulting from the pretest probability of toxicity, $p(tx+)$, and the STC.

Nonetheless, the information provided by a patient's drug level may be markedly enhanced by using decision analytic principles.

It is common in TDM to compare a patient's serum level with an arbitrary cutoff level that is used as a separator for classifying patients as toxic or nontoxic and, in other situations, therapeutic or subtherapeutic. In doing this, the serum level is applied in a manner that is analogous to using diagnostic tests in medicine. Because this approach is used so often in TDM, and because it also provides a valuable method for evaluating the usefulness of a drug's therapeutic range in classifying patients, it is discussed at length.

When serum drug concentrations are used as tests to classify or predict patient response and perhaps to modify dosage regimens, it is important to know the effectiveness of the tests. Using the serum drug level as a guide in TDM is similar to using a laboratory test in other clinical practices. The most critical question to be asked by anyone using a diagnostic test is: "How accurate is the test in identifying the true status of the patient?" So just as the precision of the assay used for measuring a serum drug level is important to know, so are the performance measures of the drug level as a diagnostic test.

The discriminatory power of a diagnostic test is its ability to distinguish between the conditions being present and absent. In TDM, clinicians may often select some maximum serum drug level and use it as a cutoff for categorizing patients as toxic or nontoxic. In practice, the top of the target concentration range usually serves, perhaps unwittingly, as a cutoff in the minds of clinicians. In other situations, a lower drug level may be chosen as a separator for classifying patients as therapeutic or subtherapeutic. In using the top of the therapeutic range as an upper limit, a patient is considered toxic or nontoxic when the serum level is above or below the cutoff, respectively. If tests functioned ideally, there would be no errors in classifying patients; those with toxicity could be clearly distinguished from those without it and those with therapeutic drug levels could be separated from those with subtherapeutic levels. But in TDM there are areas of overlap among patients, as shown in Figure 7–7, and regardless of where the cutoff value is set, some errors in classification will occur.

As a result of this overlap in classifying patients when diagnostic tests are used, eight indices, called test performance characteristics, are often used to evaluate and convey information about the effectiveness of a diagnostic test. Five of the indices are used by laboratories in determining the basic capacity of the test to accurately determine patient status: true positive, false positive, true-negative and false-negative rates, and likelihood ratio. Two indices assist the practitioner in predicting the effectiveness of the test in differentiating patients with and without the condition under consideration: positive and negative predictive values. One measure helps the practitioner to decide which test cutoff to use to minimize the classification error deemed of greatest risk to the patient: ratio of net consequences. Each of these test performance characteristics is discussed below.

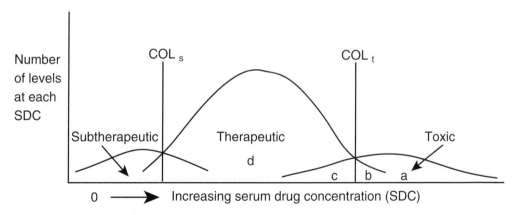

Figure 7–7. Frequency of patients with subtherapeutic, therapeutic, and toxic effects at increasing serum drug concentration (SDC). COL_s = subtherapeutic cutoff level, COL_t = toxic cutoff level. (*From Barr JT, Schumacher GE. Decision analysis and pharmacoeconomic evaluations. In: Bootman JL, Townsend RJ, McGhan WF, eds.* Principles of Pharmacoeconomics. *Cincinnati: Harvey Whitney Books Co; 1991;121.*)

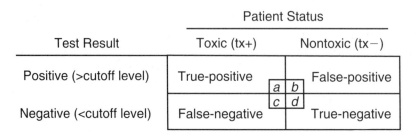

Figure 7–8. Test outcomes for toxicity using a cutoff level.

True-Positive Rate (Sensitivity) and True-Negative Rate (Specificity)

Figure 7–8 shows the testing situation described by Figures 7–6 and 7–7 in the form of a 2×2 matrix. Four classifications result from the case in which a serum drug level is used as a diagnostic test to classify patients using a drug as toxic or nontoxic. Correct classifications, called true positive (also called sensitivity) and true negative (also called specificity), reflect the test's ability to accurately identify the patient's true state. Incorrect classifications are denoted as false positive (a nontoxic patient labeled as toxic by the test because of a measured level greater than the test cutoff) and false negative (a toxic patient labeled as nontoxic by the test because the level is less than the test cutoff).

Figure 7–6 displays the testing situation in terms of a decision tree. Four possible outcomes are summarized in Table 7–6 and also discussed in Chapter 4.

When this decision process is conducted for a large number of patients using a drug, in which the serum level is measured independently of determining the true status of the patient (with the independent assessment of the patient's true state being termed the *gold standard*), the four possible outcomes are converted to probabilities or rates of occurrence that become characteristics of the drug for the test and are referred to as test performance characteristics. These characteristics are summarized in Table 7–6.

——————— **EXAMPLE 7–9** ———————————————————————————

To illustrate the meaning of these test performance characteristics, assume that 600 patients are given drug X. Of these, 100 patients experience toxicity related to the drug and 500 patients do not. Of the 100 toxic patients, 70 and 30 of the patients have positive and nega-

Test Result	Patient Status	
	Toxic (tx+)	Nontoxic (tx−)
Positive	70	100
Negative	30	400

tive tests for toxicity, respectively. Of the 500 nontoxic patients, 400 and 100 have negative and positive tests, respectively. The prevalence of toxicity, p(tx+), in the study population is 16.7% (tx+/total = 100/600).

The two test performance characteristics associated with toxic patients are the true-positive and false-negative rates:

- True-positive rate (sensitivity) of the test is 0.7 [70/(70+30)]. The test accurately classifies 70% of the toxic patients.
- False-negative rate of the test is 0.3 [30/(70+30)]. The test misclassifies 30% of the toxic patients as nontoxic.

The two test performance characteristics associated with nontoxic patients are the true-negative and false-positive rates:

- True-negative rate (specificity) of the test is 0.8 [400/(100+400)]. The test accurately classifies 80% of the nontoxic patients.
- False-positive rate of the test is 0.2 [100/(100+400)]. The test misclassifies 20% of the nontoxic patients as toxic.

These data provide laboratorians and practitioners with essential information about the effectiveness of this test and allow the quality of the test to be compared against other tests. In this case, under controlled study conditions in which patient status is known, 3 of 10 toxic patients and 2 of 10 nontoxic patients will be misclassified by the test. Overall, for this patient population, more than 1 in 5 patients will be categorized inaccurately (130/600 = 21.7%).

Sensitivity and specificity are fundamental indices that the laboratory uses to evaluate and characterize test effectiveness. When obtained by a properly conducted study, these indices are generally assumed to be constants for a given diagnostic test, and do not change when the test is used in different patient populations (eg, elderly, young, hospitalized, ambulatory) or when the underlying prevalence of the condition in the population changes.

Likelihood Ratio

A useful test performance characteristic that accompanies a positive test result comes from the ratio of the true-positive to false-positive rates and is called the likelihood ratio positive (LR+). The companion characteristic for a negative test result is the ratio of the false-negative to true-negative rates and is called the likelihood ratio negative (LR−). The likelihood ratio represents a measure of the discriminatory capacity of a diagnostic test. For patients with positive test results (values above the test cutoff level), the LR+ is the capacity of the test to differentiate the true positive (toxic in this case) from the false positive (nontoxic). For patients with negative test results (values below the test cutoff level), the LR− is the capacity of the test to differentiate the false negative (toxic in this case) from the true negative (nontoxic).

Given these two likelihood ratios, LR+ and LR−, two types of the likelihood ratio in general are discussed in this chapter, depending on the test performance characteristic being considered. The *cutoff likelihood ratio* (CLR) is used when a single test cutoff value is used to divide the test results and associated patient status into the four cells resulting from a 2 × 2 matrix, as

TABLE 7–6. DEFINITIONS FOR TEST PERFORMANCE CHARACTERISTICS IN CLASSIFYING TOXIC VERSUS NONTOXIC PATIENTS

True-positive	A truly toxic patient classified as toxic because of a positive test (level > cutoff).
True-positive rate	Proportion of toxic patients that have a positive test $[a/(a + c)]^a$ Also called sensitivity Using conditional probability notation: p(test+|tx+)
False positive	A truly nontoxic patient classified as toxic because of a positive test (level > cutoff)
False-positive rate	Proportion of nontoxic patients that have a positive test $[b/(b + d)]^a$ Also, 1 − true-negative rate Using conditional probability notation: p(test+|tx−)
True negative	A truly nontoxic patient classified as nontoxic because of a negative test (level ≤ cutoff)
True-negative rate	Proportion of nontoxic patients that have a negative test $[d/(b + d)]^a$ Also called specificity Using conditional probability notation: p(test−|tx−)
False negative	A truly toxic patient classified as nontoxic because of a negative test (level ≤ cutoff)
False-negative rate	Proportion of toxic patients that have a negative test $[c/(a + c)]^a$ Also, 1 − true-positive rate Using conditional probability notation: p(test−|tx+)
Cutoff likelihood ratio (+)	Probability that a toxic patient has a positive test (level > cutoff) divided by the probability that a nontoxic patient has a positive test
Cutoff likelihood ratio (−)	Probability that a toxic patient has a negative test (level < cutoff) divided by the probability that a nontoxic patient has a negative test
Range likelihood ratio (+)	Probability that a toxic patient has a serum drug concentration within the designated concentration range divided by the probability that a nontoxic patient has a serum drug concentration within the same range.
Range likelihood ratio (−)	Probability that a patient in a toxic condition has a serum drug concentration outside the designated concentration range divided by the probability that a patient not manifesting toxic effects has a serum drug concentration outside the same range
Positive predictive value	Proportion of patients with a positive test (drug level > cutoff) who are in a toxic condition $[a/(a + b)]^a$ Using conditional probability notation: p(tx+|test+)
Negative predictive value	Proportion of patients with a negative test (drug level ≤ cutoff) who are not manifesting toxic effects $[d/(d + c)]^a$ Using conditional probability notation: p(tx−|test−)
Ratio of net consequences	Risk of a false-positive error divided by risk of a false-negative error

[a]Using the notation for classification cells shown in Figure 7–8.

shown previously in Figure 7–8. When the term *likelihood ratio* is used in the literature without additional clarification, it usually means CLR(+) as described here in the equation

$$\text{cutoff likelihood ratio positive (CLR+)} = \frac{\text{true-positive rate}}{\text{false-positive rate}} = \frac{a/(a+c)}{b/(b+d)} = \frac{p(\text{test+}|\text{tx+})}{p(\text{test+}|\text{tx}-)} \quad (7\text{–}16)$$

Another form of the likelihood ratio, the *range likelihood ratio* (RLR), was also described previously in Equation 7–3 and later in Equation 7–17.

_____ **EXAMPLE 7–10** _____

Using the data from Example 7–9, calculate the cutoff likelihood ratio positive for the test.

$$\text{cutoff likelihood ratio positive} = \frac{\text{true-positive rate}}{\text{false-positive rate}} = \frac{0.7}{0.2} = 3.5$$

This means that a serum drug level above the test cutoff level occurs 3.5 times more often in a toxic patient than it does in a nontoxic patient. Another interpretation of CLR+ is that a patient with a positive test result will have posttest odds of toxicity that are 3.5 times greater than the pretest odds (see Equation 7–2).

In general, a likelihood ratio greater than 1 indicates that the probability of a drug level higher than the cutoff is greater in the toxic than the nontoxic patient; it also revises the probability upward so that posttest probability is greater than the pretest probability. A ratio less than 1 indicates that the probability of a level higher than the cutoff is greater in the nontoxic compared with the toxic patient and it revises the probabilities such that posttest is less than the pretest. A ratio of 1 means that the probabilities are equivalent in the toxic and nontoxic populations and that the serum level as a test does not revise the probability (posttest probability = pretest probability).

Predictive Value as a Test Performance Characteristic

Although valuable for laboratory purposes because the test characteristics are generally constant for different populations, true-positive and true-negative rates discussed above are of limited usefulness for the clinician, because these indices provide answers to the following question: "Given that the patient's condition is known, how probable is it that the test classifies the patient correctly?" Unfortunately, this is not the question clinicians are asking, for if they knew the true status of the patient, there would be no uncertainty, and there would be very little need to use a drug level for diagnostic purposes.

Clinicians are more likely to ask the following question: "Given the result of the test, how probable is it that the patient does or does not have the condition?" The most useful answer to this question is provided by the predictive value of a test. As applied in TDM for using serum drug levels as adjuncts for identifying toxic and nontoxic patients, and using the four cells (*a–d*) of the classification matrix in Figure 7–8 for reference, two predictive values are defined, as summarized in Table 7–6: positive predictive value and negative predictive value.

_____ **EXAMPLE 7–11** _____

Using the data from Example 7–9, calculate the predictive values for the test.
- Positive predictive value of the test is 0.41 [70/(70 + 100)]: 41% of the positive tests are from toxic patients.
- Negative predictive value of the test is 0.93 [400/(400 + 30)]: 93% of the negative tests are from nontoxic patients.

These values indicate to the practitioner that the diagnostic test is much more reliable in ruling out toxicity when the patient has a negative test (93% accurate) than in ruling in toxicity when the test is positive (just 41% accurate).

Make sure not to confuse positive predictive value (p[tx+|test+]) with true-positive rate (p[test+|tx+)] or negative predictive value (p[tx−|test-]) with true-negative rate (p[test-|tx−]). The conditional probabilities are not the same for these tests. Positive and negative predictive values, as the names imply, tell the probability of a patient's status *given* knowledge about the patient's result from a diagnostic test. Conversely, true-positive and true-negative rates tell the probability of a patient's test outcome *given* knowledge about the patient's status. This is why the predictive values of a test are of more use to a practitioner. These indices provide additional information useful to the practitioner in characterizing the condition of the patient whose status is not fully known.

An important caveat should be noted when using predictive values. Whereas the true-positive and true-negative rates are test performance characteristics of a serum drug level that are generally constant from population to population, predictive values are not. To the extent that the prevalence of the condition in the study patients in which the predictive values were obtained is similar to the prevalence in the actual patients in which the test is being used, predictive values are useful to clinicians in revealing the probability that a patient truly has the condition indicated by the test result. But predictive values may provide misleading estimates when the prevalences in the study and actual populations are different.[7,27]

_____ **EXAMPLE 7–12** _____

A $C_{min,ss}$ of 2 µg/mL for gentamicin and tobramycin was used as a cutoff for classifying potentially nephrotoxic from nontoxic patients in two populations: younger patients with normal baseline renal function and older patients with baseline renal insufficiency. The $C_{min,ss}$ cutoff was observed 2 to 4 days after starting treatment and the subsequent evaluation of toxicity status was made after 7 days of treatment. The prevalences of toxicity were 8% and 25% in the 300 younger patients and 200 older patients studied, respectively. The data are as follows:

	Younger Patient Status	
Test Result	Toxic (tx+)	Nontoxic (tx−)
>2 µg/mL	12	28
≤2 µg/mL	12	248

	Older Patient Status	
Test Result	Toxic (tx+)	Nontoxic (tx−)
>2 µg/mL	24	16
≤2 µg/mL	26	134

For the younger patients the following indices are calculated:

true-positive rate = 0.50,   positive predictive value = 0.30

true-negative rate = 0.90,   negative predictive value = .95

For the older patients:

true-positive rate = 0.48,   positive predictive value = 0.60

true-negative rate = 0.89,   negative predictive value = 0.84

Although the test sensitivity and specificity were essentially unchanged in the two populations, as expected, the predictive values varied with the prevalence of toxicity. Had the predictive values been determined only in the older population, and then applied to younger patients, the positive predictive value would have been markedly overestimated for the younger population with a lower prevalence of nephrotoxicity. In general, the positive predictive value increases, and the negative predictive value decreases, as the prevalence of the condition increases (nephrotoxicity here). The same result would be expected if a population of patients with normal renal function were compared with a population of renally impaired patients, regardless of age.

Ratio of Net Consequences as a Test Performance Characteristic

As diagnostic tests are intended to decrease the level of uncertainty involving patient status, misclassification errors represent the greatest liability to the use of any test. Yet it is generally inevitable, as shown in Figure 7–7, that the subpopulations of toxic and nontoxic (or therapeutic and subtherapeutic) patients overlap at all common drug cutoff levels, and this leads to some incorrect decisions resulting from false-positive and false-negative errors. For a given drug in a given situation, however, are both types of errors of equal consequence or is one more risky than the other? To answer this, it becomes important for the decision maker to assess the relative risk of each of these two types of errors to select a cutoff level for the test that minimizes, where practical, the occurrence of the error perceived to be of the greatest consequence.

Figure 7–6 describes the decision process. The probability of toxic (tx+) and nontoxic (tx−) outcomes changes as the selection of test serum drug level cutoff is varied. As the likelihood ratio characterizes a given cutoff level (eg, the true-positive and false-positive rates are defined by the choice of cutoff), it is possible to use the following equation to select a test cutoff (as represented by the associated likelihood ratio) to yield an index called the ratio of net consequences (the ratio of net risks of false-positive errors to net risks of false-negative errors) desired by the practitioner[6,7,18,22]:

$$\text{ratio of net consequences} = \frac{\text{CTN} - \text{CFP}}{\text{CTP} - \text{CFN}} = \frac{p(\text{tx}+)}{p(\text{tx}-)} \times \text{RLR}+ \qquad (7\text{--}17)$$

Here, C is the consequence assigned for true-negative (CTN), false-positive (CFP), true-positive (CTP), and false-negative (CFN) outcomes; CTN − CFP is the net consequence that results from misclassifying some truly nontoxic patients as toxic as a result of the test; CTP − CFN is the net consequence that results from misclassifying some truly toxic patients as nontoxic as a result of the test; (CTN − CFP)/(CTP − CFN) denotes the ratio of net consequences; $p(\text{tx}+)$ and $p(\text{tx}-)$ are the prevalences of toxicity and nontoxicity, respectively, in the study group; and RLR+ is the range likelihood ratio calculated as the ratio of true-positive to false-positive rates within the most narrow concentration range practical, given the available data that contain the selected cutoff value.

The use of the term *consequence* shown in Figure 7–6 and Equation 7–17 characterizes the relative risk associated with each classification outcome, as discussed previously, and values outcome in some unit like dollars, length of hospitalization, quality of life, and so on. In Equation 7–17, the numerator (CTN − CFP) and denominator (CTP − CFN) represent the cost and benefit, respectively, of the decision process, as described previously in Equations 7–10 and 7–11.

$$B_{\text{dc}} = U_{\text{dc,tx}+} - U_{\text{c,tx}+}$$

$$C_{\text{dc}} = U_{\text{c,tx}-} - U_{\text{dc,tx}-}$$

This relationship is shown in

$$\frac{\text{CTN} - \text{CFP}}{\text{CTP} - \text{CFN}} = \frac{U_{\text{c,tx}-} - U_{\text{dc,tx}-}}{U_{\text{dc,tx}+} - U_{\text{c,tx}+}} = \frac{C}{B} \qquad (7\text{--}18)$$

and allows Equation 7–17 to be rewritten as

$$\text{ratio of net consequences} = \frac{C}{B} = \frac{p(\text{tx}+)}{p(\text{tx}-)} \times \text{RLR}+ \qquad (7\text{--}19)$$

As the true-positive or true-negative outcomes are the desired correct classifications resulting from a diagnostic test and are expected to lead to proper courses of action, Equations 7–17 and 7–18 may often be simplified for most purposes by reducing (CTN − CFP)/(CTP − CFN) to CFP/CFN, a ratio that reflects the net effects of the classification errors. This is shown in

$$\text{ratio of net consequences} = \frac{\text{CFP}}{\text{CFN}} = \frac{p(\text{tx}+)}{p(\text{tx}-)} \times \text{RLR} \qquad (7\text{--}20)$$

As it is often difficult to assign a numerical value for consequence to each outcome, the task is commonly made more simple by just identifying a ratio of CFP/CFN that satisfies the comparative risk of these errors as viewed by practitioners.

_____ **EXAMPLE 7–13** _____

Using the data from Table 7–2 and Equation 7–17 or 7–20, calculate the ratio of net consequences for using a serum theophylline concentration cutoff of 20 µg/mL to represent the top of the therapeutic range (ie, serving as a separator for classifying toxic versus nontoxic patients).

$$\text{ratio of net consequences} = [p(\text{tx}+)/p(\text{tx}-)] \times \text{range likelihood ratio}$$

$$= [(39/280)/(241/280)] \times [(3/39)/(11/241)]$$

$$= 0.27$$

In the particular case of Table 7–2, the data are available more directly in the table, as the prevalence of toxicity (number of tx+ patients/total patients in study) and the range likelihood ratio are provided:

$$\text{ratio of net consequences} = [\text{prevalence}/(1 - \text{prevalence})] \times \text{range likelihood ratio}$$

$$= 0.14/0.86 \times 1.7$$

$$= 0.27$$

The ratio of net consequences of 0.27 means that for this test cutoff the net risk of committing a false-positive error is viewed as only 27% as important as the net risk of making a false-negative mistake. Stated alternatively, a false-negative error is considered nearly four times more consequential than a false-positive error. If the practitioner wants a different ratio, either to enhance the relative consequence of a false-positive (raise ratio > 0.27) or to increase the relative false-negative to false-positive risk (lower ratio < 0.27), then Equation 7–17 or 7–20 must be used to calculate new data for choosing the appropriate cutoff. To value both false-positive and false-negative errors equally, for example, rewrite Equation 7–17 or 7–20 to determine the associated range likelihood ratio:

$$\text{range likelihood ratio} = \text{ratio of net consequences} \times p(\text{tx}-)/p(\text{tx}+)$$

$$= 1.0 \times 0.86/0.14$$

$$= 6.1$$

Referring to Table 7–2, the range likelihood ratio increases with STC and is 6.4 at a cutoff of 28 µg/mL (midpoint of 27–28.9 µg/mL range). So to value the classification errors equally, a cutoff of 27–28 µg/mL is appropriate.

	Patient Status	
Test Result	Toxic (tx+)	Nontoxic (tx−)
Positive (>20 µg/mL)	26	30
Negative (≤20 µg/mL)	13	211

(Inset labels: a | b / c | d)

Figure 7–9. Theophylline outcomes using a 20 µg/mL cutoff level.

Using Theophylline Data to Illustrate Test Performance Characteristics

Our theophylline data have been discussed previously and are recorded in Table 7–2.[18] As the commonly accepted therapeutic range for theophylline is 10 to 20 µg/mL, we used the upper limit as a cutoff for evaluating the effectiveness of STC in separating toxic from nontoxic patients. To do so, refer to the data in Table 7–2, place a ruler across the middle of the STC range of 19 to 20.9 µg/mL, thereby forming a 2 × 2 matrix of toxic and nontoxic patients above and below the ruler, and fill in the totals for each cell using the form of the matrix in Figure 7–8. The numbers we used are shown in Figure 7–9.

_____ **EXAMPLE 7–14** _____

Using the data in Figure 7–9, calculate the test performance characteristics associated with using a theophylline cutoff level of 20 µg/mL.
- True-positive rate = $a/(a + c)$ = 26/(26 + 13) = 0.67.
- True-negative rate = $d/(b + d)$ = 211/(30 + 211) = 0.88.
- False-positive rate = $b/(b + d)$ = 30/(30 + 211) = 0.12.
- False-negative rate = $c/(a + c)$ = 13/(26 + 13) = 0.33.
- Cutoff likelihood ratio (positive) = true-positive rate/false-positive rate = 0.67/0.12 = 5.58.
- Positive predictive value = $a/(a + b)$ = 26/(26 + 30) = 0.46.
- Negative predictive value = $d/(d + c)$ = 211/(211 + 13) = 0.94.

These test performance characteristics for theophylline are summarized in Table 7–7. At the commonly accepted 20 µg/mL STC maximum for the target concentration range, the test is much better at accurately classifying nontoxic than toxic patients. Test sensitivity and specificity are 67% and 88%, respectively, meaning that less than 70% of the patients who are truly toxic are correctly labeled as true positive by the test, whereas nearly 90% of nontoxic patients are accurately identified as true negative by the test. Sensitivity and specificity are inversely related. View this by moving a ruler up and down the columns of data in Table 7–2. To improve the sensitivity of the test (by increasing the true positives and decreasing the false negatives), the cutoff level must be lowered (below 20 µg/mL), but this comes at the expense of decreasing the specificity (true-negative rate) of the test. The same idea applies to the false-positive and false-negative rates. At a cutoff of 20 µg/mL, 33% of the toxic patients are misclassified as false negatives, and

TABLE 7–7. TEST PERFORMANCE CHARACTERISTICS FOR THEOPHYLLINE USING A 20 µG/ML SERUM DRUG CONCENTRATION TOXICITY CUTOFF VALUE

True-positive rate (sensitivity)	0.67
True-negative rate (specificity)	0.88
False-positive rate (1 − specificity)	0.12
False-negative rate (1 − sensitivity)	0.33
Cutoff likelihood ratio	5.58
Positive predictive value	0.46
Negative predictive value	0.94
Consequence of a false-positive result/consequence of a false-negative result	0.27

12% of the nontoxic patients are misclassified as false positives. Raising the test cutoff (above 20 µg/mL) decreases the false positives but increases the false negatives. The opposite occurs when the cutoff is lowered. This observation underpins the concept of selecting a cutoff to best achieve the practitioner's desired ratio of net consequences, as discussed previously in Example 7–13.

The test likelihood ratio (+) indicates that *if a patient is toxic*, it is 5.6 times more likely that a STC greater than the test cutoff (20 µg/mL in this case) will occur than *if the patient is nontoxic*. This does not mean that there are 5.6 times more toxic patients than nontoxic patients with a STC greater than 20 µg/mL (inspection of Table 7–2 shows this not to be correct). A RLR+ of 5.6 also means that the posttest odds of toxicity, following a positive test result, will be 5.6 times the pretest odds.

The predictive values suggest that using the top of the commonly accepted therapeutic range as a test cutoff for theophylline is much more effective at ruling out toxicity than it is at ruling in toxicity. Just 46% of patients with levels greater than 20 µg/mL are correctly classified as toxic, whereas 94% of patients with levels less than 20 µg/mL are correctly identified as nontoxic. The use of the STC above the therapeutic range in predicting toxicity is mediocre, but using levels below the therapeutic range to discount toxicity is highly predictive.

Test Performance Characteristics for Commonly Monitored Drugs

Using the above approach for theophylline, we studied the test performance characteristics for additional drugs. For each drug, we varied the serum drug concentration cutoff used to define toxicity.[22] As with theophylline above, published studies were analyzed in which individual serum drug concentrations with an independent assessment of toxic or nontoxic status were reported. For each drug, only studies using similar drug-specific assessment criteria were combined. The drugs include the 280 patients who received theophylline (data pooled from six studies), as discussed above, 493 patients taking digoxin (five studies), 469 patients administered gentamicin or tobramycin (four studies), 57 patients given vancomycin (two studies), 142 patients using procainamide (one study), and 111 patients taking phenytoin (one study).

Test performance characteristics for using serum concentrations of these drugs as diagnostic tests are reported in Table 7–8. As the cutoff values were increased for the drugs, sensitivity decreased but specificity increased, as expected. When the commonly accepted test cutoff was

TABLE 7–8. TEST PERFORMANCE CHARACTERISTICS FOR VARIOUS SERUM DRUG CONCENTRATION TOXICITY CUTOFF VALUES

Drug and Cutoff Value	TPR	TNR	CLR+	PPV	NPV	CFP/CFN
Theophylline[a]						
28 µg/mL	0.33	0.98	16.50	0.70	0.89	1.00
24 µg/mL	0.46	0.95	9.20	0.56	0.92	0.57
20 µg/mL[b]	0.67	0.88	5.58	0.46	0.94	0.27
Digoxin[c]						
3.0 ng/mL	0.43	0.96	10.75	0.69	0.90	2.27
2.5 ng/mL	0.61	0.93	8.71	0.62	0.93	1.00
2.0 ng/mL[b]	0.80	0.89	7.27	0.59	0.96	0.23
Procainamide[d]						
16 µg/mL	0.27	0.99	79	0.72	0.98	2.53
12 µg/mL	0.56	0.98	28	0.49	0.99	0.29
10 µg/mL[b]	0.71	0.96	18	0.40	0.99	0.19
Phenytoin[e]						
20 µg/mL[b]	0.37	0.73	1.35	0.22	0.85	—
Gentamicin/tobramycin[f]						
2 µg/mL[b]	0.48	0.81	2.53	0.32	0.89	0.48
Vancomycin[g]						
10 µg/mL[b]	1.00	0.48	1.92	0.31	1.00	0.46

[a]Prevalence of toxicity in study group (n = 280): 0.14.
[b]Commonly used cutoff value for toxicity.
[c]Prevalence of toxicity in study group (n = 493): 0.16.
[d]Prevalence of toxicity in study group (n = 1530): 0.03.
[e]Prevalence of neurotoxicity (patient response score > 10) in study group (n = 111): 0.22.
[f]Prevalence of nephrotoxicity in study group (n = 469): 0.16.
[g]Prevalence of nephrotoxicity in study group (n = 57): 0.19.
From Schumacher GE, Barr JT. Using population-based serum drug concentration cutoff values to predict toxicity: Test performance and limitations compared with bayesian interpretation. Clin Pharm. 1990;9:788–796, with permission.

studied for each drug, sensitivity for some of the drugs appeared lower than desirable. Although vancomycin and digoxin had favorable true-positive rates (100 and 80%, respectively), less than 75% of patients with theophylline or procainamide toxicity, less than 50% of patients with aminoglycoside nephrotoxicity, and less than 40% of patients with phenytoin toxicity had serum levels above the test cutoff. These relatively low true-positive rates forecast that at commonly used cutoff values, a large fraction of false-negative classifications will occur because patients with toxicity who have drug concentrations below the cutoff will be falsely labeled as nontoxic. More than 60% of patients with phenytoin toxicity, greater than 50% of patients with aminoglycoside nephrotoxicity, and more than 25% of patients with theophylline and procainamide toxicity will have a false-negative classification, using common cutoff values. The specificity of each test at the commonly accepted cutoff levels was generally much greater than the sensitivity for most drugs studied.

As the cutoff for each drug was increased, positive predictive values increased but negative predictive values decreased, as expected. For the data we studied, the commonly accepted cutoff for each drug had a positive predictive value of less than 0.6, whereas the negative predictive value was generally greater than 0.9. This pattern of negative greater than positive predictive value for a serum drug concentration test is usually expected when the prevalence of a condition (toxicity in this case) is relatively low. As noted previously for theophylline, the greater probabilities for negative as compared with positive predictive values for these drugs confirm that these tests are much more effective at ruling out toxicity than ruling it in.

The ratio of net consequences for the drugs increased as the cutoff value increased, as expected, meaning that the selection of a higher cutoff implies that false-positive errors are weighted more heavily than false-negative errors. At the commonly accepted cutoff value for each drug, however, the ratio of net consequences was less than 0.5, indicating an implicit acceptance of a much greater consequence associated with false-negative than false-positive errors. In general, as the ratio of net consequences is fixed by the choice of cutoff value, it is usually best for the practitioner to decide on the desired ratio (or at least to determine whether the ratio should be >1, 1, or <1) and then select a drug cutoff value that yields the ratio, using Equation 7–17 or 7–20.

The Value of Knowing Test Performance Characteristics

Historically, target concentration ranges for most drugs have been developed largely on the basis of pharmacologic effect. These ranges were also introduced early in the development of TDM, when serum drug concentrations were not commonly measured, and the prevalence of toxicity was therefore higher than it usually is today. The data in Tables 7–7 and 7–8 show that when these drug levels are used as tests to assess patient status today, factors in addition to pharmacologic observation become important, such as the test performance of a drug concentration in discriminating positive from negative responses, the probabilities of correct and incorrect classifications, and the relative consequences assigned by practitioners to these outcomes.[22]

Our retrospective analysis of the usefulness of the therapeutic range for common TDM drugs bears out the value of knowing test performance characteristic data. When the commonly used maximum serum level of the therapeutic range for many drugs is used as a cutoff for separating toxic from nontoxic patients, the associated test characteristics noted in Table 7–8 show the cutoffs to be much less discriminating than desirable. Given the data available to date, passive reliance on population-based therapeutic ranges for managing individual patients is risky.

Nonetheless, our data suggest that knowledge and use of test characteristics contribute to a more informed interpretation of serum drug concentrations as adjuncts to assessing patient status. Without these data, practitioners cannot fully gauge the effectiveness of the test nor can they optimally use drug levels to assist in determining the relative merit, clinical consequences, and costs of alternative decisions in both population and patient-specific situations. Nor can the misclassification rates inherent in all diagnostic tests be appropriately applied to interpreting the TDM test results for toxic versus nontoxic and therapeutic versus subtherapeutic decisions.

The emphasis in this discussion has been on introducing the concept of test performance characteristics and in stimulating awareness of the value of using the data in TDM decision making. It is, however, important to note that the results included in Tables 7–7 and 7–8 have been calculated from retrospective analyses of published data. Prospective studies designed to collect data for TDM drugs have not been conducted to date and it is important to do so. The lack of prospective data limits the application, but it should not restrict the understanding, of test performance characteristics by the practitioner.

The Value of Using a Bayesian Rather than Cutoff Approach for Interpreting Serum Drug Levels

When drug concentrations are used as discussed above, to classify patients as positive or negative (eg, toxic versus nontoxic or therapeutic versus subtherapeutic), based on relating patient drug levels to a test cutoff, the full benefit to be gained from serum levels is not achieved.[20,22] There are two limitations to this approach. The first is the "yes or no" classification of patients that results and the underlying population-based data used for developing cutoffs. In comparing a patient's drug level with a cutoff value, a dichotomous result is achieved; the condition is classified as either present or absent. The second limitation is that cutoff levels are implicitly established based on the prevalence of disease in the general population. These underlying population-based values present limitations because each individual patient being tested may have a different pretest probability of toxicity than the fixed population prevalence value used in constructing the diagnostic test. As a result, in using a cutoff-based approach the clinician is unwittingly substituting the pretest probability of toxicity in the general population for the patient's individualized pretest probability of toxicity. So using cutoff levels results in combining a population-based, rather than a patient-specific, pretest probability of toxicity with a patient-specific serum concentration. This dilutes not only the contribution of the individualized drug level but also that of the practitioner's judgment.

Using bayesian probability for interpreting serum drug concentrations represents a more interactive and quantitative approach.[20,22] A patient-specific pretest probability of toxicity is explicitly estimated by the practitioner, then the pretest is combined with the probabilistic information contained in the patient's drug level, and this yields a revised, posttest probability of patient status. As a result, a probabilistic assessment (ranging from 0 to 1) rather than a dichotomous (yes or no) classification of patient status is achieved.

_____ **EXAMPLE 7–15** _____

Assume that a practitioner has the following two patients taking theophylline who experience adverse reactions that may be due to the drug:

	Patient A	Patient B
Pretest probability of toxicity	0.33	0.67
Serum theophylline concentration	16 µg/mL	16 µg/mL
Posttest probability of toxicity	0.26	0.59

The posttest probability for both patients was estimated from Figure 7–2. The practitioner judged the pretest probability of toxicity to be one half as great in Patient A as Patient B. For both patients the serum level measured was the same. Using the conditional probability curves results in a posttest probability of toxicity that is more than twice as great for Patient B compared with Patient A. Whereas the probability of toxicity (depending on the nature of the adverse reaction) in Patient A may be low enough for many clinicians to continue treatment, the probability of toxicity in Patient B is surely high enough to urge most physicians to reduce the dosage regimen or discontinue the drug. Yet, with the less flexible cutoff approach, using 20 µg/mL as the commonly accepted top of the therapeutic range, both patients would be classified as nontoxic. The use of a bayesian approach leads to a more informed analysis that quantifies the difference in probability of toxicity for both patients; many practitioners would continue using theophylline in Patient A, whereas most practitioners would likely give strong consideration to discontinuing the drug in Patient B.

KNOWING WHEN OBTAINING A DRUG SERUM LEVEL PROVIDES INFORMATION THAT CAN ALTER CLINICAL DECISIONS

The decision analyses described up to this point, those illustrated by Figures 7–1, 7–3, and 7–6, have all assumed that a drug level was obtained from the patient prior to selecting a decision alternative. In this section, the emphasis shifts to discussing under what conditions the serum drug level actually provides information that can alter clinical decisions.

There are a number of reasons why serum drug levels are measured in TDM: to adjust dosage regimens, individualize pharmacokinetics, occasionally check on compliance, and judge patient status. The first three applications are straightforward: The serum level assists in guiding modification of the dosage regimen, determining clearance in the patient, and assessing whether the patient's concentration is within the therapeutic range. This chapter has emphasized the latter application, to assist in determining patient status, and this application is not straightforward. There are objective reasons for measuring levels to judge patient status: when the patient's level of response is in question or when toxicity is an issue. But there are also subjective reasons for measuring levels: to fulfill a prescriber's request or as a defensive practice for inclusion in the patient's record, despite whether these reasons seem appropriate or not.

Recognizing that the variety of reasons above apply to the use of drug levels to inform about patient status, this section discusses when obtaining a level truly contributes useful information. A basic principle of decision making dictates that levels should be ordered only if test results can lead to revising pretest probabilities such that posttest probabilities may cause practitioners to change their decisions about the status of patients or the most appropriate course of action.[7(pp239–290),18,28] Specific to TDM, a drug level should be ordered only if the test result has the potential for revising the pretest probability to a posttest probability that may change the course of action. In other words, obtain a drug level only when the level has the potential for making a posttest probability cross the decision threshold, resulting in a changed decision (eg, T_{dc} for continuing versus discontinuing in Figure 7–4 or T_1 for continuing versus lowering and T_{dc} for lowering versus discontinuing in Figure 7–5). A similar case could be made, although not emphasized in this chapter, for the subtherapeutic/therapeutic decision threshold.

Using an example such as the decision to continue or discontinue drug dosage, as noted in Figure 7–10, the practitioner in TDM frequently must decide, based on an assessment of pretest probability of toxicity, whether to (1) continue without obtaining a drug level, (2) discontinue

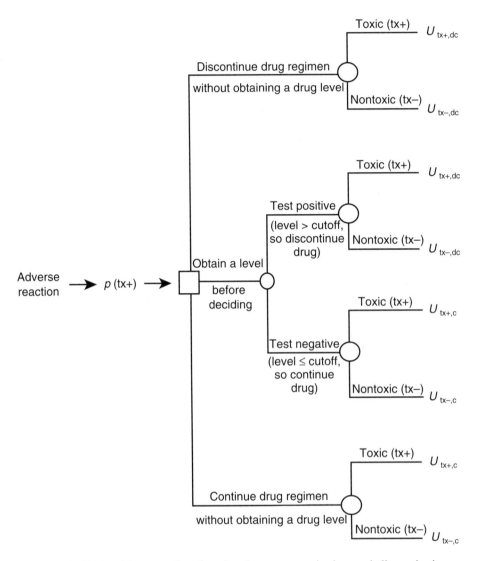

Figure 7–10. Decision tree for choosing between continuing and discontinuing a drug regimen with and without first testing the serum level. Theophylline is used as an example, with STC denoting the serum theophylline concentration and U representing the utility value assigned to each outcome.

without getting a level, or (3) order a drug level and then continue or discontinue based on the level. Figure 7–11 divides the posttest probability of toxicity continuum, derived after the pretest probability has been revised by the input of the drug level, into three regions. The threshold ($T_{c,t}$) for the continue or test decision is the probability of toxicity at which the expected values for the two decisions are equal and the decision is a tossup. Similarly, the threshold ($T_{t,dc}$) for the test or

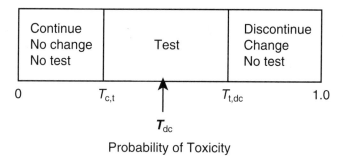

Figure 7–11. Threshold probabilities for serum drug level testing.

discontinue decision is the probability at which the expected values for these two decisions are equal.

In practice, a clinician has a perception about, or has calculated using Equation 7–13 discussed previously, the posttest probability of toxicity (the decision threshold, T_{dc}) at which it is generally expected to discontinue the drug. For an individual patient, once the pretest probability of toxicity, $p(tx+)$, is determined, the following possibilities exist, as noted in Figures 7–10 and 7–11:

- If $p(tx+)$ is below $T_{c,t}$, the regimen should be continued without seeking a drug level for additional advice. This is because a drug level cannot raise the pretest probability, when it is below the continue or test threshold ($T_{c,t}$), to a posttest probability, T_{dc}, above the decision threshold to discontinue the drug.
- If $p(tx+)$ is above $T_{c,t}$ but below $T_{t,dc}$, a drug level may contribute to changing the decision. The expected value of the "obtain a STC before deciding" decision alternative in Figure 7–10 is greater than for the other two alternatives. Obtaining a measurement is indicated: continuing the regimen if the test is negative, meaning the level is below the test cutoff (usually the top of the drug's therapeutic range), or discontinuing the drug if the test is positive, meaning the level is above the cutoff. This is because a level less than the cutoff will make the posttest probability less than T_{dc}, whereas a level greater than the cutoff will yield a posttest probability greater than T_{dc}.
- If $p(tx+)$ is above $T_{t,dc}$, the regimen should be discontinued without obtaining a drug level. This is because the level, when it is above the test or discontinue threshold ($T_{t,dc}$), cannot lower the pretest probability to a posttest probability, T_{dc}, below the decision threshold to discontinue the drug.

There are four steps in determining whether ordering a drug level in a patient has the potential to change a decision.[7(pp239–290),28] Steps 1 and 2 focus on setting the decision and testing thresholds. Steps 3 and 4 deal with setting the pretest probability and then calculating the posttest probability in the patient. As applied to the continue versus discontinue decision process:

1. Estimate the decision threshold for discontinuing treatment, T_{dc}, using intuition or Equation 7–13. In practice, intuition is used much more often than the formal utility-based approach of Equation 7–13.
2. Calculate the two testing thresholds bounding the range of pretest probabilities that con-

stitute the probability region for testing first before selecting a decision alternative. $T_{c,t}$ is the testing threshold denoting the pretest probability threshold for continuing the drug regimen or testing first, calculated using Equation 7–21. $T_{t,dc}$ is the companion threshold representing the pretest probability threshold for discontinuing the drug regimen or testing first, calculated using Equation 7–22.

$$T_{c,t} = \frac{(T_{dc})\,(\text{FPR})}{(T_{dc})\,(\text{FPR}) + (1 - T_{dc})\,(\text{TPR})} \tag{7–21}$$

$$T_{t,dc} = \frac{(T_{dc})\,(1 - \text{FPR})}{(T_{dc})\,(1 - \text{FPR}) + (1 - T_{dc})\,(1 - \text{TPR})} \tag{7–22}$$

In these equations TPR and FPR are the true-positive and false-positive rates, respectively.
3. Estimate the pretest probability of toxicity, $p(\text{tx}+)$, for the patient.
4. Relate the pretest probability estimated for the patient in Step 3 to the testing thresholds in Step 2.
   a. Do not order a drug level if $p(\text{tx}+)$ is less than $T_{c,t}$ or greater than $T_{t,dc}$. Continue the drug regimen without testing if $p(\text{tx}+)$ is less than $T_{c,t}$. Discontinue the drug without testing if $p(\text{tx}+)$ is greater than $T_{t,dc}$.
   b. Order a drug level before deciding on continuing or discontinuing if $p(\text{tx}+)$ is between $T_{c,t}$ and $T_{t,dc}$.
      i. Continue the regimen if the level is less than or equal to the test cutoff (Figure 7–10). The likelihood ratio associated with a negative test cannot lead to raising the pretest probability sufficiently to reach a posttest probability greater than T_{dc}.
      ii. Discontinue the regimen if the level is greater than the test cutoff. The likelihood ratio associated with a positive test cannot lead to lowering the pretest probability sufficiently to reach a posttest probability less than T_{dc}.

_____ EXAMPLE 7–16 _____

What are $T_{c,t}$, $T_{t,dc}$, and T_{dc} for the decision to continue or discontinue theophylline in patients, assuming the following outcome utilities are assigned to a specific type of adverse reaction in the decision tree in Figure 7–1: $U_{c,tx-} = 1.0$, $U_{dc,tx+} = 0.95$, $U_{dc,tx-} = 0.6$, and $U_{c,tx+} = 0$. Use the theophylline test performance characteristics in Table 7–7, as needed.
    Using Step 1 and Equation 7–13 above,

$$T_{dc} = \frac{U_{c,tx-} - U_{dc,tx-}}{(U_{c,tx-} - U_{dc,tx-}) + (U_{dc,tx+} - U_{c,tx+})} = \frac{1.0 - 0.6}{(1.0 - 0.6) + (0.95 - 0)} = 0.30$$

Alternately, and probably more commonly, T_{dc} is set by perception of the practitioner without formally invoking Equation 7–13.
    Using Step 2 and Equation 7–21 above,

$$T_{c,t} = \frac{(T_{dc})\,(\text{FPR})}{(T_{dc})\,(\text{FPR}) + (1 - T_{dc})\,(\text{TPR})} = \frac{(0.30)\,(0.12)}{(0.30)\,(0.12) + (0.70)\,(0.67)} = 0.07$$

Using Step 2 and Equation 7–22 above,

$$T_{t,dc} = \frac{(T_{dc})(1 - FPR)}{(T_{dc})(1 - FPR) + (1 - T_{dc})(1 - TPR)} = \frac{(0.30)(0.88)}{(0.30)(0.88) + (0.70)(0.33)} = 0.53$$

These thresholds suggest that the practitioner expects to discontinue theophylline in a patient when the posttest probability of toxicity exceeds 0.30. When the practitioner's pretest probability is less than 0.07, the regimen should be continued without ordering a theophylline level. When the pretest probability is greater than 0.07 and less than 0.53, a drug level is indicated, continuing the regimen if the level is 20 μg/mL or less and discontinuing the drug if the level is greater than 20 μg/mL. This is because a level of 20 μg/mL or less cannot raise the pretest probability to a posttest probability greater than T_{dc} (0.30), whereas a level greater than 20 μg/mL does convert the pretest probability into a posttest probability greater than T_{dc}. Above a pretest probability of 0.53, discontinuing theophylline is appropriate without ordering a drug level.

_____ **EXAMPLE 7–17** _____

A practitioner recognizes an adverse effect(s) in a patient taking theophylline that may be due to the drug and estimates the pretest probability of theophylline-induced toxicity as 0.10. Accepting the threshold values calculated above in Example 7–16, should theophylline be continued or discontinued without first ordering a serum theophylline concentration, or should a drug level be obtained before decided?

The practitioner's pretest probability is just above the $T_{c,t}$ but below the T_{dc} (see Figure 7–11). As the pretest is within the testing region (0.08–0.52), obtaining a drug level may revise the posttest probability sufficiently to increase the value above the T_{dc} of 0.30. A theophylline level is ordered and a value of 21 μg/mL is obtained, just above the theophylline cutoff of 20 μg/mL. According to Step 4, the patient's theophylline level is sufficient to increase the posttest probability of toxicity greater than the T_{dc}. Therefore, the test has been useful in modifying the decision and discontinuing theophylline is appropriate.

This decision can be checked using Bayes' formula in the form

$$\text{posttest probability} = \frac{p(tx+)(TPR)}{p(tx+)(TPR) + (1 - p(tx+))(FPR)} \qquad (7-23)$$

$$\text{posttest probability} = \frac{(0.10)(0.67)}{(0.10)(0.67) + (0.90)(0.12)} = 0.38$$

The posttest probability is greater than T_{dc} (0.30). To make a point, however: If the practitioner's pretest probability had been less than 0.07, rather than 0.10, the pretest probability would have been below the $T_{c,t}$. In that situation, continuing the regimen without resorting to ordering a level would have been the favored decision, because the level could not have raised the posttest probability above the T_{dc}.

As a final consideration about testing thresholds, note that Equations 7–21 and 7–22 depend on the selection of the decision threshold, T_{dc}. If this changes, reflecting varying severity of different adverse reactions, or changes in the number of reactions in the patient, or simply changes in the value of outcome utilities among practitioners, the calculation of T_{dc} in Equation 7–13 will vary, and this will result in changes in the testing thresholds, $T_{c,t}$ and $T_{t,dc}$.

USING RECEIVER-OPERATING CHARACTERISTIC CURVES TO COMPARE TDM SYSTEMS

Receiver-operating characteristic (ROC) curves display in graphic form the comparative effectiveness of alternative systems in identifying true-positive and true-negative patients and, in so doing, characterize the relative sensitivity and specificity of systems.[7(pp130–145),16,17] Alternative systems in TDM may refer, to cite a few examples, to different analytic approaches to measuring serum drug concentrations, to comparing total with free drug concentrations for characterizing patient status, and to comparing different procedures for TDM.

Applied specifically in TDM, an ROC curve is constructed for a given system of analyzing or monitoring drug levels by plotting the true-positive and false-positive rates for various test cutoff levels. Figure 7–12 presents three prototypical curves for three drug assay procedures used for TDM. When a number of procedures or systems are compared, the best system in terms of classification accuracy is the one displaying the curve that comes closest to the upper left portion of the graph (curve B in this example). This curve presents for each cutoff the greatest ratio of true-positive to false-positive classifications. In mathematical terms, the best system is represented by the curve with the greatest area under the curve (AUC).

Receiver-operating characteristic curves that plot substantially to the upper left of a 45-degree diagonal line represent systems that effectively discriminate between toxic and nontoxic subpopulations (or subtherapeutic and therapeutic subpopulations if the bottom of the therapeutic range is under consideration) and lead to the least number of errors in classifying patients. Curves that approach a 45-degree diagonal line represent systems that provide little useful information because the true-positive and false-positive rates for various cutoffs are similar. Curves that plot below the diagonal line, toward the lower right portion of the graph, depict hazardous systems wherein the rates for false positives exceed the true positives.

Receiver-operating characteristic curves should be applied to using drug levels as diagnostic tests, to compare new or modified analytic test systems, to monitor use of a given analytic method within an institution over time, and to compare the clinical performance of a given assay method in the therapeutic drug monitoring practices of various institutions.

As an example, we performed a retrospective analysis of studies of digoxin TDM practices in two different hospitals.[17] Aronson et al reported serum digoxin concentrations and toxicity status of 83 hospitalized patients.[29] Carruthers et al reported similar data for 101 patients at the time of hospital admission.[30] Toxicity rates were 21 and 13% for Aronson's and Carruthers' populations, respectively. In both investigations, digoxin concentration was determined by radioimmunoassay. Using their data, we calculated the true-positive and false-positive rates at various cutoff levels and constructed the ROC curves plotted in Figure 7–13. Although the digoxin test appears quite useful in the hands of Carruthers et al, it appears to offer little useful information for Aronson et al.

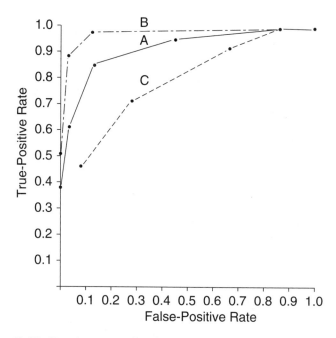

Figure 7–12. Receiver-operating characteristic (ROC) curves for a given drug. Curve A represents the total serum concentration as measured by EMIT, curve B represents the free serum concentration as measured by EMIT, and curve C represents the total serum concentration as measured by nephelometric assay. (*From Barr JT, Schumacher GE. Applying decision analysis in therapeutic drug monitoring: Using receiver-operating characteristic curves in comparative evaluations. Clin Pharm. 1986;5:239–246, with permission.*)

Institutions with TDM systems should evaluate their procedures using the ROC technique and these systems should be reassessed periodically to detect potential drifts in performance. In addition, various laboratories should compare their systems with an eye to assisting one another to improve effectiveness in monitoring.

RECOMMENDATIONS

The following recommendations are offered for the future monitoring of serum drug concentrations for drugs with narrow therapeutic ranges.[20,22] Although most practitioners recognize that these values are not infallible guides, use would be improved if a more quantitative basis were readily available for interpreting the strengths and limitations of serum levels as tests. This requires a greater interest by clinicians in adopting a more patient-specific, bayesian approach to serum drug concentrations, such as estimating the pretest probability of patient status before the drug concentration is obtained and then revising the probability based on the concentration value. It also requires understanding and using the test performance characteristic data that

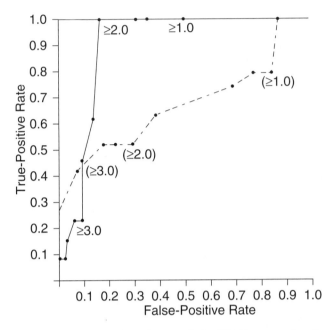

Figure 7–13. Receiver-operating characteristic (ROC) curves for digoxin. Toxicity and concentration data reported by Aronson et al[33] are represented by the dashed curve, and data reported by Carruthers *et al*[34] are represented by the solid curve. The numbers on the ROC curves denote serum digoxin concentration in ng/mL. (*From Barr JT, Schumacher GE. Applying decision analysis in therapeutic drug monitoring: Using receiver-operating characteristic curves in comparative evaluations. Clin Pharm. 1986;5:239–246, with permission.*)

describe the usefulness and limitations of serum drug levels as tests. And, because data are unavailable or are not yet analyzed with respect to test performance characteristics for many drugs of concern, a more aggressive interest in collaborating with clinical laboratorians to collect drug concentration versus outcome data is needed. These activities should involve prospective studies and well as retrospective analyses of published information.

Greater interest by practitioners and laboratorians in using decision analytic techniques in TDM should ensure that the future use of drug levels is accompanied by a better comprehension of the strengths, limitations, and alternative interpretations of such measurements; a decreasing dependence on pharmacodynamic observation as the sole criterion for decision making; and a more quantitative approach to individualizing patient assessment in general.

_____ QUESTIONS _____

1. A patient taking phenytoin 400 mg/d for 6 months starts to show some adverse effects that may or may not be induced by phenytoin, like drowsiness, visual blurring, and minor loss of coordination. The phenytoin has been effective in reducing the number

of seizures but the adverse effects are decreasing the patient's quality of life. The patient's neurologist estimates a pretest probability of phenytoin-induced toxicity of 0.5, then obtains a phenytoin level of 16 µg/mL, which results in a revised, posttest probability of toxicity of 0.33. The patient still needs some drug for his seizures so the neurologist must decide whether to (1) continue 400 mg/d and see if the adverse effects stabilize or decrease; (2) reduce the dose to 300 mg/d, risking decreased effectiveness but perhaps reducing the adverse effects; or (3) change to a different anticonvulsant.

The neurologist develops a decision tree, assigns utilities to the various possible outcomes that can result from the alternative strategies, adds the above posttest probability of toxicity to the toxic outcome branches and 1 − the posttest probability to the nontoxic outcome branches, and determines which course of action is the best choice under these conditions.

The neurologist chose the following utilities for the outcomes: 0 = continue, toxic; 1.0 = continue, nontoxic; 0.85 = reduce, toxic; 0.7 = reduce, nontoxic; 0.95 = change, toxic; 0.4 = change, nontoxic.

   a. Draw the decision tree that describes the situation and alternatives discussed above, attaching the appropriate probabilities and utilities to the tree.

   b. Calculate the best course of action, given the set of probabilities and utilities for this case.

2.   Two hundred adult epileptics taking phenytoin are monitored over 1 year. Each time a serum phenytoin concentration (SPC) is obtained from a patient, an independent assessment of patient status (nontoxic, toxic) is also obtained. Using these data, the clinicians evaluate the usefulness of a SPC of 22 µg/mL as a cutoff for separating nontoxic (tx−) from toxic (tx+) patients, wherein the toxicity is assumed to be the result of taking phenytoin: 36 patients were identified as tx+ at some time during the year; 9 of the tx+ patients had a SPC greater than 22 µg/mL at the time tx+ was assigned; 131 of the tx− patients had a SPC of 22 µg/mL or less at the time tx− was assigned.

   a. Draw the 2 × 2 matrix for these data.

   b. Calculate true-positive rate, true-negative rate, positive predictive value, negative predictive value, and cutoff likelihood ratio positive.

   c. Is the test more sensitive or specific?

   d. Is the test more correct in saying the patient is nontoxic when SPC is 22 µg/mL or less or in saying the patient is toxic when SPC is greater than 22 µg/mL?

   e. Does the test make more mistakes in classifying a patient as toxic when he or she is truly nontoxic or in classifying a patient as nontoxic when she or he is truly toxic?

   f. Critically evaluate the usefulness of 22 µg/mL as a SPC cutoff.

3.   Using the data of Eraker and Sasse[16] for relating serum digoxin concentration (SDC) to digoxin toxicity, the following test performance characteristics were calculated

using a cutoff of 2.0 ng/mL: true-positive rate = 0.8, false-positive rate = 0.11, true-negative rate = 0.89, false-negative rate = 0.2, cutoff likelihood ratio positive = 7.3, ratio of net consequences = 0.23, positive predictive value = 0.59, negative predictive value = 0.96, prevalence = 0.16. Which of the following statements are true:

a. Eighty percent of toxic patients have a SDC greater than 2 ng/mL.
b. Eighty percent of patients with a SDC greater than 2 ng/mL are toxic.
c. Eleven percent of patients with a SDC greater than 2 ng/mL are falsely classified as toxic.
d. Toxic patients are 7.3 times more likely to have an SDC greater than 2 ng/mL than are nontoxic patients.
e. At a cutoff of 2 ng/mL, falsely labeling a nontoxic patient as toxic is considered a much greater risk than falsely labeling a toxic patient as nontoxic.
f. $p(\text{tx}-|\text{SDC} \leq 2 \text{ ng/mL}) = 0.89$.
g. $p(\text{tx}+|\text{SDC} >2 \text{ ng/mL}) = 0.59$.
h. As 493 patients were evaluated in the study, 79 patients were determined to be toxic.

4. A practitioner assesses the pretest probability for digoxin toxicity in a patient as 0.33.

a. A SDC is obtained as 2.5 ng/mL. The associated range likelihood ratio for this SDC is 5.4. What is the posttest probability of toxicity in the patient?
b. Assume, instead, that the SDC is 0.8 ng/mL and the associated range likelihood ratio is 0.5. What is the posttest probability of toxicity?

5. Eraker and Sasse[16] have determined the mean utility scores among cardiologists for outcomes in the continue versus discontinue digoxin decision process when the digoxin-induced toxicity is ventricular tachycardia: $U_{c,\text{tx}-} = 1.0$, $U_{dc,\text{tx}+} = 0.91$, $U_{dc,\text{tx}-} = 0.89$, $U_{c,\text{tx}+} = 0$. What is the threshold probability (T_{dc}) for the decision process? What does the value you calculate mean?

6. Using the data in Example 7–16, what is the best decision for a practitioner who estimates a pretest probability of 0.60 for theophylline-induced toxicity in a patient?

BIBLIOGRAPHY

Barr JT, Schumacher GE. Decision analysis and pharmacoeconomic evaluations. In: Bootman JL, Townsend RJ, McGhan WF, eds. *Principles of Pharmacoeconomics.* Cincinnati: Harvey Whitney Books Co; 1991:112–133.
Sox HC, Blatt MA, Higgins MC, Marton KI. *Medical Decision Making.* Boston: Butterworths; 1988.
Weinstein MC, Fineberg HV, Elstein AS, et al. *Clinical Decision Analysis.* Philadelphia: WB Saunders; 1980.

REFERENCES

1. Ledley RS, Lusted LB. Reasoning foundations of medical diagnosis. *Science.* 1959;130:9–21.
2. Lusted LB. Decision making in patient management. *N Engl J Med.* 1971;284:416–424.
3. McNeil BJ, Keeler E, Adelstein SJ. Primer on certain elements of medical decision making. *N Engl J Med.* 1975;293:211–215.
4. Galen RS, Gambino SR. *Beyond Normality: The Predictive Value and Efficiency of Medical Diagnoses.* New York: Wiley; 1975.
5. Kassirer JP, Moskowitz AJ, Lau J, Pauker SG. Decision analysis: A progress report. *Ann Intern Med.* 1987;106:275–291.
6. Weinstein MC, Fineberg HV, Elstein AS, et al. *Clinical Decision Analysis.* Philadelphia: WB Saunders; 1980.
7. Sox HC, Blatt MA, Higgins MC, Marton KI. *Medical Decision Making.* Boston: Butterworths; 1988.
8. Einarson TR, McGhan WF, Bootman JL. Decision analysis applied to pharmacy practice. *Am J Hosp Pharm.* 1985;42:364–371.
9. Weinstein MC, Read L, MacKay DN, et al. Cost-effective choice of antimicrobial therapy for serious infections. *J Gen Intern Med.* 1986;1:351–363.
10. Kresel JJ, Hutchings HC, MacKay DN, et al. Application of decision analysis to drug selection for formulary addition. *Hosp Formul.* 1987;22:658–676.
11. Weiss JC, Melman ST. Cost effectiveness in the choice of antibiotics for the initial treatment of otitis media in children: A decision analysis approach. *Pediatr Infect Dis J.* 1988;7:23–26.
12. Callahan CW. Cost effectiveness of antibiotic therapy for otitis media in a military pediatric clinic. *Pediatr Infect Dis J.* 1988;7:622–625.
13. Reves RR, Johnson PC, Ericsson CD, DuPont HL. A cost-effectiveness comparison of the use of antimicrobial agents for treatment or prophylaxis of travelers' diarrhea. *Arch Intern Med.* 1988;148:2421–2427.
14. Mutnick AH, Szymusial-Mutnick B, Schumacher GE, Barr JT. Using decision analysis in the evaluation of drug therapy. *Pharm Times.* 1990;56 (Nov):59–66.
15. Jorgensen GM, Erramouspe J. Cost-effectiveness of selected management options for acute otitis media in ambulatory clinic patients. *Consult Pharm.* 1991;6:241–245.
16. Eraker SA, Sasse L. The serum digoxin test and digoxin toxicity: A bayesian approach to decision making. *Circulation.* 1981;64:409–420.
17. Barr JT, Schumacher GE. Applying decision analysis in therapeutic drug monitoring: Using receiver-operating characteristic curves in comparative evaluations. *Clin Pharm.* 1986;5:239–246.
18. Schumacher GE, Barr JT. Applying decision analysis in therapeutic drug monitoring: Using decision trees to interpret serum theophylline concentrations. *Clin Pharm.* 1986;5:325–333.
19. Eraker SA, Eeckhoudt LR, Vanbutsele RJM, et al. To test or not to test—To treat or not to treat: The decision-threshold approach to patient management. *J Gen Intern Med.* 1986;1:177–182.
20. Schumacher GE, Barr JT. Making serum drug levels more meaningful. *Ther Drug Monit.* 1989; 11:580–584.
21. Jordan TJ, Reichman LB. Once-daily versus twice-daily dosing of theophylline: A decision analysis approach to evaluating theophylline blood levels and compliance. *Am Rev Respir Dis.* 1989; 140:1573–1577.
22. Schumacher GE, Barr JT. Using population-based serum drug concentration cutoff values to predict toxicity: Test performance and limitations compared with bayesian interpretation. *Clin Pharm.* 1990;9:788–796.
23. Schumacher GE, Barr JT, Browne TR, et al. Test performance characteristics of the serum phenytoin concentration (SPC): The relationship between SPC and patient response. *Ther Drug Monit.* 1991; 13:318–324.

24. Drumond MF, Stoddart GL, Torrance GW. *Methods for the Economic Evaluation of Health Care Programmes.* Oxford: Oxford University Press; 1987.
25. Pauker SG, Kassirer JP. Therapeutic decision making: A cost–benefit analysis. *N Engl J Med.* 1975; 293:229–234.
26. Pauker SG, Kassirer JP. The threshold approach to clinical decision making. *N Engl J Med.* 1980; 302:1109–1117.
27. Ransohoff DF, Feinstein AR. Problems of spectrum and bias in evaluating the efficacy of diagnostic tests. *N Engl J Med.* 1978;299:926–930.
28. Schumacher GE, Barr JT. Bayesian and threshold probabilities in therapeutic drug monitoring: When can serum drug concentrations alter clinical decisions? *Am J Hosp Pharm.* 1994;51:321–327.
29. Aronson JK, Grahame-Smith DC, Wigley FM. Monitoring digoxin therapy. *Q J Med.* 1978;47: 111–122.
30. Carruthers SG, Kelly JG, McDevitt DG. Plasma digoxin concentrations in patients on admission to hospital. *Br Heart J.* 1984;36:707–712.

Chapter 8

Outcomes Assessment of Therapeutic Drug Monitoring: System and Patient Considerations

Judith T. Barr

Gerald E. Schumacher

Keep in Mind

- Outcomes assessment refers to the quantitative evaluation of certain variables that characterize the result or impact of an intervention. In this chapter, therapeutic drug monitoring (TDM) and clinical pharmacokinetic services are the interventions.

- The traditional approach of Donabedian in assessing quality of care is to characterize a combination, and occasionally the interaction, of structure, process, and outcome components. Most commonly when using this model, evaluators focus on independently measuring narrow individual variables within these components rather than recognizing and assessing the interplay among the three domains.

- This chapter emphasizes a more interactive approach to outcomes assessment of TDM by organizing the variables into two categories, system-related and patient-related measures. System-related measures focus on evaluating the administrative, procedural, and economic aspects of providing TDM. Patient-related measures focus on evaluating the effect of the intervention of TDM on the response of the patient. Examples of system-related measures include the percentage of appropriate and inappropriate assays, the percentage of samples collected at the proper time after administration of a dose, the cost of unnecessary assays, the average number of samples per patient, and the percentage of TDM results within the therapeutic range. Examples of patient-related measures for TDM drugs include the percentage of patients cured, percentage of patients exhibiting drug-induced toxic effects, and the costs of toxicity.

- A number of studies have evaluated the impact of TDM on outcomes. These studies have overwhelmingly focused on system-related outcomes. Administrative processes of care delivery variables have been most commonly studied and have often shown a positive effect of TDM on a number of variables including timing of serum drug concentration sampling, recognition of appropriate indications for TDM testing, and appropriate response to serum

191

concentration results. Administrative outcomes of care delivery have also been evaluated, most frequently with respect to the positive effect of TDM on achieving serum drug concentrations within the therapeutic range.

- Patient-related outcomes have been too infrequently studied. Although the results of TDM on improving system-related outcomes are often impressive, improvement in the proportion of TDM results within the therapeutic range (a system-related outcome) does not mean the same thing as improvement in the proportion of patients who achieve a therapeutic response without toxicity (a patient-related outcome) as a result of TDM. Although the former outcome is important, the latter outcome is more so.

- A complete examination of the economic consequences or impact of TDM requires (1) a comparison of at least two comparable populations of patients, one receiving TDM services and another, during the same period, serving as a control population and not receiving TDM care; (2) an itemization of the costs (inputs) of providing the TDM service including proportional costs of salaries and fringes, equipment, supplies, and overhead; and (3) a complete detailing of all consequences (outputs) for patients in both populations during the episode of care. When these outputs are kept in their natural units (eg, hospital days) and the differences in outputs are compared with the differences in cost of the inputs (TDM versus no TDM), a cost–effectiveness study can be performed. When the differences in outputs or benefits are converted to dollars (eg, cost of a hospital day) and compared with the differences in the cost of inputs in dollars, then a cost–benefit analysis is possible. No studies meeting these requirements have been conducted on TDM to date.

- Quality of life is a patient-centered multidimensional concept increasingly used to evaluate the health status of a patient. It includes the interrelationship of four dimensions impacting on patient status: physical, psychologic, social, and economic. Examples of the impact of TDM include the influence on the physical dimension by improving the cure rate or decreasing morbidity, on the psychologic dimension by decreasing the depressing effect of drug-induced toxicity, and on the economic dimension by reducing the days of hospitalization and the cost of cotherapy to reduce drug-induced adverse reactions.

Outcomes assessment is an important component of the evaluation of any clinical intervention or health delivery system. With limited health care dollars, clinicians as well as health administrators and policy makers need to know if tests, services, and clinical interventions are effective, if they are performed as efficiently as possible, and if they provide a benefit to the patient.

Outcomes assessment of therapeutic drug monitoring (TDM) is complicated by definitional issues. What is TDM? For some, TDM is a laboratory test, but for others, that test is part of a larger TDM system of health care delivery. As a laboratory test, it is used to determine the serum drug concentration for medications that have a narrow concentration range of therapeutic effectiveness. Following the principles of the Total Testing Process (see Chapter 3), the performance of a TDM test should incorporate an assessment of the clinical indication for testing, the timing and collection of the specimen, the performance of the analysis, the proper interpretation of the result, the initiation of indicated action, and its impact on patient care. Therapeutic drug monitoring, however, can also connote an organized system of health care delivery usually entitled a therapeutic drug monitoring service or clinical pharmacokinetic service. As a system of care, a TDM service guides or intervenes in the Total Testing Process to ensure that the serum drug concentration will have maximal positive impact on patient care. An assessment of a TDM service could include its impact not only on patient care, but also on the economic efficiency of the delivery system.

How do we assess the outcomes of therapeutic drug monitoring? In both definitions, the critical outcome measure is the effect of TDM test results or a clinical pharmacokinetic service on patient care. Patient-centered outcome measures would be the measures most directly related to the clinical effectiveness of the test or service; however, historically, studies evaluating TDM have concentrated on examining the process of TDM testing and providing TDM services, rather than assessing its impact on patient care. Also, these studies primarily have used system-related rather than patient-related outcomes in assessing the effectiveness of clinical pharmacokinetic services. Therefore, we begin this chapter with a description of these two different, but not mutually exclusive, methods of assessing quality of care: (1) the traditional structure–process–outcome method of evaluation and (2) a more patient-centered, multidimensional outcomes approach to the assessment of the effectiveness of an intervention. Then we examine, from both a system and patient perspective, the measures used to describe and evaluate the effectiveness of TDM tests and services. We conclude with recommendations of steps needed to convert the system-based structure and process TDM studies into patient-centered outcomes assessment of the clinical effectiveness of TDM tests and services.

STRUCTURE, PROCESS, AND OUTCOME

Donabedian proposed the structure–process–outcome method for the assessment of quality of care.[1] In this model, the evaluation of the *structure* component includes factors related to the structure of a health care delivery system—its buildings, equipment, and staff. This can consist of an assessment of the adequacy and quality of facilities and equipment, their conformance to building codes and other standards, qualifications and experience of staff, personnel staffing patterns, organization reporting arrangements, financing arrangements, and other structural elements. In therapeutic drug monitoring, examples of structure components include adequacy of the TDM testing equipment and facilities, qualifications of clinical and laboratory staff, presence of a TDM service, supervision, and administrative organization.

The *process* component includes the activities involved in the process of delivering health care services. These can involve actions of health care providers and patients as well as organizational processes within the health care system. Several questions that can be raised to assess the quality of the process of TDM testing center around the steps of the Total Testing Process: Is the test clinically indicated? Is the blood specimen collected at the appropriate time? Is the specimen properly labeled and processed within the laboratory? Is the TDM reported to the clinician in a timely manner? Is appropriate action taken? Is the patient adhering to the dosing schedule?

The *outcome* component examines the effect of a health care intervention on the outcome of the patient and, from a delivery system perspective, the impact on the economic performance of the health care system. The ultimate criterion to assess outcome of an intervention, such as TDM, is the health status of the individual; however, economic outcomes also can be important elements of an evaluation. The structure–process–outcome model of assessment does not include a clear definition of what is meant by *health status* to guide the evaluation of the outcome component. Generally the definition of outcomes has taken a provider-oriented approach and has focused on measures that are part of the traditional medical vocabulary. In this model, examples of outcome measures that could be used to assess the effectiveness of TDM include incidence of toxicity, cure, mortality, and cost savings associated with a TDM service.

In the structure–process–outcome model, evaluators tend to independently measure narrow individual elements rather than recognize and assess the interplay among the three components. As depicted in Figure 8–1, structure, process, and outcome interact to determine quality of care. Whether or not an outcome is achieved (reduction in toxicity) is dependent on an interaction between structural elements (presence of TDM service, staff qualifications, institutional resources, quality of facility) and process elements (specimen collection time guided by time of last dose and steady-state status, patient dosage adherence, appropriate action taken). Each of the 64 smaller cubes, some to a greater extent than others, contribute to the definition of TDM quality. For example, in the shaded cube, one asks the question: Is the incidence of toxicity related to the appropriate time-from-last-dose sampling and the presence of a TDM service? Many studies, however, including TDM examples, rely on an assessment of process variables with little attention to their impact on the other two components. Measuring improvements in process variables without linking them to changes in outcome measures or examining the implications for structure changes results in an incomplete assessment.

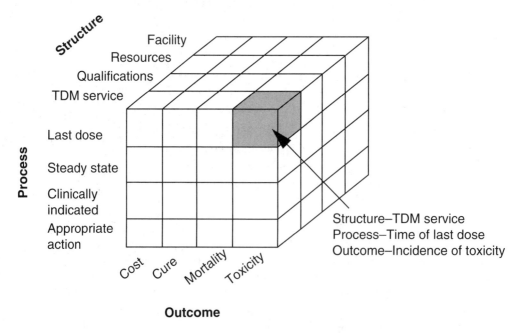

Figure 8–1. Structure, process, and outcome measures in therapeutic drug monitoring. Three-dimensional depiction of the interaction of examples of structure, process, and outcome variables used in the evaluation of therapeutic drug monitoring.

PATIENT-CENTERED OUTCOMES ASSESSMENT

Although some would say that patient-centered outcomes assessment is nothing more than an extension of the outcome component of the Donabedian structure–process–outcome model, patient-centered outcomes assessment represents a major shift in assessment content and perspective. Although the Donabedian model measures primarily *institutional* and *system* characteristics as viewed from a *medical* perspective, patient-centered outcomes assessment, as the name implies, focuses on the impact of the intervention or health delivery system on the *patient's* outcomes and, most importantly, as viewed from a *patient's* perspective. In a Continuous Quality Improvement system, the results of such outcomes-based assessment can be used to feed back into the system to identify structure and process factors that are associated with improved outcomes.

Patient-centered outcomes assessment builds on the World Health Organization's definition of health as "a complete state of physical, mental, and social well-being and not merely the absence of disease." From this perspective, outcomes assessment is now more than a biologic or pathophysiologic measurement after treatments or interventions; it is more than whether the TDM is clinically indicated, whether the serum drug concentration is within the therapeutic range, or whether a clinician takes appropriate action in response to a TDM result. As Epstein describes:

> Perhaps the most important effect of the outcomes movement has been a broadening of our focus to include a wider range of outcomes. . . . We have seen a dramatic expansion in the range of outcomes that physicians and policy makers are willing to consider valid indicators of health. These go far beyond traditional clinical indexes and include a series of variables assessed through interviews: functional status, emotional health, social interaction, cognitive function, degree of disability, and so forth. There is a growing appreciation in the medical community that instruments based on subjective data from patients can provide important information that may not be evident from physiologic measurements and may be as reliable as—or more reliable than—many of the clinical, biochemical, or physiologic indexes.[2]

Ellwood described these broader measures as "a technology of patient experience designed to help patients, payers, and providers make rational medical care-related choices based on better insight into the effect of these choices on the patient's life. It would routinely and systematically measure the functioning and well-being of patients, along with disease-specific clinical outcomes." Ellwood proposes that these types of measurements be central to the development of a longitudinal type of outcomes assessment: "The centerpiece and unifying ingredient of outcomes management is the tracking and measurement of function and well-being or quality of life" across health care locations.[3]

Quality of life is a multidimensional concept encompassing physical, psychologic, social, and economic functioning of an individual. As depicted in Figure 8–2, these quality-of-life assessments incorporate all four dimensions and sit on top of a hierarchy of progressively less comprehensive outcome measures. Quality-of-life assessments provide a complete picture of the health status of an individual. Instruments in the second level contain questions covering many characteristics of a specific dimension, and the third level consists of questions or physiologic measures of single factors within one dimension. For example, the Independent Activities of Daily Living Scale (IADL) is a comprehensive measure incorporating many patient-centered elements of physical functioning, whereas level 3 elements such as serum theophylline concentration and the forced

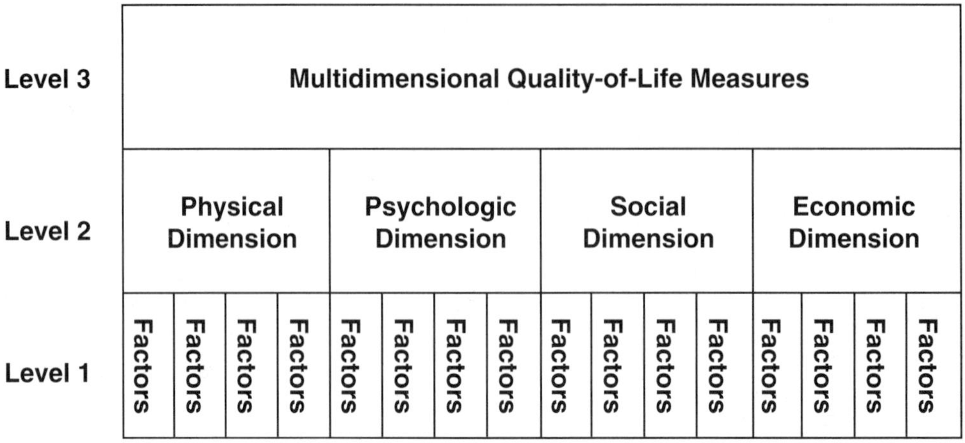

Level 3	Multidimensional Quality-of-Life Measures															
Level 2	Physical Dimension				Psychologic Dimension				Social Dimension				Economic Dimension			
Level 1	Factors	Factors	Factors	Factors	Factors	Factors	Factors	Factors	Factors	Factors	Factors	Factors	Factors	Factors	Factors	Factors

Figure 8–2. Hierarchy of patient-centered outcomes assessment measures.

expiratory capacity in 1 second (FEV_1) capture single factors within the physical functioning dimension. Measures directed only at one dimension of health or assessing only single factors within a dimension are incomplete assessments of the individual's status and provide a limited evaluation of the effectiveness of the total impact of an intervention on a patient's outcome.

Although multidimensional quality-of-life measures frequently are called *outcomes assessments,* they serve more functions than simply measuring the outcome of an intervention. They can be used to *measure* the status of a patient at a single point in time, to *monitor* the status of a patient over time and hence assess the effectiveness of clinical intervention, and then, based on the clinical effectiveness results, to *manage* future patients as well as the best allocation of limited economic resources. Determining an "outcome" implies at least a two-step process. For example, to assess the effectiveness or "outcome" of a clinical intervention, the patient must be measured both before and after a clinical intervention. Baseline or preintervention information is needed to determine patient status prior to an intervention, and then postintervention measures indicate how much the patient has changed as a result of the intervention. Clinicians can use repeated measures of multidimensional "outcomes" assessment throughout the treatment or intervention process. This helps them to better understand the impact of the intervention by profiling when and what changes appear in each of the health status dimensions.

MEASURES TO DESCRIBE AND EVALUATE THERAPEUTIC DRUG MONITORING

The goal of therapeutic drug monitoring is to maximize therapeutic effectiveness while minimizing drug-related adverse events. Therefore, it would seem logical that studies evaluating the effectiveness of TDM testing and clinical pharmacokinetic services would use clinical outcome measures that would capture the increase in therapeutic effectiveness (eg, increased rate of cure) and the decrease in such adverse drug events as nephrotoxicity and nausea and vomiting.

That has not been the case, however. Instead, therapeutic drug monitoring studies have focused primarily on the administrative processes involved in TDM testing; only a few have assessed its impact on clinical outcomes. These studies are of two general types: (1) descriptive studies, which describe the quality of the process steps in TDM testing, and (2) evaluative studies, which evaluate the effectiveness of some type of an intervention, such as the introduction of a TDM service, to improve the quality of TDM testing and the interpretation of the test results. These studies are descriptions and evaluations of elements in a system of care; few directly measure the impact of TDM on patient outcome. Although clinical pharmacists probably assume that improvements in the administrative process of care would lead to improved clinical outcomes, such assumptions rarely have been investigated.

But what measures have been used to describe or evaluate the effectiveness of TDM tests or services? Administrative measures of system efficacy dominate this literature: for example, proportion of samples that are timed correctly, proportion of serum drug concentrations within the therapeutic range, and proportion of TDM tests that were clinically indicated. These studies frequently incorporate multiple outcome measures in their study design and may assess administrative as well as economic measures such as the cost of inappropriately timed or clinically unnecessary TDM testing. Occasionally, the investigators include patient-related evaluations and examine if, as a result of TDM services, outcomes such as the incidence of toxicity have been reduced or the cure rate has been increased. None have incorporated patient-centered, quality-of-life measures in a TDM evaluation.

Table 8–1 suggests one approach to organizing this topic. First, the type of measures is divided into those that are system related and are used to describe the quality of TDM testing or to evaluate the effectiveness of a TDM service as viewed by the health care system, and those that are patient related and are used to describe the impact of TDM testing or services on factors of direct benefit to the patient. In this taxonomy, descriptors such as the percentage of TDM results within the therapeutic range, percentage of levels taken during steady state, and duration of hospital stay are classified as system-related, not patient-related, measures. These measures describe the quality of administrative aspects of care, but they serve only as proxies or indirect methods to capture the impact of TDM services on patient outcome. Patient-related outcomes include such measures as presence of toxicity, cure rate, and mortality rate.

In the next level of this taxonomy, the system-related and patient-related sections are subdivided into the Donabedian categories of structure, process, and outcome. This classification is used because most TDM reports are not "outcome" studies by either the Donabedian or patient-centered definition of outcome. Instead, TDM has been described and evaluated primarily using Donabedian's process-type measures: for example, percentage of TDM samples that were clinically indicated, percentage of samples properly timed. When outcome measures are used in the system-related studies, they are system or administrative measures that have an inferred, but not direct, link to patient outcomes.

Lastly, there is great interest in methods to assess the economic impact of health care services and to increase the economic efficacy of the health delivery system. Therefore, economic measures designed to capture the cost implications of TDM testing and services are separated from the administrative and clinical measures associated with the provision of TDM services and the assessment of its quality.

The following sections are organized following the taxonomy displayed in Table 8–1. In each area we describe the measures grouped in that section, comment on the descriptive or eval-

TABLE 8–1. TAXONOMY OF MEASURES USED IN PUBLISHED STUDIES OF THE ASSESSMENT OF THERAPEUTIC DRUG MONITORING

System-Related Measures	Patient-Related Measures
Structure	*Structure*
Process	*Process*
Administrative Process of Care Delivery Variables	Compliance
Clinically indicated	
Percentage of assays not clinically indicated	
Percentage of patients needing assay who got it	*Outcome*
Timing of specimen collection	
Steady state	*Clinical Impact on Patient Care*
Postdistribution	Incidence of toxic effects
Overall timing	Number of septic episodes
Time of phlebotomy given	Reduction of symptoms/increase in cure
Obtained within first 48 hours	Mortality
Appropriate action	*Economic*
Frequency of toxicity monitoring	
Number of dosing changes	
Economic Consequences of Administrative Processes	
Cost/savings of unnecessary samples	
Cost/savings of inappropriate samples	
Cost/savings of inappropriate action	
Cost of TDM/CPKS	

Outcome

Administrative Outcomes of Care Delivery
TDM tests
  Number of TDM tests per patient
  Percentage of TDM results within therapeutic range
    Individual monitoring parameters: toxic and therapeutic peaks, toxic and therapeutic troughs
  Percentage of patients with TDM tests within therapeutic levels in first 24 hours
Dose
Time
  Duration of therapy
  Time on intravenous dose/time to oral medication
  Length of infection
  Length of intensive care
  Length of hospital stay
Impact on further health care consumption
  Readmission
  Number of emergency room visits
  Number of hospital admission
  Number of visits
Economic Consequences of Administrative Outcomes
  Laboratory costs/day
  Cost of course of therapy
  Cost of hospital stay
  Cost of episode
  Overall costs
  Cost–benefit analysis

uative studies that used those measures, and summarize the conclusions of the studies. When no example is given below for a category in Table 8–1, for example, patient-related economic outcome, no studies have been reported.

SYSTEM-RELATED MEASURES

System evaluations rely on administrative and system-related economic measurements to describe or evaluate the structure, process, and outcome of TDM testing and TDM delivery systems. Most early TDM reports were simple descriptions documenting the poor quality of the TDM test process; some included estimations of the "wasted" dollars associated with inappropriately timed samples or unnecessary TDM tests. Later studies compared the quality of the TDM testing process before and after the introduction of a clinical pharmacokinetic service; again, economic assessments frequently were included. A few recent evaluations of clinical pharmacokinetic services have assessed their impact using the more rigorous study design of a randomized control trial.

It is important to reemphasize that the measures in this section do not directly describe the impact of TDM testing and services on patient care. They should be considered administrative measures, which have been used to describe components of the TDM testing system and methods to improve the structure, process, and outcome of that system. Although it is assumed that improvements in administrative processes and outcomes will result in improvements in patient outcomes, system studies leave unanswered larger questions concerning their impact on improving patient outcome.

Structure

Many studies have asked the system-related question: "Can clinical pharmacokinetic services improve the quality of TDM testing?"[4–56] This question is a system-related structure question: Can a change in the *structure* of the health delivery system, in this case the establishment of clinical pharmacokinetic services, improve the quality of the health care system? Although this is a structure question, process and outcome measures have been used to evaluate the services. These measures are described in the following sections, but first some comments are made about the characteristics of the structure of the clinical pharmacokinetic services that were evaluated in these studies.

Structure characteristics of a health delivery system involve such elements as physical characteristics of the facility, equipment, staff structure, administrative procedures, and professional/personnel requirements. And here lies a problem in trying to answer the question as to whether or not clinical pharmacokinetic services (CPKSs) make a difference. The CPKSs are not of uniform structure, and hence, cross-study comparisons are usually comparing apples to oranges. Some CPKSs are formal structures that require all TDM testing to pass through the service; others are informal arrangements that make only timing and dosing recommendations. Some work out of the pharmacy department; others have established separate units. Some perform their own pharmacokinetic analyses; others rely on the clinical laboratory. Some only schedule the timing of TDM samples; others also report results to the patients' floors, and others report the results with dosing recommendations. There are differences in reporting mechanisms, desired serum concentrations, serum sampling strategies, dosing methods, and other administrative procedures. Few describe the professional/personnel qualifications of the members of the CPKS.

To determine if therapeutic drug monitoring and clinical pharmacokinetic services do make a difference and to determine if different types of CPKS structure affect the answer to that question, a structured evaluation program is necessary. Structure standards for CPKS should be developed and evaluated in multiple locations. These evaluations must include both administrative and clinical outcomes assessments. Then modifications to the standards can be examined to determine which elements of the structure are essential to quality care. Although the structure of a CPKS is shaped by each institution's own characteristics, physical plant, and power hierarchy, the establishment of national, minimum guidelines for clinical pharmacokinetics services would contribute to a better understanding of the contribution that the service could provide.

Process

There are two components of system-related process measures: (1) administrative processes or actions and (2) the economic consequences of these processes. Administrative process measures are used to describe the quality of the procedural steps in the total testing process and assess the effectiveness of clinical pharmacokinetic services and pharmacy-based educational programs in improving the TDM testing process. When economic values can be assigned to the waste gener-ated by poor procedures or to process improvements associated with clinical pharmacokinetic services, then the economic consequences of traditional and CPKS delivery systems can be compared.

Early studies were simple retrospective audits documenting procedural problems in TDM testing; however, there are problems with retrospective studies. Individuals conducting audits had to rely on the written record as found in the patient's chart; generally it was incomplete and did not document all clinical reasoning or timing details. Also, the reviewer compared the documentation in the chart with a set of explicit, predetermined criteria that detailed the acceptable clinical reasons for obtaining a TDM test, the correct timing procedures for specimen collection, and the indicated action given various ranges of serum drug concentrations. Using these explicit criteria, the reviewer would interpret the chart and determine if the procedures indicated in the chart notes met the quality criteria.

The review of an incomplete chart and the application of rigid, predetermined criteria could lead to invalid conclusions. For example, the explicit criteria may state that for a patient receiving theophylline, if a properly collected serum concentration is greater than 20 µg/mL, the patient's medication should be reduced. What if a patient had a serum theophylline concentration of 24 µg/mL, was clinically stable, and had no signs of adverse drug reactions? According to the explicit written quality criteria, the reviewer could not exercise independent judgment and must conclude that the clinician did not take appropriate clinical action, even though clinical judgment indicated that the best course of action was to continue the current dose. Because this retrospective method of chart review assumed that any omission or deviation from the predetermined criteria was in error, it is possible that the use of explicit audit criteria may have biased the audits and found a poorer quality of TDM testing than actually occurred.

To reduce the bias associated with retrospective chart reviews and predetermined criteria, more sophisticated studies were performed in the late 1980s and early 1990s. These included prospective comparisons of TDM quality and the associated economic implications before and after a clinical pharmacokinetic service intervention, as well as randomized control trials with one patient population being followed by CPKS while others received traditional care.

Administrative Processes of Care

Both retrospective and prospective studies have used administrative process measures to answer three broad questions: (1) Are the TDM orders clinically indicated? (2) Are the TDM specimens correctly sampled? (3) Do TDM results lead to appropriate action relating to drug dosage? These correspond to Steps 2, 4, and 9 of the Total Testing Process (see Chapter 3). The studies and the administrative process measures used to answer these questions are summarized in Tables 8–2, 8–3, and 8–4, respectively, and in the sections that follow. Note that there are wide variations in the obtained answers. Although adequate detail is not provided to explain these differences, they may be related to the structural characteristics of the institution, unique patient populations, or differing explicit criteria for acceptable TDM testing procedures. For example, if one chart reviewer was using a digoxin level greater than 2.0 ng/mL to indicate that the dose should be reduced and another reviewer at another institution was using a concentration of 2.2 ng/mL, you can see that, if all else was the same, the first individual would conclude that her review revealed more inappropriate action because the decision threshold was set at a lower level. In this case it is the criterion that is different, not the quality of the two institutions.

Clinically Indicated. There are several approaches to answering the question: Are the TDM orders clinically indicated? The 24 studies cited in Table 8–2 report the result either as a *percentage* of the ordered TDM tests that are clinically indicated or, conversely, the *percentage* of ordered TDM tests that are clinically inappropriate. The widest variation in percentage of specimens that were judged to be clinically inappropriate was found in the 13 digoxin reports; from 18 to 82.5% were evaluated as clinically inappropriate. The variation in the four theophylline studies ranged from 7 to 41%; the three aminoglycoside reports, from 10.9 to 32.8%; and the four studies that combined all drug assessments found 17.9 to 42% clinically inappropriate TDM tests. Einarson et al, in a meta-analysis of 14 studies, found an overall average of 34.7% clinically inappropriate assays and a 27.8% inappropriate rate when the results of the 14 studies were weighted by the number of TDM tests in each study.[57] The overall unweighted average of the studies in Table 8–2, excluding that of Einarson et al, is 37.6%; this is very close to the 34.7% reported by Einarson et al.

As indicated in Table 8–2, 8 of the 24 studies evaluated the impact of some type of pharmacy-related intervention, generally the establishment of a CPKS or an educational intervention, on the rate of clinically inappropriate TDM testing. Only the investigators in the three most recent studies[37,54,75] statistically evaluated their results to determine if there was a difference in the percentage of TDM tests that were judged to be clinically unnecessary before and after the pharmacy-based intervention. All found a significant reduction in the rates of clinically inappropriate levels between the two periods.

In addition to examining the percentage of TDM tests that were not clinically indicated, another approach to answering the question, Are the TDM orders clinically indicated? is to determine the average *number of assays per patient* that were not indicated. Wing and Duff examined the question from both approaches and got different results![55] When they compared the percentage of digoxin tests that were not indicated clinically, there was no difference between the groups with and without pharmacy involvement, but when they compared the average number of digoxin assays per patient that were not indicated, the patients on floors serviced by the CPKS had

TABLE 8–2. STUDIES INCORPORATING ADMINISTRATIVE PROCESS MEASURE: CLINICALLY INAPPROPRIATE USE OF THERAPEUTIC DRUG MONITORING TESTING

First Author	Year	Percentage Inappropriate Before Pharmacy Action	Percentage Inappropriate After Pharmacy Action	Drug[a]
Goldberg (60)	1974	70.4		dig
Anderson (61)	1976	10.9		amino
Floyd (62)	1977	18.8		dig
Parker (36)	1978	37	8.3	dig
Slaughter (63)	1978	49		dig
Greenlaw (64)	1980	18		dig
Levin (30)	1981	52, 42	15, 15	dig, all
Clague (65)	1983	82.5		dig
Lampasona (66)	1983	32.8		amino
Guernsey (67)	1984	34		dig
Guernsey (68)	1984	31.9		theo
Ives (69)	1984	17.9		all
Wiser (70)	1984	>50		dig
Sargenti (71)	1985	26		theo
Farris (72)	1986	43.8		theo
Kimelblatt (26)	1986	47	35	amino
Kildoo (73)	1987	31		all
Wing (53)	1987	7–15		theo
Wing (55)	1987	74	58	dig
Karki (74)	1988	16		Li
Klamerus (27)	1988	56	47 rounds, 26 plus RN education	dig
Wing (54)[b]	1989	28	0, then 15 when stopped	phen
Pearce (37)[b]	1990	30.8	14.4	all
D'Angio (75)[b]	1990	17,62,41	3, 30, 26	amino, dig, theo
Einarson (57)	1989	34.7	average of 14 studies	
		27.8	weighted average of 14 studies	

[a]amino = aminoglycosides, dig = digoxin, li = lithium, phen = phenytoin, theo = theophylline.
[b]Statistically significant difference, at $P = 0.05$ or less, in appropriateness between before and after pharmacy action.

significantly fewer assays that were not clinically indicated than patients on floors without such a service. On the study floors, the pharmacists intervened to reduce the overall number of TDM tests. Therefore, although the percentage of clinically unnecessary TDM tests stayed the same, the average number of TDM tests as well as the average number of clinically unnecessary tests per patient decreased. This case illustrates that the framing of the question and the administrative process measure selected can influence the answer.

TABLE 8–3. STUDIES INCORPORATING ADMINISTRATIVE PROCESS MEASURES RELATED TO TIMING OF THERAPEUTIC DRUG MONITORING SAMPLES BEFORE AND WITH PHARMACY (Rx) INVOLVEMENT

| First Author | Year | Percentage of Specimens, Incorrect Timing | | | | | | Drug[a] |
| | | Steady State | | Postdistribution | | Overall | | |
		Pre-Rx	With Rx	Pre-Rx	With Rx	Pre-Rx	With Rx	
Anderson (61)	1976					52		amino
Floyd (62)	1977					48		theo
Flynn (77)	1978					51		amino
Parker (36)	1978					55.8	8.4	dig
Slaughter (42)	1978	14		4		17		dig
Greenlaw (18)[b]	1979					25.7	9.8	hep
Greenlaw (64)	1980					45		dig
Bollish (7)[b]	1981					67	5	amino
Gentry (78)	1981	36		56		59		theo
Harless (79)	1981	63		43				theo
Levin (30)	1981					44, 51	9,12	dig, all
Pasko (80)	1981					38.6		tobra
Vlasses (81)	1982	5		8				dig
Bussey (82)	1983	5		26		43		all
Clague (65)	1983	7.5		6				dig
Guernsey (67)	1984					27		dig
Guernsey (68)	1984	33		18.7				theo
Ives (69)	1984					100		all
Mason (83)	1984	42.2		27.8				all
Shaw (84)[b]	1984					30	3	amino
Tierney (46)[b]	1984			20	1.6			amino
Horn (20)[b]	1985					32	20.7	dig
Pitterle (38)[b]	1985					55	12	all
Sargenti (71)	1985	12						theo
Farris (72)	1986					56.3		theo
Gibb (85)	1986			49				dig
Kimelblatt (26)[b]	1986					89	39	amino
Winter (56)[b]	1986					82	45.8	amino, theo
Blackbourn (6)[b]	1987					42	15	theo
Kildoo (73)	1987			26				all
Wing (54)	1987					66	59	theo
Wing (55)	1987					41.5	39.5	dig
Ambrose (4)	1988					>60	1.9	all
Levine (86)	1988	72.5						phen
Karki (74)	1988					2		Li

(*continued*)

TABLE 8–3. CONTINUED

First Author	Year	Percentage of Specimens, Incorrect Timing						Drug[a]
		Steady State		Postdistribution		Overall		
		Pre-Rx	With Rx	Pre-Rx	With Rx	Pre-Rx	With Rx	
Job (23)	1989					40	5.7	all
Wing (53)	1989					75.5	66.5	phen
D'Angio (75)[b]	1990					100, 55, 59	52,53,47	amino, dig, theo
Pearce (37)[b]	1990					60.2	14.4	all
Wade (48)	1990					43.5		theo
Carroll (76)[b]	1992					79	30 (ed)	amino
Kumana (87)	1992	31.4						dig
Lynch (33)[b]	1992					38	10	amino
Einarson (57)	1989					47.2	average of 25 studies	
						42.5	weighted average of 25 studies	

[a] Drug: amino = aminoglycoside, dig = digoxin, li = lithium, phen = phenytoin, theo = theophylline.
[b] Statistically significant difference at $P = 0.05$ or lower between the period before and that after pharmacy-based action.

Although these are ways to determine if ordered tests were really needed, they do not answer a related question: What percentage of patients whose clinical condition indicated that TDM testing would be appropriate did not have levels ordered? For example, Lampasona and Crass identified all patients who were receiving aminoglycosides and then determined (1) if they had a TDM test, was it clinically indicated, or (2) if they did not have a TDM test, did they have a clinical reason why one should have been ordered.[66] Of 40 patients who met at least one criterion indicating TDM testing was appropriate, assays were ordered for only 40%; 60% did not receive a clinically indicated test. Although no information is provided as to whether these patients developed clinical complications as a result of TDM testing not being performed, this case does illustrate that a comprehensive assessment of the contribution of a CPKS to improving the process of TDM testing should examine the care of all eligible TDM patients and ask two questions: What percentage of TDM tests was clinically indicated? For what percentage of eligible patients was a TDM test indicated and obtained?

Three recent studies have asked the latter question during assessments of pharmacy-based TDM intervention and educational programs. In all studies, pharmacy-based interventions increased the percentage of patients who received clinically indicated TDM testing. Cahill et al were able to increase from 36 to 90% the percentage of patients who had an aminoglycoside determination when therapy was equal to or longer than 4 days.[10] In two other studies, a TDM service was able to increase from 43 to 83% the percentage of patients who had theophylline assays when clinically indicated,[6] and a pharmacy-based educational program increased from 48 to 76% the percentage of patients whose clinical condition indicated the need for an aminoglycoside assay and received one.[76]

TABLE 8–4. STUDIES INCORPORATING ADMINISTRATIVE PROCESS MEASURE: CLINICALLY INAPPROPRIATE ACTION IN RESPONSE TO SERUM DRUG CONCENTRATION

First Author	Year	Percentage Inappropriate Before Pharmacy Action	Percentage Inappropriate After Pharmacy Action	Drug[a]
Goldberg (60)	1974	47		dig
Wilson (52)	1974	79	66	phen
Anderson (61)	1976	80		amino
Floyd (62)	1977	80		theo
Flynn (77)	1978	78		amino
Parker (36)	1978	73.4	29.1	dig
Slaughter (42)	1978	10.8		dig
Greenlaw (18)	1979	17.7	14.5	hep
Greenlaw (88)	1979		8.5	amino
Taylor (45)	1979		28	all
Greenlaw (64)	1980	64		dig
Bollish (7)[b]	1981	86	5	amino
Levin (30)	1981	13, 16	2, 5	dig, all
Matzke (89)	1981	59		amino
Pasko (80)	1981	38	10	amino
Rich (39)[b]	1981	54.5	20	dig
Robinson (40)	1981		4, 0	dig, theo
Sketris (90)	1982	31		amino
Beardsley (91)	1983	17		anticon
Bussey (82)	1983	40		all
Clague (65)	1983	28.3		dig
Guernsey (67)	1984	13.9		dig
Guernsey (68)	1984	31.6		theo
Knodel (92)	1984	59.7		theo
Ives (69)	1984	47.8		all
Tierney (46)[b]	1984	70	16	amino
Wallace (49)	1984		17	amino
Whiting (51)	1984	28, 30, 55		dig, theo, phen
Horn (20)	1985		38.2	dig
Pitterle (38)[b]	1985	17.6	9.5	all
Quebbeman (93)	1985	76		amino
Sargenti (71)	1985	41		theo
Snidero (94)	1985	28		dig
Arroyo (95)	1986	36		amino
Cahill (10)[b]	1986	60	14	amino
Farris (72)	1986	15		theo
Gibb (85)	1986	24		dig
Winter (56)	1986	6.7	7.1	amino+theo

205

TABLE 8–4. CONTINUED

First Author	Year	Percentage Inappropriate		Drug[a]
		Before Pharmacy Action	**After Pharmacy Action**	
Blackbourn (6)[b]	1987	37	14	theo
Kildoo (73)	1987	32		all
Wing (54)[b]	1987	73.5	68	theo
Wing (55)[b]	1987	84.5	73	dig
Karki (74)	1988	21.8		li
Wing (53)	1989	87	76	phen
D'Angio (75)[b]	1990	67, 37, 35	24, 26, 8	amino, dig, theo
Destache (13)	1990	32		amino
Wade (96)	1990	>22		theo
Pearce (37)[b]	1990	47	28	all
Lynch (33)[b]	1992	74	25	amino
Tett (97)	1993	29		cyclo
Einarson (57)	1989	40.2 average of 24 studies		
		31.3 weighted average of 24 studies		

[a] Drug: amino = aminoglycoside, anticon = anticonvulsant, cyclo = cyclosporin, dig = digoxin, hep = heparin, li = lithium, theo = theophylline.
[b] Statistically significant difference at $P = 0.05$ or lower between the period before and that after pharmacy-based action.

Timing of Specimen Collection. The earliest and most frequently studied "outcome" in the assessment of TDM quality and the impact of TDM services involves the evaluation of the quality of the process steps in the timing of the specimen collection for TDM testing. Proper timing of TDM specimen collection is important to ensure that the drug concentration in the specimen is an accurate reflection of the physiologic effect at the cellular level: for example, the drug has reached steady state, and that adequate time has elapsed to ensure that postdistribution has been achieved following an oral dose. Therefore, measures used to evaluate this step have included timing of the specimen in relation to the drug's steady state, timing of the specimen in relation to the time of the last dose, and a measure of overall timing that assesses both steady-state and last dose sampling criteria.

Forty-three studies have evaluated the quality of these administrative process measures in hospitals and outpatient clinics that, at the time of the assessment, did not have pharmacy-based TDM educational or review programs in place (Table 8–3). More than 90% assessed the quality of either digoxin, theophylline, or aminoglycoside specimen collection. Occasional reports were also available for heparin, phenytoin, and lithium. Steady state, time from last dose, and overall timing quality were reported in 10, 12, and 31 studies, respectively.

As you can see in Table 8–3, the quality of TDM specimen collection varied widely from a low of only 2% incorrect timing for a lithium monitoring program in a psychiatric hospital,[74] to highs of 100% incorrect timing of aminoglycoside testing in a university medical center hospital,[75] to 100% of all TDM samples in a family practice clinic due to the lack of the time of last dose in either the chart or the test request form.[69] Based on Einarson and colleagues' meta-analysis of 25 preintervention studies,[57] the average rate of overall incorrect timing for specimen collection was 47.2% with a weighted average of 42.5%. Our average of the preintervention incorrect timing rate based on the studies reported in Table 8–3 is 52.3%.

Only one study attempted to link the quality of the TDM specimen to further clinical actions or to the clinical status of the patient. Sargenti et al did not find any relationship between incorrectly timed theophylline specimens and patient outcome.[71] Specimens taken before steady state did not result in dosage decisions that caused toxic reactions in patients.

Twenty-one of the studies evaluated the effectiveness of various forms of pharmacy-based interventions designed to improve these processes. Following the Donabedian approach to quality of care, it is probable that these investigators assumed that improvement in the process of care would translate into improvement in patient outcome. Thirteen of the interventions led to a statistically significant improvement in the timing of TDM specimen collection,[*] three from the same institution showed no improvement,[53–55] and four were not tested for statistical significance.[4,23,30,36] Also, a synthesis of 11 studies found that a larger proportion of samples were properly collected in patients monitored by a CKPS than in nonmonitored patients, but the collective improvement associated with CPKSs was not statistically significant because of the small number of studies.[59]

But did the 13 individual studies that had demonstrated significant improvements in the quality of the timing of TDM specimens lead to improvements in patient outcomes? Unfortunately, only one of the 13 studies examined if there was a link between improvements in specimen collection and improvements in the clinical outcome of the patient. In this report, as one part of an interdisciplinary protocol to improve aminoglycoside dosing, nurses obtained the specimen at the correct time and pharmacists analyzed results and recommended dosage changes. Although patients followed by this protocol tended to have fewer nephrotoxic reactions, a comparison of cure rates between groups was not reported.[33] Additionally, two studies did report that when pharmacy interventions improved the timing of the TDM specimens, more patients were in the therapeutic range than before the programs[6,76]; however, investigators in both studies did not examine if there was a relationship among improved specimen quality, therapeutic drug concentrations, and patient outcome.[6]

Although the timing of the specimen in reference to steady state and time of last dose status has been the primary process "outcome," several studies have included other measures related to specimen timing issues such as the presence of notation of the time of the specimen collection[36,69,83,87] and whether the TDM test was obtained within the first 48 hours of the dosing regimen.[33,80]

Appropriate Action. The third major process measure, which has been the object of the 50 studies listed in Table 8–4, is the assessment if appropriate action has been taken based on the TDM result and the specimen sampling information. Although specific criteria to judge if appropriate action has been taken vary among the studies, generally appropriate action in response to a properly collected specimen is defined as (1) increasing the dose if the drug concentration is below the therapeutic range, (2) decreasing or stopping the dose if the concentration is above the therapeutic range, and (3) taking no action if the concentration is within the therapeutic range.

Again, aminoglycosides, digoxin, and theophylline were the common study drugs, with

---

[*] References 6, 7, 18, 20, 26, 33, 37, 38, 46, 56, 75, 76, 84.

several studies examining clinical actions in response to lithium, phenytoin, and cyclosporine serum drug concentrations. And again, wide variation was found among the results, ranging from 11% inappropriate action in response to digoxin levels in a university teaching hospital to 87% inappropriate action in response to phenytoin levels in a community hospital. A larger percentage of clinically inappropriate actions occurred when the drug concentrations were outside the therapeutic range and dosage adjustment was not made as opposed to when the TDM result was within the therapeutic range and no action was indicated. Einarson's meta-analysis of 25 studies showed an overall average rate of 40.2% for incorrect responses to TDM results, with a weighted average of 31.3%. Based on an average of the 50 studies reported in Table 8–4, our average of the preintervention incorrect response rate is 44%.

Eighteen studies evaluated the effectiveness of a TDM educational program or CPKS in improving the clinical response to TDM results: eleven demonstrated a statistical improvement in clinical action,[*] four found no benefit,[18,53,56,81] and three did not statistically evaluate the effectiveness of the intervention.[30,36,52] Additionally, a synthesis of seven pharmacy-based interventions also reported a trend towards a larger proportion of assay results being used appropriately in pharmacy-monitored as compared with unmonitored patient populations.

As in earlier evaluations of methods to improve administrative process measures, few investigators have determined if there is a linkage between improvements in reaction to TDM results and improvements in patient outcomes. Only 4 of the 18 studies attempted to make any type of link between improvements in this step of the TDM process and impact on other outcomes. These programs improved clinical response to TDM results and were associated with more drug concentrations within the therapeutic range,[6,39] less nephrotoxicity,[33] and fewer hospital readmissions.[53]

But are the criteria selected to assess quality of responses to TDM results valid criteria? They have been based on the validity of the therapeutic range of each drug and its ability to separate toxic from nontoxic and therapeutic from subtherapeutic clinical conditions. Are these ranges valid discriminators and can they be used to answer such questions as: (1) Should dosages be reduced in all patients whose serum drug concentrations are above the therapeutic range? (2) Are pharmacists and physicians not providing good patient care if they do not decrease dosages in these situations?

New evidence indicates that it may be common for drug concentrations outside the therapeutic range not to be associated with toxic or subtherapeutic responses. For example, of a populaton of patients who were receiving theophylline and whose TDM results were above the therapeutic range, 57% were not in toxic condition.[98] If the dosages for this population were reduced, possible adverse consequences could result. For other TDM drugs also, a large percentage of concentrations above the therapeutic ranges were not associated with toxicity: aminoglycosides, 70%; digoxin, 40%; procainamide, 60%; phenytoin, more than 85%; vancomycin 70%.[99,100] And subtherapeutic levels are not always associated with subtherapeutic responses; in some cases, raising them when a patient is clinically stable can even lead to toxic reactions. For example, when seizure-free patients with subtherapeutic antiepileptic concentrations had their dosages increased until serum concentrations reached and stayed within the therapeutic range, the frequency of seizures did not change, but the incidence of neurotoxicity increased.[101]

Although the process measure "appropriate action in response to TDM results" has been used frequently as a quality indicator in TDM studies, these data suggest that basing appropriate

---

[*] References 6, 7, 10, 33, 37–39, 46, 54, 55, 75.

action criteria on where the TDM result is in respect to the therapeutic range is not a valid indicator of quality. Evaluation of responses to TDM results must combine information from the TDM result with patient-specific clinical information. If the TDM result is beyond the therapeutic range and the patient exhibits signs of toxicity, reducing the dosage would appear to be appropriate action. If, however, the TDM result is higher than the top of the therapeutic range, the patient has no signs of toxicity, and the clinical condition is under control, retaining the present dosage is very likely the correct action.

Progress in modifying TDM response criteria is being made. Two recent studies have indicated that their assessments have gone beyond having criteria linked to the therapeutic range. In a community-based rural practice setting, pharmacists are now asking if it is wrong that 63% of digoxin, theophylline, and phenytoin results are in subtherapeutic ranges and only 44% prompted increased dosages. In this outpatient environment, compliance was considered as a factor in the large proportion of subtherapeutic drug concentrations that did not prompt dosing adjustments. Mason concluded that "indications for dosing adjustments vary with both drug and patient, disallowing rigid application of criteria assessing appropriate interpretations of serum drug concentrations."[102] In the second study, criteria for response to cyclosporine levels, based on both therapeutic range and clinical indications, were used in a retrospective audit. As the authors acknowledge, the accuracy of this audit was only as good as the documented clinical reasons in the patient's report for why indicated action was not taken, but it is a first step toward tempering the traditional therapeutic range response with clinical judgment.[97]

Other Administrative Process Measures. Several other administrative processes or actions have been examined to determine the quality of TDM testing process and the contribution of clinical pharmacokinetic services. A quality-assurance audit of digoxin monitoring revealed that, in addition to problems with specimen collection, nearly 60% of digoxin results were entered in patients' charts after the patients had been discharged.[87] And in evaluating the contribution of clinical pharmacokinetic services, CPKSs were more likely to change medication dosages in patients being followed by TDM[13,38,91] and to daily monitor ototoxicity in patients receiving aminoglycosides[26] as compared with care without clinical pharmacokinetic services. Again, the connection between these process measures and patient-centered outcomes was not examined.

Overall Comments Concerning the Use of Administrative Process Measures in "Outcome" Studies. As the three main categories of administrative process measures covered in this section have been relatively easy to document and obtain, they have served as the most frequently used methods to assess the quality of TDM testing and the effectiveness of clinical pharmacokinetic services. But these "outcome" measures have many problems.

First, of course, is the fact that these are administrative process measures, not patient-centered outcome measures. Few studies have linked the quality of these administrative process measures to any variable related to patient outcome. The assumption that CPKS interventions to improve the proper timing of specimens and responses to TDM results can lead to improved patient outcome has face validity (it makes sense), but it is important to remember that it is only an assumption. To prove the link between improved administrative processes and patient-centered outcomes, the assumption must be rigorously and repeatedly tested in randomized control trials involving different patients being monitored for different medications in different types of settings.

Second is the variability in the criteria used by each institution to assess the quality of clinically appropriate testing, timing of specimens, and appropriate action. The variability issue is probably one of the major reasons for the wide range of values found in Table 8–2 to 8–4. Not only is there between-institution variability, but there also is within-institution variability. For example, when one hospital used 1.0 to 2.0 ng/mL as the therapeutic range for digoxin, only 37% of the patient care decisions were appropriate, but when it expanded the digoxin range to 0.8 to 2.2 ng/mL, the appropriate care decisions rose to 85%.[36] Some attempt at standardizing process criteria is necessary to enable the field to assess different pharmacy interventions at different types of institutions.

And third, if process criteria become modified to accommodate clinical judgment, the retrospective nature of the quality-assurance audit will be even more dependent on the quality of documentation in the patient's written record. Patients' charts are notorious for their gaps in information describing the clinical condition of the patient and supporting the type of actions taken. When pharmacists and other health care providers take action in response to TDM results that is contrary to the action indicated by explicit audit criteria (generally based on responses to being outside the therapeutic ranges), they will be required to provide more detailed written documentation so that their actions are not judged to be inappropriate.

Economic Consequences of TDM/CPKS Processes

The processes of collection, performance, and reaction to therapeutic drug monitoring tests have both direct and indirect economic implications. Twenty-nine studies have characterized the economic waste asssociated with poor TDM processes and the savings that could be achieved if clinical pharmacokinetic services implemented programs to improve the processes. The reliability of each study's conclusions is dependent on the time of the year, the length of time of the study, the assumptions behind the economic assessments, the adequacy and availability of financial information, and the comprehensiveness of the analysis. Of course, other factors such as study location (eg, intensive care unit, outpatient clinic, or selected versus all hospital floors), drug studied (eg, digoxin, aminoglycosides, theophylline, or all TDM medications), size of the institution, and case-mix severity of patients all can interact to affect the magnitude of the economic impact. For example, a hospitalwide, CPKS intervention involving all scheduling of TDM requests and interpreting of results is likely to prevent more incorrect processes, and hence prevent more wasted dollars, than a similar intervention directed at TDM processes in an outpatient clinic.

The time of year and length of the study are variables to consider when interpreting results of economic analyses. Sixteen of the results found in Table 8–5 are from studies conducted over 3 months or less and then extrapolated to 1 year to determine annual impact. These extrapolations assumed that the number, distribution, and rate of improperly performed TDM tests would be consistent over 12 months and that the pattern found in the study period would be reflective of the rest of the year. The volume and type of TDM requests are not, however, consistent throughout the year, and seasonal factors can affect the patterns of illness, which in turn can affect patterns of prescribed medications and the need for specific types of TDM testing. Therefore, studies conducted over a limited period with results generalized to the entire year may suffer from sampling bias and the extrapolated results may be inaccurate.

These caveats are particularly true in teaching hospitals where it is important to consider the time of arrival of new medical residents and the effect of their early experience on the frequency and quality of TDM testing patterns. For example, one study in a teaching hospital used the period July (when new residents commonly arrive) to November to determine the baseline

TABLE 8–5. STUDIES INCORPORATING ECONOMIC PROCESS MEASURES: YEARLY COSTS WITHOUT AND SAVINGS WITH PHARMACY INTERVENTIONS

First Author	Year	Drug[a]	Months of Study	Charge		Yearly Costs[b] with Notations
Costs (Waste) Without Pharmacy Intervention						
Anderson (61)	1976	amino	11	$21	$4,284	Incorrectly drawn, ignored, inappropriately used
Flynn (77)	1978	amino	2	15	2,500	Unused or inappropriate action
Parker (36)	1978	dig	4	16	5,424	Inappropriate use
Slaughter (42)	1978	dig	2.5	10	68,500	With $60,000 no indication and $8500 improper action
Greenlaw (88)	1979	amino	18	20	4,080	Incorrectly timed or improper action
Floyd (62)	1979	dig	1	?	5,500	Inappropriate tests
Greenlaw (64)	1980	dig	?	30	33,150	Unnecessary, incorrectly performed, or inappropriately used
Bollish (7)	1981	amino	1	30	13,440	Incorrectly timed or improper action
Sketris (90)	1982	amino	4	15	5,000	Inappropriately used results
Bussey (82)	1983	all	1	25	46,800	Inappropriately sampled and used
Guernsey (67)	1984	dig	2	34	100,900	Unnecessary, incorrectly performed, or inappropriately used
Guernsey (68)	1984	theo	2	28	77,310	Not indicated, incorrectly performed, or inappropriately used
Ives (69)	1984	all	12	23	3,737	Unusable results in outpatients
Pitterle (38)	1985	all	4	26	14,925	Incorrectly timed and inappropriate actions in outpatients
Sargenti (71)	1985	theo	1	cost 10	28,860	Not indicated, incorrectly performed, or inappropriately used
Ambrose (4)	1988	all	1	56	16,167	Waste due to incorrect sampling when pharmacists not scheduled
Karki (74)	1988	li	1	cost 12	16,632	Inappropriate testing and unnecessary orders
Wade (96)	1990	theo			12,419	Sampled inappropriately
Projected Savings with Pharmacy Intervention						
Greenlaw (18)	1979	hep	2.5	10	17,442	Savings of $15,480 inappropriate sampling, $2692 unnecessary retesting; and with cost offset of $701 for additional doses
Elenbass (15)	1980	all	6	18	14,403	Gross savings from elimination of unnecessary tests and TDM scheduling with cost offset of $1417 of personnel costs
Levin (30)	1981	all	5	20	6,005	Gross savings from inappropriate tests with cost offset of $624 for pharmacists' time
Horn (20)	1985	dig	3	20	7,920	Unnecessary tests

(continued)

TABLE 8–5. CONTINUED

First Author	Year	Drug[a]	Months of Study	Charge		Yearly Costs[b] with Notations
Wing (54)	1987	theo	3	27	5,250	Savings from reduction in tests but offset by $7500 of staff time
Wing (55)	1987	dig	3	27	5,800	Savings from reduction in tests but offset by $7500 of staff time
Ambrose (103)	1988	all	3	60	500,000	Estimated savings from improved scheduling of TDM tests
					32,299	Savings from canceled TDM orders
Klamerus (27)	1988	dig	4	cost 22	2,955	Gross cost savings from reduction in inappropriate tests but offset by $1024 of staff time plus fringes
Job (23)	1989	all	12	55	232,017	Charge savings ($175,257 inappropriate + 56,760 canceled)
				cost 20	84,360	Cost savings ($63,720 inappropriate + $20,640 canceled)
Wing (53)	1989	phen	3	27	7,618	Savings from reduction in tests but offset by $7500 of staff time
D'Angio (75)	1990	amino, dig, theo	5	43 cost 11	33,456	Charge savings from reduction in inappropriate indication, sampling, and physician action; $6708 cost savings from same

[a]Drug: amino = aminoglycoside, dig = digoxin, hep = heparin, li = lithium, phen = phenytoin, theo = theophylline.
[b]Dollar value are as reported in the study and are not adjusted for present value nor for currency exchange rate for Canadian studies.

rate of improper TDM testing and then evaluated the introduction of a CPKS scheduling program from January through May.[30] It should not be surprising that the quality of testing improved, but what part of that improvement was due to the CPKS and what part was due to the natural improvement of the residents' TDM test ordering ability was not considered.

The adequacy and availability of financial information are also important considerations. Ideally, the actual cost of a service should be used in any economic analysis. Cost information conveys the dollar value of resources actually consumed in providing a service or producing a product; however, because this information is not readily available and is difficult to generate, investigators substitute the more readily available, but less accurate, financial variable—the charge (fee) for the service—in place of actual cost information. Only 5 of the 28 studies provide cost rather than charge information[23,27,71,74,75]; two present both cost and charge analyses.[23,75] Instead of using cost information when calculating the economic consequences, the other investigators have tallied the number of incorrectly performed TDM tests and then assigned an economic value to the errors by multiplying the number of tests in error by the charge (fee) to generate the "cost" of improperly performed TDM tests. Charge information is provided in Table 8–5. Not only is this approach an inaccurate reflection of the real cost of improper testing, but it creates problems when institutions have different charge structures for different classes of payers.

Also the comprehensiveness of the analyses will influence the results. Nearly all of the studies cited in Table 8–5 examined only the charges/costs of the improperly tested TDM samples. Six included some attempt to incorporate the cost of the pharmacists' time involved in scheduling and interpreting the TDM tests. But this provides an incomplete examination of the economic consequences of poor administrative processes in TDM testing. More comprehenisve analyses would examine the consequences of poor testing on the cost of the episode of care rather than just the charges of the wasted TDM tests. In this way, process costs could be linked to economic outcome expenses. Now the analyses can be reframed to examine if the economic consequences of poor TDM quality involved more than wasted test dollars or did poor-quality testing induce additional expenses associated with more subtherapeutic or toxic responses, other complications, and longer hospital stays. Although not as numerous as the economic assessment of waste associated with poor TDM testing, several more comprehensive analyses have been performed and are summarized later under System-Related Measures: Outcome (see Economic Consequences).

Lastly, nearly all of the 29 studies reported either a combined estimate of the costs associated with clinically unnecessary tests, improperly collected specimens, and inappropriate actions in response to TDM results or the savings that could be achieved by reducing these three types of errors. Although it is clear that clinically inappropriate tests result in wasted dollars and that CPKS interventions can reduce this economic waste, it is not as straightforward that the other two types of errors will always result in waste and that CPKS efforts to correct these problems will save dollars. If a TDM test is clinically indicated but improperly performed, only the additional economic resources needed to correct the situation savings should be counted as waste and potential opportunities for cost savings. An example of these considerations is developed in the following section.

Costs Associated with Waste from Clinically Unnecessary, Inappropriate Sampling and Improper Action. When TDM tests are not clinically necessary or not sampled appropriately, or correct action is not taken in response to a result, health care dollars are wasted. Eighteen studies, summarized in Table 8–5, examined the magnitude of that waste in their institutions. All dollars are as reported from the year of the study's publication; they are not adjusted to present dollar value. Estimated annual waste ranged from $3737 involving all TDM tests in an outpatient clinic to more than $100,000 for waste associated with only digoxin serum concentrations for combined patients in the general medical units of two general teaching hospitals and a pediatric hospital.

But if clinical pharmacokinetic services were implemented, could all the waste be converted into savings? Let us examine that question by taking a closer look at the use of TDM for theophylline in one institution.[68] Guernsey et al reported a waste of $77,310 associated with the charges for clinically unnecessary, incorrectly performed, or inappropriately used theophylline serum concentration results. Although it is clear that clinically unnecessary TDM testing represented waste, in this study it consisted of only 32% of the errors or only $25,394 of the cost which could be saved by the CPKS clinical appropriateness review. The remaining 68% of the tests were clinically indicated and would have been performed, and created costs to the system, with or without CPKS scheduling and interpretation. These tests were needed and would have been performed, so the balance of these charges should not be considered potential cost savings.

In a more complete analysis, the study would have examined if faulty collection and interpretation led to additional hospital days or clinical complications and if CPKS review could have prevented these consequences; then extra expenses would be considered potential cost savings. In this analysis, however, only if these tests were recognized as being in error and repeat tests, creating additional costs, were necessary to correct the situation, could one say that this CPKS created savings through improved sampling and interpretation.

And a final consideration. In this study the pharmacists reviewed all patients receiving theophylline and identified other patients who needed theophylline tests, but for whom none had been ordered. If these tests had been performed, an additional $15,704 in expenses would have been created. Therefore, of the $77,310 of potential savings, only $25,394 of the savings was firm; an additional $15,704 of expenses would be created by the CPKS, resulting in a net potential savings of only $9690. Expenses for the CPKS were not charged against this amount, so the net savings are even lower.

Savings from Interventions to Reduce Clinically Unnecessary, Inappropriate Sampling and Improper Action. Even with the above comments, when clinical pharmacokinetic services intervene to improve the processes of therapeutic drug monitoring, savings can be realized through a reduction in waste. Of the 11 pharmacy intervention studies summarized in Table 8–5, projected estimates of annual savings ranged from $2955 for digoxin monitoring on a cardiothoracic surgery floor[27] to approximately $500,000 for an institutionwide CPKS program to review, schedule, and interpret all TDM requests.[23] Half of the studies reported the expenses associated with providing the pharmacy intervention. Three from the same institution concluded that the savings achieved by the CPKS were, at least initially, nearly equal to the cost of the pharmacists' time involved in providing the service.[53–55] Three other studies reported that savings from the CPKS exceeded the expenses associated with providing the service.[15,27,30]

Most of these studies examined the rates of inappropriately performed TDM tests before and after the introduction of a clinical pharmacokinetic service, and then converted the improvements in TDM testing to savings related to CPKS action. Not only does this introduce the error of comparing results from one period to another, but it also carries the assumption that the improvements in specimen collection and test interpretation will save the system TDM charges. As mentioned earlier, although reductions in clinically inappropriate testing will likely save expenses, the relationship among improved sampling, test interpretation, and cost savings is less straightforward. To improve our understanding of the cost-saving potential of CPKS, future evaluations must include two groups of patients (one with CPKS, one without) who are followed during the same time. Also, in addition to determining the rates of appropriate TDM testing in both populations, the clinical and economic consequences of actions that do not meet TDM guidelines must be examined and analyzed. This type of study, and others comparing the cost of providing clinical pharmacokinetic services with their economic outcome benefits, are described under System-Related Measures: Outcome (see Economic Consequences: Cost–Benefit Studies of TDM and Clinical Pharmacokinetic Services).

Cost of TDM and Clinical Pharmacokinetic Services. A cost analysis of the processes involved in providing a clinical pharmacokinetic service should include both the direct and indirect expenses of all aspects of the service. The principal direct expense is the personnel costs involved in providing the services and the associated fringe benefits. The costs of computer equipment, calculators, and supplies should also be included in direct costs after prorating for their proportional use by the CPKS and depreciating when indicated. Indirect expenses include such items as space, utilities, furniture, and other overhead expenses.

None of the studies detailing the impact of CPKS on either system- or patient-related process or outcome measures included a comprehensive cost analysis of providing such a service. Most estimated the pharmacy hours involved and then multiplied by the hourly wage. Although two studies included the fringe benefits associated with that wage,[26,27] most did not[12,13,15,30,53–55] and their inclusion was indeterminate in one.[14] Two studies by Destache and colleagues[12,13] were the only ones to include the costs of computer and office equipment, supplies, journals, and space, but they did not include fringe benefits nor overhead expenses. None of these studies determined the annual cost of offering a clinical pharmacokinetic service; instead, they limited their analyses to an estimate of only the costs involved in providing the TDM services to the patients in these reports.

Outcome

Although system-related process measures are used to assess the administrative and economic factors of TDM action steps, system-related outcome measures capture the impact of improved processes on administrative outcomes and economic resources. While getting us closer to measuring the impact of various TDM interventions on patient outcome, they still serve only as indirect measures of patient outcomes. For example, one method to assess the effectiveness of a clinical pharmacokinetic service would be to measure the success of a CPKS in improving the percentage of TDM results that are within the therapeutic range. In this method, a system-related outcome measure would be used to assess the effectiveness of an intervention to improve an administrative process, but it would not directly examine if patients were doing better because, as mentioned earlier, not all TDM results in the toxic range represent toxicity and some toxicity is present in patients who have TDM results in the therapeutic range. If, however, one asked what percentage of the patient population being followed with TDM tests experiences toxic effects, then one is directly measuring the impact on the patient. This distinction may seem like semantics, but it is the critical difference between evaluations being conducted from a health care system perspective and those being conducted from a patient perspective.

Numerous administrative outcomes have been used in the assessment of the contribution of TDM and CPKSs, but none has been as universally adopted as the administrative process measures described earlier. This leads to less uniformity in effectiveness measurement, with each investigator having different preferences for the selection of administrative outcome measures. As a result, many different types of administrative outcome measures have been used, but each is used in comparatively fewer studies than the standard administrative process measures.

Administrative Outcomes of Care

Administrative outcome measures are used to examine if improvements in processes of care have an impact on administrative outcomes. For example, does the improvement in the clinical appropriateness of TDM testing lead to a change in the number of TDM tests ordered per patient? Will improved specimen collection and responses to TDM results increase the percentage of patients who achieve serum drug concentrations within the therapeutic range and reach that concentration within a shorter period? Will clinical pharmacokinetic services shorten the duration of the hospitalization or reduce the number of admissions? All of these questions use administrative outcome measures to evaluate the effectiveness of TDM and CPKSs. To determine whether any of these are valid measures of the clinical effectiveness of TDM and CPKSs requires that evaluative studies jointly assess, and then statistically link, changes in administrative outcomes with the simultaneous changes in patient-related clinical outcomes.

TDM Tests. Several administrative outcome measures have been used to evaluate the effectiveness of CPKSs, the number of TDM tests per patient, the overall and 24-hour distribution of TDM results, and the percentage of toxic serum concentrations.

Number of TDM Tests per Patient. The ability of CPKSs to influence the number of TDM tests per patient appears to be mixed. Of the 19 studies cited in Table 8–6, 5 indicated that CPKSs reduced the number of TDM tests per patient,[20,30,33,39,53] 3 showed an increase in testing,[29,44,50] 5 showed no difference between the number of tests with and without a CPKS,[7,11,18,54,55] and 4 did not determine if there was a difference.[14,25,26,41]

In an analysis of 16 reports of the effect of therapeutic drug monitoring services on the number of serum drug assays ordered for patients, Ried and colleagues reached the following conclusions:

> Overall, TDM has no effect on the number of serum drug assays (SDAs) ordered per patient. However, there were a number of moderator variables that influenced the results. In studies utilizing control groups for comparisons, TDM service-monitored patients were ordered fewer SDAs than nonmonitored patients. When data from the same institution were collected before and after implementation of a TDM service, there was an increase in the number of SDAs per patient. Aminoglycoside patients monitored by a TDM service were ordered more SDAs and nonaminoglycoside monitored patients were ordered fewer SDAs than nonmonitored patients. When the pharmacy department determined when the SDAs were to be collected and adjusted the dose, monitored patients were ordered fewer SDAs than nonmonitored patients. However, when the pharmacy department did not have control of these parameters, the TDM patients were ordered more SDAs than nonmonitored patients.[58]

The number of TDM tests per patient has been, and will continue to be, a difficult outcome measure to use in assessing the effectiveness of clinical pharmacokinetic services. Early studies concluded that CPKSs could be justified because, by reviewing the clinical appropriateness of TDM requests, the service could eliminate unnecessary orders and their associated charges; however, as Ried indicated, "a good TDM service should decrease the number of inappropriate TDM determinations, yet it also may increase the number of appropriate measurements." Examples of such situations include patients needing TDM tests who previously had been unmonitored and other patients, particularly those receiving aminoglycosides, for whom insufficient TDM tests had been ordered to adequately follow their courses of therapy. Both are examples where CPKS review would lead to additional, not reduced, TDM testing. Overall, the net result of CPKS intervention could be a decrease, increase, or no change in the number of TDM determinations.

Whether or not the number of TDM tests per patient is a valid measure of the effectiveness of a clinical pharmacokinetic service requires studies including both this administrative outcome measure and such clinical outcome measures as improvement in therapeutic response, cure, reduction of toxicity, and survival.

TABLE 8–6. STUDIES INCORPORATING ADMINISTRATIVE OUTCOME MEASURES RELATED TO NUMBER OF THERAPEUTIC DRUG MONITORING (TDM) TESTS AND PERCENTAGE IN THERAPEUTIC RANGE WITH AND WITHOUT PHARMACY (Rx) INVOLVEMENT

First Author	Year	Number of TDM Tests Per Patient		Percentage of TDM Results in Therapeutic Range		Drug[a]
		No Rx	With Rx	No Rx	With Rx	
Greenlaw (18) ns[b]	1979	6.36	5.76			hep
Taylor (45) nt	1979			33	94	all
Bollish (7) ns	1981	2.2	6.2			amino
Fröscher (17) nt	1981			67	66	anticonv
Levin (30)[c]	1981	2.4, 2.2	1.7, 1.9			dig, all
Rich (39)[c]	1981	1.96	1.68	45	80	dig
Lehmann (29)[c]	1982	1.48	3.03			theo
Mungall (34)[c]	1983			41	82	theo
Privitera (104)	1984			58.3		anticonv
Shaw (85) nt	1984			38	83	amino
Squire (105)	1984			22.5		antiarrhy
Whiting (51)[c]	1984			29.5	62.8	dig, theo, phen
Burton (9) nt	1985			33.1	86.1	amino
Horn (20)[c]	1985	2.02	1.58	23	55	dig
Kearns (25) nt	1985	4.44	3.94			amino
Saya (41) nt	1985	10.5	6.96	25.8	76.9	hep
Sveska (44)[c]	1985	1.5	4.4			amino
Hurley (21)[c]	1986			44.4	71.1	theo
Kimelblatt (26)	1986	0.19	0.69			amino
Blackbourn (6)[c]	1987			17	47	theo
Crist (11)	1987	3.12	3.84			amino
Smith (43)	1987	2.63	3.63			amino
Wing (55)	1987	1.2	0.75			dig
Wing (54)	1987	2.36	1.84			theo
Ionnides (22)[c]	1988			40	80	anticonv
Klamerus (106)	1988	5.1	3.2			dig
Destache (14)	1989	3.69	4.22			amino
Hoffa (19)[c]	1989			32	96	amino
Wing (53)[c]	1989	2.28	0.95			phen
Burton (107)	1991			60.3	82.9	amino
Whipple (50)[c]	1991	4	8	53	77	amino
Carroll (76)	1992			43	68	amino
Lynch (33)[c]	1992	4.2	2.8	20	61	amino

[a]Drug: amino = aminoglycoside, anticonv = anticonvulsant, antiarrhy = antiarrhythmics, dig = digoxin, hep = heparin, li = lithium, phen = phenytoin, theo = theophylline.

[b]ns, not significant; nt, not tested for statistical significance.

[c]Statistically significant difference, at $P = 0.05$ or less, in appropriateness between before and after pharmacy action.

Percentage of TDM Results Within the Therapeutic Range. Seventeen studies summarized in Table 8–6 reported an increase in the proportion of serum drug concentrations that fell within the therapeutic range as a result of CPKS policies. At baseline prior to CPKS interventions, the studies averaged 38.0% of TDM results within the therapeutic range. CPKS review and dosing recommendations increased the average proportion of TDM concentrations within the desired range to 74.6%, more than doubling the preintervention level. This increase was found with all medications studied and occurred in both outpatient and hospital patient settings. Ried et al also concluded that clinical pharmacokinetic services had a positive effect on maintaining serum drug concentrations within an acceptable range based on a synthesis of 12 studies.[59]

Again, an important caution is indicated. Although the preceding results are impressive, improvement in the proportion of TDM results within the therapeutic range does not mean the same thing as improvement in the proportion of patients who achieve a therapeutic response without toxicity. The first is an administrative outcome measure; the latter is a patient-related outcome measure. It does not directly translate that all serum concentrations that were moved into the therapeutic range resulted in clinical condition improvement in the patient. Some patients may require serum drug concentrations above the therapeutic range to achieve a clinical improvement. In these cases, the reduction of patients' medications in an effort to achieve drug concentrations within the therapeutic range is likely to result in deterioration of their clinical condition. Just as dosing regimens are tailored to the patient's individual pharmacokinetics, it might be necessary to individualize the response to serum drug concentrations beyond the therapeutic range. For optimal patient care, responses to TDM results above the therapeutic range must be tempered with clinical judgment.

Ried et al[59] have also examined the effect of clinical pharmacokinetic review on the achievement of therapeutic peaks[6,9,11,12,17,34,41,43,49,51] and troughs,[6,11,35,43,49,51] and the prevention of toxic peaks[6,17,34,35,49,43,51] and troughs.[6,18,34,35,43,49,51] Results from an analysis of these four sets of studies indicate that clinical pharmacokinetic services reduce the frequency of toxic trough concentrations, but although improvements were seen in the other three individual monitoring parameters, they were not statistically significant.

Percentage of Patients with TDM Concentrations Within the Therapeutic Range Within Protocol Time. Several descriptions of pharmacokinetic dosing protocols included an assessment of their effectiveness in achieving a therapeutic serum drug concentration within a stated period. A larger proportion of patients followed by a CPKS using dosing protocols achieved target peak aminoglycoside concentrations within 48 hours[33] and therapeutic levels of anticoagulation[41] within 12 hours than those not receiving such care. Logically, achieving early therapeutic levels should contribute to improved patient care. In fact, Moore and colleagues found that, in patients with bacteremia, 97.6% of those who had a therapeutic peak concentration 1 hour postinfusion survived, whereas 20.9% died who did not achieve this early drug concentration.

In these two studies, however, the investigators focused on process rather than outcome measures to assess the effectiveness of the dosing protocol. Neither group of investigators examined whether the improvement in dosing led to improvement in survival or to a reduction in the length of hospitalization; however, the financial impact of the new heparin protocol was considered. Both did determine if the period of therapy was affected and reached opposite conclusions; the period of anticoagulation was shortened, but there was no effect on the duration of aminoglycoside therapy.

As protocols and guidelines become a more common part of health care practices, they must be evaluated to determine their safety, effectiveness, and efficiency with all patient types. These assessments must be comprehensive and include system- and patient-related measures from administrative, economic, and clinical categories. Limiting protocol evaluations to the percentage of specimens that are properly sampled and the percentage of results that are within the therapeutic range does not adequately assess the impact of the protocol on a range of clinical and economic outcomes.

Dose. A good clinical pharmacokinetic service should strive to achieve the maximal therapeutic effect with the minimum amount of drug. In some institutions that might mean increasing the traditional institutional dose; in another, it might mean decreasing it. Comparative dosing data provide useful descriptive information, but their significance can be determined only by interpreting them in light of clinical outcome data such as therapeutic effectiveness, cure, and mortality rates.

Of the various dosing descriptors, total dose and number of dosage changes were the two principal administrative outcome measures used to assess the effectiveness of clinical pharmacokinetic services. The majority of the studies evaluating the impact of CPKSs on the total medication dose determined that the total dose of aminoglycosides,[11,109] vancomycin,[110] heparin,[41] and maintenance doses of digoxin[31] was significantly less in the CPKS-monitored population than in the traditionally treated group. Total aminoglycoside dose in a CPKS-monitored population has also been described as being slightly higher than in patients followed with empiric therapy.[24] Also, as indicated in several studies of critically ill patients, higher doses may be necessary to increase survival.[50] Although the total aminoglycoside dose did not differ between critically ill patients who were and were not followed by a CPKS, the patients receiving CPKS care had higher daily doses, achieved a therapeutic peak earlier, and had an increased survival rate.[50]

The total number of dose changes that occur during a course of therapy is one measure of the responsiveness of clinicians to information provided by the serum drug concentrations. Using this measure as an outcome variable, however, yields results that vary: dosages were adjusted more often,[6,12] less often,[5] or as often[14] in CPKS-monitored patients as compared with nonmonitored patients.

Daily dose, dosing intervals, number of doses, and number of days before the initial dosing regimen was changed are other dosing characteristics, primarily describing the process of care, that have been used in evaluation studies. At best, these and the two other principal dosing variables can be used to describe differences between approaches to care, not to conclude that one approach is better than another. The significance of these findings can be interpreted only in light of additional information concerning the clinical outcome of the patient.

Time. Time has been used as an outcome measure of efficiency in TDM studies. It is based on the assumptions that shorter duration of therapy, less time on intravenous medication and correspondingly shorter time to oral medication, fewer days of infection, fewer days in the intensive care unit, and shorter length of hospital stay are desirable outcomes and represent efficient delivery of care. These appear to be reasonable assumptions as long as the groups being compared are composed of patients with similar demographic characteristics and clinical conditions and that clinical outcome measures such as mortality rates are also included in the evaluation. Remember that a shorter period may not always indicate the best outcome. A population with a high mortality rate may have a shorter duration of therapy, fewer days of infection, and fewer hospital days than a population with a higher survival rate.

Duration of Therapy. Nine studies included duration of therapy as an outcome measure with varying results. Eight involved the treatment of serious infections with aminoglycosides,[8,11,12–14,26,44,108] and the ninth evaluated the use of heparin.[41] In patients followed by clinical pharmacokinetic services, the duration of therapy was shorter than,[11,13,14,26,44,109] longer than,[8] or not significantly different from[12,41] that of patients not followed by such a service. In the one CPKS-monitored population that had a longer period of antibiotic use,[8] the survival rate also was higher in the patients followed by the CPKS, implying that the therapy increased survival and hence extended the duration of treatment. In one study, the CPKS-monitored population had a better survival rate.[44] In the remaining four evaluations, the mortality rates of the two groups were similar. Again, by linking a clinical outcome measure (mortality) to an administrative outcome measure (duration of therapy), one can now suggest that the shorter duration of therapy was associated with increased efficiency and not an increased death rate in the CPKS-monitored patients.

Time on Intravenous Dose/Time to Oral Medication. Four theophylline dosing programs have used the length of time on intravenous (IV) therapy as one of their outcome measures to judge the effectiveness of a CPKS. One of three early assessments found that lower theophylline doses extended the course of IV therapy as compared with patients receiving higher doses and who had higher theophylline concentrations.[112] The other two programs had conflicting results, with one program directed at patients in a Veterans Administration hospital having longer IV therapy when followed by a CPKS[29] and another program based in a medical intensive care unit in a teaching hospital having a shorter IV course.[34] A more recent evaluation of a dosing program in a teaching hospital found no difference in length of theophylline IV therapy in patients with and without therapeutic drug monitoring program.[54]

Length of Infection. The goal of antibiotic therapy is to cure the infection in as short a period as possible. Length of infection is an administrative process measure; the percentage of patients cured of the infection is a clinical outcome measure. Not all studies using the length of infection outcome measure provided information concerning the cure rate, a measure more reflective of the patient's actual outcome.

Four studies evaluated the impact of a CPKS on the effectiveness of aminoglycoside therapy for the treatment of serious Gram-negative infections using length of infection as one of the outcome variables. Destache et al defined the length of infection as the time required to return to baseline values of temperature, heart rate, and respiratory rate,[12–14] whereas in the fourth study, length of infection was undefined.[8]

The burn patients followed by the CPKS in Bootman and colleagues' study[8] had a longer period of infection than those treated empirically. The latter population had a higher mortality rate and hence fewer days of life after the initiation of antibiotic therapy. In all three studies by Destache et al, patients followed by a CPKS had shorter lengths of infections, but in one report the mortality rate was higher in the CPKS-monitored population than in the regularly treated patients.[12]

One of the studies by Destache et al is an interesting examination of whether process variables affect outcomes.[13] Patients who were initially followed by a CPKS, but whose physicians did not follow the CPKS dosing recommendations, were compared with those patients whose physicians followed 100% of the recommendations. Did patients whose process of care devi-ated from CPKS criteria have an adverse outcome? Although patient characteristics and infecting organisms could explain some of the variation between groups, there was a striking difference in the shortened length of infection in the patient population with 100% compliance to dosing recommendations. Additional studies to duplicate these results and better control for case-mix characteristics are needed.

Length of Intensive Care Stay. Only one study used the number of days in the intensive care unit (ICU) as an administrative outcome variable. Patients who were admitted to the ICU, received theophylline, and were followed by the CPKS had significantly fewer ICU days (6.6 days) than those with similar conditions who had been treated empirically (12.4 days).[34]

Length of Hospital Stay. Table 8–7 lists the 18 studies that incorporated length of hospital stay as an outcome variable into the assessment of the effectiveness of clinical pharmacokinetic services. Ten of the studies had a significant difference in length of stay between CPKS-monitored and unmonitored patients.[11,13,14,20,21,44,107,108] In eight evaluations, the CPKS group had a shorter length of stay; in two evaluations, patients in the CPKS group had a longer length of stay.[8,29]

Mortality rates are also displayed in Table 8–7 and provide a means to link system- and patient-related outcomes. For example, in the Bootman et al study, the large number of additional hospital days experienced by the CPKS-monitored patients contrasts with all other results. But when you link the length of stay information with the mortality data, you can begin to see what happened. Although the other studies that included mortality data showed no differences between the patient populations, the CPKS-monitored patients in the Bootman et al study had a significantly lower mortality rate. This unusual finding of a shorter hospital stay in non-CPKS-monitored patients was related to the increased mortality in that population. Linking system and patient outcomes provides insight into the complete impact of a CPKS.

When the impact of CPKSs on hospital length of stay is studied, it is best to broaden the assessment to include other measures. Although length of stay is potentially a good measure of therapeutic efficiency, it is affected by many factors. Perhaps the patient is ready for discharge, but home care or nursing home care is not available. Now discharge is delayed and length of stay is extended. On the other hand, a patient may be discharged too early in an unstable condition. In this case the hospital stay is shortened, but the probability of readmission increases. Through the use of a large randomized study designs incorporating comprehensive outcome measures, these problems should be equally spread between the CPKS- and non-CPKS-monitored patients to decrease the possibility that these factors will confuse an evaluation of CPKS efforts.

Critically ill patients pose unique problems. In this population, a short length of stay generally could be associated with increased mortality rather than increased therapeutic efficiency. Therefore, length of stay studies in critically ill populations should be supported with other outcome measures such as time to cure and rates of cure, toxicity, and mortality.

Impact on Future Health Care Consumption. After discharge or during the chronic care of patients, what effects do clinical pharmacokinetic services have on patients' needs for future care? Although this question is not common in the TDM literature, four studies (three from the anticonvulsant literature) do provide some answers by examining readmission rates and determining the number of hospital admissions and office and emergency room visits in patients with and without CPKS care.

TABLE 8–7. STUDIES INCORPORATING ADMINISTRATIVE AND CLINICAL OUTCOME MEASURES: HOSPITAL LENGTH OF STAY AND MORTALITY IN PATIENTS FOLLOWED WITH AND WITHOUT A CLINICAL PHARMACOKINETIC SERVICE (CPKS)

First Author	Year	Length of Stay (Days)		Percentage Mortality		Drug[a]
		Without CPKS	With CPKS	Without CPKS	With CPKS	
Bootman (8)	1979	72.3	93.2[b]	66.7	36.4[b]	amino
Lehmann (29)	1982	6.2	8.6[b]	0	3.3	theo
Mungall (34)	1983	22.3	15.4			theo
Horn (20)	1985	15.3	11.6[b]	7.5	8.7	dig
Kearns (25)	1985	16.6	14.1			tobra
Sveska (44)	1985	35	27[b]	42	12[b]	amino
Kimelblatt (26)	1986	36.0	30.5	18.9	24.6	amino
Hurley (21)	1986	8.7	6.3[b]	4.7	0	theo
Winter (56)	1986	8.4	10.2			all
Crist (11)	1987	11.8	8.4[b]	1.7	1.0	amino
Smith (43)	1987	21.6	18.9			amino
Wing (54)	1987	12.2	11.9			theo
Begg (5)	1989			4.5	22	amino
Dillon (109)	1989	15.8	11.3[b]	2.4	2.4	amino
Destache (14)	1989	19.1	13.1[b]	13.0	13.0	amino
Destache (12)	1990	18.4	13.2	10.0	18.7	amino
Destache (13)	1990	29.1	13.4[b]			amino
Burton (107)	1991	20.3	16.0[b]	4	1.4	amino
Jorgenson (24)	1991	14.4	12.4			amino
Whipple (50)	1991			62.5	12.5[b]	amino

[a]Drug: amino = aminoglycoside, dig = digoxin, hep = heparin, theo = theophylline, tobra = tobramycin.
[b]Statistically significant difference, at $P = 0.05$ or less, in appropriateness between before and after pharmacy action.

In a population of patients taking anticonvulsant medication, Beardsley,[91] Ionnides-Demos,[22] Wing,[53] and their co-workers assessed the impact of therapeutic drug monitoring and clinical pharmacokinetic services on some aspects of future health care consumption. Beardsley et al found that the introduction of serum anticonvulsant levels into an outpatient population resulted in increased number of office visits and dosage adjustments.[91] Also in a similar outpatient population, the CPKS significantly reduced the number of seizures (a clinical outcome measure) and also reduced, but not as substantially, the number of emergency room visits and hospital admissions during the study period.[22] In a hospitalized population, Wing and Duff found that there were fewer seizure-related readmissions in the CPKS-monitored patients as compared with those without CPKS care.[53] In an earlier study examining theophylline monitoring in an inpatient population, however, Wing and Duff found no difference in readmission rates between those who did and did not have CPKS care.[54]

The inclusion of measures of future health care consumption creates a fuller picture of the contribution of CPKSs. Both inpatients and outpatients could be randomized to CPKS or non-CPKS care and then followed longitudinally over time. Computerized insurance claims and clinic records could provide data sources for this type of assessment.

Economic Consequences

The economic aspects of clinical pharmacokinetic services have been the topic of at least four recent review articles.[113-116] We approach this subject by describing some of the basic principles of economic evaluation of health care programs, examining how the CPKS economic studies have been conducted, and then analyze the conclusions of the studies in light of the quality of the economic analyses.

A complete examination of the system-related economic consequences or impact of a clinical pharmacokinetic service requires (1) a comparison of at least two comparable populations of patients, one receiving clinical pharmacokinetic services and another, during the same period, serving as a control population and not receiving CPKS care, but who in all other ways receives similar treatment; (2) an itemization of the costs (inputs) of providing the CPKS, including proportional costs of pharmacists' salaries and fringe benefits, equipment, supplies, and overhead; and (3) a complete detailing of all consequences (outputs) for patients in both populations during the episode of care.

As a measure of economic outcome, the analysis should examine the total impact of the CPKS intervention and not focus on change in one of the process components. Using the health care system perspective, this should include at a minimum the lengths of hospital and intensive care unit stays, total drug dose, duration of drug therapy, TDM tests, and adverse drug reactions. When these outputs are kept in their natural units (eg, hospital days) and the differences in outputs are compared with the differences in cost of the inputs (CPKS versus no CPKS), a cost–effectiveness study can be performed. When the differences in outputs or benefits are converted to dollars (eg, cost of a hospital day) and compared with the differences in the cost of inputs in dollars, then a cost–benefit analysis is possible or a simple "net savings" (subtracting the costs of the CPKS from the dollar benefits) can be calculated.

How well do the published CPKS economic studies meet these three requirements? Several problems are common. Concerning the first requirement, although lack of a comparison population was found,[117] most did use patient controls so that the differences in economic inputs and outputs between CPKS and control populations could be determined in each study. However, the larger problems concern the comparability of the CPKS and control populations and the timing of patient care; for example, the two groups were not studied during the same period. These issues affect not only the economic, but also the administrative and clinical outcomes. Some studies compared patients at different times (before and after the introduction of a CPKS),[8] whereas others attempted to match CPKS and control patients.[14] Neither method is satisfactory; instead randomization of patients to CPKS and control populations is recommended.

What about the second requirement—an itemization of the costs or inputs of providing the CPKS, including proportional costs of pharmacists' salaries and fringe benefits, equipment, supplies, and overhead? As mentioned earlier in reference to the economic consequences of administrative process measures, none of the studies completely includes all the information necessary to accurately arrive at the total costs of providing clinical pharmacokinetic services. Occasionally, even the proportion of the pharmacist's time devoted to the CPKS was excluded,[110] but more commonly salaries, fringe benefits, equipment, supplies, and overhead were omitted from the determination of CPKS costs.

And how well do the studies meet the third requirement—a complete detailing of all consequences or outputs in both population during the episode of care and their conversion into the appropriate unit of measurement for the selected economic assessment? This requirement presented many problems. In some cases, attempts were made to patch together components of the economic picture that in aggregate would approximate all consequences resulting from CPKS interventions. For example, in comparing patients for whom physicians requested a CPKS consult and a matched group of patients with pneumonia and sepsis with no CPKS care, Destache et al approximated the total difference in the cost of an episode of care by adding the differences in charges for TDM assays, total drug, and hospital days.[14] Additional economic components such as the differences between the groups in costs associated with toxicity or administration of drug were not included.

Investigators have used numerous economic measures, with various degrees of comprehensiveness, to compare the benefits or outputs of CPKS- and non-CPKS-monitored populations. They include, ranked in decreasing magnitude of completeness, overall costs, cost of episode of care, cost of hospital stay, cost of course of therapy, and laboratory costs per day. Estimated net savings between CPKS and non-CPKS populations have been measured in yearly savings. Savings range from Kimelblatt's and co-workers' $55,000 per year savings in drug usage without the subtraction of the cost of the CPKS review[26] to Destache and colleagues' estimated savings of $2,263,000 per year if CPKS provided care and the aminoglycoside recommendations were followed.[13] As the total savings depend on the number of patients that the service can reach, other investigators have reported their economic impact in terms of net savings per patient. Burton,[107] Crist,[11] Smith,[43] and their co-workers calculated that the CPKS saved $1311, $725, and $491 per patient, respectively. Lehmann and Leonard, however, estimated that the CPKS increased the cost of care by $700 per patient, primarily due to increased length of hospitalization.[29]

Cost–Benefit Studies of TDM and Clinical Pharmacokinetic Services. A cost–benefit study is a form of economic analysis that compares the economic benefits or savings (outputs) of an intervention with the costs of performing the intervention (inputs) and is used to produce a benefit-to-cost ratio. A benefit-to-cost ratio of 1.0 means that the economic benefits equaled the economic costs, a ratio less than 1.0 indicates that the costs exceed the benefits, and a ratio greater than 1.0 indicates that the benefits exceed the cost. Bootman,[8] Burton,[107] Destache,[12] and their colleagues estimated benefit-to-cost ratios of 8.7:1, 4.09:1, and 52.25:1, respectively.

PATIENT-RELATED MEASURES

The majority of the evaluations of the impact of therapeutic drug monitoring and the assessment of the contributions of clinical pharmacokinetic services are conducted with a relatively narrow administrative focus. The improvement in quality of the testing process, appropriateness of TDM ordering, and interpretation of results coupled with an emphasis on the reduction of length of hospital stay, total dosage amounts, and number of TDM orders all are part of the system-based administrative review. In this section we consider those measures that directly reflect a patient's action or condition.

Structure

Relatively few studies have asked the patient-related question, Can clinical pharmacokinetic services improve patient outcome?, as compared with the companion question, asked in more than 50 studies, Can clinical pharmacokinetic services improve the quality of TDM testing? The concerns about the varying structures of clinical pharmacokinetic services remain the same, however. More sophisticated questions about the structure and contribution of CPKS have not been asked, but would make important contributions: Should there be different CPKS structural characteristics for different TDM drugs? For patient conditions of different severity? For different locations? Should CPKS offer services that are specific for selected units and clinics or is a general, all-purpose service adequate?

Process

Patients can control part of the process of their care; namely, they can or cannot be compliant with their medication regimen. Only two studies explicitly considered the impact of TDM on patient compliance. Can the therapeutic drug monitoring of medication in an outpatient environment increase patient compliance? Beardsley et al indicated that after the introduction of TDM for anticonvulsant agents, compliance rose from 23 to 32%.[91] In another outpatient population, this time receiving antiarrhythmic agents, Squire et al found that patients who were being monitored also had high rates of noncompliance.[105] When the technology is approved for home testing, it will be interesting to watch the introduction of self-monitoring into the home, and examine whether the patient who has control of the testing process and directly performs and receives the TDM results is more compliant.

Outcomes

The clinical and economic impact of TDM and clinical pharmacokinetic services on patient-related measures is considered in this section. The principal reason for therapeutically monitoring medication—to optimize therapeutic effectiveness while preventing toxicity—is directly assessed by clinical outcome measures such as incidence of toxicity, reduction of symptoms/increase in cure, and mortality. These variables are directly related to patient outcome.

Clinical Impact on Patient Care

Incidence of Toxicity. Table 8–8 lists 26 studies that examined the incidence of various toxic effects in patients who were receiving medications with narrow therapeutic windows. Early investigators examined digoxin toxicity and, with the use of serum digoxin concentrations, were able to improve patient dosing and reduce the toxicity rate.[118,119] With the value of digoxin monitoring established, later studies examined other medications and whether individualization of patient doses by clinical pharmacokinetic services further contributed to reduction in toxicity. Twenty studies compared the incidence of toxic effects in patients who were being followed with

TABLE 8–8. STUDIES INCORPORATING PATIENT-RELATED OUTCOME MEASURES: INCIDENCE OF TOXICITY IN PATIENTS FOLLOWED WITH AND WITHOUT THERAPEUTIC DRUG MONITORING (TDM) AND WITH AND WITHOUT A CLINICAL PHARMACOKINETIC SERVICE (CPKS)

			Percentage of Patients with Toxicity			
First Author	**Year**	**Type of Toxicity**	**No TDM/CPKS**	**With TDM**	**With TDM + CPKS**	**Drug**[a]
Duhme (118)	1974	Toxicity	10	4		dig
Koch-Weser (119)	1974	Toxicity	13.9	5.9		dig
Lewis (31)	1976	Toxicity		50.1	22.9[b]	dig
Bootman (8)	1976	Nephrotoxicity		7	0	amino
Gannaway (120)	1981	Ataxia, diplopia, dysarthria		44		pheny
Lehmann (29)	1982	Nausea, vomiting, cardiac		14.8	10	theo
Beardsley (91)	1983	Toxicity		nd[c]	nd	anticonv
Coodley (122)	1983	Toxicity		21.4	12.3	dig
Mungall (34)	1983	Nausea, vomiting, cardiac		50	15.7	theo
Horn (20)	1985	Toxicity		11.1	2.2[b]	dig
Sveska (44)	1985	Nephrotoxicity		21.7	7.1[b]	amino
Arroyo (95)	1986	Nephrotoxicity	8	15		amino
Cahill (10)	1986	Nephro- and ototoxicity			0	amino
Kimelblatt (26)	1986	Nephro- and ototoxicity		14	14	vanco
Winter (56)	1986	Nephrotoxicity, adverse drug reactions		nd	nd	amino, theo
Eisenberg (121)	1987	Nephrotoxicity	14.7	7		amino
Ionnides-Demos (22)	1988	Adverse drug reactions		21.1	14.8	anticonv
Begg (5)	1989	Nephrotoxicity		nd	nd	amino
Dillon (109)	1989	Nephrotoxicity		2.4	7.3	amino
Hoffa (19)	1989	Nephrotoxicity		7.3	0	amino
Destache (14)	1989	Nephrotoxicity		11.6	8.7	amino
Destache (13)	1990	Nephrotoxicity		14.3	8	amino
Wade (48)	1990	Nephrotoxicity			0	amino
Burton (107)	1991	Nephrotoxicity		9.7	5.1	amino
Lynch (33)	1992	Nephrotoxicity		12	3	amino
Bertino (123)	1993	Nephrotoxicity		19.2	7.9	amino

[a]Drug: amino = aminoglycoside, anticonv = anticonvulsant, dig = digoxin, pheny = phenytoin, theo = theophylline, vanco = vancomycin.
[b]Statistically significant difference, at $P = 0.05$ or less, in toxicity between TDM and TDM + CPKS.
[c]nd = no difference, but actual value not given.

only serum drug concentrations (TDM) or by a CPKS ordering the TDM tests and interpreting the results. In 15 studies, CPKS-monitored patients had a lower incidence of toxic reactions than those followed by TDM alone, but only 3 of the 15 showed a significant improvement with CPKS over TDM. The small sample size may have prevented more of the studies from detecting a significant difference.

Ried et al conducted a meta-analysis of 14 studies to determine the effect of a CPKS on the occurrence of toxic drug reactions.[124] When all 14 studies were combined, a monitoring service was able to reduce the rate of toxicity and appeared to be more beneficial for patients taking digoxin and theophylline.

Number of Septic Episodes. Only one study used the number of septic episodes as an outcome variable and the results may appear counterintuitive. Nearly 23% of the CPKS-followed burn patients had two or more septic episodes, whereas only 7.7% of the non-CPKS-monitored group had multiple septic episodes. Because the CPKS patients lived longer and had a higher survival rate, however, they had more opportunities to develop septic episodes.

Reduction of Symptoms/Increase in Cure. Given that TDM leads to a certain level of reduction of symptoms and achievement of cure, two questions are examined in this section: (1) Does the monitoring of serum drug concentrations (TDM) incrementally add to the benefit (symptom relief or cure) of these drugs? (2) Does the scheduling and interpretation of TDM results and the initiation of appropriate action in response to the results provide additional benefit as compared with routine TDM testing? These topics are discussed with respect to cure of infections and seizure control.

Cure of Infections. Given that an association exists between serum aminoglycoside concentrations (SACs) and clinical outcome,[125] does knowledge of the SAC improve the cure rate? And does the CPKS offer additional benefit over the SAC information alone? No studies were found that compared the cure rate in two similar populations where the clinicians for one group of patients received SAC information while the others did not. In a recent review article, however, six studies were cited as examining the hypothesis that individualized aminoglycoside dosing has a positive effect on outcome[126]; three involved a formalized CPKS.[13,14,44] None of the latter three directly stated the cure rate of the patients while they were receiving aminoglycosides and were followed or not followed by a CPKS. Instead, proxies such as hours of fever, duration of therapy, and survival rates were used to express the therapeutic effectiveness of the CPKS. These are indirect measures of CPKS effectiveness because a number of factors (eg, change of medication type) could also be captured by these factors.

A distinction made by the Burton et al study can be used to illustrate the points made in the preceding paragraph.[107] Burton and co-workers defined cure rate as absence of fever for 4 days and the response rate as the same criterion but with another antibiotic being administered after aminoglycoside was discontinued. When comparing patients followed by a bayesian dosing program and those followed by physician choice, they found a difference in the response rate but not in the cure rate. The measures one uses in asking a question can influence the conclusions reached when answering the question.

Two studies did use cure rate as an outcome measure,[95,107] and a third used "failure rate."[127] No differences were found in the cure rate between CPKS- and non-CPKS-monitored patients in either study; however, patients with perforated and gangrenous appendicitis had a 1.6% failure rate with CPKS and a 11.3% failure rate without CPKS, a difference that was significant.

Seizure Control. On the basis of studies demonstrating a relationship between increasing anticonvulsant drug concentrations and decreasing seizure frequency,[128,129] serum drug concentration determinations became common for phenytoin and other anticonvulsant medications. In one clinic, Beardsley et al found that new TDM information did not directly link to improved seizure control; rather, it was mediated by whether or not clinicians took appropriate action based on the TDM result. When appropriate action was taken, 51% of the patients improved as compared with only 5% when physicians made an inappropriate response.[91] Also, in a randomized trial, Fröscher et al were not able to detect a difference in the patients followed by clinicians who did receive TDM results and those who did not[17]; however, they did not examine the quality of the response to the TDM results.

These studies suggest that information in the form of a TDM result is not sufficient to increase seizure control; rather, appropriate response to the result is necessary. Can CPKSs improve the appropriate response rate and reduce symptoms? Two studies indicate that they can have some effect. In the first, Ionnides-Demos et al detected a decrease in toxic clonic seizures from 36.7 to 24.3% following the introduction of a CPKS in an outpatient epilepsy clinic.[22] In the second example, in an inpatient environment, when patients were followed by a CPKS, they had fewer seizure-related readmissions than patients who were randomized to non-CPKS care.[53] Woo et al, however, do caution that an appropriate response must combine TDM results with clinical judgment. Patients who were well controlled on subtherapeutic doses received no additional benefit when their drug concentration was raised to a therapeutic level and even suffered increased neurotoxicity with the increased drug concentration.[101]

Mortality. Thirteen studies examined the impact of a CPKS on the decrease in mortality (see Table 8–7). Only the three studies with the largest differences in mortality rates between the CPKS- and non-CPKS-monitored patients resulted in significant mortality differences.[8,44,50] Mortality in a burn population followed by a CPKS was 36.4% as compared with 66.7% in an earlier burn population treated without a CPKS.[8] In pneumonia and sepsis patients, mortality was 12% in the presence of the CPKS, but it was 42% in a matched control group of patients who were treated at the same time without a CPKS.[44] And in severely ill surgery patients, mortality was 12.5% in the patients randomized to receive CPKS monitoring; patients not being followed by the CPKS had a 62.5% mortality rate.[50] These studies on burn and severe surgical patients as well as other reports on severely ill patient populations suggest that early and higher dose treatment increases survival.[108,125,130]

Although the incidence of toxic effects, cure, and mortality have been included as outcome measures in the assessment of the clinical effectiveness of therapeutic drug monitoring and clinical pharmacokinetic services, true patient-centered outcomes such as multidimensional health status and quality-of-life measures have not. Although that may be acceptable in the assessment of the treatment of acute, life-threatening conditions, the lack of such measures in the evaluation of the effectiveness of therapeutic drug monitoring in a chronic care population unnecessarily restricts the assessment to the views of the measures of health care professionals.

There is room for quality-of-life measures and patient preference determinations in the evaluation of the clinical effectiveness of TDM and CPKSs in a chronic care population (and, some would say, even in acute care). From the patient's perspective, other things are more important than whether the TDM samples were collected properly or whether the drug concentration is within the therapeutic range. Although these factors may ultimately impact on the quality of life of the patient, it is also possible that even through the specimen was collected properly and the result is within the therapeutic range, the patient's quality of life is adversely affected because of the toxicity of the medication that accompanies the therapeutic response. Or maybe there is a trade-off between maximal therapeutic effectiveness and increasing side effects. Should not the point of view of the patient and the patient's preferences be incorporated into the determination of the effectiveness of dosing recommendations? As more drugs are chronically monitored by TDM technology and the technology evolves to permit self-monitoring, the perspective of the patient must be included in future assessments of TDM protocols, testing methodologies, and CPKS effectiveness.

Economic Consequences

None of the economic assessments to date have taken a patient or societal perspective. Instead the analyses have adopted the traditional health care view and have examined the health care dollars wasted in poor TDM testing or the cost savings in shorter hospital stays. An economic assessment from the patient perspective requires that all costs to the patient be identified and incorporated. Do patients have additional costs and savings related to their TDM care? If they need to have frequent TDM testing, does that interrupt their jobs, affect their salaries, and create transportation expenses? This is certainly an issue that needs to be examined as new TDM technology is developed to permit self-monitoring of serum drug concentrations. And what is the economic impact to patients if a toxic reaction develops requiring additional hospital days and time lost from work?

Perhaps patients have adequate sick days and do not lose wages when undergoing TDM testing, but society has an economic productivity loss when individuals are away from their work. A societal perspective requires that all costs—whether health care, patient, or societal costs—be included in an economic analysis. In cost–benefit studies, that means that an economic value must be placed on lost work productivity as well as the death of a patient. As society is uncomfortable in placing a value on human life and because that value is difficult to determine, cost–effectiveness studies may be a better economic approach. Clinical pharmacokineticists should collaborate with health care economists to conduct more sophisticated, patient-centered and societal economic and cost–effectiveness studies of TDM in general and of their services in particular.

RECOMMENDATIONS

Although therapeutic drug monitoring assays have been performed for more than 20 years and clinical pharmacokinetic services have been offered by most teaching hospitals for nearly 10 years, more studies with improved study designs and increased use of patient-centered outcome assessments are needed to evaluate both the use of therapeutic drug monitoring and the contribution of clinical pharmacokinetic services.

On the basis of comments made earlier in this chapter and earlier suggestions from an insightful review article on the problems involved in evaluating therapeutic drug monitoring services,[131] the following recommendations are made to define and improve the clinical and economic contributions of therapeutic drug monitoring and clinical pharmacokinetic services:

 I. Conduct studies to link the processes of TDM and CPKS interventions to changes in patient and economic outcomes.
   A. Prospective studies with control population(s), preferably patients randomized to test and control populations.
   B. Studies of sufficient size to detect clinically significant differences between patients not monitored, monitored with TDM only, and monitored with TDM and CPKS.
   C. Studies of sufficient size to detect differences in response between patients with diseases of differing severity.
   D. Studies targeted to assessing the impact on one drug, or of sufficient size to detect if TDM and CPKS make differential contributions within the therapeutically monitored drugs.
   E. Studies including patient-centered outcomes and quality-of-life measures.
   F. Studies identifying and determining the economic value of all inputs and outputs of TDM testing and CPKS care.
   G. Studies examining relationships between structure, process, and clinical and economic outcome measures.
 II. Develop TDM audit criteria that allow for inclusion of clinical judgment in response to TDM results.
   A. Examine the validity of the present therapeutic ranges.
   B. Develop and evaluate methods to individualize response to TDM results.
III. Develop and adhere to a common set of process and outcome measures that, at the minimum, would be included in all studies. This would not preclude the use of additional measures within a particular study.
IV. Require adequate description of the nature of the CPKS intervention to enable comparison of different CPKS structures and processes and their impact on outcome.

———— QUESTIONS ————————————————————————————————

 1. Differentiate system-related from patient-related outcome measures in TDM.

 2. Give three examples of system-related and three examples of patient-related outcome measures.

 3. What is meant by the structure–process–outcome method proposed by Donabedian for the assessment of quality of care?

 4. Give an example of the interaction of a set of structure, process, and outcome variables (using the Donabedian approach) that applies to the evaluation of TDM. Include both system-related and patient-related measures.

 5. Identify three common system-related measures that have frequently been used to evaluate the effectiveness of TDM services.

6. The pharmacy department in your hospital initiates a system of various audits that includes the fraction of patients whose serum concentrations are within the therapeutic range for TDM drugs. What are the value and limitations of this type of audit?

7. What has been the principal limitation in applying outcomes assessment in TDM to date?

8. Give an example of how you would evaluate whether an organized TDM service improved patient-related measures of outcome.

9. What is meant by the term *quality of life?* How may TDM impact on a patient's quality of life?

REFERENCES

1. Donabedian A. Evaluating the quality of medical care. *Milbank Memorial Fund Q.* 1966;44:166–206, Part 2.
2. Epstein AM. The outcomes movement—Will it get us where we want to go? *N Engl J Med.* 1990;323:266–270.
3. Ellwood PM. Outcome management: A technology of patient experience. *N Engl J Med.* 1988; 318:1549–1556.
4. Ambrose PJ, Nitake M, Kildoo CW. Impact of pharmacist scheduling of blood-sampling times for therapeutic drug monitoring. *Am J Hosp Pharm.* 1988;45:380–382.
5. Begg EJ, Atkinson HC, Jeffery GM, et al. Individualized aminoglycoside dosage based on pharmacokinetic analysis is superior to dosage based on physician intuition at achieving target plasma drug concentrations. *Br J Clin Pharmacol.* 1989;28:137–141.
6. Blackbourn J, Sunderland VB. Impact of pharmacist intervention on oral theophylline therapy in adult inpatients. *Drug Intell Clin Pharm.* 1987;21:811–816.
7. Bollish SJ, Kelly WN, Miller DE, et al. Establishing an aminoglycoside pharmacokinetic monitoring service in a community hospital. *Am J Hosp Pharm.* 1981;38:73–76.
8. Bootman JL, Wertheimer AI, Zaske D, Rowland C. Individualized gentamicin dosage regimens in burn patients with Gram-negative septicemia: A cost–benefit analysis. *J Pharm Sci.* 1979;68:267–272.
9. Burton ME, Brater DC, Chen PS, et al. Bayesian feedback method of aminoglycoside dosing. *Clin Pharmacol Ther.* 1985;37:349–357.
10. Cahill RJ, Myers RM, Bauer LA, Alston RM. Impact of aminoglycoside kinetic service on aminoglycoside use in a community hospital. *Hosp Pharm.* 1986;21:734ff.
11. Crist KD, Nahata MC, Ety J. Positive impact of a therapeutic drug-monitoring program on total aminoglycoside dose and cost of hospitalization. *Ther Drug Monit.* 1987;9:306–310.
12. Destache CJ, Meyer SM, Bittner MJ, et al. Impact of a clinical pharmacokinetic service on patients treated with aminoglycosides: A cost–benefit analysis. *Ther Drug Monit.* 1990;12:419–427.
13. Destache CJ, Meyer SM, Rowley KA. Does accepting pharmacokinetic recommendations impact hospitalization? A cost–benefit analysis. *Ther Drug Monit.* 1990;12:427–433.
14. Destache CJ, Meyer SM, Padomek MJ, et al. Impact of a clinical pharmacokinetic service on patients treated with aminoglycosides for Gram-negative infections. *Drug Intell Clin Pharm: Ann Pharmacother.* 1989;23:33–38.
15. Elenbass RM, Payne VW, Bauman JL. Influence of clinical pharmacist consultations on the use of drug level tests. *Am J Hosp Pharm.* 1980;37:61–64.

16. Fox J, Hicks P, Feldman BR, et al. Theophylline blood levels as a guide to intravenous therapy in children. *Am J Dis Child.* 1982;136:928–930.
17. Fröscher W, Eichelbaum M, Gulger R, et al. A prospective randomized trial on the effect of monitoring plasma anticonvulsant levels in epilepsy. *J Neurol.* 1981;224:193–201.
18. Greenlaw CW, Henrietta GC, Stolley SN. Standardized heparin dosage schedule using pharmacokinetic principles. *Am J Hosp Pharm.* 1979;36:920–923.
19. Hoffa DE. Serial pharmacokinetic dosing of aminoglycosides: A community hospital experience. *Ther Drug Monit.* 1989;11:574–579.
20. Horn JR, Christensen DB, deBlaquiere PA. Evaluation of a digoxin pharmacokinetic monitoring service in a community hospital. *Drug Intell Clin Pharm.* 1985;19:45–52.
21. Hurley SF, Dziukas LJ, McNeil JJ, et al. A randomized controlled clinical trial of pharmacokinetic theophylline dosing. *Am Rev Respir Dis.* 1986;134:1219–1224.
22. Ionnides-Demos LL, Horne MK, Tong N, et al. Impact of a pharmacokinetic consultation service on clinical outcomes in an ambulatory-care epilepsy clinic. *Am J Hosp Pharm.* 1988;45:1549–1551.
23. Job ML, Ward ES, Murphy JE. Seven years of experience with a pharmacokinetic service. *Hosp Pharm.* 1989;24:512–519.
24. Jorgenson JA, Rewers RF. Justification and evaluation of an aminoglycoside pharmacokinetic dosing service. *Hosp Pharm.* 1991;26:609–611, 615.
25. Kearns GL, Jimenez JF, Brown AL, et al. Evaluation of clinical pharmacokinetic services provided to children and adolescents with cystic fibrosis. *J Ark Med Soc.* 1985;82:215–219.
26. Kimelblatt BJ, Bradbury K, Chodoff L, et al. Cost–benefit analysis of an aminoglycoside monitoring service. *Am J Hosp Pharm.* 1986;43:1205–1209.
27. Klamerus KJ, Munger MA. Effect of clinical pharmacy services on appropriateness of serum digoxin concentration monitoring. *Am J Hosp Pharm.* 1988;45:1887–1893.
28. Koren G, Soldin SJ, MacLeod SM. Organization and efficacy of a therapeutic drug monitoring consultation service in a pediatric hospital. *Ther Drug Monit.* 1985;7:295–298.
29. Lehmann CR, Leonard RG. Effect of theophylline pharmacokinetic monitoring service on cost and quality of care. *Am J Hosp Pharm.* 1982;39:1656–1662.
30. Levin B, Cohen SS, Birmingham PH. Effect of pharmacist intervention on the use of serum drug assays. *Am J Hosp Pharm.* 1981;38:845–851.
31. Lewis KP, Cooper JW, McKercher PL. Pharmacists' effect on digoxin usage and toxicity. *Am J Hosp Pharm.* 1976;33:1272–1276.
32. Liebiszewski D. The development of a drug-dose adjustment service for patients with renal impairments. *J Clin Hosp Pharm.* 1981;6:39–49.
33. Lynch TJ, Possidente CJ, Cioffi WG, et al. Multidisciplinary protocol for determining aminoglycoside dosage. *Am J Hosp Pharm.* 1992;49:109–115.
34. Mungall D, Marshall J, Penn D, et al. Individualizing theophylline therapy: The impact of clinical pharmacokinetics on patient outcomes. *Ther Drug Monit.* 1983;5:95–101.
35. Norris S. Evaluation of gentamicin prescribing after drug review. *Am J Hosp Pharm.* 1982; 39:1529–1530.
36. Parker WA, Reid LW. Serum digoxin level utilization review. *Can J Hosp Pharm.* 1978;31:97–99.
37. Pearce GA, Day RO. Compliance with criteria necessary for effective drug concentration monitoring. *Ther Drug Monit.* 1990;12:250–257.
38. Pitterle ME, Sorkness CA, Wiederholt JB. Use of drug concentrations in outpatient clinics. *Am J Hosp Pharm.* 1985;42:1547–1552.
39. Rich DS, Mahoney CD, Jeffrey LP, et al. Evaluation of a computerized digoxin pharmacokinetic consultation service. *Hosp Pharm.* 1981;16:23–27.
40. Robinson JD. Pharmacokinetics service for ambulatory patients. *Am J Hosp Pharm.* 1981; 38:1713–1716.

41. Saya FG, Coleman LT, Martinoff JT. Pharmacist-directed heparin therapy using a standard dosing and monitoring protocol. *Am J Hosp Pharm.* 1985;42:1965–1969.

42. Slaughter RL, Schneider PJ, Visconti JA. Appropriateness of the use of serum digoxin and digitoxin assays. *Am J Hosp Pharm.* 1978;35:1376–1379.

43. Smith M, Murphy JE, Job ML, et al. Aminoglycoside monitoring: Use of a pharmacokinetic service versus physician recommendation. *Hosp Formul.* 1987;22:92–102.

44. Sveska KJ, Roffe BD, Solomon DK, Hoffmann RP. Outcome of patients treated by an aminoglycoside pharmacokinetic dosing service. *Am J Hosp Pharm.* 1985;42:2472–2478.

45. Taylor JW, McLean AJ, Leonard RG, et al. Initial experience of clinical pharmacology and clinical pharmacy interactions in a clinical pharmacokinetics consultation service. *J Clin Pharmacol.* 1979; 19:1–7.

46. Tierney MG, Braden LA. An evaluation of a pharmacy nased aminoglycoside monitoring service. *Can J Hosp Pharm.* 1984;37:135–137.

47. Vozeh S, Uematsu T, Ritz R, et al. Computer-assisted individualized lidocaine dosage: Clinical evaluation and comparison with physician performance. *Am Heart J.* 1987;113:928–933.

48. Wade WE, McCall CY. Therapeutic drug monitoring in a community hospital. *Ther Drug Monit.* 1990;12:79–81.

49. Wallace SM, Gesy K, Gorecki DKJ. Establishing a clinical pharmacokinetic service for gentamicin in a community hospital. *Can J Hosp Pharm.* 1984;37:10–14.

50. Whipple JK, Ausman RK, Franson T, Quebbeman EJ. Effect of individualized pharmacokinetic dosing on patient outcome. *Crit Care Med.* 1991;19:1480–1485.

51. Whiting B, Kelman AW, Bryson SM, et al. Clinical pharmacokinetics: A comprehensive system for therapeutic drug monitoring and prescribing. *Br Med J.* 1984;288:541–545.

52. Wilson JT, Wilkinson GR. Delivery of anticonvulsant drug therapy in epileptic patients assessed by plasma level analyses. *Neurology.* 1974;24:614–623.

53. Wing DS, Duff HJ. The impact of a therapeutic drug monitoring program for phenytoin. *Ther Drug Monit.* 1989;11:32–37.

54. Wing DS, Duff HJ. Evaluation of a therapeutic drug monitoring program for theophylline in a teaching hospital. *Drug Intell Clin Pharm.* 1987;21:702–706.

55. Wing DS, Duff HJ. Impact of a therapeutic drug monitoring program for digoxin. *Arch Intern Med.* 1987;147:1405–1408.

56. Winter ME, Herfindal ET, Bernstein LR. Impact of a decentralized pharmacokinetics consultation service. *Am J Hosp Pharm.* 1986;43:2178–2184.

57. Einarson TR, Segal HJ, Mann JL. Serum drug level utilization: A literature analysis. *Can J Hosp Pharm.* 1989;42:63–68.

58. Ried LD, McKenna DA, Horn JR. Effect of therapeutic drug monitoring services on the number of serum drug assays ordered for patients: A meta-analysis. *Ther Drug Monit.* 1989;11:253–263.

59. Ried LD, McKenna DA, Horn JR. Meta-analysis of research on the effect of clinical pharmacokinetics services on therapeutic drug monitoring. *Am J Hosp Pharm.* 1989;46:945–951.

60. Goldberg GA, Abbott JA. Explicit criteria for use of laboratory tests. *Ann Intern Med.* 1974; 81:857–858.

61. Anderson AC, Hodges GR, Barnes WG. Determination of serum gentamicin sulfate levels, ordering patterns and use as a guide to therapy. *Arch Intern Med.* 1976;136:785–787.

62. Floyd RA, Cohen JL. Application of clinical pharmacokinetics in the assessment of theophylline therapy. *Am J Hosp Pharm.* 1977;34:402–407.

63. Slaughter RL, Schneider PJ, Visconti JA. Appropriateness of the use of serum digoxin and digitoxin assays. *Am J Hosp Pharm.* 1978;35:1376–1379.

64. Greenlaw CW, Geiger GS, Haug MT. Use of digoxin serum assays in a nonteaching hospital. *Am J Hosp Pharm.* 1980;37:1466–1470.

65. Clague HW, Twum-Barima Y, Carruthers SG. An audit of requests for therapeutic drug monitoring of digoxin: Problems and pitfalls. *Ther Drug Monit.* 1983;5:249–254.

66. Lampasona V, Crass RE. Patient selection for serum gentamicin levels. *Ther Drug Monit.* 1983;5:255–262.

67. Guernsey BG, Hokanson JA, Ingrim NB, et al. A utilization review of digoxin assays: Sampling patterns and use. *Hosp Pharm.* 1984;19:187–200.

68. Guernsey BG, Ingrim NB, Hokanson JA, et al. A utilization review of theophylline assays: Sampling patterns and use. *Drug Intell Clin Pharm.* 1984;18:906–912.

69. Ives TJ, Parry JL, Gwyther RE. Serum drug level utilization review in a family medicine residency program. *J Fam Pract.* 1984;19:507–512.

70. Wiser TH, Michocki RJ, Knapp DA, et al. Audit of digoxin prescribing in ambulatory patients. *Hosp Pharm.* 1984;19:811–816.

71. Sargenti C, Zelman L, Beauclair T, et al. Evaluation of appropriateness and interpretation of serum theophylline assays. *Drug Intell Clin Pharm.* 1985;19:380–384.

72. Farris CR, Stanaszek WF, Kashner TM, et al. Dealing with DRGs: Analysis of serum theophylline assays in Medicare patients. *Hosp Pharm.* 1986;21:39ff.

73. Kildoo CW, Bolger PB, Ambrose PH, et al. Use of serum drug concentrations in a private outpatient clinic. *Am J Hosp Pharm.* 1987;44:1410–1411.

74. Karki SD, Holden JMC. Appropriateness of the use of serum lithium assays. *Drug Intell Clin Pharm.* 1988;22:151–153.

75. D'Angio RG, Stevenson JG, Lively BT, et al. Therapeutic drug monitoring: Improved performance through educational intervention. *Ther Drug Monit.* 1990;12:173–181.

76. Carroll DJ, Austin GE, Stajich, et al. Effect of education on the appropriateness of serum drug concentration determination. *Ther Drug Monit.* 1992;14:81–84.

77. Flynn TW, Revonka MP, Yost RL, et al. Use of serum gentamicin levels in hospitalized patients. *Am J Hosp Pharm.* 1978;35:806–808.

78. Gentry SM, Keith TD, McMillan DM, et al. Evaluation of the ordering of serum theophylline concentrations. *Am J Hosp Pharm.* 1981;38:1937–1939.

79. Harless GR. Clinical use of serum theophylline assays in a community hospital. *Am J Hosp Pharm.* 1981;38:901–902.

80. Pasko MT, Mylotte JM, Boh LE. Evaluation of the use of laboratory tests in monitoring tobramycin therapy. *Am J Hosp Pharm.* 1981;38:1956–1957.

81. Vlasses PH, DiPiro CR, Chalupa D, et al. Appropriateness of sampling time for selected serum drug assays. *Hosp Pharm.* 1982;17:371–373.

82. Bussey HI, Hoffman EW. A prospective evaluation of therapeutic drug monitoring. *Ther Drug Monit.* 1983;5:245–248.

83. Mason GD, Winter ME. Appropriateness of sampling times for therapeutic drug monitoring. *Am J Hosp Pharm.* 1984;41:1796–1801.

84. Shaw MA, Russell WL, Bradham DD. Quality assurance in a clinical pharmacy program. *Qual Rev Bull.* 1984;10:87–89.

85. Gibb I, Cowan JC, Parnham AJ, et al. Use and misuse of a digoxin assay service. *Br Med J.* 1986;293:678–680.

86. Levine M, McCollom R, Chang T, Orr J. Evaluation of serum phenytoin monitoring in an acute care setting. *Ther Drug Monit.* 1988;10:50–57.

87. Kumana CR, Chan YM, Kou M. Audit exposes flawed blood sampling for "digoxin levels." *Ther Drug Monit.* 1992;14:155–158.

88. Greenlaw CW, Blough SS, Haugen RK. Aminoglycoside serum assays restricted through a pharmacy program. *Am J Hosp Pharm.* 1979;36:1080–1083.

89. Matzke GR, Lloyd CW, Lucarotti RL. Evaluation of the use of serum aminoglycoside concentrations. *Hosp Pharm.* 1981;16:145–152.

90. Sketris IS, Parker WA, Noble MA. Compliance with guidelines for monitoring aminoglycoside therapy. *Can J Hosp Pharm.* 1982;35:179–183.

91. Beardsley RS, Freeman JM, Appel FA. Anticonvulsant serum levels are useful only if the patient appropriately uses them: An assessment of the impact of providing serum level data to physicians. *Epilepsia.* 1983;24:330–335.

92. Knodel AR, Covelli HD, Beekman JF. Outpatient theophylline determinations. *West J Med.* 1984;140:741–744.

93. Quebbeman XJ, Franson TR, Whipple JE, et al. Quality control analysis in aminoglycoside management. *Arch Surg.* 1985;120:1069–1071.

94. Snidero M, Traina GL, Bonati M. Is ambulatory therapeutic digoxin monitoring useful? *Drug Intell Clin Pharm.* 1985;18:660–661.

95. Arroyo JC, Milligan WL, Davis J, et al. Impact of aminoglycoside serum assays on clinical decision and renal toxicity. *South Med J.* 1986;79:272–276.

96. Wade WE, Waite WW, McCall CY. Evaluation of empiric dosing of theophylline by physicians in a nontertiary care regional referral center. *Curr Ther Res.* 1990;47:1009–1016.

97. Tett S, Espinos E, Weekes L. Who is ordering all those cyclosporin concentrations and how do they use them? An audit of cyclosporin therapeutic drug monitoring. *Ther Drug Monit.* 1993;15:195–198.

98. Schumacher GE, Barr JT. Making serum drug levels more meaningful. *Ther Drug Monit.* 1989;11:580–584.

99. Schumacher GE, Barr JT. Using population-based serum drug concentration cutoff values to predict toxicity: Test performance and limitations compared with bayesian interpretation. *Clin Pharm.* 1990;9:88–96.

100. Schumacher GE, Barr JT, Browne TR, et al. Test performance characteristics of the serum phenytoin concentration (SPC): The relationship between SPC and patient response. *Ther Drug Monit.* 1991;13:318–324.

101. Woo E, Chan YM, Chan YW, Huang CY. If a well-stabilized epileptic patient has a subtherapeutic antiepileptic drug level, should the dose be increased? A randomized prospective study. *Epilepsia.* 1988;29:129–139.

102. Mason BJ. Subtherapeutic serum drug concentration and compliance. *Drug Intell Clin Pharm.* 1991;25:103–104.

103. Ambrose PJ, Smith WE, Palarea ER. A decade of experience with a clinical pharmacokinetic service. *Am J Hosp Pharm.* 1988;45:1879–1886.

104. Privitera MD. Dosing accuracy of antiepileptic drug regimens as determined by serum concentrations in outpatient epilepsy clinic patients. *Ther Drug Monit.* 1989;11:647–651.

105. Squire A, Goldman ME, Kupersmith J, et al. Long-term antiarrhythmic therapy: Problem of low drug levels and patient noncompliance. *Am J Med.* 1984;77:1035–1036.

106. Klamerus KJ, Munger MA. Effect of clinical pharmacy services on appropriateness of serum digoxin concentration monitoring. *Am J Hosp Pharm.* 1988;45:1887–1893.

107. Burton ME, Ash CL, Hill DP, et al. A controlled trial of the cost benefit of a computerized bayesian aminoglycoside administration. *Clin Pharmacol Ther.* 1991;49:685–694.

108. Moore RD, Smith CR, Lietman PS. The association of aminoglycoside plasma levels with mortality in patients with Gram-negative bacteremia. *J Infect Dis.* 1984;149:443–448.

109. Dillon KR, Dougherty SH, Casner P, Polly S. Individualized pharmacokinetic versus standard dosing of amikacin: A comparison of therapeutic outcomes. *J Antimicrob Chemother.* 1989;24:581–589.

110. McCormack JP, Lynd LD, Pfeifer NM. Vancomycin cost containment through a therapeutic and pharmacokinetic drug monitoring service. *Can J Hosp Pharm.* 1989;42:3–9.

111. Franson TR, Quebbeman EJ, Whipple J, et al. Prospective comparison of traditional and pharmacokinetic aminoglycoside dosing methods. *Crit Care Med.* 1988;16:840–843.

112. Vozeh S, Kewitz G, Perruchoud A, et al. Theophylline serum concentration and therapeutic effect in severe acute bronchial obstruction: The optimal use of intravenously administered aminophylline. *Am Rev Respir Dis.* 1982;125:181–184.

113. Destache CJ. Economic aspects of pharmacokinetic services. *PharmacoEconomics.* 1993;3:433–436.

114. Destache CJ. Use of therapeutic drug monitoring in pharmacoeconomics. *Ther Drug Monit.* 1993;15:608–610.

115. Gardner DM, Hardy BG. Cost-effectiveness of therapeutic drug monitoring. *Can J Hosp Pharm.* 1990;43:7–12.

116. Gentry CA, Rodvold KA, Bertino JS. Methods of minimizing the cost of aminoglycoside therapy to hospitals. *PharmacoEconomics.* 1993;3:228–243.

117. Schloemer JH, Zagozen JJ. Cost analysis of an aminoglycoside pharmacokinetic dosing program. *Am J Hosp Pharm.* 1984;41:2347–2351.

118. Duhme DW, Greenblatt DJ, Koch-Weser J. Reduction of digoxin toxicity associated with measurement of serum levels. *Ann Intern Med.* 1974;80:516–519.

119. Koch-Weser J, Duhme DW, Greenblatt DJ. Influence of serum digoxin concentration measurements on frequency of digitoxicity. *Clin Pharm Ther.* 1974;16:284–287.

120. Gannaway DJ, Mawer GE. Serum phenytoin concentration and clinical response in patients with epilepsy. *Br J Clin Pharmacol.* 1981;12:833–839.

121. Eisenberg JM, Koffer H, Glick HA, et al. What is the cost of nephrotoxicity associated with aminoglycosides? *Ann Intern Med.* 1987;107:900–909.

122. Coodley EL, Rodriguez J. The pharmacokinetic consultation service: A new approach to digoxin therapy. *Drug Ther.* 1983;13:82–85.

123. Bertino JS, Booker LA, Franck PA, et al. Incidence of and significant risk factors for aminoglycoside-associated nephrotoxicity in patients dosed by using individualized pharmacokinetic monitoring. *J Infect Dis.* 1993;167:173–179.

124. Ried LD, Horn JR, McKenna DA. Therapeutic drug monitoring reduces toxic drug reactions: A meta-analysis. *Ther Drug Monit.* 1990;12:72–78.

125. Moore RD, Smith CR, Lietman PS. Association of aminoglycoside plasma levels with therapeutic outcome in Gram-negative pneumonia. *Am J Med.* 1984;77:657–662.

126. McCormack JP, Jewesson PJ. A critical reevaluation of the "therapeutic range" of aminoglycosides. *Clin Infect Dis.* 1992;14:320–329.

127. Gill MA, Cheetham TC, Chenella FC, et al. Matched case–control study of adjusted versus nonadjusted gentamicin dosing in perforated and gangrenous appendicitis. *Ther Drug Monit.* 1986; 8:451–456.

128. Gram L, Flachs H, Würtz-Jørgensen A, et al. Sodium valproate, serum level and clinical effect in epilepsy: A controlled study. *Epilepsia.* 1979;20:303–312.

129. Reynolds EH, Shorvon SD, Galbraith AW, et al. Phenytoin monotherapy for epilepsy: A long-term prospective study, assisted by serum level monitoring in previously untreated patients. *Epilepsia.* 1981;22:475–488.

130. Zaske DE, Bootman JL, Solem LB, et al. Increased burn patient survival with individualized dosages of gentamicin. *Surgery.* 1982;91:142–149.

131. Reents S, Hatton R. Influence of methods on the evaluation of therapeutic drug-monitoring services. *Am J Hosp Pharm.* 1991;48:1553–1559.

Chapter 9

Aminoglycosides

S. James Matthews

Keep in Mind

- When designing a dosing regimen, be sure to review the patient's chart for disease-related factors that may affect the pharmacokinetics of the aminoglycoside antibiotics.
- Base doses on lean body mass or actual body weight, whichever is less. (Exceptions are the obese patient and the patient with ascites.)
- Monitor serum creatinine and BUN every 3 days unless renal function is changing.
- Monitor ototoxicity using the patient's subjective statements, patient observation, or audiometry in patients with preexisting conditions.
- If using a multiple-dose regimen, obtain peak and trough serum concentrations after the third dose and adjust the dosage regimen if needed.
- If using single-dose therapy, peak concentrations are not necessary; however, trough samples or random concentrations should be obtained. Concentration determinations should be obtained initially and then every 4 days during therapy.
- When determining serum concentrations, be sure to run the levels using the same assay technique.
- Review the patient's medications to determine possible drug interactions and effects these may have on interpretation of assay results.

The aminoglycoside antibiotics have been a mainstay for the therapy of community and hospital-acquired Gram-negative and select Gram-positive organisms since the first agent became available in 1944. The emergence of resistant strains of bacteria and the introduction of newer, less toxic antibiotics with similar spectra of action have begun to relegate these agents to secondary status. This is especially true as the cost of the newer agents decreases and our understanding of their place in therapy improves. Although the use of these antibiotics is decreasing, they remain an important class of drugs, especially for the treatment of resistant organisms. Recent identification of multi-drug-resistant organisms associated with the use of third-generation cephalosporins has raised questions on the use of these antibiotics as single therapy in serious Gram-negative infections. Resistance of *Enterobacter* spp may emerge less frequently during therapy with an aminoglycoside antibiotic than with a third-generation cephalosporin.[1]

With reduced use of the aminoglycoside antibiotics it is especially important to keep current in the dosing and monitoring of these medications. The less frequent use of these antibiotics also puts the pharmacist in a position to be of maximal assistance in the development of dosage regimens, monitoring of therapy, and prevention of the toxic effects of these medications.

CLINICAL PHARMACOLOGY AND THERAPEUTICS

Spectrum of Activity and Clinical Use

The aminoglycoside antibiotics are a group of medications whose basic compounds contain amino sugars. They are produced by fungi of the order Actinomycetales. Streptomycin, kanamycin, neomycin, paromomycin, and tobramycin are products of *Streptomyces* spp. Gentamicin and sisomicin are from *Micromonospora* spp. Semisynthetic varieties have been made and include amikacin from kanamycin and netilmicin from sisomicin. These agents have been extremely important in the treatment of serious infections caused by Gram-negative bacilli.

Streptomycin was the first aminoglycoside and was discovered in 1944. Emergence of resistant Gram-negative organisms has relegated it to adjunct use with other antibiotics to treat *Mycobacterium tuberculosis* and enterococcal endocarditis. Newer drugs are replacing streptomycin for the management of enterococcal endocarditis. It is considered half a drug when used to treat tuberculosis because it is active in the blood but not intracellularly. It is administered intramuscularly; however, intravenous use is possible but not recommended.[2]

Neomycin was discovered in 1949, and is a combination of neomycins B and C. Initial parenteral use of this drug resulted in ototoxicity (deafness, irreversible) and nephrotoxicity (usually reversible), and it is now indicated for topical use only. These uses include presurgical gut sterilization, treatment of hepatic encephalopathy, ophthalmic infections, and bladder irrigation.

Paromomycin was introduced in 1956, and its major use has been to treat intestinal amebiasis and hepatic encephalopathy. Its use in the treatment of diarrhea in patients with AIDS with cryptosporidia has potential.[3]

Kanamycin (1957) was used extensively for neonatal sepsis which occurred within the first 5 days of life and in gynecologic infections. Because of the emergence of resistant organisms and the availability of newer agents, it is no longer used.

Gentamicin (1969 IM, 1971 IV), tobramycin (1975), and amikacin (1976) are the most widely used aminoglycoside antibiotics. All have activity against *Pseudomonas aeruginosa*, with tobramycin being the most active. Gentamicin is the most active against *Serratia* spp, and amikacin's major use occurs when gentamicin- or tobramycin-resistant organisms are documented or suspected.

Amikacin has in vitro activity against some strains of *Mycobacterium tuberculosis*. Atypical strains of *Mycobacterium chelonei* and *Mycobacterium fortuitum* may also be susceptible to amikacin. Amikacin has been found to be effective as part of a multidrug regimen for the treatment of disseminated *Mycobacterium avium* complex infection.[4] Gentamicin liposome injection has been granted orphan drug status by the FDA for the management of *M. avium* complex infection and is undergoing clinical study to assess efficacy.

Netilmicin, released in 1983, has an antibacterial spectrum similar to that of gentamicin; however, it is less active against *Pseudomonas aeruginosa*. It may be effective against some gentamicin-resistant, Gram-negative bacilli. Sisomicin, isepamicin, dactimicin, ribostamycin, and dibekacin are currently under investigation.

Combinations of the broad-spectrum penicillins (ie, ticarcillin, piperacillin) or antipseudomonal third-generation cephalosporins with the aminoglycosides act synergistically against many strains of *Pseudomonas aeruginosa*.[5] *Serratia marcescens*, *Escherichia coli*, *Klebsiella* spp, and *Proteus mirabilis* may also be affected favorably by such combinations;

however, because of the high activity of the third-generation cephalosporins for Gram-negative organisms, synergy may not be noted with combined use.

Some Gram-negative organisms may exhibit a postantibiotic effect (PAE) when incubated with the aminoglycoside antibiotics.[6] Postantibiotic effect refers to the period after complete removal of the drug when there is no growth of the study organism. In one study, the PAE of tobramycin on *Pseudomonas aeruginosa* was 2 to 7.5 hours.[7] If the PAE is found to be clinically significant in human studies, more rational dosing regimens may result.[6]

The aminoglycosides have activity in vitro against other Gram-negative organisms (ie, *Haemophilus influenzae, Listeria monocytogenes*); however, more active and less toxic agents are available.

In vitro, the aminoglycoside antibiotics appear to have good activity against *Staphylococcus aureus* and *Staphylococcus epidermidis*; however, in vivo infections may not be cured when these drugs are used alone. Therapy of Gram-positive infections (staphylococcus, streptococcus) is limited to synergistic combinations with other antibiotics. The mechanism of this synergy (penicillin, cephalosporin) is thought to result from enhanced penetration of the bacterium by the aminoglycoside as a result of damage to the cell wall by the beta-lactam antibiotic.

The aminoglycosides have no activity against strict anaerobes (ie, bacteroides, fusobacteria, clostridia), as these organisms lack the oxygen-requiring enzymes to transport the antibiotics into the cell.

Although these agents have been of great value in the therapy of Gram-negative infections, the emergence of resistant strains of bacteria, drug toxicity (ototoxicity, nephrotoxicity), and the development of newer antibiotics have altered their use.

MECHANISM OF ACTION

The aminoglycoside antibiotics are bactericidal and act by binding to a particular protein or proteins of the 30 S subunit of bacterial ribosomes, resulting in a misreading of messenger RNA (mRNA) codons. This leads to the production of defective proteins. The detachment of ribosomes from mRNA results in rapid cell death.

Aminoglycosides are transported into the cell in two phases. In the first phase, the drug is bound to respiratory energization complexes, and the rate of killing is concentration dependent. In vitro studies have shown that the aminoglycoside antibiotics eradicate organisms best when the serum concentration peak-to-minimum inhibitory concentration (MIC) ratios are greater than 8.[8,9] The second phase involves an oxygen-generated active transport mechanism that is not concentration dependent.

MECHANISM OF RESISTANCE

The emergence of resistant strains of bacteria has severely limited the usefulness of the aminoglycoside antibiotics. Resistance occurs through three mechanisms. The first involves an alteration in the 30 S subunit of the bacteria. Because of the change, the aminoglycoside is unable to bind to the site. This mechanism of resistance is uncommon.

The second and most common reason for resistance is the elaboration by the organism of enzymes that modify and inactivate the antibiotic. These enzymes are found in the bacterial membrane, at or near sites of drug transport into the cell. The ability to produce inactivating enzymes is plasmid mediated and can be transferred among Gram-negative organisms. These enzymes either acetylate amino groups or phosphorylate or adenylate hydroxyl groups of the aminoglycoside. Amikacin is the most resistant to bacterial enzyme inactivation, which accounts for its activity against gentamicin-, netilmicin-, and tobramycin-resistant strains.

The third type of resistance is a result of the failure of the aminoglycoside to penetrate the bacterial cell (permeability resistance). This mechanism is an important cause of amikacin resistance. Permeability resistance is not plasmid mediated. Resistance by this mechanism generally precludes the use of all aminoglycoside antibiotics.

A reversible form of penetration resistance (adaptive resistance) has been noted in vitro.[10] A decreased rate of killing is noted in those organisms that survive an initial exposure to an aminoglycoside antibiotic. A drug-free period is needed to reverse the effect. If the organisms are exposed to another dose of an aminoglycoside before recovery has occurred, bacterial killing is impaired. This effect provides a rationale for less frequent administration of these agents (see Single-Dose Therapy).

CLINICAL PHARMACOKINETICS

General Properties

The aminoglycoside antibiotics are highly polar basic compounds. They are relatively insoluble in lipids and their antimicrobial properties are enhanced by an alkaline pH environment. Binding to serum protein under normal conditions has been estimated to be between 0 and 30%.[11]

Absorption

Aminoglycoside antibiotics are poorly absorbed after oral administration; however, absorption may be appreciable if the antibiotics are applied topically to large wounds or to the peritoneal space. They are well absorbed (virtually completely) after intramuscular administration, producing peak serum levels in from 30 to 90 minutes. Patients with diabetes may absorb amikacin more slowly after intramuscular injection.[12] Seriously ill patients should not receive aminoglycoside antibiotics by the intramuscular route because of concerns about the reliability of absorption in these subjects.

Administration of the aminoglycoside antibiotics by the intraperitoneal route in patients undergoing continuous ambulatory peritoneal dialysis has been shown to result in therapeutic serum concentrations.[13-15] Mean absolute systemic bioavailability varies from 49 to 84% after a 4- to 6-hour dwell time.[13,15-18] Absorption is good regardless of the presence or absence of peritonitis.[13,15,16,18] The presence of peritonitis has been found to increase significantly the absorption of tobramycin in patients undergoing intermittent peritoneal dialysis.[19] Absorption from the peritoneal cavity is variable and monitoring of serum aminoglycoside concentrations is warranted.

Endotracheally administered aminoglycoside antibiotics have been employed in an attempt to treat Gram-negative pneumonias that are unresponsive or poorly responsive to systemically administered antimicrobial agents.[20,21] Endotracheal administration of antibiotic may increase serum concentration of the agent being given by vein. A range of systemic absorption of 1.5 to 34% in patients receiving gentamicin or tobramycin by the endotracheal route has been noted.[20] The degree of absorption is highly variable and some patients absorb significant amounts of aminoglycoside. In administration of aminoglycosides by the endotracheal route, close monitoring of serum concentration is necessary, especially if these antibiotics are also being administered systemically.[21]

The absorption characteristics of gentamicin mixed in bone cement used in total hip joint arthroplasties have been studied.[22] Local concentrations of drug are high; however, serum levels are negligible in patients with normal renal function.

Distribution

Aminoglycoside antibiotic distribution is best described by a modified two-compartment or three-compartment open model, although a one-compartment system is most often used. In the two-compartment model the apparent volume of the central compartment (V_c) approximates the extracellular fluid volume (about 20–30% of lean body weight in the adult) (Table 9–1).

Following intravenous administration, distribution to highly perfused organs and extracellular fluid is rapid, with the distribution phase (α) half-life varying from 5 to 15 minutes. The distribution phase is usually completed in 25 to 75 minutes. After the rapid phase, a second slower period (β) of serum concentration decline begins. During the second phase the drug is being eliminated from the body and taken up by tissue. A third phase (γ) has also been noted (three-compartment model).

The aminoglycoside antibiotics do not pass into the cerebrospinal fluid in therapeutic concentrations, even with inflamed meninges. Intralumbar or intraventricular injections may be needed to treat a Gram-negative meningitis.[47] With the development of the third-generation cephalosporins with improved spectra of activity and cerebrospinal fluid penetration, the use of the aminoglycoside antibiotics for this indication has decreased.

Concentrations of the aminoglycoside antibiotics between 14 and 66% of serum may be found in pleural and bronchial secretions.[48,49] Bronchial secretion concentrations increase in conjunction with increases in serum concentration. The use of an aminoglycoside alone to treat Gram-negative pneumonias is generally inadequate because of the inability to achieve therapeutic drug concentrations at the site of infection. In these cases combination therapy is indicated. The presence of infection may enhance tobramycin penetration into bronchial secretions.[49]

Aminoglycoside levels in the synovial fluid are usually adequate to treat septic arthritis after parenteral administration and direct instillation is not necessary.[50,51] Synovial fluid concentrations of gentamicin or tobramycin may exceed by 50% simultaneous serum levels.[51]

Aminoglycoside penetration into the bile is dependent on the drug as well as the degree of obstruction.[52] Concentrations in bile are generally lower than those found in the serum and usually do not greatly exceed the minimum inhibitory concentration of potential infecting organisms. When total obstruction is present no antibiotic levels can be detected, and adequate serum levels are needed to treat hepatobiliary infection.

The aminoglycosides do not penetrate the eye, and intraocular injections are necessary for treatment of endophthalmitis.[53–55] Concentrations in tears are also minimal after parenteral administration.[55]

TABLE 9–1. PHARMACOKINETIC PARAMETERS IN PREMATURE INFANTS,[a] CHILDREN, AND ADULTS

Antibiotic and Age	Weight (kg)	V_d (L/kg)	$t_{1/2}$ (h)	Reference
Premature Infants				
Gentamicin				
<28 wk[b]	0.883	0.52	10.71	23
	(1.36)	(0.19)	(2.92)	
	0.937[c]	0.65	8.8	24
	(0.07)	(0.11)	(0.70)	
28–34 wk[b]	1.435	0.51	8.25	23
	(0.62)	(0.09)	(2.94)	
	1.336	0.60	7.8	24
	(0.05)	(0.07)	(1.1)	
> 34 wk[b]	3.01	0.50	6.04	23
	(0.76)	(0.09)	(1.24)	
	2.661	0.58	6.2	24
	(0.225)	(0.05)	(0.5)	
Netilmicin				
28–34 wk[b]	1.293	0.57	8.44	25
	(0.28)	(0.20)	(2.1)	
Amikacin				
28–34 wk[b]	1.38	0.57	8.42	26
	(0.47)	(0.11)	(2.55)	
Tobramycin				
28–34 wk[b]	0.834	0.61	10.0	27
	(0.07)	(0.09)	(1.6)	
	1.25	0.93	9.49	28
	(0.19)	(0.18)	(3.72)	
	1.72	0.69	7.48	28
	(0.16)	(0.16)	(1.61)	
>34 wk[b]	2.83	0.61	5.64	28
	(0.47)	(0.14)	(1.2)	
Children and Adults				
Amikacin				
Term infants		0.59 ± 0.14	4.76 ± 1.5	29
		NR[d]	4.6 ± 1.7	30
1.2–16 y		0.26 ± 0.02	1.24 ± 0.09	31
7–15 y		27.3 ± 5.1%[e]	1.64 ± 0.41	32
19.7 ± 7.0 y		0.22 ± 0.08	1.40 ± 0.4	33
48.8 ± 14.8 y		0.23 ± 0.09	3.70 ± 2.9	33
Gentamicin				
Term infants		0.42 ± 0.09	4.93 ± 1.6	34
		NR	5.54 ± 0.36	25
		52 ± 22%[e]	3.30 ± 1.3	35
2.5 mo[f]		NR	2.9	36
8.7 mo[f]		NR	2.7	36

Antibiotic and Age	Weight (kg)	V_d (L/kg)	$t_{1/2}$ (h)	Reference
11.1 mo[f]		NR	2.3	36
29.4 ± 13.6		0.18 ± 0.08	1.60 ± 1.2	37
39.0 ± 10.0		0.35 ± 0.17	2.48 ± 0.72	38
76.5 ± 7.9		0.23 ± 0.12	4.43 ± 3.78	39
80.0 ± 6.0		0.37 ± 0.11	4.11 ± 1.39	38
>80		0.22 ± 0.09	4.0 ± 2.7	37
Netilmicin				
Term infants		0.51	4.1	40
0.25–13 y		0.21 ± 0.09[g]	2.54 ± 1.19	41
15–20 y		0.21 ± 0.79	1.25 ± 0.79	42
21–30 y		0.18 ± 0.03	1.21 ± 0.29	42
37–59 y		0.19 ± 0.06	2.30 ± 1.4	42
54 ± 5 y		NA[h]	2.3 ± 0.7	43
60–88 y		0.26 ± 0.11	2.39 ± 0.88	42
66 ± 13 y		NA	2.1 ± 0.5	43
Tobramycin				
Term infants		0.36 ± 0.491	4.4 ± 1.9	44
2–8 y		0.49 ± 0.06	2.0 ± 0.23	45
11–18 y		0.40 ± 0.04	1.4 ± 0.10	45
16.2 ± 7.2 y		0.21 ± 0.08	1.4 ± 0.60	46
64.6 ± 15.5y		0.22 ± 0.09	3.0 ± 1.8	46

[a]Numbers in parentheses are standard deviations.
[b]Postconceptional age = gestational age + postnatal age.
[c]Less than 30 wk.
[d]Not reported.
[e]Percentage of body weight.
[f]Mean age values.
[g]Represents volume of the central compartment.
[h]Not available.

Studies of the pharmacokinetics of the aminoglycoside antibiotics in patients with ascites are limited, and usually involve single doses.[56–58] Available data, however, indicate that aminoglycoside concentrations in ascites rise slowly, achieving peak levels 2 to 6 hours after a dose. These agents achieve therapeutic concentrations in ascites[56,57]; however, aminoglycoside levels in ascites are close to the minimum inhibitory concentration for Gram-negative bacteria. Two to four hours after a dose the serum and ascites concentrations appear to be comparable.[56,57]

Penetration of the aminoglycoside antibiotics after intravenous administration into peritoneal dialysate during peritoneal dialysis is variable.[37,39,42,59] This is true regardless of the presence or absence of peritonitis.[39,59] Concentrations in dialysate have been shown to be subtherapeutic or low therapeutic after single and multiple doses of gentamicin and tobramycin.[39,42,59] Dialysate concentrations increase as serum concentrations increase over time.[59]

The aminoglycosides concentrate in renal cortical tissue to levels 10 to 50 times serum concentrations. The kidney may account for up to 40% of the total antibiotic (ie, gentamicin) in the body.[60] Tobramycin may accumulate to a lesser extent than gentamicin.[61] Animal studies have shown that kidney cortical uptakes of gentamicin, tobramycin, and netilmicin are saturable, whereas kidney uptake of amikacin appears saturable at low concentrations and linear at high serum levels.[62] Preliminary data indicate that the same relationship exists for humans, and single doses of gentamicin, tobramycin, amikacin, and netilmicin result in lower kidney tissue accumulation than the same dose administered by continuous infusion.[62–64]

The distribution of the aminoglycoside antibiotics into placental and fetal tissue has been investigated.[65,66] High concentrations of drug are noted in the placenta and in fetal urine, kidney, and spleen. These drugs should be avoided in pregnancy because of the risk of toxic effects in the developing fetus.

Penetration of the aminoglycosides into bone has not been well studied. Preliminary data indicate poor penetration into noninfected bone.[50,67,68]

Penetration into human peritoneal tissue and small bowel has been investigated.[69,70] Tobramycin and amikacin appear to enter uninflamed peritoneal tissue better than netilmicin.[69] Therapeutic small bowel tissue concentrations of gentamicin have been noted within 2 hours of a dose in patients undergoing abdominal surgery.[70]

Elimination

The aminoglycoside antibiotics are not metabolized and are excreted unchanged in the urine. They are cleared by glomerular filtration, and some proximal tubular reabsorption occurs. Following the administration of an aminoglycoside antibiotic, serum concentrations decline in three phases. The rapid phase (α) represents distribution. The second phase (β) has a half-life of 2 to 3 hours in adults with normal renal function (see Table 9–1). The second-phase half-life ($t_{1/2}$) increases in proportion to a decrease in creatinine clearance (Cl_{cr}), with $t_{1/2}$ reported to vary from 17 to 150 hours in patients with Cl_{cr} values less than 10 mL/min.[11,71] The third-phase (γ) half-life represents the release of the aminoglycoside from tissue stores, which explains the incomplete recovery of drug from the urine if collection is not continued long enough.[60,72] Mean half-lives in this phase have been reported for amikacin (mean ± SD, 187.7 ± 62.5 h); gentamicin (mean, 112 h [range 27–693 h]); tobramycin (mean, 146 h [range 33–428 h]); and netilmicin (range, 33–432 h).[60,72–74] The aminoglycoside antibiotics are also concentrated in the urine and levels may be 30 to 100 times those found in serum.

The effects of peritoneal dialysis, hemofiltration, hemodialysis, hemodiafiltration, extracorporeal membrane oxygenation, plasma exchange, exchange transfusion, and cardiopulmonary bypass on the elimination of the aminoglycoside antibiotics have been investigated.[13–15,17,59,75–82]

There are two basic types of peritoneal dialysis: continuous ambulatory peritoneal dialysis (CAPD) and intermittent peritoneal dialysis (IPD). The effect of peritoneal dialysis on the elimination of aminoglycoside antibiotics depends on the dialysis conditions. These conditions include type of dialysis (CAPD, IPD), dialysate composition, dwell time, dialysate volume, dialysate outflow rate, and presence of peritonitis. In patients undergoing CAPD, the dialysis clearance accounts for approximately 15 to 50% of the total body clearance.[13,15,17] The half-life of these antibiotics does not appear to be appreciably altered by CAPD. On the other hand, IPD with rapid exchanges can significantly enhance the elimination of the aminoglycosides.[75–78] Increasing the dialysate glucose concentration from 1.5 to 4.0% has been shown to increase significantly the clearance of gentamicin during IPD.[78] An increased clearance of gentamicin in patients with peritonitis undergoing IPD has been reported[59]; however, the number of patients was too small to determine the significance of this observation.

The clearance of the aminoglycoside antibiotics by continuous hemofiltration is dependent on the type of filter used and ultrafiltration rates.[79–81] Armendariz et al noted no effect of hemofiltration on the half-life of amikacin at an ultrafiltration flow rate of 10 mL/min.[80] Robert et al, however, reported a marked effect of hemofiltration on amikacin half-life at an ultrafiltration rate of 19.2 mL/min.[81] Aminoglycoside clearance values during hemofiltration have varied from 0.7 to 1.3 L/h depending on the study conditions.[79–82]

The aminoglycoside antibiotics are significantly removed by hemodialysis. A supplemental dose is necessary after dialysis. Hemodialysis clearance of these agents varies with the type of artificial kidney used, flow rates of blood and dialysate, and hemofiltration rate (Table 9–2). Length of dialysis also affects the fraction of drug removed during the procedure. One should become familiar with the type of dialyzer used in your institution.[86,89]

A rebound of serum concentrations of the aminoglycoside antibiotics after the end of hemodialysis has been noted.[88,90] The maximum increase in concentration occurs from 1 to 2 hours after the completion of hemodialysis. Mean maximal postdialysis increase in serum concentrations of gentamicin, tobramycin, and netilmicin are (0.42, 0.73), 0.37, and 0.54 µg/mL, respectively.[88,90] The rebound phenomenon may be due to more rapid elimination of drug from the serum versus a slower rate of redistribution from tissues sites to the serum during hemodialysis. An alternate explanation involves decreased tissue clearance of the antibiotic during hemodialysis.

TABLE 9–2. HEMODIALYSIS OF THE AMINOGLYCOSIDE ANTIBIOTICS

Medication	$t_{1/2}$ (h) Interdialysis	Intradialysis	$C_{dialysis}$[a] (mL/min)	Percentage Removed	Reference
Amikacin	28	3.75	NR[b]	53	83
	86.5[c]/44.3[d]	5.6	21.5[e]	NR	76
	53.3	7.2	37.5	21	84
Gentamicin	37.9	4.4	NR	NR	85
	52.7	5.5	31.9	NR	86
	52.7	7.8	27.2	NR	86
Netilmicin	44	3.4	87.3	56.1	87
	46	NR	60.8	50.2	88
	40.8	5.0	46.3	45	89
	40.8	2.87	109.0	62	89
Tobramycin	57.8	4.3	39.4	NR	86
	57.8	6.3	31.4	NR	86
	58.1	NR	54.7	49.9	88

[a] Dialysis clearance.
[b] Not reported.
[c] Anephric patients.
[d] Minimal residual kidney function.
[e] mL/min/m^2.

The effect of hypertonic hemodiafiltration versus standard hemodialysis on the disposition of netilmicin has been investigated.[91] Hemodiafiltration markedly increased netilmicin clearance and decreased the drug's half-life when compared with hemodialysis. Hemodiafiltration significantly increases netilmicin clearance when compared with conventional hemodialysis.

Infants treated with extracorporeal membrane oxygenation (ECMO) exhibit changes in the pharmacokinetics of gentamicin.[92,93] ECMO significantly increases the volume of distribution (V_d) and decreases the elimination of gentamicin. Dosage adjustments of gentamicin and probably the other aminoglycosides are necessary in infants undergoing ECMO.[92,93]

The effect of exchange transfusions on the pharmacokinetics of gentamicin in neonates has been studied.[94] Exchange transfusion resulted in a decrease in gentamicin serum concentrations and an increase in elimination rate. Only 4.6% of a single dose was removed during exchange transfusion. Exchange transfusion should be performed near the end of a dosage interval to minimize the effect on aminoglycoside serum concentrations.

Plasma exchange does not appear to alter significantly the pharmacokinetics of tobramycin.[95] The renal clearance of netilmicin is decreased during cardiopulmonary bypass.[96]

Special Populations

Age
At birth, the newborn renal function is significantly decreased as compared with the adult.[97] Glomerular and tubular function may require several months to reach adult values. The rate of renal development is slower for the preterm infant, especially if gestational age is less than 34 weeks.[97] Aminoglycoside clearance has been found to correlate with creatinine clearance in premature and full-term newborns.[98–100] Preterm infants less than 1 month and term infants less than 2 weeks of age have aminoglycoside clearances 20 to 40% those of adults with normal renal function. Half-life (younger—longer, lighter—longer) varies inversely with age (postconceptional [gestational age + postnatal age], gestational) and body weight[23,24,27,28,30,40,41,101–103] (see Table 9–1). Half-life correlates better with postconceptional age than with postnatal age.[101] A significant decrease in aminoglycoside half-life may be noted in newborns after postnatal day 7.[25,26] Pons et al reported that the half-life of gentamicin was not significantly different between postnatal days 1 and 2 when compared with day 0.[104] The half-life decreased in premature and term infants from postnatal days 3–7 when compared with days 0 to 2. In premature infants, the half-life decreased from 6.6 hours on days 0–2 to 4.23 hours on days 3–7. In term infants, the half-life decreased from 4.96 hours on days 0–2 to 3.4 hours on days 3–7.[104] Kildoo et al, however, in a study of premature, very low birth weight infants, found that gentamicin renal clearance did not increase significantly until 30 days of life.[98]

Total body clearance varies directly with postconceptional age, gestational age, and birth weight.[103,105,106] Children generally clear the aminoglycosides faster than adults and have a shorter half-life[31,32] (see Table 9–1).

The volume of distribution is larger in the neonate than the adult and may average nearly 50% of total body weight[107] (see Table 9–1). There is no correlation between volume of distribution and postconceptional age.[105,106] A high degree of variability in all pharmacokinetic parameters is noted in this patient population. As the physiologic and metabolic processes in term and premature, low-birth-weight infants change rapidly in the first weeks of life, serum levels of aminoglycosides should be measured frequently to ensure the presence of therapeutic and non-toxic concentrations.

It has been determined that creatinine clearance decreases with advancing age. Interestingly, serum creatinine remains in the normal range because the decrease in creatinine clearance is proportional to a concurrent decrease in creatinine production that occurs with aging. For this reason serum creatinine becomes less reliable as a measure of renal function in the elderly.[38,39] Additional factors such as the presence of malnutrition and chronic illness further compromise the usefulness of serum creatinine in the assessment of renal function. It is important to note that a small increase in serum creatinine may represent a change in renal function in these patients and warrant serial creatinine determinations to establish a trend. An existing abnormal serum creatinine in an elderly patient may also indicate a greater decrease in renal function than reflected by the observed creatinine concentration. As the aminoglycoside antibiotics are eliminated similarly to creatinine, their elimination also decreases with age[37-39] (see Table 9-1). These factors must be taken into consideration when using an aminoglycoside in the elderly to avoid potential overdose.

Cystic Fibrosis

The effects of cystic fibrosis on the pharmacokinetics of the aminoglycoside antibiotics have been extensively studied.[32,108-116] Investigations in patients with severe cystic fibrosis indicate an increase in total body clearance and volume of distribution when compared with subjects without cystic fibrosis.[32,108-110] Patients with mild to moderate cystic fibrosis, however, do not appear to have significant increases in total body clearance or volume of distribution when compared with patients without cystic fibrosis.[113-115] Malnutrition, severity of pulmonary disease, cor pulmonale, or cardiac disease (ie, right-sided congestive heart failure) may be responsible for the altered pharmacokinetics of the aminoglycosides in patients with severe cystic fibrosis.[115] Considerable variability in the pharmacokinetics of the aminoglycoside antibiotics exists within the cystic fibrosis population. Patients with cystic fibrosis must be monitored carefully to ensure the presence of therapeutic concentrations.

Congestive Heart Failure

Acute or uncontrolled congestive heart failure affects aminoglycoside antibiotic disposition.[37] The fluid retention noted in these patient results in an increase in volume of distribution. The decreased cardiac output results in a decrease in renal perfusion and a decreased glomerular filtration rate. As a result, an increase is noted in the half-life of these antibiotics. Increased doses and prolonged administration intervals may be necessary. As heart failure is reversed, dosage regimens will need to be adjusted accordingly.

Liver Disease and Ascites

The volume of distribution of the aminoglycosides is significantly increased in cirrhotic patients with ascites.[58,116-118] The ascites appears to be a part of the central compartment.[58] The mean volume of distribution after the first dose of tobramycin has been reported to be 0.32 L/kg.[116] Half-life is not affected by the presence of ascites.[117] Studies performed at our institution found a similar mean volume of distribution of 0.33 L/kg for tobramycin in patients with ascites.[118] Because of the enlarged volume of distribution, the loading dose of the aminoglycoside antibiotics should be based on actual body weight to ensure immediate therapeutic peak concentrations.[118,119]

Although maintenance dose recommendation are not available, it is likely from our preliminary data that the dose should also be based on actual body weight. The difficulty arises in determining the maintenance interval. We have found that routine methods of estimating half-life from patients' serum creatinine levels give results that underestimate the actual observed half-life. This observation can be explained by the fact that creatinine production is decreased in patients with liver disease, regardless of the degree of renal function. The use of serum creatinine as a means of determining a maintenance interval for these agents in patients with ascites would result in higher than expected trough serum concentrations. The increased volume of distribution and the unreliability of serum creatinine as a tool for kinetic dosing in these patients makes careful blood level monitoring imperative. Patients with liver disease appear to be more sensitive to the nephrotoxic effects of these antibiotics.[120] Aminoglycoside antibiotics should be avoided, when possible, in patients with liver disease.

Obesity

The effects of obesity on the pharmacokinetics of the aminoglycoside antibiotics have been studied.[121–123] Obesity does not appear to affect the half-life of these drugs.[121] Alterations in the volume of distribution of the aminoglycosides in obese patients are noted and are due to a decreased distribution into adipose tissue. Dosing based on actual body weight may result in overdose, whereas dosing based on ideal body weight may result in underdose. Studies have found that the aminoglycoside "dosing weight" can be normalized in obese patients by the use of a correction factor.[121–123] This factor is based on the understanding that adipose tissue contains approximately 45 to 50% as much extracellular fluid by weight as does nonadipose tissue.[121] As aminoglycosides distribute into extracellular fluid, the content of this fluid in fat tissue should be included in dosing considerations. To determine the dosing weight one does the following:

1. Calculate ideal body weight (IBW) from one of these formulas.[124]

$$\text{Males} \qquad \text{IBW} = 50 \text{ kg} + 2.3 \text{ (inches} > 5 \text{ ft)} \qquad (9\text{--}1)$$

$$\text{Females} \qquad \text{IBW} = 45 \text{ kg} + 2.3 \text{ (inches} > 5 \text{ ft)} \qquad (9\text{--}2)$$

2. Weigh the patient to determine actual body weight (ABW).
3. Subtract IBW from ABW.

$$\text{ABW} - \text{IBW} = \text{fat weight (FW)} \qquad (9\text{--}3)$$

4. Multiply fat weight by 40% and add the figure to IBW, which gives you the aminoglycoside dosing weight.[121]

$$\text{IBW} + 0.4 \text{ (FW)} = \text{dosing weight} \qquad (9\text{--}4)$$

5. To derive an estimated volume of distribution (V_d) for use in calculations, take the average V_d for a population and multiply by the dosing weight.

$$0.26 \text{ L/kg} \times \text{dosing weight} = \text{normalized } V_d \qquad (9\text{--}5)$$

Blouin et al reported a different factor for tobramycin, namely, 58%.[123] Most sources use the 40% figure, however.

These adjustments are likely to be adequate for initial dosing; however, because of the large patient variability in observed volumes of distribution, serum levels should be obtained to ensure the presence of therapeutic concentrations.

Burns

The effect of a burn on the pharmacokinetics of the aminoglycoside antibiotics depends on the severity of the burn and the overall condition of the patient. The acute phase of a burn is characterized by decreased blood flow to the kidney, and creatinine clearance is subsequently decreased. In the early phase, the volume of distribution of the aminoglycoside antibiotics may be decreased and the half-life of elimination increased. After about 48 hours, patients with severe burns enter a hypermetabolic phase and are often hemodynamically unstable. Hypervolemia occurs and is constant in the initial period after the burn. In this situation an increase in aminoglycoside volume of distribution is noted. A decrease in the half-life of tobramycin has been reported in some burn patients.[125] This is a result of a supranormal increase in glomerular filtration rate. Patients may require more frequent dosing to maintain adequate serum concentrations. It is important to realize that the condition of a burn patient may change rapidly. Renal failure is not uncommon in severely burned patients and adjustments of aminoglycoside dosages must be done as needed. Also, as a patient comes out of renal failure, the kinetics will also change. Because of the variability in volume of distribution and half-life resulting from changes in patient status, diligent attention to aminoglycoside dosing is indicated.

Renal Function

The half-life of the aminoglycoside antibiotics increases as renal function worsens. Urine levels also decrease as renal function deteriorates. The volume of distribution of the aminoglycoside antibiotics is not affected by the degree of kidney function unless fluid overload is present.[13,77,60,72,88] The pharmacokinetics of gentamicin and tobramycin are similar in patients with varying degrees of kidney function[126]; however, in patients with renal insufficiency (creatinine clearance < 80 mL/min), differences exist between these agents and netilmicin.[88,126] The volume of distribution of netilmicin is significantly larger than that of tobramycin in these patients. The half-life of netilmicin is also significantly longer than that of gentamicin or tobramycin in patients with renal insufficiency.[88,126]

Miscellaneous Factors

Hydration Status. As the aminoglycoside antibiotics are distributed in extracellular fluids, any change in body fluid status would affect the volume of distribution. Overhydration would increase and dehydration would decrease the volume of distribution. The clinical correlate would be that an ill patient may be dehydrated on admission to the hospital and kinetic evaluation would yield a lower volume of distribution as compared with a follow-up, days later when the patient is well hydrated.

Hypoxemia. Hypoxemia may result in a prolonged aminoglycoside half-life.[30,127] The effect of perinatal asphyxia on the pharmacokinetics of gentamicin has been investigated.[127] A mean gentamicin half-life of 14.55 hours in a perinatal asphyxia group versus 8.2 hours in the nonasphyxia group was noted. The volume of distribution was not affected by the presence or absence of asphyxia. A similar finding has been noted with amikacin[30]; however, when birth weight and gestational age were taken into consideration the effect of hypoxemia on half-life was not significant in infants less than 4 days old. The increase in half-life may result from a hypoxemia-induced decrease in renal blood flow and a subsequent decrease in glomerular filtration rate.[30,127]

Malnutrition. In patients with severe protein malnutrition the production of creatinine is decreased. The use of serum creatinine becomes unreliable for monitoring, making dosage calculations based on average patient data inaccurate. Renal function may also be decreased in the presence of severe protein calorie malnutrition.[128]

A significantly increased aminoglycoside volume of distribution has been noted in nutritionally deficient patients.[129,130] The increased volume may result from an observed increase in extracellular water in patients with severe nutritional deficiency.

Fever. Febrile patients have been reported to have lower gentamicin levels when compared with controls.[107,131] The effect on serum concentrations of gentamicin was due to a decreased half-life in one study.[107] The increased elimination may be a result of improved renal blood flow and glomerular filtration secondary to the increased heart rate and cardiac output induced by fever.

Hematocrit. An inverse relationship between hematocrit and gentamicin peak levels has been reported.[132] As the hematocrit decreased, the levels increased. Others have not been able to replicate these results.[107] Schentag et al found no relationship between the volume of the central compartment and the volume of distribution at steady state for gentamicin and tobramycin and the hematocrit.[60,72] Barza et al noted a significant correlation between the half-life of gentamicin and the reciprocal of hematocrit.[133] The clinical significance of the hematocrit effect on the pharmacokinetics of aminoglycoside antibiotics is unknown.

Gender. In one study women eliminated gentamicin more rapidly than men.[37] The mean distribution volume was also significantly lower in women.

Pregnancy. Circulating plasma volume and cardiac output increase throughout pregnancy. Total body water increases an average of 7 to 8 L at term (80% extracellular). Renal blood flow and glomerular filtration rate increase by 50% in early pregnancy and slowly return to normal values after birth of the child. As a result of these physiologic changes, the volume of distribution and elimination rate of the aminoglycoside antibiotics are increased in pregnancy and the postpartum period.[134]

Spinal Cord Injury. A statistically significant increase in the volume of distribution of gentamicin and amikacin has been reported in quadriplegic and paraplegic individuals.[135,136] Segal et al also noted an increase in half-life and mean residence time of amikacin in patients with chronic spinal cord injury.[135] The observed increase in volume of distribution is a result of an increase in extracellular volume. A significant decrease in the rate of absorption of gentamicin has been found after intramuscular administration into paralyzed muscle of spinal cord-injured patients.[136] Bioavailability is not affected.

Hematologic Malignancy. Zeitany et al compared the pharmacokinetics of amikacin and gentamicin in febrile neutropenic patients with hematologic malignancy with those of a control group with no underlying cancer.[137] They noted a significantly elevated volume of distribution in the study group relative to the control group. A shorter half-life and an increased total body clearance were also found in subjects with a malignancy. Other studies in children and adults have not found similar results when age, body weight, and renal function are considered.[9,138,139] Differences in study design, including patient characteristics and type of malignancy, may explain the difference in results. A subset of patients with malignancy may have altered aminoglycoside pharmacokinetics.

Patent Ductus Arteriosus. Watterberg et al studied the effect of patent ductus arteriosus on the pharmacokinetics of gentamicin in very low birth weight infants.[140] Patients with patent ductus arteriosus had a significantly increased volume of distribution and half-life when compared with a control group. Gentamicin total body clearance was not significantly different between the two groups. The volume of distribution decreased toward control values after closure of the patent ductus arteriosus.

Critical Illness. Intuitively, the critically ill patient is likely to exhibit altered pharmacokinetics of the aminoglycoside antibiotics.[141–143] Many of the preceding factors (ie, cardiac and kidney failure) are often present in these patients, making monitoring of aminoglycoside therapy extremely important. Traditional monitoring parameters such as serum creatinine may not be reliable for dosing or toxicity considerations in the critical care setting.[141] Rapid changes in patient status (worsen or improve) require diligent attention, to avoid inappropriate dosing.[142,143]

PHARMACODYNAMICS

Adverse Reactions

The major limiting factors in the use of the aminoglycoside antibiotics are their potential ototoxicity and nephrotoxicity (Table 9–3).

Ototoxicity
Ototoxicity may be either vestibular or cochlear and results from an antibiotic-induced loss of sensory hair cells in the cochlea and vestibular labyrinth. The aminoglycosides differ in their site

TABLE 9–3. AMINOGLYCOSIDE-INDUCED ADVERSE REACTIONS

Ototoxicity
Nephrotoxicity
Neuromuscular blockade
Electrolyte disturbances
Skin rash
Anaphylaxis

of toxicity. Gentamicin and streptomycin are primarily vestibulotoxic.[144,145] Amikacin, neomycin, and netilmicin cause primarily cochlear damage.[146–148] Tobramycin affects vestibular and cochlear function equally.[149] The incidence of symptomatic auditory disturbances is low (Table 9–4).

Symptoms of toxicity may appear between the first and second weeks of therapy or as early as the third day of treatment.[144,149] Delayed toxicity occurring 10 to 14 days after stopping gentamicin therapy in patients with renal impairment has been reported.[145] Delayed vestibular toxicity presenting 3 and 6 weeks after completion of a course of gentamicin therapy has been reported.[151] Early damage may be reversible but if the antibiotic is continued it may be permanent. Damage can be mixed (vestibular and cochlear) and is usually bilateral.[144]

Vertigo, ataxia, nystagmus, nausea, and vomiting may be noted in vestibulotoxic patients. Vestibular dysfunction may be reversible in up to 50% of patients, and visual and proprioceptive mechanism can help compensate for the deficit.[144,145,149] Symptoms may not be apparent if the patient is bedridden, critically ill, or receiving antiemetic agents.

Initially, cochlear damage occurs as a subclinical loss of high-frequency (>4000 Hz) hearing. Hearing loss is usually irreversible and may progress to deafness, even after drug discontinuation.[149] Tinnitus, mild high-frequency loss noted on audiograms, conversational hearing loss, and deafness may be noted. Patients may also report a feeling of pressure or fullness in the ears during or shortly after an infusion of drug. Neomycin is the most ototoxic of the aminoglycoside antibiotics and is indicated for topical use only. Neomycin-associated ototoxicity has been reported after bowel and wound irrigation, aerosolization, topical application, and oral administration to patients with hepatic failure.[147,152–154] When neomycin is used orally in patients with decreased kidney function, absorption (0.6–3%) may be sufficient to cause deafness, worsen renal function, or both.[147] Deafness from neomycin is often irreversible.[147] Its use should be avoided in patients with kidney failure.

A review of reports of comparative, prospective, and randomized studies on ototoxicity of the aminoglycosides has been published.[155] In these studies, audiometry was used to assess cochlear toxicity. Brain stem auditory evoked response (BAER) has been used to assess eighth nerve and cochlear function in newborn and young infants. Vestibular function can be assessed by electronystagmograms and caloric and balance tests. From the available data, netilmicin

TABLE 9–4. RELATIVE INCIDENCE OF OTOTOXICITY WITH THE AMINOGLYCOSIDE ANTIBIOTICS[a]

| Antibiotic | Clinical Toxicity (%)[b] | | Reference |
	Cochlear	Vestibular	
Amikacin	0.52	0.65	146
Gentamicin	0.4	2.0	145
Tobramycin	0.4	0.4	150
Netilmicin	1.6	0.6	148

[a]Compilations of patient experience.
[b]Clinically apparent hearing loss.

appears to be significantly less ototoxic than amikacin and tobramycin; however, a wide range in confidence limits is noted.

The risk factors associated with the use of the aminoglycoside antibiotics are listed in Table 9–5. Elderly patients and possibly those with preexisting hearing deficit appear to be at risk of manifesting ototoxicity.[149,156,157] The decrease in kidney function with age may predispose the patient to more sustained serum concentrations of the aminoglycoside, resulting in higher accumulation in the ear. These agents should be used cautiously in patients with preexisting ear disease. Further aminoglycoside-induced damage may be noticed more readily in these patients. The incidence of ototoxic effects in neonates is lower than in adults.[158]

Duration of treatment greater than 10 days and total dose are risk factors in that the drug can accumulate and remain in contact with ear structures longer and cause damage.[146,149,150,156,157] Prior exposure to the drugs is important because much of the damage is subclinical and repeated treatment courses, especially if given shortly after each other, encourage new or continued damage.[144,156,159]

The existence of renal impairment is a risk factor for aminoglycoside ototoxicity.[144,145,149] Kidney failure may encourage accumulation of these agents in the ear.

When aminoglycoside therapy is used in conjunction with ethacrynic acid, ototoxicity may be more likely.[160] The use of ethacrynic acid during concurrent aminoglycoside therapy should be avoided. Furosemide can be used safely with an aminoglycoside antibiotic.[161]

Although we attempt to keep peak levels of the aminoglycoside antibiotics below those listed in Table 9–5, the importance of serum levels to ototoxicity is unclear.[162] Jackson et al recommended that peak gentamicin concentrations of 12 µg/mL be avoided.[144] They found that 53% of subjects with ototoxic effects had peak concentrations of 8 µg/mL or greater, and 7 of the 10 patients had gentamicin levels between 16 and 40 µg/mL. Interestingly, 22% of non-toxic patients had peak concentrations of 8 µg/mL or greater and 6% had peak levels of 16 µg/mL or greater. Mawer et al observed an association of a trough gentamicin concentration greater than 4 µg/mL with ototoxicity.[163] Black et al noted amikacin-induced ototoxic effects in patients with peak and trough concentrations greater than 32 µg/mL and greater than 10 µg/mL, respectively.[156] Trough levels of amikacin and gentamicin did not, however, correlate with ototoxicity

TABLE 9–5. RISK FACTORS FOR AMINOGLYCOSIDE-INDUCED OTOTOXICITY

1. Age
2. Duration of treatment greater than 10 days
3. Prior exposure to aminoglycosides
4. Renal impairment
5. Concurrent use of diuretic—ethacrynic acid
6. Total dose of drug
7. High serum levels, rough guidelines, absolute importance of peak or trough levels is not clear

Antibiotic	Peak Level to Avoid
Gentamicin, tobramycin, netilmicin	>12 µg/mL
Amikacin	>32 µg/mL

TABLE 9–6. AMINOGLYCOSIDE OTOTOXICITY: ONCE DAILY DOSES VERSUS MULTIPLE DAILY DOSES

Antibiotic	Toxicity (%)		Significance[a]	Reference
	Daily	Multiple		
Amikacin	20	30	NS	165
	3	3	NS	166
	1.2	1.3	NS	167
	9	7	NS	168
Gentamicin	8	11	NS	169
	25	27	NS	170
Netilmicin	6	3	NS	171
	16	58	S	165
	0	0	NS	169
	7	0	NS	172
	0	0	NS	173

[a]NS, no significant difference; S, significant difference.

in a study by Lau et al.[164] In a study of patients on chronic hemodialysis, the risk of gentamicin-induced vestibular dysfunction was associated with age, total dose received per kilogram, and duration of therapy.[157] The mean peak and trough gentamicin concentrations did not differ between patients with and without toxic effects. Toxicity may correlate better with area under the serum concentration-versus-time curve than with serum concentration.[163] It is evident that patients with "therapeutic" peak and trough levels may manifest ototoxicity, and a clear association between peak or trough level and ototoxicity is not demonstrable.

Studies comparing the administration of single total daily dose versus the same dose given in divided doses have found comparable ototoxicity (Table 9–6).[165–174] Proctor et al reported no significant difference in vestibular toxicity in a group of volunteers receiving either single or three-times-daily doses of tobramycin.[175] Once-daily dose administration achieves peak serum concentrations much higher than we are used to seeing (ie, amikacin peak, 53.8 ± 10.1 µg/mL) and yet toxicity is either reduced or identical to that resulting from divided-dose regimens.[165–174]

Monitoring of therapy should include a dynamic assessment of risk factors, attention to subjective statements by the patients, and serum level monitoring. Baseline audiometry and follow-up studies would also be helpful, especially if prolonged therapy is contemplated. Unfortunately, such testing may not be possible in a clinical setting. When a single-dose regimen is used, peak levels are not necessary and trough or random serum (see Single-Dose Dosing Considerations) levels can be obtained.[176] Gentamicin, tobramycin, and netilmicin concentrations should be less than 2 µg/mL and amikacin less than 5 µg/mL prior to the next dose. A visual test for vestibular function has been proposed to assist in monitoring aminoglycoside therapy.[177]

Nephrotoxicity
The aminoglycoside antibiotics are intrinsically nephrotoxic. The mechanism of aminoglycoside-induced nephrotoxicity has been extensively reviewed.[178,179] These antibiotics are filtered by the glomerulus and bind to the brush border of the proximal convoluted tubules at the same

negatively changed binding sites that attract basic amino acids. The number of amino groups available for binding to these receptors correlates somewhat with their nephrotoxic potential. Neomycin (most nephrotoxic) has six; gentamicin, tobramycin, amikacin, and netilmicin have five; and streptomycin (least nephrotoxic) has two free amino groups.

After binding to the brush border, absorptive pinocytosis and lysosomal processing occur. An increase in phospholipid content in the renal cortex occurs as a result of aminoglycoside-induced inhibition of lysosomal phospholipase activity. The continued increase in lysosomal phospholipid content results in the rupture or dysfunction of the lysosome. The end result of these processes is proximal tubular necrosis. Proximal tubular resorptive function becomes defective and glomerular filtration stops to prevent massive fluid loss. Only after a significant number of nephrons cease to function does serum creatinine begin to rise. An alternate hypothesis to explain the observed decrease in glomerular filtration rate during aminoglycoside therapy has been proposed.[179] Aminoglycoside antibiotics have been shown to inhibit phosphatidylinositol phospholipase C (PI-lipase C) and sodium–potassium ATPase activity. Inhibition of PI-lipase C may result in decreased production of vasodilating prostaglandins. Inhibition of sodium–potassium ATPase could result in an increase in renin activity and adrenergic tone. These combined effects would result in vasoconstriction and a fall in glomerular filtration rate. It is most likely that a combination of effects are responsible for the observed nephrotoxic effects of these antibiotics.

The definition of aminoglycoside nephrotoxicity is usually based on a change in the patient's baseline serum creatinine. For toxicity to be considered, a patient with normal renal function should have an increase in creatinine of 0.5 mg/dL or more. Patients with elevated baseline serum creatinine levels between 2.0 and 4.9 mg/dL and between 5.0 and 10 mg/dL should have increases of 1.0 mg/dL or higher and 1.5 mg/dL or higher, respectively.

Review of published studies indicates that gentamicin is more nephrotoxic than amikacin and tobramycin, and netilmicin is less nephrotoxic than tobramycin.[155] Schentag et al have stated that tobramycin may be less nephrotoxic because of its lower accumulation in the kidney versus gentamicin.[180,181]

The initial manifestation of aminoglycoside nephrotoxicity is enzymuria. These enzymes may arise from the loss of brush border membranes of the proximal tubule. Urinary excretion of lysosomal enzymes can also be seen. As damage continues, tubular resorptive function is affected and tubular proteinuria (ie, β_2-microglobinuria), aminoaciduria, glycosuria, and magnesium and potassium wasting are noted. Urine sodium concentrations also increase. Polyuria and nephrogenic diabetes insipidus develop in early nephrotoxicity. Typically, aminoglycoside nephrotoxicity does not become evident until the patient has been receiving the drug for 5 to 7 days. The patient is usually nonoliguric, with normal or increased urine output. Oliguric renal failure is less common and can be acute or follow the nonoliguric variety. Renal failure often progresses even after a decrease in dose or drug withdrawal. It may also become evident after drug discontinuation. The renal deficit is usually reversible; however, weeks to months may pass before return of baseline function.

Laboratory tests have been developed that detect proximal tubule damage up to 5 to 10 days prior to elevation of serum creatinine in patients receiving aminoglycoside antibiotics. These include tests for urinary enzymes, urinary β_2-microglobulin, and urinary cast excretion.[182–184] These tests, however, are not specific enough to always differentiate drug- versus disease-induced kidney damage and remain research tools.

Risk factors associated with the potential for experiencing aminoglycoside nephrotoxicity

TABLE 9–7. RISK FACTORS FOR NEPHROTOXICITY IN PATIENTS RECEIVING AMINOGLYCOSIDE ANTIBIOTICS

1. Age
2. Prolonged therapy
3. Preexisting kidney disease
4. Presence of liver disease
5. Volume depletion
6. Concomitant use of other nephrotoxic drugs:

Cephalothin	Amphotericin
Vancomycin	Methoxyflurane
Cisplatin	Cyclosporine A

7. Shock
8. Prolonged high trough levels, rough guidelines: importance of trough level not clearly defined

Antibiotic	Trough Level to Avoid (µg/mL)
Amikacin	>10
Gentamicin, tobramycin, netilmicin	>2

are listed in Table 9–7. In many studies, one or more of these factors were found to significantly impact on the risk of nephrotoxicity.[146,150,151,185] Some researchers dispute the predictive value of these risk factors.[185–187]

The older patient may be at greater risk of manifesting nephrotoxicity, because if dosage adjustments are made solely on the serum creatinine value, more sustained serum concentrations may be present. The effect of age as a risk factor has not been a consistent finding, however.[146,150,164,186]

The risk of nephrotoxicity increases with prolonged therapy and in patients receiving repeated courses separated by a few days or weeks.[146,186] This is most likely a result of the increased time for accumulation in kidney tissue. Not all studies noted an increase in nephrotoxicity related to duration of therapy.[164,188] Preexisting kidney disease may be important because the kidney reserve is decreased and further damage by the aminoglycoside is exaggerated.

Liver disease is considered a risk factor for the development of nephrotoxicity.[120,185,188] If possible, an aminoglycoside antibiotic should not be used to treat infections in patients with chronic liver disease.

Dehydration resulting from overuse of diuretics or clinical condition of the patient may predispose to nephrotoxicity. Dehydration causes concentration of the urine and may enhance the tissue accumulation of the aminoglycosides in the kidney. Diuretic therapy per se is not a major risk factor for nephrotoxicity, as long as close attention is given to a patient's fluid status.[161]

Increased risk of toxicity has been noted with concomitant drug therapy. The combination of cephalothin with an aminoglycoside has been reported to result in a significant increase in nephrotoxicity when compared with combinations of an aminoglycoside with other antibiotics.[185,189,190] Although the exact mechanism of combined toxicity is unknown, one study suggests that the aminoglycoside exerts a potentiating action on the nephrotoxicity of cephalosporins and that the cephalosporin is the principal nephrotoxin.[191]

Concurrent use of vancomycin and the aminoglycosides may potentiate nephrotoxicity.[185,192,193] The incidence of nephrotoxicity during combined therapy has been reported to vary between 5.7 and 35%. The incidence of nephrotoxicity from vancomycin alone ranges from 5 to 15%.[192,193] Risk factors identified for nephrotoxicity with combined therapy include increased age, vancomycin peak and trough (> 10 µg/mL) concentrations, length of combined therapy, concurrent use of amphotericin B, and presence of liver disease and peritonitis.[192,193]

Reports of synergistic nephrotoxicity between cisplatin and aminoglycosides often involve cases in which patients received combined cephalothin–aminoglycoside therapy.[194] Cisplatin–aminoglycoside combinations have been reported to result in a higher incidence of nephrotoxic effects than cisplatin alone.[195] Toxic effects are usually mild and manageable.[195,196] The available clinical data indicate that aminoglycosides can be used safely in patients receiving cisplatin as long as therapy is carefully monitored.[196]

The proposed interaction between amphotericin B and the aminoglycoside antibiotics has not been well documented. One study noted deterioration of kidney function in four patients receiving gentamicin when amphotericin B therapy was initiated.[197] The authors felt that the rapid increase in serum creatinine on initiation of amphotericin B indicated synergistic nephrotoxicity. The toxicity noted may have been due to the aminoglycoside alone. Also, amphotericin B can cause an elevation of serum creatinine soon after initiation of therapy in salt-depleted patients. Although the aminoglycoside–amphotericin B combination may show increased nephrotoxicity, more study is needed to document the interaction.

There have been miscellaneous reports of increased nephrotoxicity from combined use of aminoglycoside antibiotics and other agents.[185,198–200] Combined use of methoxyflurane anesthesia and the aminoglycoside antibiotics has been reported to increase the risk of methoxyflurane-induced kidney failure.[198] The risk of renal toxicity may be additive. In one study of kidney transplant patients, the combination of cyclosporine A with gentamicin and lincomycin increased the incidence of acute tubular necrosis from 5 to 67% compared with the use of gentamicin and lincomycin alone.[199] Increased nephrotoxicity has been associated with combined gentamicin–clindamycin therapy.[185,200] Review of three cases indicates that the decrease in kidney function may be attributed to gentamicin alone.[200] Use of the aminoglycoside antibiotics with methoxyflurane and cyclosporine A should be avoided if possible.

The presence of shock has been associated with an increased risk of aminoglycoside nephrotoxicity. In one study in which aminoglycoside serum levels were closely monitored, the effects of shock and aminoglycoside administration were found to be additive.[201]

The relationship between serum aminoglycoside concentrations and nephrotoxicity has been reviewed.[202] Controversy exists over the importance of peak and trough concentrations as risk factors for nephrotoxicity. In one study, the initial 1-hour peak serum concentration was significantly correlated with the risk of toxicity.[203] Dahlgren et al noted that 36% of patients with nephrotoxic effects had trough gentamicin concentrations greater than 2 µg/mL.[204] No patient with trough concentrations below 2 µg/mL had an increase in serum creatinine. In contrast, 64% of patients with trough concentrations greater than 2 µg/mL showed no deterioration of kidney function. In another study, a trough gentamicin concentration of 4 µg/mL or greater was associated with nephrotoxicity.[205] Smith et al noted that 25% of patients with a trough amikacin concentration greater than 10 µg/mL manifested nephrotoxicity.[206] Patients with trough

TABLE 9–8. RANGE OF PEAK AND TROUGH CONCENTRATIONS

Antibiotic	Peak (µg/mL)	Trough (µg/mL)
Gentamicin	5–10	0.5–<2
Tobramycin	5–10	0.5–<2
Netilmicin	6–10	0.5–2
Amikacin	15–35	5.0–10

concentrations below 10 µg/mL had no change in kidney function. When determining the importance of trough serum levels it is not possible to tell whether elevated predose serum levels are a result of nephrotoxicity or a risk for it. The generally accepted safe trough concentrations are listed in Table 9–8. Alterations in kidney function can occur in the presence of therapeutic concentrations.[202] As with ototoxicity, a clear association between serum concentration and nephrotoxicity has not been established[186]; however, a significantly increased rate of rise and size of increase of trough gentamicin concentrations over time in patients with nephrotoxic effects versus subjects without effects has been noted.[207]

Studies comparing administration of a single total daily dose of the aminoglycoside antibiotics with administration of the same dose in divided doses have found comparable incidences of nephrotoxicity (Table 9–9).[165–174,208,209] Prins et al noted a significant increase in nephrotox-

TABLE 9–9. AMINOGLYCOSIDE NEPHROTOXICITY: ONCE DAILY DOSES VERSUS MULTIPLE DAILY DOSES

Antibiotic	Toxicity (%)[a]		Significance[b]	Reference
	Daily	Multiple		
Amikacin	0	0	NS	165
	10	3	NS	166
	5.5	7.4	NS	167
	3	2	NS	168
Gentamicin	14	33	NS	169
	5	24	S	170
Netilmicin	0	0	NS	165
	7	7.6	NS	169
	15	17	NS	171
	3.8	13.6	NS	172
	2.8	0	NS	173
	3	3	NS	174
	0	0	NS	208
	5	7	NS	209

[a] Based on defined change in serum creatinine.
[b] NS, no significant difference; S, significant difference.

icity when gentamicin was administered three times daily versus once daily.[170] Although the overall incidences of nephrotoxicity were identical, TerBraak et al noted that patients with nephrotoxic effects receiving once-daily doses of netilmicin had a significantly greater increase in serum creatinine than subjects without nephrotoxic effects receiving multiple daily doses.[171] The mean maximal trough concentration was greater in the patients with than in patients without nephrotoxic effects receiving once-daily therapy. These trough concentrations were 2.8 and 1.1 µg/mL, respectively. No association between nephrotoxicity and peak serum concentration was found in either group. Single-dose therapy must be monitored carefully because nephrotoxicity and ototoxicity have resulted from such therapy. Peak aminoglycoside concentration determinations are not necessary; however, trough gentamicin, tobramycin, and netilmicin levels should be less than 2 µg/mL and amikacin less than 5 µg/mL prior to the next dose[176] (see Single-Dose Dosing Considerations).

Monitoring considerations to prevent nephrotoxicity should include a dynamic assessment of risk factors, careful monitoring of renal function, and serum trough concentration determinations. As the disposition of the aminoglycoside antibiotics follows multicompartment pharmacokinetics, trough concentrations will rise during therapy regardless of changes in kidney function. Serum trough concentrations should be obtained every 3 to 4 days during therapy. Patients receiving multiple daily doses should have their regimen manipulated to keep trough levels below 2 µg/mL for gentamicin, tobramycin, and netilmicin and between 5 and 10 µg/mL for amikacin. With close attention to these guidelines, gentamicin nephrotoxicity in one study occurred in only 13 of 1640 patients (0.9%).[37]

Neurotoxicity

The aminoglycosides have been associated with adverse neurologic effects. These reactions are most commonly manifested as muscular paralysis and respiratory depression. The neuromuscular blocking potency in order of decreasing effect is neomycin and netilmicin > streptomycin > amikacin > gentamicin and tobramycin. Neuromuscular blockade has occurred after oral, intrapleural, intraperitoneal, intravenous, intramuscular, topical, intraluminal, and retroperitoneal administration. These agents differ in their effect on neuromuscular function; however, basically they interfere with the presynaptic release of acetylcholine or postsynaptically decrease the response to acetylcholine. Patients with myasthenia gravis, Parkinson's disease, or severe hypocalcemia, infants with botulism, and those receiving neuromuscular blocking agents are at risk.[210–212] The duration of neuromuscular blockade is prolonged when aminoglycoside antibiotics are administered concurrently with neuromuscular blocking agents. Neuromuscular irritability and seizure activity can occur secondary to hypomagnesemia and hypocalcemia induced by gentamicin.[213] The intravenous administration of calcium gluconate and neostigmine has been used to reverse the neuromuscular blockade. Corticoneural toxicity following gentamicin and tobramycin has also been reported.[214,215] Acute organic brain syndrome and delirium may be noted.

Increased mortality in infants receiving intraventricular gentamicin for the treatment of Gram-negative meningitis has been reported.[216] This increased mortality may be partially explained by an observed increase in inflammatory response (increased ventricular cerebrospinal fluid concentration of endotoxin and interleukin-1β) to the intraventricular administration of gentamicin.[217]

Hypomagnesemia, hypokalemia, and hypocalcemia have been reported during aminoglycoside administration.[213,218] Hypomagnesemia may occur in up to 38% of patients and occurs early in therapy.[218] Risk factors associated with hypomagnesemia include NPO (nothing per mouth) status, poor dietary intake, and lack of magnesium supplementation. Hypomagnesemia results from aminoglycoside-induced renal Mg^{2+} wasting.[213,218] Hypokalemia and hypocalcemia are a consequence of hypomagnesemia and can be corrected by Mg^{2+} administration. Potassium is lost in the urine. Hypocalcemia results from parathyroid gland malfunction and peripheral resistance to parathyroid hormone in hypomagnesemic patients. A case of Fanconi syndrome has also been reported in a 14-year-old boy undergoing gentamicin therapy.[219]

Other Adverse Reactions

Other adverse reactions include anaphylaxis, loss of sense of smell after intranasal instillation, alopecia, thrombocytopenia, and skin rash (urticaria, maculopapular).[145,150,220–223]

Drug–Drug Interactions

The aminoglycoside antibiotics have been reported to interact with a number of other medications (Table 9–10). Agents that may potentiate ototoxicity and nephrotoxicity have been discussed under Adverse Reactions (see Tables 9–5 and 9–7).

The aminoglycoside antibiotics have been shown to potentiate the action of nondepolarizing muscle relaxants. Prolongation of action of neuromuscular blockers or recurrence of neuromuscular blockade after the block has been reversed has been reported.[224] No significant effect on the neuromuscular blocking effect of atracurium and d-tubocurarine by gentamicin or tobramycin has been noted.[225,226] Vecuronium neuromuscular blockade is prolonged in patients receiving gentamicin and tobramycin.

Miconazole administration has been associated with a significant increase in the apparent volume of distribution and clearance of tobramycin.[227] These parameters returned to baseline on substitution of amphotericin B for miconazole. The exogenous lipids (polyethoxylated castor oil vehicle of miconazole) may potentiate the entry of tobramycin into cells, causing the observed increase in volume of distribution.

Zarfin et al have found significant increases in peak and trough concentrations of amikacin

TABLE 9–10. DRUG INTERACTIONS WITH THE AMINOGLYCOSIDE ANTIBIOTICS

Drug or Drug Type	Nature of Effect
Neuromuscular blocking agents	Prolonged neuromuscular blockade or recurrence of blockade
Miconazole	Increased apparent V_d and clearance
Indomethacin	Reduced renal elimination of aminoglycoside
Penicillins	Inactivation of the aminoglycoside antibiotic
Penicillin V	Decreased extent of absorption of penicillin V^a
Digoxin	Decreased rate and extent of absorption of digoxin[a]
Methotrexate	Decreased extent of absorption of methotrexate[b]

[a]Concurrent administration with oral neomycin.

[b]Mixture of orally administered nonabsorbable antimicrobial agents.

and gentamicin in patients with patent ductus arteriosus treated with indomethacin.[228] This effect may be due to a decrease in glomerular filtration rate induced by indomethacin in these patients. Reduced aminoglycoside dosage may be warranted prior to indomethacin administration.

Carbenicillin, ticarcillin, azlocillin, mezlocillin, and piperacillin inactivate the aminoglycoside antibiotics when they are mixed together in vitro.[229–231] Ampicillin and moxalactam also inactivate tobramycin.[231,232] The reaction is concentration, temperature, and time related, and appears to be a result of a nucleophilic opening of the beta-lactam ring of the penicillin by a methylamino group of the aminoglycoside.[233] The reaction results in inactivation of both agents. Tobramycin is most inactivated, followed by gentamicin. Amikacin and netilmicin are the least inactivated. Mezlocillin, azlocillin, and piperacillin cause less inactivation of tobramycin and gentamicin than does carbenicillin.[229] The microbiologic assay detects the most inactivation, possibly because of continued drug inactivation during the assay procedure. The enzyme-multiplied immunoassay (EMI) assay technique detects the least inactivation because it measures both active and inactive aminoglycoside.[229,234] Fluorescence polarization immunoassay and radioimmunoassay assays are equal in their ability to detect the interaction.

The interaction is not significant in vivo except in patients with severely diminished renal function.[235] In this situation, aminoglycoside serum half-life (except for amikacin and netilmicin) may decrease significantly, making more frequent dosing necessary to maintain therapeutic serum concentrations.

When aminoglycoside serum concentrations are determined in patients receiving these beta-lactam antibiotics, it is extremely important to remember that if the assay cannot be performed quickly (ie, within 10 hours), the serum should be frozen (-20 to $-70°C$) to prevent interaction-induced low aminoglycoside concentrations.[229,231,236] It is also advisable to obtain peak and trough levels of the aminoglycoside when the penicillin level is a trough. Administration of the penicillin can be delayed when drawing levels. Interaction is most significant when the beta-lactam is present with gentamicin or tobramycin.

The extent of absorption of penicillin V and digoxin is significantly decreased during concurrent administration with oral neomycin.[237,238] The rate of absorption of digoxin is also significantly decreased.[238] Spacing out doses may not be effective in overcoming the interaction. Concurrent administration of methotrexate with nonabsorbable antimicrobial agents (paromomycin, polymyxin B, nystatin, vancomycin) has been shown to decrease the oral absorption of methotrexate by more than 30%.[239] The rate of absorption of 5-fluorouracil was decreased by the concurrent administration of neomycin; however, the clinical significance of the finding is unknown.[240]

Therapeutic Range and Efficacy

The therapeutic ranges of the aminoglycoside antibiotics are somewhat correlated with achievable serum concentrations and the average minimum inhibitory concentration (MIC) of a sensitive organism versus levels that may be associated with toxicity. Generally accepted desirable peak and trough concentrations for the parenterally administered agents are listed in Table 9–8. As a range is provided, lower levels in the range are used for less serious infections such as urinary tract infection without sepsis. The higher levels in the range are used in more seriously ill patients or when infection is present in a poorly accessible area, such as the lung.

To justify the need for therapeutic drug monitoring there must be a correlation between measured drug concentrations and therapeutic or toxic outcome. This section discusses the data documenting the need for therapeutic drug monitoring (TDM) as it relates to therapeutic outcome (see Adverse Reactions for discussion of toxicity).

Noone et al were one of the first groups to attempt to correlate clinical efficacy with peak concentration of gentamicin.[241] They noted that of 20 episodes of urinary tract infection, in all 17 episodes that resulted in cure, peak serum concentrations of 5 µg/mL were achieved in the first 3 days of treatment. A similar finding was noted in patients with sepsis. In patients with Gram-negative pneumonia, a favorable outcome was associated with a peak concentration of 8 µg/mL or higher.

Anderson et al studied patients with persistent or recurrent bacteremia despite more than 24 hours of antibiotic therapy.[242] Subinhibitory gentamicin serum concentrations were noted in 3 of 9 patients with early and 7 of 18 subjects with late "breakthrough" bacteremia. Early and late breakthrough bacteremia was defined as bacteremia occurring between 24 and 72 hours and after 72 hours of antibiotic therapy, respectively. They encouraged the use of a loading dose of gentamicin in septic patients and the monitoring of serum concentrations to ensure therapeutic levels early in therapy. Interestingly, another group of patients who did not have persistent or recurrent bacteremia had a similar rate of subinhibitory levels, indicating that other host factors in addition to antibiotic concentrations were important in the success or failure of therapy.

Moore et al reported their results of a retrospective review of effect of peak aminoglycoside concentrations on outcome of therapy in patients with Gram-negative bacteremia and pneumonia.[243,244] In the bacteremia study, the early peak plasma concentration of more than 5 µg/mL for gentamicin or tobramycin and of more than 20 µg/mL for amikacin was associated with a significant improved survival.[243] No correlation between trough levels and survival was noted.

In the Gram-negative pneumonia review, the maximal peak plasma aminoglycoside concentration throughout therapy of 7 µg/mL or greater for gentamicin or tobramycin and of 28 µg/mL or greater for amikacin was significantly associated with improved patient outcome.[244] Achieving an adequate peak concentration was the most important factor associated with a favorable outcome.

Deziel-Evans et al investigated the correlation of five pharmacokinetic factors with therapeutic outcome in adult patients with bacterial infections receiving aminoglycoside antibiotics.[245] Significant correlation was found between the five factors and the patients' clinical response; however, the steady-state peak serum concentration ($C_{max,ss}$)/MIC ratio appeared to be the most clinically useful. A $C_{max,ss}$/MIC ratio greater than 4 resulted in a cure rate of 83%, and a ratio greater than 8 yielded a cure rate of 91%.

In a retrospective study, Moore et al reviewed the correlation of plasma aminoglycoside concentrations with MIC.[246] Results indicated that the maximal peak/MIC ratio and the mean peak/MIC ratio are significantly associated with clinical outcome.

Single-Dose Therapy

The above studies and the fact that these agents exhibit concentration-dependent killing of Gram-negative bacilli followed by a prolonged postantibiotic effect have increased interest in dosage regimens that incorporate less frequent administration of these agents.[6,8,9] These regimens are predicated on the idea that high peak antibiotic concentrations increase bacterial killing and that low trough levels result in less nephrotoxicity and ototoxicity while taking advantage of the postantibiotic effect. As the nephrotoxicity of the aminoglycoside antibiotics is associated with the accumulation of the agent in the renal cortex, it is logical to assume that techniques that will minimize such accumulation may be associated with lower toxicity. A washout period may also be important to allow sufficient time for ear fluid levels to decrease to avoid ototoxicity. Studies show that single doses of aminoglycosides result in lower kidney accumulation than continuous infusions or multiple doses.[62–64,247,248] Regimens in which the total daily dose of the aminoglycoside antibiotic is administered in a single dose have been compared with those in which the same dose is administered two or three times daily in humans.[165–174,208,209] Studies have shown equal efficacy and either reduced or identical toxicity. Single-dose aminoglycoside therapy is usually combined with other antimicrobial agents. Combination therapy is especially important if single-dose therapy is used in neutropenic patients.[168,249] Concerns that prolonged periods of low or undetectable concentrations of the aminoglycoside would result in regrowth of the infecting organism are addressed by combination therapy.

Aminoglycoside Blood Sampling and Assay Considerations

To perform effective therapeutic drug monitoring, the data used must be as accurate as possible. In this section, we discuss the appropriate blood sampling issues and select assay considerations that make TDM possible.

Blood Sampling Considerations. For the aminoglycoside antibiotics, drug concentrations are usually obtained as either peak or trough levels. Peak concentrations should be drawn after distribution is complete (30 to 60 minutes after the completion of the intravenous infusion). Typical infusions are 30 to 60 minutes in duration. The sampling schedule for peak concentrations takes into consideration the typical distribution time of the aminoglycoside antibiotics of 25 to 75 minutes. In some patient populations, the distribution time may be prolonged and sampling of peak concentrations should be delayed to make sure distribution has been completed. In our experience, peak aminoglycoside concentrations should be obtained at least 2 hours after completion of an infusion (60 minutes) in patients with ascites from cirrhosis. Patients receiving intramuscular administration can have peak concentrations obtained from 1 to $1^1/_2$ hours after the dose is injected. In some patient populations, the peak levels may be delayed when the aminoglycoside is given intramuscularly. Delayed absorption has been noted in patients with diabetes, spinal cord injury (when injected into paralyzed muscle), and septic shock.[36,136]

A trough concentration is defined as the level obtained prior to the next dose (typically within 30 minutes of the next dose). Blood samples should be obtained in the arm opposite the one in which the drug is being infused. This maneuver avoids the possible false elevation of a serum concentration due to backflow of antibiotic into the vein being sampled.

Although a one-compartment model is most often used to characterize the pharmacokinetics of these antibiotics, a multicompartment system best reflects the disposition of the agents. Peak and trough concentrations rise during therapy regardless of change in kidney function. The increase reflects tissue accumulation of these antibiotics. For this reason, peak and trough concentrations are best obtained at steady state. Steady state is usually achieved after the medication has been administered for about five half-lives. An increase or decrease in dose will require the same amount of time to reach a new steady state.

Once dosing is initiated, a peak and trough pair may be obtained at steady state. These samples are used to document the presence of therapeutic peak and nontoxic trough concentrations. If a regimen change is indicated, a follow-up peak/trough pair should be obtained after a new steady state has been reached (three to five doses) to document the effect of the new dosage. Follow-up concentrations should be obtained every 3 to 4 days for monitoring purposes. Should the patient condition change, more frequent monitoring of serum concentrations should be undertaken. The serum creatinine should be obtained every 2 to 3 days in the stable patient and every other day in the patient with risk factors for toxicity or changing clinical condition.

To be able to interpret the serum concentration data appropriately, the exact sampling time, infusion time, and time of last dose must be available. Unfortunately, these times are very difficult to obtain in clinical settings and individual attention to these issues is often required. Drawing of the levels oneself and education of the house staff and nursing personnel with respect to the importance of these times are methods of obtaining this information. Inaccurate data as they relate to the time of blood sampling and infusions can result in inaccurate dosing recommendations, and their importance to successful TDM cannot be overestimated.

Recent information indicates that aminoglycoside pharmacokinetics may vary depending on the time of day.[250,251] Lucht et al noted a significant increase in mean netilmicin concentrations drawn at 5 AM and trough concentrations obtained at 9 AM versus mean and trough concentrations obtained at other times of the day.[250] Peak concentrations did not vary significantly throughout the day. Elting et al found similar results in that they noted significantly higher amikacin concentrations obtained at 7 AM and 3 PM when compared with those obtained at 9 PM.[251] The observed effects can be explained by the known increase in glomerular filtration rate (GFR) during the day and the decrease in GFR during the night. Aminoglycoside serum concentrations should be obtained around a set dose to minimize the effect of diurnal variation in aminoglycoside disposition.

Inaccurate documentation of infusion times may result in erroneous dosage regimen changes. A rapid infusion in a patient with normal renal function will result in a higher observed serum peak concentration than would a slower infusion of the same dose. If the slower infusion rate is considered when in fact the faster infusion rate was used, erroneous dosage regimens may be recommended. The opposite is also true. The effect of infusion time on peak concentration decreases as renal function decreases. Aminoglycosides are administered intravenously by either gravity flow or infusion pump. Serum concentrations obtained by these different methods of infusion appear to vary significantly.[252,253] It is important not to use different methods of administration in the same patient.

One should also become familiar with the assay technique used by the clinical laboratory and the minimal amount of serum/plasma needed to run the sample. This issue is important when multiple samples are necessary to monitor the patient. Multiple blood samples of large volumes combined with routine blood drawing for clinical monitoring can result in anemia.

Single-Dose Sampling Considerations. Peak aminoglycoside concentration determinations are not necessary; however, trough or random serum levels (see Single-Dose Dosing Considerations) should be obtained soon after starting therapy.[176] Trough concentrations prior to the next dose should be less than 2 µg/mL for gentamicin, tobramycin, and netilmicin and less than 5 µg/mL for amikacin. Sampling should be repeated every 4 days during therapy. More frequent determination is necessary if kidney function is changing.

Assay Considerations. Therapeutic drug monitoring relies heavily on the laboratory assessment of aminoglycoside concentrations. Without dependable assay results, the monitoring and dosage recommendations would be impossible. In addition to the accurate timing of dosing and sampling, the need for reliable assay results cannot be overstated. Antibiotic concentrations to be used to make dosage recommendations should be assayed at the same time to avoid between-run assay variability.

One issue that arises in clinical discussions of drug levels is whether there is a difference between serum and plasma concentration values. When a fluorescence polarization immunoassay or EMIT assay for gentamicin and tobramycin is used, serum and plasma are interchangeable.[254,255] Arterial serum gentamicin concentrations are comparable to those obtained by heel stick in neonates weighing greater than 1000 g.[256]

Various methods are available for the assessment of aminoglycoside levels. The microbiologic, radioimmunoassay (RIA), enzyme-multiplied immunoassay (EMI,EMIT), and fluorescence polarization immunoassay (FPI,FPIA) are the most commonly used clinically for TDM. These assays are highly specific for these antibiotics; however, other aminoglycosides present in the same sample may cross-react.[257]

Assessment of the available assay techniques indicates that they are not interchangeable, and results from one assay procedure may be different from those of another. The EMIT assay system yields lower aminoglycoside concentrations when compared with RIA, microbiologic assay, and FPIA.[257,258]

The effects of assay procedure on the calculation of pharmacokinetic variables of gentamicin and amikacin have been studied.[259–261] When RIA is compared with EMIT, mean values for the pharmacokinetic parameters (V_d, $t_{1/2}$, and TBC) were significantly higher when EMIT-derived gentamicin concentration data were used.[259] Dosage recommendations to achieve a desired peak concentration were also significantly higher when EMIT-derived data were used. A similar finding was noted when pharmacokinetic parameters from data derived by RIA and FPIA were compared.[260] Dosages calculated using FPIA data are significantly higher than those determined using RIA-derived parameters.[260] Bleske et al compared the pharmacokinetic parameters derived from EMIT with those from FPIA of amikacin.[261] They noted a significant difference in volume of distribution and dosage recommendations when using EMIT data versus FPIA. Similarly, Boyce et al noted that mean EMIT-derived values for the elimination rate constant (k), volume of distribution, total body clearance, and dose were significantly higher than when FPIA-generated parameters were used.[262] None of the studies used a more specific assay than the RIA or presented data on toxicity. These data indicate that EMIT will give significantly different pharmacokinetic parameters than FPIA and RIA. Also, it is important not to switch between assays when monitoring aminoglycoside antibiotics.

Special contaminating substances and their effects on assay results are worth noting. Exogenously administered fluorescein can interfere with FPIA assays for the aminoglycoside antibiotics.[263] FPIA uses fluorescein-labeled antigen, which competes with exogenous antigen for binding sites on antibody molecules. High serum concentrations of fluorescein can cause a false elevation of aminoglycoside concentrations. Guidelines for handling samples in the presence of fluorescein have been developed.[263]

Heparin in high concentrations (ie, 100 U/mL) has been shown to cause a falsely low concentration of the aminoglycoside antibiotics when measured by microbiologic, enzyme, and radioenzymatic immunoassays.[264,265] These high levels may be encountered when aminoglycoside levels are improperly obtained through heparinized intravenous catheters or when a heparinized collection tube is not completely filled with sample. Samples obtained from patients receiving heparin for therapeutic purposes do not contain enough heparin to interfere with the assays.[264] Heparin does not affect RIA or FPIA.[264,265]

THERAPEUTIC REGIMEN DESIGN

Approach to the Patient

When consulting on a patient for aminoglycoside dosing one should become acquainted with the overall clinical situation of the subject. A problem list should be made to ascertain the presence of disease states that may affect aminoglycoside dosing (ie, congestive heart failure, ascites, kidney failure). The degree of activity or severity of these problems must also be considered. Congestive heart failure that is under control is not the same as uncontrolled congestive heart failure. The clinician must also review all other medications the patient is receiving to determine appropriateness of dose, presence or absence of adverse drug reactions or interactions, and the like.

Once these issues have been addressed it is time to determine the proper therapy for the patient's infectious disease. The appearance of the patient is important in determining how aggressive therapy should be. Is the patient in coma or sitting in bed reading a newspaper? Knowledge of the site of infection and possible offending organisms is vital to the choice of antibiotic regimen. The site of infection can be ascertained from the patient's symptoms, such as a productive cough (pneumonia), complaints of frequency and dysuria (urinary tract infection), and discussion with the medical team. Diagnostic tests such as cultures of blood, urine, and sputum and radiologic tests are also helpful in determining the organisms involved and the source of infection. Culture results and sensitivity testing will help tailor therapy.

From the available data, the appropriateness of therapy must be considered. Once the clinician has determined that the antibiotic therapy, in general, and the use of an aminoglycoside, in particular, are appropriate, the dosing and monitoring of these agents can begin. After appropriate therapy is initiated the patient's response to treatment must be followed. Temperature, white blood cell count, repeat cultures, and chest x-ray (patient with pneumonia) are a few examples of factors to follow. Serum concentration monitoring can also begin as discussed above.

Empiric Dosing Considerations

The goal of therapy when using the aminoglycoside antibiotics is to ensure the presence of both therapeutic and nontoxic serum concentrations throughout therapy (see Tables 9–5, 9–7, and 9–8). Whether a patient responds favorably to such therapy depends on the many factors that determine outcome, such as underlying disease states and severity, nutritional status, drainage of an abscess, and relief of an obstruction. Patients may experience toxic effects even when therapeutic, "nontoxic" concentrations are maintained; however, the dose-related toxicity should be preventable with close attention to monitoring of serum concentrations, kidney function, presence of concurrent disease states, and so on.[37] This section discusses initial empiric dosing considerations for select situations. Dosing based on pharmacokinetic principles is discussed in the next section.

Infants and Children

The pharmacokinetics of the aminoglycoside antibiotics are highly variable in premature and term infants. Kidney function is decreased in the newborn compared with the adult.[97] This is especially true for the premature, low-birth-weight infant. Various empiric dosage regimens for these antibiotics have been developed for the newborn (Tables 9–11, 9–12, and 9–13). Lopez-Samblas et al have compared several of the more popular guidelines and have proposed dosing recommendations for gentamicin based on postconceptional age[267] (see Table 9–11). No significant difference in the ability of the studied regimens to achieve peak concentrations in the therapeutic range was noted; however, the ability to produce trough concentrations less than 2 μg/mL was best with their dosage guidelines. The manufacturer of netilmicin suggests caution

TABLE 9–11. EMPIRIC DOSING CHART: GENTAMICIN AND TOBRAMYCIN

Patient Group	Dosage Regimen	Reference
Neonate[a]		
<28 wk GA[b]	2.5 mg/kg q24h	266
28–34 wk GA	2.5 mg/kg q18h	
>34 wk GA	2.5 mg/kg q12	
Neonate[b]		
<28 wk GA	2.5 mg/kg q18h	
28–34 wk GA	2.5 mg/kg q12h	
>34 wk GA	2.5 mg/kg q8h	
Neonate[d]		
<30 wk PCA[e]	3.0 mg/kg q24h	267
30–37 wk PCA	2.5 mg/kg q18h	
Children		
	6–7.5 mg/kg/24 h	266
	(in 3 doses)	
Cystic fibrosis		
Children[d]	3 mg/kg q6h	268
(3 mo–17 y)		
Adult[d]	3 mg/kg q8h	
(≥18 y)		
Adults[f]		
Loading dose	1.75–2.0 mg/kg	
Maintenance dose	3–5.0 mg/kg/24 h	
Dialysis[g]		
Loading dose	1.75–2.0 mg/kg	
Maintenance dose		
Dialysis three times weekly[h]	1–1.5 mg/kg after dialysis	
Dialysis daily	0.5–0.75 mg/kg after dialysis	

[a]First week of life only.
[b]GA = gestational age.
[c]After 1 week of life.
[d]Guidelines for gentamicin.
[e]PCA = postconceptional age (gestational age + neonatal age).
[f]Normal kidney function.
[g]Hemodialysis.
[h]Monday, Wednesday, Friday.

TABLE 9–12. EMPIRIC DOSING CHART: NETILMICIN

Patient Group	Dosage Regimen	Reference
Neonate[a] (<6 wk)	4.0–6.5 mg/kg/q24 h (2 divided doses)	269
Children and infants (6 wk–12 y)	5.5–8.0 mg/kg/24 h (2 or 3 divided doses)	269
Cystic fibrosis	10 mg/kg/24 h (3 divided doses)	270
Adults[b]		
Loading dose	1.75–2.0 mg/kg	269
Maintenance dose	4.0–6.5 mg/kg/24 h (2 or 3 divided doses)	
Dialysis[c]		
Loading dose	1.75–2.0 mg/kg	
Maintenance dose		
Dialysis three times weekly[d]	1–1.5 mg/kg after dialysis	
Daily dialysis	0.5–0.75 mg/kg after dialysis	

[a]Caution must be exercised in neonates and children due to the presence of benzyl alcohol in the diluent.
[b]Normal kidney function.
[c]Hemodialysis.
[d]Monday, Wednesday, Friday.

when the product is used in neonates and children because the product contains benzyl alcohol.[269] Premature neonates have experienced neurotoxic effects (gasping syndrome) after large daily doses of benzyl alcohol. Whichever dosage guidelines are used, follow-up peak and trough concentrations should be obtained and dosage adjustments made if indicated.

Patients With Cystic Fibrosis

The pharmacokinetics of these antibiotics vary in patients with cystic fibrosis based on the severity of the disease and age.[32,108–115,268] Subjects with mild to moderate cystic fibrosis may have pharmacokinetic parameters similar to those of patients without cystic fibrosis,[113–115] whereas more severely ill cystic fibrosis patients have marked increases in volume of distribution and total body clearance when compared with subjects without cystic fibrosis.[32,108–110] Hendeles et al have recommended initial dosing regimens for children and adults with cystic fibrosis receiving gentamicin (see Table 9–11). Similar guidelines are likely to apply for tobramycin and netilmicin, as well[271] (see Tables 9–11 and 9–12). Peak concentrations of 8 to 12 µg/mL and trough concentrations less than 2 µg/mL are recommended for gentamicin, tobramycin, and netilmicin. Initial dosing recommendations for cystic fibrosis patients receiving amikacin are listed in Table 9–13. Peak concentrations of 25 to 30 µg/mL and trough concentrations of 5 to 10 µg/mL are recommended for amikacin. Because of the great variability in the pharmacokinetics of aminoglycoside antibiotics in these patients, initial dosage regimens should be followed up with serum concentration evaluations.

TABLE 9–13. EMPIRIC DOSING CHART: AMIKACIN

Patient Group	Dosage Regimen	Reference
Neonate[a]		
<28 wk GA[b]	7.5 mg/kg q24h	266
28–34 wk GA	7.5 mg/kg q18h	
>34 wk GA	7.5 mg/kg q12h	
Neonate[c]		
<28 wk GA	7.5 mg/kg q18h	
28–34 wk GA	7.5 mg/kg q12h	
>34 wk GA	7.5 mg/kg q8h	
Children	15–22.5 mg/kg/24 h	266
	(in 2 or 3 doses, maximum dose 1.5 g/24 h)	
Cystic fibrosis	30 mg/kg/24 h	270
	(in 3 doses)	
Adults[d]		
Loading dose	7.5 mg/kg	
Maintenance dose	15 mg/kg/24 h	
	(in 2 or 3 divided doses)	
Dialysis[f]		
Loading dose	7.5 mg/kg	
Maintenance dose		
Dialysis three times weekly[f]	5 mg/kg after dialysis	
Dialysis daily	2.5 mg/kg after dialysis	

[a]First week of life only. Dose should be infused over 1–2 hours.
[b]GA = gestational age.
[c]After 1 week of life.
[d]Normal kidney function.
[e]Hemodialysis.
[f]Monday, Wednesday, Friday.

Adults

Normal Kidney Function. In seriously ill patients, the rapid attainment of therapeutic serum concentrations is beneficial. These concentrations can be obtained by administering a loading dose (see Tables 9–11, 9–12, and 9–13). Loading doses of 1.75 to 2.0 mg/kg based on actual body weight (ABW) for gentamicin, tobramycin, and netilmicin and of 7.5 mg/kg ABW for amikacin should be sufficient. Loading doses of 2.5 to 3.0 mg/kg have been proposed in select populations of critically ill patients receiving gentamicin and tobramycin because of the increase in volume of distribution.[272,273] Doses should be infused over 30 to 60 minutes.

Morbidly obese patients may experience high peak levels after dosing based on ABW; however, because of the variability in volume of distribution noted in these patients, some would be underdosed if the adjustment factor method were used initially. The initial dose should be based on ABW in morbidly obese patients. Patients with ascites should receive loading doses based on ABW, as well.[118,119]

In the seriously ill patient, the risk of an undertreated infection is far greater than the risk of aminoglycoside toxicity. The loading dose is also extremely important in patients with decreased kidney function, to whom the subsequent maintenance doses may not be administered for long periods (ie, dialysis patients). If a loading dose is not given, considerable time may elapse until therapeutic concentrations are attained. When a single-dose regimen is used, every dose is like a loading dose.

Maintenance doses are based on ideal body weight (IBW) or ABW (exceptions: patients with ascites and morbid obesity), whichever is less. The IBW can be determined using Equations 9–1 and 9–2 (see discussion under Obesity).

Recommended daily doses in adults with normal kidney function vary from 3 to 5 mg/kg in divided doses for gentamicin and tobramycin, to 4 to 6.5 mg/kg for netilmicin, to 15 mg/kg in two or three divided doses for amikacin. In one study, however, the gentamicin dosages needed to achieve therapeutic, nontoxic serum concentrations varied from 0.7 to 25.8 mg/kg/d.[37] Such variability explains the intrinsic error involved in assuming that standard dosage regimens are appropriate for all patients.

End Stage Kidney Disease. Patients with end-stage kidney disease may be managed with peritoneal or hemodialysis. Peritoneal dialysis can be either intermittent (IPD) or continuous (CAPD). Dosing considerations for aminoglycoside antibiotics in subjects on peritoneal dialysis depend on, among other things, the type of dialysis, amount of residual kidney function, and site of infection (ie, presence of peritonitis with or without systemic infection).

In patients with systemic infection without peritonitis it is important to develop a dosing regimen that maintains therapeutic serum concentrations during and between dialysis periods. IPD removes the aminoglycoside more efficiently than CAPD.[76,77] As the volume of distribution is similar to that of patients with normal renal function, loading doses are the same as those mentioned above. For example, a patient undergoing IPD twice weekly would receive a tobramycin loading dose of 1.75 to 2.0 mg/kg by vein, followed by a maintenance dose of 1.0 mg/kg every 3 days.[274] Similar regimens would apply for gentamicin and netilmicin. In patients receiving amikacin, a loading dose of 7.5 mg/kg is followed by a 5 mg/kg dose after 3 to 4 days.[76] Because of the varied frequency of dialysis and degree of residual kidney function, individualized regimens must be developed, guided by serum concentration monitoring.

Patients on peritoneal dialysis are at increased risk of experiencing peritonitis during therapy. Patients without systemic symptoms may be treated by instillation of the aminoglycoside intraperitoneally. This can be accomplished by adding a desired therapeutic concentration (ie, tobramycin, 5–10 µg/mL) into each dialysis exchange. Alternate regimens have been proposed to minimize the risk of ototoxic effects in patients on CAPD.[15,17] An initial intraperitoneal tobramycin loading dose of 3 or 4 mg/kg followed by a single daily dose of 1.2 or 1.5 mg/kg IP has been proposed for patients undergoing CAPD.[15,17] These regimens allow the serum concentrations to fall between doses. These dosing methods may lessen the theoretical risk of ototoxic effects from constant serum concentrations noted during continuous intraperitoneal administration of antibiotic. If the patient is systemically ill, intravenous administration of the antibiotic can be added to intraperitoneal therapy. This would involve giving a loading dose identical to that in patients with normal renal function. Systemic doses can then be adjusted based on serum concentration determination. To reduce the risk of toxicity, courses of aminoglycoside therapy in this setting should not exceed 2 to 3 weeks if possible.

Initial dosing guidelines for patients on hemodialysis are listed in Tables 9–11, 9–12, and 9–13. Doses should be administered after dialysis. Dosage regimens should be individualized by monitoring serum concentrations. Levels obtained prior to and at the end of dialysis can be used to determine the percentage by which the serum concentration is decreased by dialysis. Ideally, trough concentrations should be obtained 2 hours after the end of dialysis, and peak concentrations, 30 to 60 minutes after a dose.[88] This delay takes into consideration the redistribution phenomenon noted with these antibiotics. The delay in sampling and dosing may not be practical in the clinical setting, however.

Application of Pharmacokinetic Principles to Dosing

Several methods have been developed to assist in adjusting aminoglycoside dosing based on renal function. The various dosing methods (from the simplest to more advanced) and their advantages and disadvantages are discussed now.

Variable-Dose and Fixed-Interval Method

The first method used to adjust for renal function is one in which the dosage is reduced as renal function decreases and the maintenance interval is kept constant. The maintenance interval in this method for gentamicin, tobramycin, and netilmicin is 8 hours, and the interval for amikacin is 12 hours. For example, instead of giving gentamicin 80 mg every 16 hours in a patient with a creatinine of 2.0 mg/dL, one would give 40 mg every 8 hours. Serum levels oscillate markedly when renal function is normal; however, little fluctuation in peak and trough concentrations occurs in patients with marked decreases in renal function. This method may not result in therapeutic peaks or nontoxic troughs in such patients.[205,275] The variable-dose regimen may result in almost constant blood levels as renal function worsens and is potentially more toxic. This dosing method is not recommended.

Variable-Interval Method

The second dosing technique is the variable-interval method. This method involves giving the usual maintenance dose and adjusting the interval based on assessment of renal function. The variable-interval method takes into consideration the need to achieve therapeutic peak concentrations (concentration-dependent killing) and the issue of postantibiotic effect. Various dosing adjustment techniques have been developed using this concept.

Rule of 8's

One such method, the rule of 8's, is the one used by most physicians when dosing adults and is the easiest to use.[205] The loading dose and maintenance dose are chosen as mentioned above. The dosage interval is then based on a multiple of the measured serum creatinine. The dosage interval is determined by multiplying the observed serum creatinine by 8 for gentamicin, tobramycin, and netilmicin. The observed serum creatinine is multiplied by 9 to determine the interval for amikacin. The dosing interval is rounded off to the nearest convenient period. The technique is a simple way to adjust for renal function. An every-8-hour interval is most often used for gentamicin, tobramycin, and netilmicin in patients with "normal" renal function.

Amikacin is dosed initially at 5.0 mg/kg every 8 hours or 7.5 mg/kg every 12 hours in patients with "normal" kidney function.

The use of this technique results in marked variation between peak and trough levels. In the older patient, the tendency is toward overdose due to age-related factors. These factors may include diminished kidney function without an appreciable change in serum creatinine, presence of ascites as a result of liver disease, and malnutrition. In these patients, the serum creatinine may be unreliable for use in dosing considerations.

Concurrently administered medications may also affect the measurement of the serum creatinine level. Patients receiving cimetidine or trimethoprim may experience an increase in serum creatinine with no change in glomerular filtration rate.[276,277] A small increase in serum creatinine may be noted in from 10 to 59% of patients receiving cimetidine at doses of 300 mg qid.[276,278] Elevations of 2 mg/dL or more have been noted during the administration of cimetidine. Whether the new dosage regimens of cimetidine will cause similar degrees of creatinine elevation is unknown.

In one study, trimethoprim-induced increase in serum creatinine was significant only in patients with preexisting kidney failure.[277] The increase in serum creatinine noted in patients receiving cimetidine or trimethoprim results from a competitive inhibition of the tubular secretion of creatinine by the kidney. The change in serum creatinine is reversed when these agents are discontinued. The effect of these medications on serum creatinine should be considered during aminoglycoside therapy, especially if the increase in serum creatinine occurs soon after cimetidine or trimethoprim is added to therapy.

Cephalothin, cefoxitin, ceforanide, and flucytosine can falsely elevate serum creatinine, depending on their serum concentration, the assay procedure used, and preexisting kidney failure.[279–281] Cephalothin, cefoxitin, and ceforanide can falsely elevate serum creatinine values at achievable serum concentrations.[279,280] To avoid potential false elevations of serum creatinine by these agents, the serum creatinine level should be obtained prior to administration of cephalothin, cefoxitin, and ceforanide.

Flucytosine can falsely elevate serum creatinine levels if the old two-slide method with the Kodak Ektachem analyzer is used.[281] If a patient is receiving flucytosine, the Jaffé method or the newer Kodak unit should be used for creatinine determinations.

To use the rule of 8's, one must be cognizant of its deficiencies and follow up with serum concentration measurements. With this method, peak and trough levels would be obtained around a dose, preferably after steady state had been achieved. Dosage regimen adjustments are made depending on the result (Table 9–14). This technique may be referred to as the best guess

TABLE 9–14. DOSAGE REGIMEN MANIPULATION: PEAK AND TROUGH LEVELS

Level Parameter	Manipulation
Peak too high, trough OK	Decrease dose
Peak too low, trough OK	Increase dose
Peak OK, trough too high	Increase interval
Peak OK, trough too low	Decrease interval
Peak too high, trough too high	Decrease dose, increase interval
Peak too low, trough too low	Increase dose, decrease interval

method. In general, the dose and infusion time determine the peak and the interval determines the trough. It is, however, obvious that both factors affect each other. For example, if the peak level is too high and the trough level is OK, then the dose should be decreased. For gentamicin or tobramycin a decrease of 10 mg would result in a decrease in peak of about 1 µg/mL. If the peak is OK and the trough is too high, the interval is lengthened. Usual intervals using this technique are: 8, 12, 16, 24, 36, and 48 hours. The interval is decreased if the peak is OK and the trough is too low. Many such manipulations are possible depending on the observed levels.

Nomogram Methods

Another popular method used to develop aminoglycoside dosage regimens employs a nomogram.[282–287] Advantages are ease of use and ready availability. The disadvantage of nomograms is that they were developed using a limited number of patients and are applicable to adult subjects only. They also rely on measurement of creatinine clearance or estimation by standard formulas for regimen development, both of which are fraught with potential inaccuracies. It has also been determined that only 38% of the variance in elimination rate of gentamicin is explained by differences in creatinine clearance.[285] Nomogram methods are also inaccurate if renal function is changing. As nomograms are designed to achieve fixed peak and trough concentrations, they do not allow individualization of dosages based on severity of infection and risk of toxicity. They cannot be used to adjust dosage regimens based on measured serum concentrations. In addition, they rely on mean pharmacokinetic data and are not adaptable to patients who do not conform to these values.

Nomograms cannot account for the wide patient variability in aminoglycoside disposition; however, they serve as a reasonable guide to initial choice of dosing. The Sarubbi–Hull nomogram is easy to use and is widely available. As with other nomograms, the therapeutic peak levels required to treat seriously ill patients may not be achieved.[285,287] Follow-up serum level determinations are mandatory to ensure the presence of therapeutic, nontoxic concentrations when using nomograms.

Individualized Methods

General Considerations

The preceding methods require little understanding of pharmacokinetic concepts and formula manipulation. They are easy to use and are likely to be adequate for initiation of therapy. The dosage adjustment based on serum levels may be based on clinical experience or the use of pharmacokinetic concepts and formulas. Because of the wide variability in the pharmacokinetics of aminoglycoside antibiotics, and the narrow therapeutic range, efforts have been made to individualize therapy based on pharmacokinetic principles. These efforts may include the use of population data to develop initial dosage regimens (loading and maintenance dosing) to be followed by measurement of serum levels and dose adjustment.

Much discussion has been generated regarding the most appropriate pharmacokinetic model to use for dosing considerations. As discussed previously, the aminoglycoside antibiotics are best described by a three-compartment model; however, as this model is quite cumbersome, a two-compartment and more frequently a one-compartment model have been employed in dosing. The two-compartment model developed by Schentag et al adequately accounts for the observed increase in peak and trough levels with no apparent change in renal function noted with repeated dosing of the aminoglycoside antibiotics.[60,72,73,181] The one-compartment model does not take this rise into consideration. The validity of the Schentag et al two-compartment model has been documented in that it accurately predicts tissue accumulation in vivo.[60] Few direct comparisons on the validity in dosing between the one- and two-compartment models have been undertaken.[288,289] No significant difference in prediction of trough concentrations of tobramycin was noted between one-compartment and two-compartment models in one study.[288] The Schentag et al two-compartment models tended to overestimate the trough concentrations. When using the one-compartment model for dosing, one must be cognizant of the fact that an observed increase in peak and trough concentrations is a normal consequence of repeated dosing of these agents. The advantage of using the two-compartment model is that an increase above the predicted trough levels may indicate increased tissue accumulation and risk of toxicity.[207] Increased observation of the patient and monitoring would thus be indicated. Taking these cautionary notes into consideration, the one-compartment model is adequate for routine dosing and monitoring of these antibiotics.

Determining Loading and Maintenance Doses

All individualized methods begin by calculating an initial loading dose and maintenance dose. These doses are out of necessity based on initial parameters estimated from population data (see Table 9–1). The regimen is initiated and serum concentrations are obtained. Individualized dosing is then performed on the basis of the observed results. The following discussion focuses on methods used to determine loading and maintenance doses of the aminoglycoside antibiotics with one-compartment pharmacokinetic principles. Initial assessment of the patient as mentioned above should be entertained. The patient data needed include age, gender, weight, height, BUN, and serum creatinine or, if available, creatinine clearance. Choice of aminoglycoside and site and severity of infection assist in determining target peak concentrations.

Loading Dose. Let us do this by running through a practice case. You are asked to provide an initial loading dose and maintenance regimens for a 65-year-old gentleman with a presumed Gram-negative pneumonia. He weighs 155 pounds and is 5 ft 7 in. tall. His serum creatinine is 1.2 mg/dL. No other information is available at this time except that the physician wants to use gentamicin. Assuming that his renal function is stable we can begin by calculating a creatinine clearance (Cl_{cr}). Refer to Table 9–15 for description of pharmacokinetic terms.

Calculate ideal body weight using Equation 9–1. Using this equation, the patient's IBW is 66.1 kg: [(ABW in kg) − (weight in pounds)]/2.2 lb/kg = 70.4 kg. Calculate Cl_{cr} using the following formula developed in patients 18 to 92 years of age.[290]

$$\text{Males} \quad Cl_{cr} = (140 - \text{age})(\text{IBW})/72 \times S_{cr}(\text{mg/dL}) \qquad (9\text{–}6)$$

$$\text{Females} \quad Cl_{cr} = 0.85(Cl_{cr} \text{ males}) \qquad (9\text{–}7)$$

Using Equation 9–6, his creatinine clearance is 57.4 mL/min.

A formula for estimating glomerular filtration rate (GFR) from birth to age 21 has been investigated.[291]

$$\text{GFR} = kL/P_{cr} \qquad (9\text{–}8)$$

Glomerular filtration rate is expressed in mL/min/1.73 m^2, k (a proportionality constant) is a

TABLE 9–15. DEFINITIONS OF PHARMACOKINETIC TERMS

S_{cr}	Serum creatinine
Cl_{cr}	Creatinine clearance
GFR	Glomerular filtration rate
D	Dose
$t_{1/2}$	Half-life of elimination (h)
V_d	Volume of distribution (L)
Cl	Clearance
TBC	Total body clearance
C_{max}	Serum concentration at end of infusion (µg/mL)
C_{min}	Serum concentration prior to start of infusion (µg/mL)
$C_{max,ss}$	Maximum steady-state concentration
$C_{min,ss}$	Minimum steady-state concentration
C_{post}	Measured serum concentration after end of infusion
C_{pre}	Measured serum concentration prior to dose at which C_{post} is measured
t'	Duration of infusion (h)
τ	Dosing interval (h)
t_1	Period between end of infusion and time when C_{post} is obtained
t_2	Period between when C_{pre} was drawn and beginning of infusion

function of urinary creatinine elimination per unit of body size, L refers to body length in centimeters, and P_{cr} represents plasma creatinine. k can be determined by measuring the GFR and solving Equation 9–8, or average population data can be used. The estimates of GFR can be used in place of Cl_{cr} to generate the pharmacokinetic parameters mentioned below for this age group.

Once the Cl_{cr} is calculated there are various methods to calculate the half-life. We use the method of Sarubbi and Hull.[284]

$$t_{1/2} = 0.693/[0.0024(Cl_{cr}) + 0.01] \qquad (9\text{–}9)$$

Using Equation 9–9, his $t_{1/2}$ is 4.69 hours.

Next we need to calculate the volume of distribution (Equation 9–5) for this patient. Using a population value of 0.26 L/kg we arrive at a value of 17.2 L (66.1 kg × 0.26 L/kg). Now we can determine the loading dose (LD) for our patient using

$$LD\ (mg) = C_{max}(0.693/t_{1/2})\ V_d\ t'/(1 - e^{-(0.693/t_{1/2})\,t'}) \qquad (9\text{–}10)$$

to achieve a peak level in the range 8 to 10 µg/mL based on severity of disease and penetration issues discussed above for infection in the lung. Let us pick a level of 8 µg/mL for our initial dose. For this simulation let us use a t' of 1 hour and a C_{max} of 8 µg/mL. Running through the calculation, the recommended loading dose is 148 mg. After rounding to the nearest 10 mg you would recommend a loading dose of 150 mg of gentamicin, infused over 1 hour.

Maintenance Dose. Now let us calculate a maintenance dose to maintain the peak concentration of 8 μg/mL and trough level of 1.0 μg/mL. To calculate the maintenance dose and interval we start by calculating the dosing interval:

$$\tau = [(-1/0.693/t_{1/2}) \ln C_{min,ss}/C_{max,ss}] + t' \qquad (9\text{--}11)$$

Using a t' of 1 hour, the calculated dosage interval would be 15.1 hours. Rounding to the nearest reasonable interval (6, 8, 12, 16, 24), we choose a 16-hour dosing schedule.

With this completed, we plug the information into the steady-state intermittent intravenous infusion equation (assume t' is 1 hour):

$$\text{dose (mg)} = C_{max,ss} \, V_d \, (0.693/t_{1/2}) \, t'[1-e^{-(0.693/t_{1/2})\tau}]/[1-e^{-(0.693/t_{1/2})t'}] \qquad (9\text{--}12)$$

The maintenance dose is 134 μg/mL administered every 16 hours. Rounding the dose to the nearest 10 mg results in a maintenance dose of gentamicin 130 mg every 16 hours. Because the loading dose, maintenance dose, and dosing interval are rounded off, the predicted levels will be different from the ones you picked. To calculate the actual predicted concentrations, you can use the following equations. To calculate the C_{max} after the loading dose (150 mg), plug the known information into

$$C_{max} \, (\mu g/mL) = LD[1-e^{-(0.693/t_{1/2})t'}]/0.693/t_{1/2} \, V_d \, t' \qquad (9\text{--}13)$$

Solving this equation would give a peak of 8.1 μg/mL after a loading dose of 150 mg. Calculate the $C_{max,ss}$ and $C_{min,ss}$ expected from this maintenance regimen (130 mg q16h):

$$C_{max,ss} \, (\mu g/mL) = \text{dose}[1-e^{-(0.693/t_{1/2})t'}]/V_d \, (0.693/t_{1/2}) \, t'[1-e^{-(0.693/t_{1/2})\tau}] \qquad (9\text{--}14)$$

$$C_{min,ss} \, (\mu g/mL) = C_{max,ss} \, e^{-(0.693/t_{1/2})(\tau-t')} \qquad (9\text{--}15)$$

The maintenance dose of 130 q16h is predicted to yield an approximate steady-state peak and trough of 7.8 and 0.85 μg/mL, respectively. Follow-up peak and trough concentrations can be obtained after three to five doses.

Follow-up Serum Concentration Manipulations
Results of follow-up concentrations (peak and trough) can be used to further individualize the pharmacokinetic variables with the following equations. First obtain peak and trough levels at steady state. Note times of trough, time of start and stop of the infusion, infusion dose, time of last dose, and time the peak was drawn in relation to the end of the infusion. These times are crucial to the proper use of the formulas. Having obtained correctly timed samples and infusion times, we can proceed. First determine the aminoglycoside half-life:

$$t_{1/2} = 0.693[\tau - (t_1 + t_2 + t')]/\ln(C_{post}/C_{pre}) \qquad (9\text{--}16)$$

Then calculate C_{max} and C_{min}:

$$C_{max} = C_{post}/e^{-(0.693/t_{1/2})t_1} \qquad (9\text{--}17)$$

$$C_{min} = (C_{pre})(e^{-(0.693/t_{1/2})t_2}) \qquad (9\text{--}18)$$

Now we can estimate a volume of distribution from the observed data:

$$V_d = (D/t'/0.693/t_{1/2}) \, [1-e^{-(0.693/t_{1/2})t'}]/C_{max} - C_{min}e^{-(0.693/t_{1/2})t'} \qquad (9\text{--}19)$$

With these new parameters, dosage adjustments can be made using Equations 9–11 and 9–12 to determine a new interval and dose to achieve desired values. Of course, if the observed levels are in the desired range no adjustment is necessary and monitoring for therapeutic response (ie, resolution of infection) and adverse reactions can continue.

Fitted Method

The fitted method involves the use of population data for initial dosage determination.[292] A trough and peak pair is then obtained at steady state. A set volume of distribution is used throughout the model and a $t_{1/2}$ that best fits into the following Equations to predict the observed serum trough level is determined. This half-life is then used to determine subsequent dosing regimens for the aminoglycoside antibiotics.

$$C_{max} = \{D[1-e^{-(0.693/t_{1/2})t'}]/(0.693/t_{1/2})V_d\} + C_{min}e^{-(0.693/t_{1/2})t'} \tag{9–20}$$

$$C_{min} = C_{max}e^{-(0.693/t_{1/2})(\tau-t')} \tag{9–21}$$

As discussed under Nomogram Methods, which also incorporates population data, the fitted method compares favorably with the Sawchuk–Zaske method.[286] The procedure requires a hand-held programmable calculator or similar device to be clinically useful. The exact times of all administered doses up to the time the trough concentration was obtained must be recorded. Such reliable record keeping may not be available at all institutions. To use this method, kidney function must be stable.

Sawchuk–Zaske Method

Sawchuk and Zaske developed a method to individualize aminoglycoside therapy by obtaining serial serum concentrations around a dose and determining the actual pharmacokinetic parameters for the individual patient.[293] Serial samples can be obtained after the first dose or after multiple doses. Three samples are obtained after the first dose, including a sample at the end of the distribution phase (0.5–1 hour after the end of the infusion; 1 to 2 hours in patients with a creatinine clearance less than 45 mL/min or with ascites).[294] Samples 2 and 3 are obtained over a period that allows the serum concentrations to fall through a minimum of one estimated half-life. Four samples are obtained if the patient is already receiving aminoglycoside antibiotics. Samples are as after the first dose, with the exception of a sample prior to the dose to be studied.

A one-compartment open linear pharmacokinetic model with first-order elimination is used. Nonlinear regression analysis is used to estimate the patient's half-life, C_{max}, and C_{min}. Data points can also be plotted on semilogarithmic paper and the $t_{1/2}$, C_{max}, and C_{min} taken from the graph. V_d is then calculated using Equation 9–19. The $C_{min}e^{-(0.693/t_{1/2})t'}$ portion of the equation is omitted if first-dose data are obtained. The resulting individualized $t_{1/2}$ and V_d are then used to generate a new dosing regimen using Equations 9–11 and 9–12 in that order. Individualized pharmacokinetic parameters are generated every 3 days during aminoglycoside administration. This technique provides an accurate method to assist in dosing patients.[286] Toxicity is also low, with only 0.9% of 1640 patients experiencing nephrotoxicity during gentamicin therapy monitored by this method.[37]

The method is labor intensive and expensive, and requires multiple samples throughout the course of therapy. The volume of distribution determined by this method is larger than that generated by the area method. The fact that these antibiotics conform to a multicompartmental pharmacokinetic model is reflected in a general underprediction of trough concentration when the Sawchuk–Zaske method is used.[295] The use of first-dose pharmacokinetics to predict subsequent serum concentrations may explain the observed results.[296,297] The Sawchuk–Zaske technique is extremely valuable in seriously ill patients with changing clinical status or renal function and is the method of choice in such situations.

Studies on the effect of decreasing the number of postinfusion levels on the pharmacokinetic parameters of these antibiotics have been published.[294,298] In general, no apparent clinically significant difference in pharmacokinetic data has been noted when two postinfusion samples are compared with three. If a two-point method is used it is imperative that very close attention be paid to obtaining the first postinfusion level after distribution is completed. Exact timing of doses, infusion duration, and times of sample collection is also imperative.

Single-Dose Dosing Considerations

Single-dose aminoglycoside dosing has the potential to revolutionize the way these agents are administered. In most studies, the standard dose is administered once daily in patients with normal kidney function. Doses of 4 to 5 mg/kg for gentamicin and tobramycin, 5 to 6.6 mg/kg for netilmicin, and 15 to 20 mg/kg for amikacin have been employed. Gilbert et al have suggested a nomogram for single-dose therapy in patients with varying degrees of kidney function.[299] They suggest a reduction of dose in patients with decreased kidney function. The problem with this approach is that it may not take full advantage of the concentration-dependent killing activity of the aminoglycoside antibiotics as kidney function deteriorates. A dosing method using pharmacokinetic principles has been developed by Nicolau et al.[176] It is based on the observation that aminoglycosides kill effectively when peak concentrations are more than eight times the MIC of the organism involved.[8,9] Their model for dosing involves a standard loading dose for gentamicin and tobramycin of 7 mg/kg and a dosing interval designed to allow the serum concentration to fall below 2 µg/mL prior to the next dose. The dose is based on their population pharmacokinetics and a desire to achieve a peak concentration of approximately 20 µg/mL gentamicin and tobramycin (10 times the MIC for *Pseudomonas aeruginosa* at their hospital). The dose is placed in 50 mL of fluid and infused over 60 minutes. The initial dosing interval is determined based on estimates of creatinine clearance. A patient with a creatinine clearance of 60 mL/min or greater would receive the dose every 24 hours; with a clearance of 40 to 59 mL/min, every 36 hours; and with a clearance of 20 to 39 mL/min, every 48 hours. A patient with a creatinine clearance less than 20 mL/min would have serum concentrations monitored until the level was less than 2 µg/mL.

Nicolau et al have developed a nomogram to assist in determining the dosing interval once serum concentration information is available (Figure 9–1). Serum concentrations are obtained approximately 6 to 14 hours after the start of an infusion and the result is plotted on the nomogram. If the level is within the q24h, q36h, or q48h area, that dosing interval is chosen. If the result is on the line, the longer interval is chosen. If the level falls off the nomogram, the serum concentration will need to be monitored until it falls below 2 µg/mL. For amikacin a dose of 15 mg/kg is used and a level obtained as described above. The observed level is divided in half and the result placed on the nomogram. More frequent monitoring of serum levels is necessary in patients with changing renal function. Serum concentrations should be repeated every 4 days. Results for the first 31 patients on this regimen have been published and no untoward events were noted.[176] More than 1000 patients have been studied to date (personal communication).

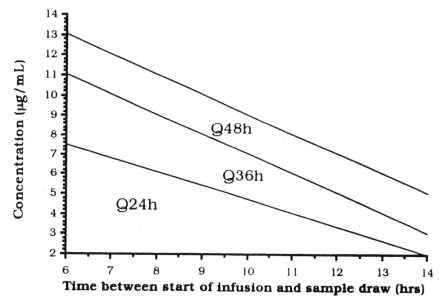

Figure 9–1. Single-dose aminoglycoside nomogram. (*From Nicolau D, Quintiliani R, Nightingale CH. Once-daily aminoglycosides.* Conn Med. *1992;56:561–563, with permission.*)

Nephrotoxicity has been noted in 1.2% of subjects and ototoxicity in less than 1%. Current data are not sufficient to recommend the use of single-dose therapy in children; in patients with burns, ascites, or previous hearing loss; in dialysis patients; or in those patients in whom the aminoglycoside is being used for synergy (ie, endocarditis).

Bayesian Method

The newest technique for individualizing dosing of the aminoglycoside antibiotics is based on the principles of bayesian forecasting.[300] The technique allows the use of statistical considerations of probability in pharmacokinetic monitoring. Initial dosage regimens are based on population-derived estimates of volume of distribution and clearance, as mentioned above (Determining Loading and Maintenance Doses). Input of serum aminoglycoside concentrations obtained in the patient triggers the bayesian feedback loop to adjust the population-derived volume of distribution and clearance to fit the observed levels. The relative adjustment of the two parameters is affected by the population standard deviations. The program also weighs serum drug concentrations such that the most recently obtained level receives the most weight. The program then uses these new pharmacokinetic parameters to develop new dosage regimens. Other parameters, such as variability in drug assay, can be included in the analysis. The validity of bayesian forecasting has been well studied and compares favorably with the Sawchuk–Zaske method.[301–304] A major advantage over the Sawchuk–Zaske method is that the bayesian technique requires fewer blood samples while maintaining similar precision and accuracy.

The use of specific patient population pharmacokinetics has been shown to improve the predictive performance of bayesian analysis.[305,306] Bayesian forecasting has also been applied to low-birth-weight infants.[307]

SUMMARY

Use of the aminoglycoside antibiotics has been decreasing over the last few years. Although they have been supplanted by newer, less toxic agents, they remain an important part of our antibiotic armamentarium. The new single-dose regimens appear to be safe and effective. Less frequent dosing may decrease cost of therapy in that monitoring is simplified and nursing and pharmacist time may be conserved. The need to prepare the individual doses must be factored in, however. Development of resistance to the third-generation antibiotics is becoming worrisome and the aminoglycoside agents may be an alternative. Diligent attention to their correct use and monitoring must be continued, so when they are needed their benefit will be maximized.

_____ QUESTIONS _____

1. A 30-week-old premature infant born at 28 weeks' gestation requires gentamicin for suspected Gram-negative sepsis. The infant is initiated on a dose of 2.5 mg/kg every 8 hours. The regimen was chosen from dosing guidelines based on postnatal age. The patient's kidney function is normal. You are asked to follow up and monitor the patient's aminoglycoside levels.
   a. Is an initial dosing regimen based on postnatal age appropriate for the patient?
   b. Based on your dosing and monitoring recommendations, follow-up peak and trough aminoglycoside concentrations are 2.5 and 2.7 µg/mL, respectively. The timing and labeling of the blood samples are appropriate. What is your assessment of these results? What would you recommend?

2. J.F. is a 9-year-old, 30-kg male patient admitted for pulmonary exacerbation of his cystic fibrosis. Sputum cultures from his previous admission, 2 months earlier, indicated the presence of *Pseudomonas aeruginosa*. His WBC is 13.7, and his BUN/S_{cr} are 10 mg/dL/0.5 mg/dL. He is empirically placed on tobramycin 90 mg IV every 8 hours and ceftazidime 1.5 g IV every 6 hours based on the organism's previous sensitivity.
   a. Explain some of the possible reasons why dosing of aminoglycoside antibiotics is high in cystic fibrosis patients when compared with dosing in subjects without cystic fibrosis.
   b. Peak and trough tobramycin serum concentrations are obtained around the third dose. The results are reported as a peak of 27 µg/mL and a trough of 0.3 µg/mL. Explain these results.
   c. In the above situation how is drug sampling best handled to provide interpretable results?

I am indebted to Barbara Maas, University of Massachusetts Medical Center, for her contribution of Questions 1 and 2.

3. R.D. is a 55-year-old man who presented to the hospital with a chief complaint of neck pain for 3 weeks. Computed axial tomography of the neck revealed the presence of an extramedullary tumor. He underwent a cervical laminectomy and, 3 days after surgery, was found to have aspirated mouth contents. He was begun on cefuroxime and clindamycin. Culture of sputum grew out *Serratia marcescens* and the patient's antibiotics were switched to tobramycin 120 mg q8h and piperacillin 2 g q4h. The patient weighs 222 pounds and is 5 ft 10 in. tall. His serum creatinine is 1.0 mg/dL.

    a. How would you monitor this case?
    b. Peak and trough serum concentrations are drawn 30 minutes after and before a dose. The infusion time was also 30 minutes. The observed peak and trough were 9.4 and 5.0 µg/mL, respectively. How can you explain these levels in a patient with a creatinine of 1.0 mg/dL?
    c. You suggest a dosage regimen change to achieve a peak of 8 to 10 µg/mL and trough of 1.5 µg/mL. Because of the possibility of synergy with the piperacillin and a concern for ototoxicity, the physician wants peaks around 7 µg/mL. The patient is also responding nicely to the therapy. Suggest a dosage regimen.

4. E.K. is a 69-year-old man with acute myelogenous leukemia undergoing chemotherapy. During a cycle of chemotherapy, he spikes a fever and is found to have a WBC of 400 mg/cm^3. He is begun on tobramycin and piperacillin therapy. Three days later, peak and trough tobramycin serum concentrations are obtained and they are 1.0 and 0 µg/mL, respectively. The physician increases the dose of tobramycin and orders repeat peak and trough concentrations. These levels come back as 1.2 and 0 µg/mL, respectively. You are asked to comment.

REFERENCES

1. Chow JW, Fine MJ, Shlaes DM, et al. Enterobacter bacteremia: Clinical features and emergence of antibiotic resistance during therapy. *Ann Intern Med.* 1991;ll5:585–590.
2. Kim-Sing A, Kays MB, James VE, et al. Intravenous streptomycin use in a patient infected with high-level, gentamicin-resistant *Streptococcus faecalis. Ann Pharmacother.* 1993;27:712–714.
3. Fichtenbaum CJ, Ritchie DJ, Powderly WG. Use of paromomycin for treatment of cryptosporidiosis in patients with AIDS. *Clin Infect Dis.* 1993;16:298–300.
4. Jorup-Ronstrom C, Julander I, Petrini B. Efficacy of triple drug regimen of amikacin, ethambutol and rifabutin in AIDS patients with symptomatic *Mycobacterium avium* complex infection. *J Infect.* 1993;26:67–70.
5. Rolston KV, Chandrasekar PH, LeFrock JL, et al. The activity of ceftazidime, other β-lactams, and aminoglycosides against *Pseudomonas aeruginosa. Chemotherapy.* 1984;30;31–34.
6. Vogelman B, Gudmundsson S, Turnidge J, et al. In vivo postantibiotic effect in a thigh infection in neutropenic mice. *J Infect Dis.* 1988;157:287–298.
7. Zhanel GG, Hoban DJ, Harding KM. The postantibiotic effect: A review of in vitro and in vivo data. *Drug Intell Clin Pharm.* 1991;25:153–163.
8. Nilsson L, Sörén L, Rådberg G. Frequencies of variants resistant to different aminoglycosides in *Pseudomonas aeruginosa. J Antimicrob Chemother.* 1987;20:255–259.

9. Blaser J, Stone BB, Groner MC, et al. Comparative study with enoxacin and netilmicin in a pharmacodynamic model to determine importance of ratio of antibiotic peak concentration to MIC for bactericidal activity and emergence of resistance. *Antimicrob Agents Chemother.* 1987;31:1054–1060.

10. Daikos GL, Lolans VT, Jackson GG. First-exposure adaptive resistance to aminoglycoside antibiotics in vivo with meaning for optimal clinical use. *Antimicrob Agents Chemother.* 1991;35:117–123.

11. Pechere J-C, Dugal R. Clinical pharmacokinetics of aminoglycoside antibiotics. *Clin Pharmacokinet.* 1979;4:170–199.

12. García G, de Vidal EL, Trujillo H. Serum levels and urinary concentrations of kanamicin, bekanamicin, and amikacin (BB-K8) in diabetic children and a control group. *J Int Med Res.* 1977;5:322–329.

13. Smeltzer BD, Schwartzman MS, Bertino JS. Amikacin pharmacokinetics during continuous ambulatory peritoneal dialysis. *Antimicrob Agents Chemother.* 1988;32:236–240.

14. Neale TJ, Malani J, Humble M. Netilmicin in the treatment of clinical peritonitis in chronic renal failure patients managed by continuous ambulatory peritoneal dialysis. *NZ Med J.* 1987;100:374–377.

15. Walshe JJ, Morse GD, Janicke DM, et al. Crossover pharmacokinetic analysis comparing intravenous and intraperitoneal administration of tobramycin. *J Infect Dis.* 1986;153:796–799.

16. Pancorbo S, Comty C. Pharmacokinetics of gentamicin in patients undergoing continuous ambulatory peritoneal dialysis. *Antimicrob Agents Chemother.* 1981;19:605–607.

17. Bunke CM, Aronoff GR, Brier ME, et al. Tobramycin kinetics during continuous ambulatory peritoneal dialysis. *Clin Pharmacol Ther.* 1983;34:110–116.

18. Somani P, Shapiro RS, Stockard H, et al. Unidirectional absorption of gentamicin from the peritoneum during continuous ambulatory peritoneal dialysis. *Clin Pharmacol Ther.* 1982;32:113–121.

19. Rubin J, Deraps GD, Walsh D, et al. Protein losses and tobramycin absorption in peritonitis treated by hourly peritoneal dialysis. *Am J Kidney Dis.* 1986;8:124–127.

20. Crosby SS, Edwards D, Brennan C, et al. Systemic absorption of endotracheally administered aminoglycosides in seriously ill patients with pneumonia. *Antimicrob Agents Chemother.* 1987;31:850–853.

21. Stillwell PC, Kearns GL, Jacobs RF. Endotracheal tobramycin in gram-negative pneumonitis. *Drug Intell Clin Pharm.* 1988;22:577–581.

22. Bunetel L, Segui A, Cormier M, et al. Comparative study of gentamicin release from normal and low viscosity acrylic bone cement. *Clin Pharmacokinet.* 1990;19:333–340.

23. Bloome MR, Warren AJ, Ringer L, et al. Evaluation of an empirical dosing schedule for gentamicin in neonates. *Drug Intell Clin Pharm.* 1988;22:618–622.

24. Miranda JC, Schimmel MM, James LS, et al. Gentamicin kinetics in the neonate. *Pediatr Pharmacol.* 1985;5:57–61.

25. Kuhn RJ, Nahata MC, Powell DA, et al. Pharmacokinetics of netilmicin in premature infants. *Eur J Clin Pharmacol.* 1986;29:635–637.

26. Kenyon CF, Knoppert DC, Lee SK, et al. Amikacin pharmacokinetics and suggested dosage modifications for the preterm infant. *Antimicrob Agents Chemother.* 1990;34:265–268.

27. Nahata MC, Powell DA, Durrell DE, et al. Tobramycin pharmacokinetics in very low birth weight infants. *Br J Clin Pharmacol.* 1986;21:325–327.

28. Nahata MC, Powell DA, Gregoire RP, et al. Clinical and laboratory observations. Tobramycin kinetics in newborn infants. *J Pediatr.* 1983;103:136–138.

29. Sardemann H, Colding H, Hendel J, et al. Kinetics and dose calculations of amikacin in the newborn. *Clin Pharmacol Ther.* 1976;20:59–66.

30. Myers MG, Roberts RJ, Mirhij NJ. Effects of gestational age, birth weight and hypoxemia on pharmacokinetics of amikacin in serum of infants. *Antimicrob Agents Chemother.* 1977;11:1027–1032.

31. Cleary TG, Pickering LK, Kramer WG, et al. Amikacin pharmacokinetics in pediatric patients with malignancy. *Antimicrob Agents Chemother.* 1979;16:829–832.

32. Vogelstein B, Kowarski AA, Lietman PS. The pharmacokinetics of amikacin in children. *J Pediatr.* 1977;91:333–339.

33. Zaske DE, Strate RG, Kohls PR. Amikacin pharmacokinetics: Wide interpatient variation in 98 patients. *J Clin Pharmacol.* 1991;31:158–163.
34. Kalenga M, Devos D, Moulin D, et al. The need for pharmacokinetic monitoring of gentamicin therapy in critically ill neonates. *Dev Pharmacol Ther.* 1984;7(suppl 1):130–133.
35. Paisley JW, Smith AL, Smith DH. Gentamicin in newborn infants. Comparison of intramuscular and intravenous administration. *Am J Dis Child.* 1973;126:473–477.
36. McCracken GH. Clinical pharmacology of gentamicin in infants 2 to 24 months of age. *Am J Dis Child.* 1972;124:884–887.
37. Zaske DE, Cipolle RJ, Rotschafer JC, et al. Gentamicin pharmacokinetics in 1,640 patients: Method for control of serum concentrations. *Antimicrob Agents Chemother.* 1982;21:407–411.
38. Lackner TE, Birge S. Accuracy of pharmacokinetic dose determination of gentamicin in geriatric patients. *Drug Intell Clin Pharm.* 1990;24:29–32.
39. Zaske DE, Irvine P, Strand LM, et al. Wide interpatient variations in gentamicin dose requirements for geriatric patients. *JAMA.* 1982;248:3122–3126.
40. Siegel JD, McCracken GH, Thomas ML, et al. Pharmacokinetic properties of netilmicin in newborn infants. *Antimicrob Agents Chemother.* 1979;15:246–253.
41. Bergan T, Michalsen H. Pharmacokinetic assessment of netilmicin in newborns and older children. *Infection.* 1982;10:153–158.
42. Rotschafer JC, Crossley KB, Zaske DE, et al. Clinical use of a one-compartment model for determining netilmicin pharmacokinetic parameters and dosage recommendations. *Ther Drug Monit.* 1983;5:263–267.
43. Welling PG, Baumueller A, Lau CC, et al. Netilmicin pharmacokinetics after single intravenous doses to elderly male patients. *Antimicrob Agents Chemother.* 1977;12:328–334.
44. Yoshioka H, Takimoto M, Fujita K, et al. Pharmacokinetics of tobramycin in the newborn. *Infection.* 1979;7:180–182.
45. Hoecker JL, Pickering LK, Swaney J, et al. Clinical pharmacology of tobramycin in children. *J Infect Dis.* 1978;137:592–596.
46. Cipolle RJ, Seifert RD, Zaske DE, et al. Systematically individualizing tobramycin dosage regimens. *J Clin Pharmacol.* 1980;20:570–580.
47. Donauer E, Drumm G, Moringlane J, et al. Intrathecal administration of netilmicin in gentamicin-resistant ventriculitis. *Acta Neurochir.* 1987;86:83–88.
48. Valcke Y, Pauwels R, Van Der Straeten M. Pharmacokinetics of antibiotics in the lungs. *Eur Respir J.* 1990;3:715–722.
49. Alexander MR, Schoell J, Hicklin G, et al. Bronchial secretion concentrations of tobramycin. *Am Rev Respir Dis.* 1982;125:208–209.
50. Schurman DJ, Wheeler R. Gram-negative bone and joint infection: Sixty patients treated with amikacin. *Clin Orthop.* 1978;134:268–274.
51. Dee TH, Kozin F. Gentamicin and tobramycin penetration into synovial fluid. *Antimicrob Agents Chemother.* 1977;12:548–549.
52. Bermúdez RH, Lugo A, Ramírez-Ronda CH, et al. Amikacin levels in human serum and bile. *Antimicrob Agents Chemother.* 1981;19:352–354.
53. Barza M. Treatment of bacterial infections of the eye. In: Remington JS, Swartz MN, eds. *Current Clinical Topics in Infectious Disease, 1.* New York: McGraw Hill; 1980:158–194.
54. Orr WM, Jackson WB, Colden K. Intraocular penetration of netilmicin. *Can J Ophthalmol.* 1985;20:171–175.
55. Woo FL, Johnson AP, Insler MS, et al. Gentamicin, tobramycin, amikacin, and netilmicin levels in tears following intravenous administration. *Arch Ophthalmol.* 1985;103:216–218.
56. Gerding DN, Wendell HH, Schierl EA. Antibiotic concentrations in ascitic fluid of patients with ascites and bacterial peritonitis. *Ann Intern Med.* 1977;86:708–713.

57. Fevery J, Zachee P, Verbist L. Concentrations of gentamicin in ascitic fluid after intravenous infusion. *Neth J Med.* 1983;26:191–192.

58. Lanao JM, Dominguez-Gil A, Macias JG, et al. The influence of ascites on the pharmacokinetics of amikacin. *Int J Clin Pharmacol Ther Toxicol.* 1980;18:57–61.

59. Smithivas T, Hyams PJ, Matalon R, et al. The use of gentamicin in peritoneal dialysis. I. Pharmacologic results. *J Infect Dis.* 1971;124(suppl):77–83.

60. Schentag JJ, Jusko WJ, Vance JW, et al. Gentamicin disposition and tissue accumulation on multiple dosing. *J Pharmacokinet Biopharm.* 1977;5:559–577.

61. Whelton A, Carter GG, Craig TJ, et al. Comparison of the intrarenal disposition of tobramycin and gentamicin: Therapeutic and toxicologic answers. *J Antimicrob Chemother.* 1978;4(suppl A):13–22.

62. De Broe ME, Giuliano RA, Verpooten GA. Choice of drug and dosage regimen. Two important risk factors for aminoglycoside nephrotoxicity. *Am J Med.* 1986;80(suppl 6B):115–118.

63. De Broe ME, Verbist L, Verpooten GA. Influence of dosage schedule on renal cortical accumulation of amikacin and tobramycin in man. *J Antimicrob Chemother.* 1991;27(suppl C):41–47.

64. Verpooten GA, Giuliano RA, Verbist L, et al. Once-daily dosing decreases renal accumulation of gentamicin and netilmicin. *Clin Pharmacol Ther.* 1989;45:22–27.

65. Bernard B, Abate M, Thielen PF, et al. Maternal–fetal pharmacological activity of amikacin. *J Infect Dis.* 1977;135:925–932.

66. Bernard B, Garcia-Caizares, Ballard SJ, et al. Tobramycin: Maternal–fetal pharmacology. *Antimicrob Agents Chemother.* 1977;11:688–694.

67. Smilack JD, Flittie WH, Williams TW. Bone concentrations of antimicrobial agents after parenteral administration. *Antimicrob Agents Chemother.* 1976;9:169–171.

68. Rosin H, Rosin A-M, Krämer J. Determination of antibiotic levels in human bone. I. Gentamicin levels in bone. *Infection.* 1974;2:3–6.

69. Serour F, Dan M, Gorea A, et al. Penetration of aminoglycosides into human peritoneal tissue. *Chemotherapy.* 1990;36:251–253.

70. Thadepalli H, Lou MA, Prabhala RH, et al. Human intestinal tissue antibiotic concentrations. Clindamycin, gentamicin, and mezlocillin. *Am Surg.* 1990;56:655–658.

71. Burkle WS. Comparative evaluation of the aminoglycoside antibiotics for systemic use. *Drug Intell Clin Pharm.* 1981;15:847–862.

72. Schentag JJ, Lasezkay G, Cumbo TJ, et al. Accumulation pharmacokinetics of tobramycin. *Antimicrob Agents Chemother.* 1978;13:649–656.

73. French MA, Cerra FB, Plaut ME, et al. Amikacin and gentamicin accumulation pharmacokinetics and nephrotoxicity in critically ill patients. *Antimicrob Agents Chemother.* 1981;19:147–152.

74. Edwards DJ, Mangione A, Cumbo TJ, et al. Predicted tissue accumulation of netilmicin in patients. *Antimicrob Agents Chemother.* 1981;20:714–717.

75. Matzke GR, Salem N, Bockbrader H, et al. The effect of peritoneal dialysis on the pharmacokinetics of amikacin. *Proc Clin Dial Transplant Forum.* 1980;10:302–304.

76. Regeur L, Colding H, Jensen H, et al. Pharmacokinetics of amikacin during hemodialysis and peritoneal dialysis. *Antimicrob Agents Chemother.* 1977;11:214–218.

77. Kojarern S, Arkaravichien W, Indraprasit S, et al. Dosing regimen of gentamicin during intermittent peritoneal dialysis. *J Clin Pharmacol.* 1989;29:140–143.

78. Indraprasit S, Ukaravichien V, Pummangura C, et al. Gentamicin removal during intermittent peritoneal dialysis. *Nephron.* 1986;44:18–21.

79. Thomson AH, Grant AC, Stuart R, et al. Gentamicin and vancomycin removal by continuous venovenous hemofiltration. *Drug Intell Clin Pharm.* 1991;25:127–129.

80. Armendariz E, Chelluri L, Ptachcinski R. Pharmacokinetics of amikacin during continuous venovenous hemofiltration. *Crit Care Med.* 1990;18:675–676.

81. Robert R, Rochard E, Malin F, et al. Amikacin pharmacokinetics during continuous veno-venous hemofiltration. *Crit Care Med.* 1991;19:588–589.

82. Zarowitz BJ, Anandan JV, Dumler F, et al. Continuous arteriovenous hemofiltration of aminoglycoside antibiotics in critically ill patients. *J Clin Pharmacol.* 1986;26:686–689.

83. Madhavan T, Yaremchuk K, Levin N, et al. Effect of renal failure and dialysis on the serum concentration of the aminoglycoside amikacin. *Antimicrob Agents Chemother.* 1976;10:464–466.

84. Armstrong DK, Hodgman T, Visconti JA, et al. Hemodialysis of amikacin in critically ill patients. *Crit Care Med.* 1988;16:517–520.

85. Melby MJ, Heissler JF, Grochowski EC, et al. Predicting serum gentamicin concentrations in patients undergoing hemodialysis. *Clin Pharm.* 1985;4:74–77.

86. Matzke GR, Halstenson CE, Keane WF. Hemodialysis elimination rates and clearance of gentamicin and tobramycin. *Antimicrob Agents Chemother.* 1984;25:128–130.

87. Herrero A, Ruiz Alarcó F, García Díez, JM, et al. Pharmacokinetics of netilmicin in renal insufficiency and hemodialysis. *Int J Clin Pharmacol Ther Toxicol.* 1988;26:84–87.

88. Halstenson CE, Berkseth RO, Mann HJ, et al. Aminoglycoside redistribution phenomenon after hemodialysis: Netilmicin and tobramycin. *Int J Clin Pharmacol Ther Toxicol.* 1987;25:50–55.

89. Herrero A, Ruiz Alarcó F, García-Díez JM, et al. Pharmacokinetics of netilmicin during hemodialysis: Comparison of four artificial kidneys. *Int J Clin Pharmacol Ther Toxicol.* 1988;26:605–609.

90. Catolico MM, Campbell S, Jones WN, et al. Time course of gentamicin serum concentration rebound following hemodialysis. *Drug Intell Clin Pharm.* 1987;21:46–49.

91. Basile C, DiMaggio A, Curino E, et al. Pharmacokinetics of netilmicin in hypertonic hemodiafiltration and standard hemodialysis. *Clin Nephrol.* 1985;24:305–309.

92. Bhatt-Mehta V, Johnson CE, Schumacher RE. Gentamicin pharmacokinetics in term neonates receiving extracorporeal membrane oxygenation. *Pharmacotherapy.* 1992;12:28–32.

93. Cohen P, Collart L, Prober CG, et al. Gentamicin pharmacokinetics in neonates undergoing extracorporeal membrane oxygenation. *Pediatr Infect Dis J.* 1990;9:562–566.

94. Bertino JS, Kliegman RM, Myers CM, et al. Alterations in gentamicin pharmacokinetics during neonatal exchange transfusion. *Dev Pharmacol Ther.* 1982;4:205–215.

95. Ouellette SM, Visconti JA, Kennedy MS. A pharmacokinetic evaluation of the effect of plasma exchange on tobramycin disposition. *Clin Exp Dial Apheresis.* 1983;7:225–233.

96. Klamerus KJ, Rodvold KA, Silverman NA, et al. Effect of cardiopulmonary bypass on vancomycin and netilmicin disposition. *Antimicrob Agents Chemother.* 1988;32:631–635.

97. Arant BS. Developmental patterns of renal functional maturation compared in the human neonate. *J Pediatr.* 1978;92:705–712.

98. Kildoo C, Modanlou HD, Komatsu G, et al. Developmental pattern of gentamicin kinetics in very low birth weight (VLBW) sick infants. *Dev Pharmacol Ther.* 1984;7:345–356.

99. McCracken GH, West NR, Horton LJ. Urinary excretion of gentamicin in the neonatal period. *J Infect Dis.* 1971;123:257–262.

100. Arbeter AM, Saccar CL, Eisner S, et al. Tobramycin sulfate elimination in premature infants. *J Pediatr.* 1983;103:131–135.

101. Kasik JW, Jenkins S, Leuschen MP, et al. Postconceptional age and gentamicin elimination half-life. *J Pediatr.* 1985;106:502–505.

102. Granati B, Assael BM, Chung M, et al. Clinical pharmacology of netilmicin in preterm and term infants. *J Pediatr.* 1985;106:664–669.

103. Nahata MC, Powell DA, Durrell DE, et al. Effect of gestational age and birth weight on tobramycin kinetics in newborn infants. *J Antimicrob Chemother.* 1984;14:59–65.

104. Pons G, d'Athis P, Rey E, et al. Gentamicin monitoring in neonates. *Ther Drug Monit.* 1988;10:421–427.

105. Husson C, Chevalier JY, Jezequel M, et al. Pharmacokinetic study of gentamicin in preterm and term neonates. *Dev Pharmacol Ther.* 1984;7(suppl 1):125–129.

106. McCracken GH, Jones LG. Gentamicin in the neonatal period. *Am J Dis Child.* 1970;120:524–533.

107. Siber G, Echeverria P, Smith A, et al. Pharmacokinetics of gentamicin in children and adults. *J Infect Dis.* 1975;132:637–651.

108. Kearns GL, Hilman BC, Wilson JT. Dosing implications of altered gentamicin disposition in patients with cystic fibrosis. *J Pediatr.* 1982;100:312–318.

109. Levy J, Smith AL, Koup JR, et al. Disposition of tobramycin in patients with cystic fibrosis: A prospective controlled study. *J Pediatr.* 1984;105:117–124.

110. Michalsen H, Bergan T. Pharmacokinetics of antibiotics in children with cystic fibrosis with particular reference to netilmicin. *Acta Pediatr Scand.* 1982;(suppl 301):101–105.

111. Kelly HB, Menendez R, Fan L, et al. Pharmacokinetics of tobramycin in cystic fibrosis. *J Pediatr.* 1982;100:318–321.

112. Delage G, Desautels L, Legault S, et al. Individualized aminoglycoside dosage regimens in patients with cystic fibrosis. *Drug Intell Clin Pharm.* 1988;22:386–389.

113. Autret E, Marchand S, Breteau M, et al. Pharmacokinetics of amikacin in cystic fibrosis: A study of bronchial diffusion. *Eur J Clin Pharmacol.* 1986;31:79–83.

114. Kildoo CW, Harralson AF, Folli HL, et al. Direct determination of tobramycin clearance in patients with mild-to-moderate cystic fibrosis. *Drug Intell Clin Pharm.* 1987;21:639–642.

115. MacDonald NE, Anas NG, Peterson RG, et al. Renal clearance of gentamicin in cystic fibrosis. *J Pediatr.* 1983;103:985–990.

116. Sampliner R, Perrier D, Powell R, et al. Influence of ascites on tobramycin pharmacokinetics. *J Clin Pharmacol.* 1984;24:43–46.

117. Gill MA, Kern JW. Altered gentamicin distribution in ascitic patients. *Am J Hosp Pharm.* 1979;36:1704–1706.

118. Matthews SJ, Viscidi R, O'Brien J, et al. First dose recommendations for gentamicin and tobramycin in patients with ascites. Presented at the 15th Annual ASHP Midyear Clinical Meeting and Exhibits; December 7–11, 1980; San Francisco.

119. Spicehandler JR, Bernhardt L, Simberkoff MS, et al. Pharmacokinetics of amikacin and netilmicin in cirrhotic subjects. Presented at the 11th International Congress of Chemotherapy and 19th Interscience Congress of Antimicrobial Agents and Chemotherapy; October 1–5, 1979; Boston.

120. Desai TK, Tsang T-K. Aminoglycoside nephrotoxicity in obstructive jaundice. *Am J Med.* 1988;85:47–50.

121. Schwartz SN, Pazin GJ, Lyon JA, et al. A controlled investigation of the pharmacokinetics of gentamicin and tobramycin in obese subjects. *J Infect Dis.* 1978;138:499–505.

122. Bauer LA, Blouin RA, Griffen WO, et al. Amikacin pharmacokinetics in morbidly obese patients. *Am J Hosp Pharm.* 1980;37:519–522.

123. Blouin RA, Mann HJ, Griffen WO, et al. Tobramycin pharmacokinetics in morbidly obese patients. *Clin Pharmacol Ther.* 1979;26:508–512.

124. Devine BJ. Gentamicin therapy. *Drug Intell Clin Pharm.* 1974;8:650–655.

125. Loirat P, Rohan J, Baillet AL, et al. Increased glomerular filtration rate in patients with major burns and its effect on the pharmacokinetics of tobramycin. *N Engl J Med.* 1978;299:915–919.

126. Matzke GR, Millikin P, Kovarik JM. Variability in pharmacokinetic values for gentamicin, tobramycin, and netilmicin in patients with renal insufficiency. *Clin Pharm.* 1989;8:800–806.

127. Friedman CA, Parks BR, Rawson JE. Gentamicin disposition in asphyxiated newborns: Relationship to mean arterial blood pressure and urine output. *Pediatr Pharmacol.* 1982;2:189–197.

128. Buchanan N, Davis MD, Eyberg C. Gentamicin pharmacokinetics in kwashiorkor. *Br J Clin Pharmacol.* 1979;8:451–453.

129. Zarowitz BJ, Pilla AM, Popovich J. Expanded gentamicin volume of distribution in patients with indicators of malnutrition. *Clin Pharm.* 1990;9:40–44.

130. Longley JM, Pittman DG, Newby FD. Altered aminoglycoside volume of distribution in patients with acquired immunodeficiency syndrome. *Clin Pharm.* 1991;10:784–786.

131. Pennington JE, Dale DC, Reynolds, HY, et al. Gentamicin sulfate pharmacokinetics: Lower levels of gentamicin in blood during fever. *J Infect Dis.* 1975;132:270–275.

132. Riff LJ, Jackson GG. Pharmacology of gentamicin in man. *J Infect Dis.* 1971;124(suppl):98–105.

133. Barza M, Brown RB, Shen D, et al. Predictability of blood levels of gentamicin in man. *J Infect Dis.* 1975;132:165–174.

134. Gardner DK, Schneider PJ. Gentamicin dosage requirements in postpartum patients. *Clin Pharm.* 1984;3:416–418.

135. Segal JL, Brunnemann SR, Gordon SK, et al. Amikacin pharmacokinetics in patients with spinal cord injury. *Pharmacotherapy.* 1988;8:79–81.

136. Segal JL, Brunnemann SR, Gray DR. Gentamicin bioavailability and single-dose pharmacokinetics in spinal cord injury. *Drug Intell Clin Pharm.* 1988;22:461–465.

137. Zeitany RG, El Saghir NS, Santhosh-Kumar CR, et al. Increased aminoglycoside dosage requirements in hematologic malignancy. *Antimicrob Agents Chemother.* 1990;34:702–708.

138. Kramer WG, Cleary T, Frankel LS, et al. Multiple-dose amikacin kinetics in pediatric oncology patients. *Clin Pharmacol Ther.* 1979;26:635–640.

139. Bianco TM, Dwyer PN, Bertino JS. Gentamicin pharmacokinetics, nephrotoxicity, and prediction of mortality in febrile neutropenic patients. *Antimicrob Agents Chemother.* 1989;33:1890–1895.

140. Watterberg KL, Kelly HW, Johnson JD, et al. Effect of patent ductus arteriosus on gentamicin pharmacokinetics in very low birth weight (< 1,500 g) babies. *Dev Pharmacol Ther.* 1987;10:107–117.

141. Fuhs DW, Mann JH, Kubajak CAM, et al. Intrapatient variation of aminoglycoside pharmacokinetics in critically ill surgery patients. *Clin Pharm.* 1988;7:207–213.

142. Triginer C, Izquierdo I, Fernández R, et al. Gentamicin volume of distribution in critically ill septic patients. *Intensive Care Med.* 1990;16:303–306.

143. Triginer C, Fernández I, Rello J, et al. Gentamicin pharmacokinetic changes related to mechanical ventilation. *Drug Intell Clin Pharm.* 1989;23:923–924. Letter.

144. Jackson GG, Arcieri G. Ototoxicity of gentamicin in man: A survey and controlled analysis of clinical experience in the United States. *J Infect Dis.* 1971;124(suppl):130–137.

145. Hewitt WL. Gentamicin toxicity in perspective. *Postgrad Med J.* 1974;50(suppl 7):55–61.

146. Lane AZ, Wright GE, Blair DC. Ototoxicity and nephrotoxicity of amikacin: An overview of phase II and phase III experience in the United States. *Am J Med.* 1977;62:911–918.

147. Masur H, Whelton PK, Whelton A. Neomycin toxicity revisited. *Arch Surg.* 1976;111:822–825.

148. Lane AZ. Clinical experience with netilmicin. *J Antimicrob Chemother.* 1984;13(suppl A):67–72.

149. Neu HC, Bendush CL. Ototoxicity of tobramycin: A clinical overview. *J Infect Dis.* 1976;134(suppl):206–218.

150. Bendush CL, Weber R. Tobramycin sulfate: A summary of worldwide experience from clinical trials. *J Infect Dis.* 1976;134(suppl):219–234.

151. Tjernström Ö, Banck G, Belfrage S, et al. The ototoxicity of gentamicin. *Acta Pathol Microbiol Scand.* 1973;81 (suppl 241):73–78.

152. Deafness after topical neomycin. *Br Med J.* 1969;4:181–182. Editorial.

153. Berk DP, Chalmers T. Deafness complicating antibiotic therapy of hepatic encephalopathy. *Ann Intern Med.* 1970;73:393–396.

154. Ward KM, Rounthwaite FJ. Neomycin ototoxicity. *Ann Otol Rhinol Laryngol.* 1978;87:211–215.

155. Buring JE, Evans DA, Mayrent SL, et al. Randomized trials of aminoglycoside antibiotics: Quantitative overview. *Rev Infect Dis.* 1988;10:951–957.

156. Black RE, Lau WK, Weinstein RJ, et al. Ototoxicity of amikacin. *Antimicrob Agents Chemother.* 1976;9:956–961.

157. Gailiunas P, Dominguez-Moreno M, Lazarus JM, et al. Vestibular toxicity of gentamicin. Incidence in patients receiving long-term hemodialysis therapy. *Arch Intern Med.* 1978;138:1621–1624.

158. McCracken GH. Aminoglycoside toxicity in infants and children. *Am J Med.* 1986;80(suppl 6B):172–178.

159. McRorie TI, Bosso J, Randolph L. Aminoglycoside ototoxicity in cystic fibrosis: Evaluation of high-frequency audiometry. *Am J Dis Child.* 1989;143:1328–1332.

160. Meriwether WF, Mangi RJ, Serpick AA. Deafness following standard intravenous dose of ethacrynic acid. *JAMA.* 1971;216:795–798.
161. Smith CR, Lietman PS. Effect of furosemide on aminoglycoside-induced nephrotoxicity and auditory toxicity in humans. *Antimicrob Agents Chemother.* 1983;23:133–137.
162. Barza M, Lauerman M. Why monitor serum levels of gentamicin? *Clin Pharmacokinet.* 1978;3: 202–215.
163. Mawer GE, Ahmad R, Dobbs S, et al. Prescribing aids for gentamicin. *Br J Clin Pharmacol.* 1974;1: 45–50.
164. Lau WK, Young LS, Black RE, et al. Comparative efficacy and toxicity of amikacin/carbenicillin versus gentamicin/carbenicillin in leukopenic patients. *Am J Med.* 1977;62:959–966.
165. Tulkens PM. Pharmacokinetics and toxicological evaluation of a once-daily regimen versus conventional schedules of netilmicin and amikacin. *J Antimicrob Chemother.* 1991;27(suppl C):49–61.
166. Giamarellou H, Yiallouros K, Petrikkos G, et al. Comparative kinetics and efficacy of amikacin administered once or twice daily in the treatment of systemic gram-negative infections. *J Antimicrob Chemother.* 1991;27(suppl C):73–79.
167. Maller R, Ahrne H, Holmen C, et al. Once- versus twice-daily amikacin regimen: Efficacy and safety in systemic gram-negative infections. *J Antimicrob Chemother.* 1993;31:939–948.
168. The International Antimicrobial Therapy Cooperative Group of the EORTC. Efficacy and toxicity of single daily doses of amikacin and ceftriaxone versus multiple daily doses of amikacin and ceftazidime for infection in patients with cancer and granulocytopenia. *Ann Intern Med.* 1993;119: 584–593.
169. Nordström L, Ringberg H, Cronberg S, et al. Does administration of an aminoglycoside in a single daily dose affect its efficacy and toxicity? *J Antimicrob Chemother.* 1990;25:159–173.
170. Prins JM, Abuller HR, Kuijper EJ, et al. Once versus thrice daily gentamicin in patients with serious infections. *Lancet.* 1993;341:335–339.
171. TerBraak EW, VeVries PJ, Bouter KP, et al. Once-daily dosing regimen for aminoglycoside plus β-lactam combination therapy of serious bacterial infections: Comparative trial with netilmicin plus ceftriaxone. *Am J Med.* 1990;89:58–66.
172. Van der Auwera P, Meunier F, Ibrahim S, et al. Pharmacodynamic parameters and toxicity of netilmicin (6 milligrams/kilogram/day) given once daily or in three divided doses to cancer patients with urinary tract infection. *Antimicrob Agents Chemother.* 1991;35:640–647.
173. Sturm AW. Netilmicin in the treatment of gram-negative bacteremia: Single daily versus multiple daily dosage. *J Infect Dis.* 1989;159:931–937.
174. Vigano A, Principi N, Brivio L, et al. Comparison of 5 milligrams of netilmicin per kilogram of body weight once daily versus 2 milligrams per kilogram thrice daily for treatment of gram-negative pyelonephritis in children. *Antimicrob Agents Chemother.* 1992;36:1499–1503.
175. Proctor L, Petty B, Thakor R, et al. A study of potential vestibulotoxic effects of once daily versus thrice daily administration of tobramycin. *Laryngoscope.* 1987;97:1443–1449.
176. Nicolau D, Quintiliani R, Nightingale CH. Once-daily aminoglycosides. *Conn Med.* 1992; 56:561–563.
177. Longridge NS, Mallinson AI. A discussion of the dynamic illegible "E" test: A new method of screening for aminoglycoside vestibulotoxicity. *Otolaryngol Head Neck Surg.* 1984;92:671–677.
178. Laurent G, Kishore BK, Tulkens PM. Aminoglycoside-induced renal phospholipidosis and nephrotoxicity. *Biochem Pharmacol.* 1990;40:2383–2392.
179. Lipsky JJ, Lefkowith J, Lietman PS. Cytoplasmic and membrane effects of aminoglycosides. In: Solez K, Whelton A, eds. *Acute Renal Failure—Correlation Between Morphology and Function.* New York: Marcel Dekker; 1984:261–271.
180. Plaut ME, Schentag JJ, Jusko WJ. Aminoglycoside nephrotoxicity: Comparative assessment in critically ill patients. *J Med.* 1979;10:257–266.

181. Adelman M, Evans E, Schentag JJ. Two-compartment comparison of gentamicin and tobramycin in normal volunteers. *Antimicrob Agents Chemother.* 1982;22:800–804.

182. Adelman RD, Halsted CC, Jordan GW, et al. Use of urinary enzyme activities in the early detection of aminoglycoside nephrotoxicity: A study in children and adults receiving gentamicin or netilmicin. *Proc West Pharmacol Soc.* 1981;24:261–264.

183. Schentag JJ, Sutfinta, Plaut ME, et al. Early detection of aminoglycoside nephrotoxicity with urinary beta-2-microglobulin. *J Med.* 1978;9:201–210.

184. Schentag JJ, Gengo FM, Plaut ME, et al. Urinary casts as an indicator of renal tubular damage in patients receiving aminoglycosides. *Antimicrob Agents Chemother.* 1979;16:468–473.

185. Bertino J, Booker LA, Franck PA, et al. Incidence of and significant risk factors for aminoglycoside-associated nephrotoxicity in patients dosed by using individualized pharmacokinetic monitoring. *J Infect Dis.* 1993;167:173–179.

186. Schentag JJ, Cerra FB, Plaut ME. Clinical and pharmacokinetic characteristics of aminoglycoside nephrotoxicity in 201 critically ill patients. *Antimicrob Agents Chemother.* 1982;21:721–726.

187. Gatell JM, SanMiguel JG, Araujo V, et al. Prospective randomized double-blind comparison of nephrotoxicity and auditory toxicity of tobramycin and netilmicin. *Antimicrob Agents Chemother.* 1984;26:766–769.

188. Garrison MW, Rotschafer JC. Clinical assessment of a published model to predict aminoglycoside-induced nephrotoxicity. *Ther Drug Monit.* 1989;11:171–175.

189. Mannion JC, Bloch R, Popovich NG. Cephalosporin–aminoglycoside synergistic nephrotoxicity: Fact or fiction. *Drug Intell Clin Pharm.* 1981;15:248–256.

190. The EORTC International Antimicrobial Therapy Project Group. Three antibiotic regimens in the treatment of infection in febrile granulocytopenic patients with cancer. *J Infect Dis.* 1978;137:14–29.

191. Gibey R, Dupond J-L, Henry J-C. Urinary *N*-acetyl-beta-D-glucosaminidase (NAG) isoenzyme profiles: A tool for evaluating nephrotoxicity of aminoglycosides and cephalosporins. *Clin Chim Acta.* 1984;137:1–11.

192. Farber BF, Moellering RC. Retrospective study of the toxicity of preparations of vancomycin from 1974 to 1981. *Antimicrob Agents Chemother.* 1983;23:138–141.

193. Rybak MJ, Albrecht LM, Boike SC, et al. Nephrotoxicity of vancomycin, alone and with an aminoglycoside. *J Antimicrob Chemother.* 1990;25:679–687.

194. Salem PA, Jabboury KW, Khalil MF. Severe nephrotoxicity: A probable complication of cis-dichlorodiammine platinum (II) and cephalothin-gentamicin therapy. *Oncology.* 1982;39:31–32.

195. Haas A, Anderson L, Lad T. The influence of aminoglycosides on the nephrotoxicity of cis-diamminechloroplatinum. *J Infect Dis.* 1983;147:363.

196. Cooper BW, Creger RJ, Soegiarso W, et al. Renal dysfunction during high-dose cisplatin therapy and autologous hematopoietic stem cell transplantation: Effect of aminoglycoside therapy. *Am J Med.* 1993;94:497–504.

197. Churchill DN, Seely J. Nephrotoxicity associated with combined gentamicin amphotericin B therapy. *Nephron.* 1977;19:176–181.

198. Mazze RI, Cousins MJ. Combined nephrotoxicity of gentamicin and methoxyflurane anaesthesia in man. *Br J Anaesth.* 1973;45:394–398.

199. Termeer A, Hoitsma AJ, Koene RAP. Severe nephrotoxicity caused by the combined use of gentamicin and cyclosporine in renal allograft recipients. *Transplantation.* 1986;42:220–221.

200. Butkus DE, de Torrente A, Terman DS. Renal failure following gentamicin in combination with clindamycin. *Nephron.* 1976;17:307–313.

201. Ambinder RF, Moore RD, Smith CR, et al. Lack of evidence for interaction between tobramycin and shock in their effect on renal function. *Antimicrob Agents Chemother.* 1985;27:217–219.

202. Yee GC, Evans WE. Reappraisal of guidelines for pharmacokinetic monitoring of aminoglycosides. *Pharmacotherapy.* 1981;1:55–75.

203. Moore RD, Smith CR, Lipsky JJ, et al. Risk factors for nephrotoxicity in patients treated with amino-glycoside. *Ann Intern Med.* 1984;100:353–357.

204. Dahlgren JG, Anderson ET, Hewitt WL. Gentamicin blood levels: A guide to nephrotoxicity. *Antimicrob Agents Chemother.* 1975;8:58–62.

205. Goodman EL, Van Gelder J, Holmes R, et al. Prospective comparative study of variable dosage and variable frequency regimens for administration of gentamicin. *Antimicrob Agents Chemother.* 1975;8:434–438.

206. Smith CR, Maxwell RR, Edwards CQ, et al. Nephrotoxicity induced by gentamicin and amikacin. *Johns Hopkins Med J.* 1978;142:85–90.

207. Schentag JJ, Cumbo TJ, Jusko WJ, et al. Gentamicin tissue accumulation and nephrotoxic reactions. *JAMA.* 1978;240:2067–2069.

208. Hollender LF, Bahnini J, DeManzini N, et al. A multicentric study of netilmicin once daily versus thrice daily in patients with appendicitis and other intra-abdominal infections. *J Antimicrob Chemother.* 1989;23:773–783.

209. Rozdzinski E, Kern WV, Reichle A, et al. Once-daily versus thrice-daily dosing of netilmicin in com-bination with β-lactam antibiotics as empirical therapy for febrile neutropenic patients. *J Antimicrob Chemother.* 1993;31:585–598.

210. Holtzman JL. Gentamicin and neuromuscular blockade. *Ann Intern Med.* 1976;84:55.

211. L'Hommedieu C, Stough R, Brown L, et al. Potentiation of neuromuscular weakness in infant botu-lism by aminoglycosides. *J Pediatr.* 1979;95:1065–1070.

212. L'Hommedieu CS, Huber PA, Rasch DK. Potentiation of magnesium-induced neuromuscular weak-ness by gentamicin. *Crit Care Med.* 1983;11:55–56.

213. Patel R, Sauage A. Symptomatic hypomagnesemia associated with gentamicin therapy. *Nephron.* 1979;23:50–52.

214. Byrd GJ. Acute organic brain syndrome associated with gentamicin therapy. *JAMA.* 1977;238:53–54.

215. McCartney CF, Hately LH, Kessle JM. Possible tobramycin delirium. *JAMA.* 1982;247:1319.

216. McCracken GH, Mize SG, Threlkeld N. Intraventricular gentamicin therapy in gram-negative bacil-lary meningitis of infancy. Report of the Second Neonatal Meningitis Cooperative Study Group. *Lancet.* 1980;1:787–791.

217. Mustafa MM, Mertsola J, Ramilo O, et al. Increased endotoxin and interleukin-1β concentrations in cerebrospinal fluid of infants with coliform meningitis and ventriculitis associated with intraventric-ular gentamicin therapy. *J Infect Dis.* 1989;160:891–895.

218. Zaloga GP, Chernow B, Pock A, et al. Hypomagnesemia is a common complication of aminoglyco-side therapy. *Surg Gynecol Obstet.* 1984;158:561–565.

219. Russo JC, Adelman RD. Gentamicin-induced Fanconi syndrome. *J Pediatr.* 1980;96:151–153.

220. Hall FJ. Anaphylaxis after gentamicin. *Lancet.* 1977;2:455.

221. Jojart GY. Sense of smell after gentamicin nose-drops. *Lancet.* 1992;339:313. Letter.

222. Yoshioka H, Matsuda I. Loss of hair related to gentamicin therapy. *JAMA.* 1970;211:123.

223. Chen JH, Wiener L, Distenfeld A. Immunologic thrombocytopenia induced by gentamicin. *NY State J Med.* 1980;80:1134–1135.

224. Kronenfeld MA, Thomas SJ, Turndorf H. Recurrence of neuromuscular blockade after reversal of vecuronium in a patient receiving polymyxin/amikacin sternal irrigation. *Anesthesiology.* 1986;65:93–94.

225. Dupuis JY, Martin R, Tétrault J-P. Atracurium and vecuronium interaction with gentamicin and tobramycin. *Can J Anaesth.* 1989;36:407–411.

226. Lippmann M, Yang E, Au E, et al. Neuromuscular blocking effects of tobramycin, gentamicin, and cefazolin. *Anesth Analg.* 1982;61:767–770.

227. Hatfield SM, Crane LR, Duman K, et al. Miconazole-induced alteration in tobramycin pharmacoki-netics. *Clin Pharm.* 1986;5:415–419.

228. Zarfin Y, Koren G, Maresky D, et al. Possible indomethacin–aminoglycoside interaction in preterm infants. *J Pediatr.* 1985;106:511–513.

229. Pfaller MA, Granich GG, Valdes R, et al. Comparative study of the ability of four aminoglycoside assay techniques to detect the inactivation of aminoglycosides by β-lactam antibiotics. *Diagn Microbiol Infect Dis.* 1984;2:93–100.

230. Pickering LK, Gearhart P. Effect of time and concentration upon interaction between gentamicin, tobramycin, netilmicin, or amikacin and carbenicillin or ticarcillin. *Antimicrob Agents Chemother.* 1979;15:592–596.

231. O'Bey KA, Jim LK, Gee JP, et al. Temperature dependence of the stability of tobramycin mixed with penicillins in human serum. *Am J Hosp Pharm.* 1982;39:1005–1008.

232. Spruill WJ, McCall CY, Francisco GE. In vitro inactivation of tobramycin by cephalosporins. *Am J Hosp Pharm.* 1985;42:2506–2509.

233. Henderson JL, Polk RE, Kline BJ. In vitro inactivation of gentamicin, tobramycin, and netilmicin by carbenicillin azlocillin, or mezlocillin. *Am J Hosp Pharm.* 1981;38:1167–1170.

234. Dalmady-Israel C, Green PJ, Sloskey GE, et al. Ticarcillin and assay of tobramycin. *Ann Intern Med.* 1984;100:460–461.

235. Halstenson CE, Hirata CAI, Heim-Duthoy KL, et al. Effect of concomitant administration of piperacillin on the dispositions of netilmicin and tobramycin in patients with end-stage renal disease. *Antimicrob Agents Chemother.* 1990;34:128–133.

236. Polk RE, Kline BJ. Mail order tobramycin serum levels: Low values caused by ticarcillin. *Am J Hosp Pharm.* 1980;37:920–922.

237. Cheng SH, White A. Effect of orally administered neomycin on the absorption of penicillin V. *N Engl J Med.* 1962;267:1296–1297.

238. Lindenbaum J, Maulitz RM, Butler VP. Inhibition of digoxin absorption by neomycin. *Gastroenterology.* 1976;71:399–404.

239. Cohen MH, Creaven PJ, Fossieck BE, et al. Effect of oral prophylactic broad spectrum nonabsorbable antibiotics on the gastrointestinal absorption of nutrients and methotrexate in small cell bronchogenic carcinoma patients. *Cancer.* 1976;38:1556–1559.

240. Bruckner HW, Creasey WA. The administration of 5–fluorouracil by mouth. *Cancer.* 1974;33:14–18.

241. Noone P, Parsons TMC, Pattison JR, et al. Experience in monitoring gentamicin therapy during treatment of serious gram-negative sepsis. *Br Med J.* 1974;1:477–481.

242. Anderson ET, Young LS, Hewitt WL. Simultaneous antibiotic levels in "breakthrough" gram-negative rod bacteremia. *Am J Med.* 1976;61:493–497.

243. Moore RD, Smith CR, Lietman PS. The association of aminoglycoside plasma levels with mortality in patients with gram-negative bacteremia. *J Infect Dis.* 1984;149:443–448.

244. Moore RD, Smith CR, Lietman PS. Association of aminoglycoside plasma levels with therapeutic outcome in gram-negative pneumonia. *Am J Med.* 1984;77:657–662.

245. Deziel-Evans LM, Murphy JE, Job ML. Correlation of pharmacokinetic indices with therapeutic outcome in patients receiving aminoglycosides. *Clin Pharm.* 1986;5:319–324.

246. Moore RD, Lietman PS, Smith CR. Clinical response to aminoglycoside therapy: Importance of the ratio of peak concentration to minimal inhibitory concentration. *J Infect Dis.* 1987;155:93–99.

247. Powell SH, Thompson WL, Luthe MA, et al. Once-daily vs. continuous aminoglycoside dosing: Efficacy and toxicity in animal and clinical studies of gentamicin, netilmicin, and tobramycin. *J Infect Dis.* 1983;147:918–932.

248. Bergeron MG, Beauchamp D, Poirier A, et al. Continuous vs. intermittent administration of antimicrobial agents: tissue penetration and efficacy in vivo. *Rev Infect Dis.* 1981;3:84–97.

249. Meunier F, Van der Auwera P, Aoun M, et al. Empirical antimicrobial therapy with a single daily dose of ceftriaxone plus amikacin in febrile granulocytopenic patients: A pilot study. *J Antimicrob Chemother.* 1991;27(suppl C):129–139.

250. Lucht F, Tigaud S, Esposito G, et al. Chronokinetic study of netilmicin in man. *Eur J Clin Pharmacol.* 1990;39:199–201.
251. Elting L, Bodey GP, Rosenbaum B, et al. Circadian variation in serum amikacin levels. *J Clin Pharmacol.* 1990;30:798–801.
252. Bosch DE, Williams DN. Comparison of serum aminoglycoside concentrations produced by two infusion methods. *Clin Pharm.* 1990;9:777–780.
253. Lane JR, Murray WE, Willenborg NL, et al. Controlled release infusion kinetics of tobramycin. *Ther Drug Monit.* 1989;11:264–268.
254. Ebert SC, Leroy M, Darcey B. Comparison of aminoglycoside concentrations measured in plasma versus serum. *Ther Drug Monit.* 1989;11:44–46.
255. Knight D, Ukena T. Heparin does not affect enzyme immunoassay of gentamicin. *Clin Chem.* 1981;27:640.
256. Bosso JA, Mead RA, Matsen JM, et al. Agreement between capillary and arterial serum gentamicin concentrations in neonates. *Pediatr Infect Dis.* 1985;4:142–144.
257. Fukuchi H, Yoshida M, Tsukiai S, et al. Comparison of enzyme immunoassay, radioimmunoassay, and microbiologic assay for amikacin in plasma. *Am J Hosp Pharm.* 1984;41:690–693.
258. Witebsky FG, Sliva CA, Selepak ST, et al. Evaluation of four gentamicin and tobramycin assay procedures for clinical laboratories. *J Clin Microsc.* 1983;18:890–894.
259. Rotschafer JC, Morlock C, Strand L, et al. Comparison of radioimmunoassay and enzyme immunoassay methods in determining gentamicin pharmacokinetic parameters and dosages. *Antimicrob Agents Chemother.* 1982;22:648–651.
260. Rotschafer JC, Berg HG, Nelson RB, et al. Observed differences in gentamicin pharmacokinetic parameters and dosage recommendations determined by fluorescent polarization immunoassay and radioimmunoassay methods. *Ther Drug Monit.* 1983;5:443–447.
261. Bleske BE, Larson TA, Rotschafer JC. Observed differences in amikacin pharmacokinetic parameters and dosage recommendations determined by enzyme immunoassay and fluorescence polarization immunoassay. *Ther Drug Monit.* 1987;9:48–52.
262. Boyce EG, Lawson LA, Gibson GA, et al. Comparison of gentamicin immunoassays using univariate and multivariant analyses. *Ther Drug Monit.* 1989;11:97–104.
263. Toler SM, Porter WH, Chandler MHH. Evaluation of precision and accuracy of a fluorescence polarization immunoassay system after dilution of serum samples containing fluorescein dye. *Ther Drug Monit.* 1990;12:300–302.
264. Walters MI, Roberts WH. Gentamicin/heparin interactions: Effects on two immunoassays and on protein binding. *Ther Drug Monit.* 1984;6:199–202.
265. Krogstad DJ, Granich GG, Murray PR, et al. Heparin interferes with the radioenzymatic and homogenous enzyme immunoassay for aminoglycosides. *Clin Chem.* 1982;28:1517–1521.
266. Johnson KB, ed. *The Harriet Lane Handbook.* 13th ed. St. Louis: Mosby-Year Book; 1993.
267. Lopez-Samblas AM, Torres CL, Wang H, et al. Effectiveness of a gentamicin dosing protocol based on post conceptional age: Comparison to published neonatal guidelines. *Drug Intell Clin Pharm.* 1992;26:534–538.
268. Hendeles L, Lafrate RP, Stillwell PC, et al. Individualizing gentamicin dosage in patients with cystic fibrosis: Limitations to pharmacokinetic approach. *J Pediatr.* 1987;110:303–310.
269. Netromycin package insert. Kenilworth, NJ: Schering Corp; January 1987.
270. Mouton JW, Kerrebijn KF. Antibacterial therapy in cystic fibrosis. *Med Clin North Am.* 1990;74:837–850.
271. Winnie GB, Cooper JA, Witson J, et al. Comparison of 6 and 8 hourly tobramycin dosing intervals in treatment of pulmonary exacerbations in cystic fibrosis patients. *Pediatr Infect Dis J.* 1991;10:381–386.
272. Chelluri L, Warren J, Jastremski MS. Pharmacokinetics of a 3 mg/kg body weight loading dose of gentamicin or tobramycin in critically ill patients. *Chest.* 1989;95:1295–1297.

273. Townsend PL, Fink MP, Stein, KL, et al. Aminoglycoside pharmacokinetics: Dosage requirements and nephrotoxicity in trauma patients. *Crit Care Med.* 1989;17:154–157.

274. Paton TW, Cornish WR, Manuel MA, et al. Drug therapy in patients undergoing peritoneal dialysis. Clinical pharmacokinetic considerations. *Clin Pharmacokinet.* 1985;10:404–426.

275. Schumacher GE. IV: Gentamicin blood level versus time profiles of various dosage regimens recommended for renal impairment. *Am J Hosp Pharm.* 1975;32:299–308.

276. Dubb JW, Stote RM, Familiar FG, et al. Effect of cimetidine on renal function in normal man. *Clin Pharmacol Ther.* 1978;24:76–83.

277. Myre SA, McCann J, First MR, et al. Effect of trimethoprim on serum creatinine in healthy and chronic renal failure volunteers. *Ther Drug Monit.* 1987;9:161–165.

278. Kruss DM, Littman A. Safety of cimetidine. *Gastroenterology.* 1978;74:478–486.

279. Hyneck ML, Berardi RR, Johnson RM. Interference of cephalosporins and cefoxitin with serum creatinine determination. *Am J Hosp Pharm.* 1981;38:1348–1352.

280. Guay DRP, Meatherall RC, Macaulay PA. Interference of selected second and third generation cephalosporins with creatinine determination. *Am J Hosp Pharm.* 1983;40:435–438.

281. Kennedy CA, Goetz MB, Mathisen GE. Artifactual elevation of the serum creatinine in patients receiving flucytosine for cryptococcal meningitis. *J Infect Dis.* 1991;163:421. Letter.

282. Chan RA, Benner EJ, Hoeprich PD. Gentamicin therapy in renal failure: A nomogram for dosage. *Ann Intern Med.* 1972;76:773–778.

283. Cutler RE, Gyselynck A-M, Fleet WP, et al. Correlation of serum creatinine concentration and gentamicin half-life. *JAMA.* 1972;219:1037–1041.

284. Sarubbi FA, Hull JH. Amikacin serum concentrations: Prediction of levels and dosage guidelines. *Ann Intern Med.* 1978;89(pt 1):612–618.

285. Lesar TS, Rotschafer JC, Strand LM, et al. Gentamicin dosing errors with four commonly used nomograms. *JAMA.* 1982;248:1190–1193.

286. Platt DR, Matthews SJ, Sevka MJ, et al. Comparison of four methods of predicting serum gentamicin concentrations in adult patients with impaired renal function. *Clin Pharm.* 1982;1:361–365.

287. Thomson AH, Campbell KC, Kelman AW. Evaluation of six nomograms using a bayesian parameter estimation program. *Ther Drug Monit.* 1990;12:258–263.

288. Hatton RC, Massey KL, Russell WL. Comparison of the predictions of one- and two-compartment microcomputer programs for long-term tobramycin therapy. *Ther Drug Monit.* 1984;6:432–437.

289. Murray KM, Bauer LA, Koup JR. Predictive performance of computer dosing methods for tobramycin using two pharmacokinetic models and two weighting algorithms. *Clin Pharm.* 1986; 5:411–414.

290. Cockcroft DW, Gault MH. Prediction of creatinine clearance from serum creatinine. *Nephron.* 1976;16:31–41.

291. Schwartz GJ, Brion LP, Spitzer A. The use of plasma creatinine concentration for estimating glomerular filtration rate in infants, children, and adolescents. *Pediatr Clin North Am.* 1987; 34:571–590.

292. Chow M, Deglin J, Harralson A, et al. Prediction of gentamicin serum levels using a one-compartment open linear pharmacokinetic model. *Am J Hosp Pharm.* 1978;35:1078–1081.

293. Sawchuk RJ, Zaske DE. Pharmacokinetics of dosing regimens which utilize multiple intravenous infusions: Gentamicin in burn patients. *J Pharmacokinet Biopharm.* 1976;4:183–195.

294. Jameson JP, Lewis JA. Three-point versus two-point method for early individualization of aminoglycoside doses. *Drug Intell Clin Pharm.* 1991;25:635–637.

295. Sawchuk RJ, Zaske DE, Cipolle RJ, et al. Kinetic model for gentamicin dosing with the use of individual patient parameters. *Clin Pharmacol Ther.* 1977;21:362–369.

296. Evans WE, Taylor RH, Feldman S, et al. A model for dosing gentamicin in children and adolescents that adjusts for tissue accumulation with continuous dosing. *Clin Pharmacokinet.* 1980;5:295–306.

297. Horner GW, Stempel DA. Tobramycin elimination rate change from first to later doses in older cystic fibrosis patients. *Drug Intell Clin Pharm.* 1987;21:276–278.
298. Tores MJ, Kern JW, Gill MA, et al. Comparison of serum sampling methods for estimating gentamicin pharmacokinetic variables. *Clin Pharm.* 1983;2:353–355.
299. Gilbert DN, Bennett WM. Use of antimicrobial agents in renal failure. *Infect Dis Clin North Am.* 1989;3:517–531.
300. Schumacher GE, Barr JT. Bayesian approaches in pharmacokinetic decision making. *Clin Pharm.* 1984;3:525–530.
301. Burton ME, Chow MSS, Platt DR, et al. Accuracy of bayesian and Sawchuk–Zaske dosing methods for gentamicin. *Clin Pharm.* 1986;5:143–149.
302. Rodvold KA, Blum RA. Predictive performance of Sawchuk–Zaske and bayesian dosing methods for tobramycin. *J Clin Pharmacol.* 1987;27:419–427.
303. Godley PJ, Black JT, Frohna PA, et al. Comparison of a bayesian program with three microcomputer programs for predicting gentamicin concentrations. *Ther Drug Monit.* 1988;10:287–291.
304. Lacarelle B, Granthil C, Manelli JC, et al. Evaluation of a bayesian method of amikacin dosing in intensive care unit patients with normal and impaired renal function. *Ther Drug Monit.* 1987;9:154–160.
305. Okamoto MP, Chin A, Gill MA, et al. Comparison of two microcomputer bayesian pharmacokinetic programs for predicting serum gentamicin concentrations. *Clin Pharm.* 1990;9:708–711.
306. McClellan SD, Farringer JA. Bayesian forecasting of aminoglycoside dosing requirements in obese patients: Influence of subpopulation versus general population pharmacokinetic parameters as the internal estimates. *Ther Drug Monit.* 1989;11:431–436.
307. Lui K, Bryson SM, Irwin DB, et al. Evaluation of bayesian forecasting for individualized gentamicin dosage in infants weighing 1000 g or less. *Am J Dis Child.* 1991;145:463–467.

Chapter 10

Antiarrhythmics

Alan H. Mutnick
Timothy G. Burke

Keep in Mind

- In general, the therapeutic range for each of the antiarrhythmic agents discussed, using serum drug concentrations, is less well defined than previously assumed.

Lidocaine
- Monitor serum concentrations for all patients dosed longer than 24 hours.
- Modify dosage regimens, if necessary, for patients with congestive heart failure and liver disease.
- If the patient has breakthrough arrhythmias, consider an additional bolus dose in addition to an increase in infusion rate.

Amiodarone
- Assess baseline electrocardiogram, ophthalmologic, and thyroid function values before starting treatment.
- Check and adjust for drug interactions when adding the drug to other regimens.
- The effect on other drugs may last weeks to months after discontinuation of amiodarone.

Procainamide
- Order serum concentration measurements judiciously, weighing the costs of testing against the benefits to patient care.
- Compare baseline electrocardiogram and duration of QRS segment prior to and after starting the drug.
- Consider whether there are predisposing factors that increase the likelihood for an adverse drug reaction (eg, systemic lupus erythematosus, Torsade de pointes).
- Do not design a dosage regimen (eg, q3–4h) that promotes patient noncompliance.

Quinidine
- Compare baseline electrocardiogram and duration of QRS segment prior to and after starting the drug.
- Consider whether there are predisposing factors that increase the likelihood for an adverse drug reaction (eg, drug–drug interactions, Torsade de pointes, previous quinidine-induced syncope).
- Be sure of the type of assay used in the laboratory for evaluating serum drug concentrations.

The antiarrhythmics, as a group, pose an interesting dilemma to the practicing physician. Of initial concern in each individualized patient will be the selection of the correct antiarrhythmic for each specific situation. A second concern involves the most appropriate way to use the selected agent once a choice has been made.

Most of the available antiarrhythmic agents are characterized by a narrow therapeutic index and a direct relationship between their pharmacologic response and plasma concentrations. The efficacy of these agents is frequently difficult to determine because of the marked variability in arrhythmia events. Analysis of the original pharmacokinetic data does reveal that therapeutic and toxic levels are not as well defined as oftened assumed. Lack of standardized sampling sizes, unreliable assay procedures, small numbers of patients, and inadequate arrhythmia documentation help explain the reasons for such concerns.

Of additional concern today is the fact that all antiarrhythmics do not lend themselves to the steps required to conduct appropriate therapeutic drug monitoring:

1. There must be a relationship between blood level and therapeutic effect.
2. Serum drug level determinations must be drawn after the steady state is attained.
3. Once steady state is attained, serum drug levels must be determined after the drug has completed its distributive phase.
4. When serum drug level determinations are evaluated, they must be related to those levels used in the literature in the same circumstances.

In this chapter, we identify four antiarrhythmic agents, which through their historical use, readily available pharmacokinetic database, uniqueness in pharmacokinetic disposition, and potential to produce major adverse drug effects and drug interactions form a basis for our discussion on therapeutic drug monitoring. The agents to be discussed are amiodarone, lidocaine, procainamide, and quinidine.

Table 10–1 has been developed to help the reader identify the currently available agents and the respective classes into which the agents are categorized.

LIDOCAINE

Clinical Pharmacology and Therapeutics

Use of lidocaine as an antiarrhythmic was first reported in 1950 in a pregnant woman who developed ventricular fibrillation during cardiac catheterization.[1] After intravenous procaine failed to facilitate electrical defibrillation, the physicians reached for the next local anesthetic on the shelf and administered 2 mL of 1% lidocaine with epinephrine into the left ventricle. Defibrillation was then successful and lidocaine was identified as a useful antiarrhythmic agent. In this case, the active drug may well have been the epinephrine; however, lidocaine soon was in widespread use for the treatment and prevention of ventricular arrhythmias.[1,2] Thus, discovered through serendipity, this useful antiarrhythmic agent has been in use in coronary care units and prehospital settings for more than 40 years.

Lidocaine is indicated for the treatment of life-threatening ventricular tachycardia and ventricular fibrillation. It may also be used post-myocardial infarction in the prehospital or hospital setting for the prevention of primary ventricular tachycardia and fibrillation, although this indi-

TABLE 10–1. CURRENTLY AVAILABLE ANTIARRHYTHMICS

Class IA	*Class II*	
Quinidine	Propranolol (beta-adrenergic blockers)	
Procainamide		
Disopyramide		
Class IB	*Class III*	
Lidocaine	Amiodarone	
Mexiletine	Bretylium	
Tocainide	Sotalol	
Phenytoin		
Class IC	*Class IV*	*Other Agents*
Flecainide	Verapamil	Adenosine
Propafenone	Diltiazem	Atropine
Moricizine	Nifedipine	Digoxin

cation remains controversial.[3,4] At therapeutic concentrations, lidocaine has little or no effect on the firing of the sinoatrial (SA) node and on conduction through the atrium.

Lidocaine is classified as a IB antiarrhythmic because of its effect on the fast sodium channel during phase 0 of the myocardial action potential.[5]

Lidocaine is a safe and effective agent when properly administered and monitored. The drug exhibits unique pharmacokinetics; serum levels continue to rise for 24 to 48 hours after apparent steady state has been reached. This continuous upward trend in serum levels coupled with a low therapeutic index makes the potential for toxicity very real for every patient on the drug. The patients at greatest risk of manifesting toxicity are, of course, the most severely ill. Those with large myocardial infarctions, congestive heart failure, or liver disease and the elderly are all at the greatest risk because of their diminished capacity for metabolism. In this chapter, we discuss the absorption, distribution, metabolism, excretion, adverse reactions, and methods of safe administration of this useful agent.

Clinical Pharmacokinetics

Absorption

Lidocaine is poorly bioavailable orally because of extensive first-pass metabolism. The oral bioavailability of lidocaine is approximately 35% in patients with normal liver function. Oral doses large enough to elicit therapeutic serum levels result in central nervous system and gastrointestinal toxic effects because of the accumulation of metabolites.[6] This low bioavailability in normal patients is due mainly to hepatic clearance, as the bioavailability of lidocaine orally in patients with cirrhotic liver disease approaches 90%.[7]

The drug is well absorbed over a period of 15 to 30 minutes when administered by intramuscular injection. This absorption is more rapid when given in the deltoid (absorption $t_{1/2} = 12$ minutes) than the gluteus (absorption $t_{1/2} = 26$ minutes).[8,9]

Lidocaine is well absorbed when given by the endotracheal (ET) route. Absorption is rapid and therapeutic serum levels are obtained in less than 1 minute.[10] Although the actual mechanism of absorption is unknown, therapeutic serum levels are obtained when 2 mg/kg lidocaine diluted to a total of 10 mL is administered endotracheally. Serum levels of 1.6 to 2.0 mg/L are obtained when lidocaine is diluted in normal saline.[11]

Lidocaine is absorbed when administered intranasally, with about 50% of the administered dose reaching the systemic circulation.[12] A serum level of approximately 2 mg/L was obtained when 300 mg of a topical lidocaine solution was administered to the vocal cords.[13] This must be kept in mind not from a therapeutic standpoint, but from the realization that toxic effects can result from topical administration. Toxic reaction has also been reported to the administration of topical lidocaine to cutaneous skin lesions. Serum levels as high as 21 mg/L, resulting in seizures and cardiac arrest, have been reported in a patient with extensive (60%) body surface area erosions receiving 5% lidocaine topical preparations.[14] Toxic reactions can also occur when lidocaine is administered as a local anesthetic for breast and muscle biopsies. The total dose of lidocaine relative to the patient's body weight must always be kept in mind.

Distribution

Lidocaine's distribution has been described as a two-compartment open model[15] with an initial distribution phase of 8 minutes. Lidocaine may best be described as a three-compartment model with an initial small central volume.[16] Lidocaine initially accumulates in those tissues with a high blood flow and affinity for the drug. These tissues include the brain, heart, kidney, and lung. These organs plus the blood constitute the initial volume of distribution (V_i). Bolus doses of lidocaine exert therapeutic effects based on V_i alone. This must be taken into account when loading doses are calculated using volumes of distribution. Lidocaine has a high affinity for pulmonary tissue. A large proportion of the bolus dose is initially sequestered in the lung which will attenuate peak concentrations.[16] In patients with right-to-left shunts or pulmonary arteriovenous fistulas, greater than normal concentrations can occur after boluses and may precipitate symptoms of toxicity. Although this phenomenon occurs in adults, it does not appear to be significant in children with right-to-left cardiac shunts.[17]

Muscle and fat are the major sites of lidocaine distribution, with only about 6% of total body stores at steady state being located in the blood.[16]

The volume of distribution is altered in disease states, with heart failure and cardiogenic shock decreasing the V_d and liver disease increasing the V_d.[3,6,16,18,19] The initial volume of distribution in patients with normal cardiac output is 0.5 L/kg, whereas it is 0.3 L/kg for those with heart failure and 0.6 L/kg for those with cirrhosis. The V_d in patients with normal cardiac output is 1.6 L/kg, whereas it is 0.88 L/kg for patients with congestive heart failure[20] and 2.3 L/kg for those with hepatic failure. It must be remembered that these are population-based parameters and wide variations can occur between individuals. The volume of distribution is reduced during cardiopulmonary resuscitation (CPR) ($V_i = 0.3$ L/kg and $V_d = 1.6$ L/kg) as this should be considered a severe low-cardiac-output state.[21] It has been recommended that in patients undergoing CPR, maintenance infusions not be done until spontaneous circulation returns, as the extreme low cardiac output state substantially reduces both the volume of distribution and metabolism of lidocaine.[2]

Lidocaine is approximately 70% protein bound at therapeutic serum levels (2–5 mg/L); at

6 to 10 mg/L, the protein binding decreases to about 60%.[16,22] This excess unbound drug can cross into the central nervous system and elicit toxic reactions. Central nervous system toxicity associated with lidocaine is related to the amount of unbound drug in the blood, with the exception of those symptoms that can occur immediately postbolus. Here, protein-bound lidocaine is partially available to cross the blood–brain barrier on the first pass and the symptoms observed are independent of unbound drug concentration.[23] The clinician must keep this in mind and administer licocaine boluses at a rate no faster than 50 mg/min to reduce the chance of deleterious side effects.

As the alpha phase of lidocaine is 8 minutes, it is possible to administer a bolus, begin an infusion, and still have subtherapeutic blood levels 10 to 15 minutes after the bolus is given. To prevent this, it is recommended that one-half the original bolus be administered 10 minutes after the first in patients who have had ventricular tachycardia or ventricular fibrillation.[2]

During the first 7 days after myocardial infarction, one of the principal proteins to which lidocaine is bound, α_1-acid glycoprotein (AAGP), doubles or triples in serum concentration. This increase in AAGP results in redistribution of lidocaine out of the red blood cells and tissue stores. This increase in total lidocaine levels is an indication of increased protein binding, not an indicator of toxicity. It has been recommended that lidocaine clearance be calculated on the basis of the free lidocaine.[23] This requires knowledge of AAGP levels which, in most institutions, take longer than 48 hours to assay. Because of the delay in laboratory time, the usefulness of calculating unbound lidocaine clearance is at present questionable in most clinical situations. Lidocaine clearance also decreases over time because of a number of mechanisms, which are discussed later.

Metabolism

Lidocaine is metabolized in the liver to two identified metabolites: monoethylglycinexylidide (MEGX) and glycinexylidide (GX). Both of these metabolites exhibit antiarrhythmic and convulsant activity.[24] MEGX has pharmacologic activity similar to that of lidocaine, is hepatically metabolized, and has a $t_{1/2}$ of approximately 2 hours. GX is approximately one fourth as potent as lidocaine as an antiarrhythmic and convulsant, has a $t_{1/2}$ of 10 hours, and is both renally and hepatically eliminated.[24] Accumulation of these metabolites may contribute to the symptoms seen in lidocaine toxicity.

Lidocaine's apparent clearance decreases with continuing maintenance infusions. This upward trend in concentrations may be due to disease states, reduced cardiac output, post-myocardial infarction, changes in plasma protein binding, presence of a third compartment, other changes in the volume of distribution, or the ability of lidocaine to inhibit its own metabolism via inhibition of the P450 cytochrome oxidase system.[15,16,20,25–29] Whatever the cause, the potential for toxicity is very real for every patient on lidocaine infusions longer than 24 hours, as the half-life can double or triple during this time with corresponding increases in the serum level. This upward trend in serum concentrations requires the monitoring of serum levels in all patients on the drug longer than 24 hours.

Elimination

Lidocaine is a weak base (pK_a = 7.85) and the urinary excretion is dependent on urinary pH. Maximal excretion of lidocaine in an acid urine is about 10% of an administered dose.[19,30] The rest is eliminated via progressive metabolism and excretion via the bile.[2] Thus, it would appear that renal disease would have little effect on the elimination of lidocaine or the active metabolite MEGX.[24]

Special Populations

Congestive Heart Failure. A decrease in cardiac output will cause an increase in lidocaine serum levels through more than one mechanism. As cardiac output decreases, blood is shunted away from the peripheral tissues and can result in a decrease in the volume of distribution of lidocaine.[18] Second, decreased blood flow to the liver can result in accumulation of both lidocaine and the metabolite MEGX.[20] The half-life of lidocaine can be prolonged to as much as 72 hours in patients with severe heart failure.[16,20] It would appear that the average half-life of lidocaine in patients with cardiac dysfunction is 4.6 hours.[23] This increase in half-life must be taken into account when studies such as electrophysiology are performed. If the infusion is discontinued 3 to 4 hours prior to electrophysiologic testing, the patient may still have therapeutic lidocaine levels during the study. This will, of course, alter the results of the study and result in an unnecessary expensive procedure.[28] To prevent this, lidocaine should be discontinued for as long as possible prior to electrophysiologic testing.

Liver Failure. Severe liver failure also results in an increase in lidocaine serum levels through a decrease in clearance, even though the volume of distribution is increased.[27] The clearance of lidocaine decreases by approximately 40% to 6 mL/kg/min and the half-life increases to 6.6 hours in patients with hepatic failure. Both the initial and total volumes of distribution increase to 0.6 and 2.3 L/kg, respectively.[27]

Age. Lidocaine clearance is decreased in the elderly despite their increased volume of distribution compared with young and middle-aged persons. The average elimination half-life initially in the elderly is 2.3 hours, compared with 1.7 hours in younger patients.[31] As with all patients one would expect the lidocaine serum levels to increase with prolonged infusions. The initial volume of distribution of lidocaine in the elderly appears to be somewhat larger than that seen in younger patients.[31] Decreases in body weight and functioning liver mass may play a role in the observed decrease in lidocaine clearance.

The pharmacokinetic parameters for lidocaine are summarized in Table 10–2.

Pharmacodynamics

Adverse Reactions

Lidocaine toxicity is a very real concern in clinical medicine, with the incidence of toxic reactions ranging up to 40% in some patient populations studied.[26] When the elderly and those patients with severe cardiac and liver disease are excluded, the incidence of toxic reactions may still be as high as 15 to 19%.[26,32] In one group, 25% of those patients in whom the drug was toxic, by serum levels, had morbid events including hypotension, syncope, severe agitation requiring restraints, coma, and cardiac arrest.[26] The majority of the symptoms seen in lidocaine toxicity are related to the central nervous and cardiovascular systems.

Sinus arrest, third-degree atrioventricular block, an accelerated ventricular rate during atrial fibrillation or flutter, hypotension, and cardiac arrest are cardiac events that have been reported in lidocaine toxicity.[33–37]

TABLE 10–2. SUMMARY OF PHARMACOKINETIC PARAMETERS FOR LIDOCAINE

| | | | | Therapeutic serum level | 1–5 µg/mL |
| Toxicity symptoms | | | | | >5 µg/mL |

Patient Subset	V_i (L/kg)	V_d (L/kg)	$t_{1/2\alpha}$ (min)	$t_{1/2\beta}$ (h)	Cl (mL/min/kg)
Normal cardiac output	0.5	1.6	8	1.7	7–10
Normal cardiac output with infusion longer than 24 hours	0.5	1.6	8	1.5–4.3	3–10
Congestive heart failure	0.3	0.88	8	1.7–72	See below
Liver disease	0.6	2.3	8	5–7	4–6

Clearance in Congestive Heart Failure Patients

NYHA Class	Symptoms	Cardiac Index (total)
I	Asymptomatic	10 mL/min/kg
II	S_3 gallop	
	Pulmonary rales	5 mL/min/kg
III	Pulmonary edema	2.1 mL/min/kg
IV	Cardiogenic shock	2.1 mL/min/kg

V_i, central volume distribution; V_d, total volume distribution; $t_{1/2\alpha}$, distribution half-life; $t_{1/2\beta}$, elimination half-life

Toxic reactions related to the central nervous system include severe agitation, tinnitus, visual disturbances, confusion, and paresthesias; these are often seen before more serious symptoms develop. These symptoms would be very hard to evaluate in an already seriously ill patient, and it would appear that proper dosing and careful monitoring of the serum level would be the only safe way to manage the patients.

If symptoms do develop, treatment involves, first, discontinuing the lidocaine and, then, giving supportive treatment. In patients with seizures, treatment with barbiturates or benzodiazepines seems to be the most effective. The clinician must always keep in mind that the half-life of lidocaine may be markedly prolonged at this point and treatment may be required up to 24 hours or longer.

Drug–Drug Interactions

The coadministration of beta-adrenergic blocking drugs can decrease lidocaine clearance by an average of 20%.[2,38,39] This has been demonstrated with the drugs metoprolol, nadolol, and propranolol. Atenolol and pindolol appear to decrease the clearance by around 10%.[2] The exact mechanism of this interaction is controversial but is probably related to a combination of decreased blood flow to the liver and inhibition of metabolism.[38,39] A reasonable approach to lidocaine dosing in a patient on concomitant beta blockers would be to reduce the infusion rate by 20%.

Cimetidine reduces lidocaine clearance by approximately 20% through inhibition of metabolism.[40] This drug interaction is not seen with ranitidine.[41] Again, a reasonable approach is to reduce the lidocaine maintenance dose by 20% when the patient is receiving concomitant cimetidine.

Phenytoin does not appear to have an effect on lidocaine metabolism. This may be due to the fact that lidocaine is already extensively metabolized in the liver, and enzyme induction does not further increase the ability of the liver to metabolize the drug.[2]

Dosing Considerations

Intravenous is the preferred route of administration of lidocaine in emergency situations, although the intramuscular and endotracheal routes can be employed. Intramuscular administration has the distinct disadvantages of slow absorption and slow onset of action, both of which would be deleterious in a life-threatening situation. Endotracheal administration requires that the patient be intubated. This route is effective in the intubated patient in whom an intravenous line cannot be established. The maximum amount of fluid that can be given endotracheally at any one time is 10 mL.

Effective serum concentrations show great interpatient variability as does the relationship between toxicity symptoms and serum levels. It is generally felt that the minimum effective concentration of lidocaine is 1 to 2 mg/L, whereas toxicity symptoms can be seen at serum levels greater than 5 mg/L. In some cases, serum levels higher than 5 mg/L may be required to control life-threatening ventricular arrhythmias. As can be seen, there is overlap between the therapeutic and toxic effects of lidocaine. The clinician should always keep this in mind and use the lowest effective dose of lidocaine when treating ventricular arrhythmias.

If lidocaine is used for prophylaxis post-myocardial infarction, the infusion should be stopped after 24 hours. At this time the greatest risk of ventricular arrhythmias has passed and the risk of lidocaine toxicity increases. Stopping the infusion after 24 hours avoids the dosing adjustments that are necessary in prolonged infusions.

There is little or no rationale for the common practice of tapering lidocaine infusions rather than simply shutting them off. Because of the long half-life of the drug, lidocaine "tapers itself." The differences in serum levels, whether the infusion is shut off or tapered slowly, would be negligible.

Therapeutic Regimen Design

At present there are three methods of calculating the lidocaine bolus and maintenance infusions used in clinical medicine. One is a general dosing guideline as recommended by the American Heart Association's Advanced Cardiac Life Support Program, the second is prospective using population-based volumes of distribution and clearances, and the last is retrospective, calculating patient-specific parameters via the use of two separate serum level determinations. We discuss all three with sample calculations of each.

Method 1

The first method, based on the guidelines recommended in AHA's Advanced Cardiac Life Support Program, recommends giving a 1 to 1.5 mg/kg "bolus" at a rate no faster than 50 mg/min and repeating with one-half this amount every 8 to 10 minutes until the arrhythmia is abolished or a total of 3 mg/kg has been administered. The recommendations for the maintenance infusion are as follows: If the dysrhythmia is abolished after a 1 mg/kg bolus, begin the infusion at 2 mg/min; if a total of 2 mg/kg was needed to abolish the arrhythmia, begin the infusion at 3 mg/min; and if the maximum, or 3 mg/kg, was needed to abolish the dysrhythmia, begin the infusion at 4 mg/min. In all these cases, if the patient has heart failure, give one-half the total bolus and begin the infusion at one-half the recommended rate. If the patient has liver disease or is elderly, give the recommended bolus and begin the infusion rate at one-half the normal rate. During CPR give bolus doses only. As CPR constitutes an extremely low output state, hepatic metabolism of lidocaine will be severely limited. During CPR it is advisable to repeat boluses with 25 to 50 mg when arrhythmias recur. A maintenance infusion may be started after spontaneous circulation returns.

_____ **EXAMPLE 10–1**_____

The patient is a 55-year-old, 70-kg man with no hepatic disease or cardiac failure. Assume three bolus doses are needed; then start an infusion.

The first bolus would be 70 mg (1 mg/kg); each subsequent bolus would be 0.5 mg/kg, or 35 mg. This patient would receive a total of 140 mg of lidocaine in bolus dosing.

A total of 2 mg/kg was given in bolus dosing. Begin the infusion rate at 3 mg/min.

_____ **EXAMPLE 10–2**_____

The patient is a 55-year-old, 70-kg woman with congestive heart failure. Assume a total of three bolus doses are needed; then start an infusion.

As the patient has congestive heart failure, we would give one-half the normal bolus dose each time to account for the decreased volume of distribution seen. The first bolus dose would be 35 mg, followed by two bolus doses of 17.5 mg each. A total of 70 mg would be given.

A total of three boluses were given. In a patient without hepatic disease or cardiac failure the infusion rate would be 3 mg/min. Because this patient has heart failure, the infusion rate is begun at one-half the usual rate to take into account the reduced metabolic capabilities secondary to reduced blood flow to the liver. The infusion rate would be 1.5 mg/min.

_____ **EXAMPLE 10–3**_____

The patient is a 55-year-old, 70-kg man with cirrhosis. Assume a total of three bolus doses are needed and start an infusion.

The bolus doses remain the same: 1 mg/kg for the first bolus (70 kg), then one-half that amount for each subsequent bolus (35 mg). A total of 140 mg or 2 mg/kg will be given.

A total of three bolus doses (2 mg/kg) were given. In a patient without liver failure the infusion rate would be 3 mg/min. In liver failure the infusion rate is started at one-half the normal rate, or 1.5 mg/min. This takes into account the reduced metabolic capabilities of the liver.

Method 2

The second method uses population-based parameters as listed here:

Patient Subset	V_i (L/kg)	V_d (L/kg)	$t_{1/2}$ min	$t_{1/2}$ h	Cl (mL/min/kg)
Normal cardiac output	0.5	1.6	8	1.7	7–10
Normal cardiac output with infusion longer than 24 hours	0.5	1.6	8	1.5–4.3	3–10
Congestive heart failure	0.3	0.88	8	1.7–72	See below
Liver disease	0.6	2.3	8	5–7	4–6

V_i refers to the central volume of distribution and V_d refers to the total volume of distribution; $t_{1/2\alpha}$, distribution half-life; $t_{1/2\beta}$, elimination half-life.

Clearance in Congestive Heart Failure Patients

NYHA Class	Symptoms	Cardiac Index, Total (mL/min/kg)
I	Asymptomatic	10
II	S_3 gallop Pulmonary rales	5
III	Pulmonary edema	2.1
IV	Cardiogenic shock	2.1

_____ EXAMPLE 10–4 _____

The patient is a 55-year-old, 70-kg woman with no cardiac failure or liver disease.

As the effective blood concentration of lidocaine is between 2 and 5 mg/L it would be best to attempt to obtain a blood level in the middle of the therapeutic range. It is hoped this will provide a therapeutic effect without eliciting any toxic reactions.

Because the parameters are all population-based with a wide interpatient variance, it would also be advisable to use those parameters in the middle to decrease the chance of grossly over- or underdosing the patient.

$$V_i = 0.5 \text{ L/kg (70 kg)} = 35 \text{ L}$$

$$C^0 = \text{Dose}/V_i = 3 \text{ mg/L}$$

Rearranging the equation leads to $C^0 V_i = \text{dose}$.

$$35 \text{ L (3 mg/L)} = 105 \text{ mg to be given as a bolus}$$

$$K_0 = C_{ss} \text{ (Cl)}$$

$$C_p \text{ (desired)} = 3 \text{ mg/L}$$

$$\text{Cl} = 7\text{–}10 \text{ mL/kg/min (we use 8 mL/min/kg)}$$

$$8 \text{ mL/min/kg (70 kg)} = 560 \text{ mL/min}$$

$$K_0 = 560 \text{ mL/min (3 mg/L)} = 1680 \text{ μg/min, or 1.68 mg/min}$$

────────── **EXAMPLE 10–5** ──────────────────────────────

The patient is a 55-year-old, 70-kg man with class III congestive heart failure.

$$\text{Target } C_p = 3 \text{ mg/L}$$

$$V_i = 0.3 \text{ L/kg (70 kg)} = 21 \text{ L}$$

$$21 \text{ L (3 mg/L)} = 63 \text{ mg to be given as a bolus}$$

$$K_0 = 3 \text{ mg/L (Cl)}$$

$$\text{Cl} = 2.1 \text{ mL/min/kg (70 kg)} = 147 \text{ mL/min}$$

$$K_0 = 3 \text{ mg/L (147 mL/min)} = 441 \text{ μg/min} = 0.44 \text{ mg/min}$$

────────── **EXAMPLE 10–6** ──────────────────────────────

The patient is a 55-year-old, 70-kg woman with cirrhotic liver disease.

$$\text{Target } C_p = 3 \text{ mg/L}$$

$$V_i = 0.6 \text{ L/kg (70 kg)} = 42 \text{ L}$$

$$\text{Cl} = 5 \text{ mL/min/kg (70 kg)} = 350 \text{ mL/min}$$

$$K_0 = 3 \text{ mg/L (350 mL/min)} = 1050 \text{ μg/min} = 1.05 \text{ mg/min}$$

Method 3

The third method uses patient-specific clearances and population-based volumes of distribution (Chiou equation). The patient-specific clearance is calculated using two serum levels drawn approximately 0.5 to 1 hour (first level) and 3 to 6 hours (second level) after the infusion is begun. This method relies on population-based volumes of distribution as do the other methods. The Chiou equation has been shown to maintain serum levels under the toxic range. It does appear to underestimate clearance somewhat (ie, serum levels will be lower than predicted). This, however, is safer than overestimating clearance, which can lead to potentially toxic blood levels. Remember, it is always easier to increase an infusion rate than it is to treat drug toxicity!

The discrepancies in predicted versus actual serum levels may be due in part to the fact that the first serum level is drawn before the drug reaches steady state. At the time of the first blood draw there will still be lidocaine in the blood from the bolus. This causes the initial level to be higher than it would without the bolus and, thus, underestimates the total clearance.

_____ **EXAMPLE 10–7** _____

The patient is a 55-year-old, 70-kg man with no cardiac or hepatic failure.

$$K_0 = 3 \text{ mg/min} = 180 \text{ mg/h}.$$

$T_1 = 1$ hour after infusion started $\qquad C_{p1} = 3.4$ mg/L

$T_2 = 6$ hours after infusion started $\qquad C_{p2} = 2.6$ mg/L

$$C_1 = \frac{2K_0}{C_1 + C_2} + \frac{2V_d(C_1 - C_2)}{(C_1 + C_2) \times (T_2 - T_1)}$$

$$V_d = 1.6 \text{ L/kg} (70 \text{ kg}) = 112 \text{ L}$$

$$C_1 = \frac{2(180)}{3.4 + 2.6} + \frac{224(3.4 - 2.6)}{(3.4 + 2.6)(6 - 1)} = \frac{360}{6} + \frac{224(0.8)}{6(5)}$$

$$= 60 + \frac{179.2}{30} = 65.97 \text{ L/h} = \frac{65,970 \text{ mL/h}}{60 \text{ min/h}} = 1099 \text{ mL/min}$$

$$K_0 = C_1 (C_p \text{ desired}) = 1099 \text{ mL/min } (3 \text{ μg/mL}) = 3298 \text{ μg/min})$$

$$= 3.3 \text{ mg/min}$$

_____ **EXAMPLE 10–8** _____

The patient is a 55-year-old, 70-kg woman with class III heart failure.

$$K_0 = 1.5 \text{ mg/min} = 90 \text{ mg/h}$$

$T_1 = 1$ hour after infusion started $C_{p1} = 3.9$ mg/L

$T_2 = 6$ hours after infusion started $C_{p2} = 3.7$ mg/L

$V_d = 0.88$ L/kg (70 kg) $= 61.6$ L

$$C_1 = \frac{2(90)}{3.9 + 3.7} + \frac{2(61.6)(3.9 - 3.7)}{(3.9 + 3.7)(6 - 1)}$$

$$= \frac{180}{7.6} + \frac{123.2(0.2)}{(7.6)(5)}$$

$$= 23.68 + \frac{24.64}{38} = 23.68 + 0.648$$

$$= 24.32 \text{ L/h} = \frac{24{,}320 \text{ mL/h}}{60 \text{ min/h}} = 405 \text{ mL/min}$$

$K_0 = 405$ mL/min (3 µg/mL) $= 1216$ µg/min $= 1.22$ mg/min

_____ **EXAMPLE 10–9** _____

The patient is a 55-year-old, 70-kg man with cirrhotic liver disease.

$K_0 = 1.5$ mg/min $= 90$ mg/h

$T_1 = 1$ hour after infusion started $C_{p1} = 2.7$ mg/L

$T_2 = 6$ hours after infusion started $C_{p2} = 3.1$ mg/L

$V_d = 2.3$ L/kg (70 kg) $= 161$ L

$$C_1 = \frac{2(90)}{2.7 + 3.1} + \frac{2(161)(2.7 - 3.1)}{(2.7 + 3.1)(6 - 1)}$$

$$= \frac{180}{5.8} + \frac{322(-0.4)}{(5.8)(5)}$$

$$= 31.03 + \frac{-128.8}{29} = 31.03 - 4.44$$

$$= 26.59 \text{ L/h} = \frac{26{,}590 \text{ mL/h}}{60 \text{ min/h}} = 443 \text{ mL/min}$$

$K_0 = 443$ mL/min (3 µg/mL) $= 1329.5$ µg/min $= 1.33$ mg/min

AMIODARONE

Clinical Pharmacology and Therapeutics

Amiodarone was originally developed in Belgium as an antianginal agent[42] and later was found to have antiarrhythmic properties. This drug is efficacious in 75% of patients who have failed other antiarrhythmic therapy.[43,44]

Amiodarone has a number of potentially serious side effects and up to 85% of people on amiodarone 4 years or longer will experience at least one side effect.[44] There are a number of potentially serious drug interactions that require careful monitoring by the clinician. Amiodarone is unique among antiarrhythmics with the unusual pharmacokinetic parameters it exhibits.

Clinical Pharmacokinetics

Absorption

Oral amiodarone is absorbed slowly with high interpatient variability. This low bioavailability (average 50%, range 22–86%) is thought, in part, to be due to intestinal mucosal cell dealkylation before the drug reaches the portal circulation.[45–47] Presystemic hepatic clearance and poor tablet dissolution do not seem to play a role in the poor bioavailability.[48,49] Although therapeutic effects may be seen quickly with the intravenous form, oral amiodarone has an onset of action of 2 to 3 days in a few individuals and of 1 to 3 weeks in most. The maximum antiarrhythmic effect is seen in 1 to 5 months.[50] Because of high tissue binding, various loading schemes have been developed to fill the body stores while trying to prevent unwanted side effects. The most commonly employed regimen consists of giving 800 to 1600 mg daily for 1 to 3 weeks, then 600 to 800 mg daily for 1 month, then the chronic maintenance dose of 200 to 400 mg per day. Another oral dosing schedule for the treatment of ventricular arrhythmias is 2 g on day 1, followed by 1.4 g per day for 3 days, and 1 g per day for 7 days; 800 mg per day is given for another 1 to 2 weeks before the dose is reduced to 400 mg per day. It has been suggested that for supraventricular tachycardias, the aforementioned regimen be reduced by 50% (1 g for 1 day, then 700 mg for 3 days, etc) because of the increased sensitivity of supraventricular arrhythmias to amiodarone.[42] Adverse gastrointestinal side effects can occur in greater than 50% of the patients during the loading phase.[50] For this reason it is recommended that the drug be given in three or four divided doses, with food, throughout the day. Once steady-state plasma levels have been reached, there does seem to be a dose–serum level relationship with the 200 and 400 mg/d doses producing serum levels of 1 and 2 µg/mL, respectively.[51] We must note that although "therapeutic serum levels" have been defined, the efficacy and toxicity of amiodarone may be determined more by extensive tissue deposition than by its serum concentration. This tissue deposition may continue for months once the therapy is initiated.[52] The lowest effective dose should be used, as the incidence of pulmonary fibrosis increases in patients with total daily amiodarone doses greater than 400 mg.[53–55]

Distribution

The complex nature of amiodarone's distribution initially caused confusion among the clinicians studying the drug. The distribution half-life is usually measured in minutes, but in the case of amiodarone it is measured in days. The distribution half-life of amiodarone ranges from 2 to 10 days.[46]

Amiodarone has a very large volume of distribution, indicating vast tissue accumulation.[47] Concentrations 300 to 400 times those found in the serum can be found in fat stores and in the liver. Because of the drug's lipid solubility, approximately 40% of the body stores are located in adipose tissue. One would expect that the onset of action during the loading phase in obese individuals would be prolonged. Other tissues in which amiodarone levels are greater than in serum include the lungs (200 times serum level), heart (40 times serum level), thyroid (15 times serum level), and brain (10 times serum level).[56,57] The drug does cross the placenta at approximately one-fourth the maternal serum concentration. Amiodarone is found in the breast milk at 2.5 to 9 times the maternal blood level.[58] It is recommended that women not breastfeed if they are or have been taking amiodarone within the last 6 months to 1 year. If administration of amiodarone during pregnancy is unavoidable, it is recommended that the infant be monitored for hypothyroidism and given replacement therapy until the thyroid function resolves (usually weeks).[58]

Amiodarone is 96% protein bound, mainly to albumin and, to a lesser extent, to a beta-lipoprotein.[59] This high protein binding prevents the removal of the drug by either hemo- or peritoneal dialysis.[60]

Metabolism

The exact metabolic pathways of amiodarone are not fully known. It appears to be extensively metabolized, mainly in the liver and intestinal mucosa, to at least one major metabolite. The metabolite, N-desethylamiodarone, is formed through N-dealkylation. N-Desethylamiodarone may have some antiarrhythmic activity in animals but it is uncertain whether it has any activity in humans.[46,61,62] Another metabolite, di-N-desethylamiodarone, has been identified in animals but not in humans.[63] N-Desethylamiodarone levels will usually be found in a 1:1 ratio in humans once steady state has been reached.

Elimination

Amiodarone and N-desethylamiodarone appear to be excreted by the feces via the bile. The drug may undergo enterohepatic circulation, but this has not been clearly established.[47]

The pharmacokinetic parameters for amiodarone are summarized in Table 10–3.

TABLE 10–3. SUMMARY OF PHARMACOKINETIC PARAMETERS FOR AMIODARONE

Therapeutic serum levels	1–2.5 µg/mL
Principal metabolite	N-Desethyl amiodarone
Route of metabolism	Hepatic
Distribution half-life	2–10 d
Elimination half-life	26–107 d (av 53 d)
Protein binding	96%
Time to peak (oral)	5 h
Removed by hemo- or peritoneal dialysis?	No
Bioavailability (oral)	22–86%
Volume of distribution at steady state, $V_{d,ss}$	18–144 L/kg (av 66 L/kg)

Pharmacodynamics

Drug–Drug Interactions

When discussing drug interactions, we are always talking about the possibility of a certain interaction occurring. With amiodarone, we can speak with certainty of the interaction occurring. Amiodarone interacts with a number of cardiac drugs that may be given concurrently, and these interactions require careful evaluation by the clinician monitoring the drug therapy. In light of the fact that amiodarone has a half-life of 53 days in most individuals, the potential for drug interactions can continue months after the drug is discontinued. This must be kept in mind when drugs with fairly narrow therapeutic indexes, such as warfarin and digoxin, are initiated. The long half-life also makes evaluation of therapeutic serum levels of a number of antiarrhythmics very difficult if they are initiated after the drug is discontinued. Monitoring of serum levels and dosage adjustments may take months.

The amiodarone–digoxin interaction is complex and may involve a number of mechanisms. Amiodarone seems to decrease the renal and nonrenal clearance of digoxin, may increase digoxin's oral bioavailability, and displaces digoxin from tissue stores.[60,64] As a result of the last mechanism, the digoxin level may rise for weeks to months in patients previously on digoxin who had amiodarone instituted. The digoxin serum level may double in adults and may increase as much as eightfold in children. Amiodarone-induced changes in thyroid function may also play a role in the interaction.[65] Digoxin elimination is decreased as thyroid function decreases and increased as thyroid function increases. The amiodarone-induced increases in serum digoxin serum concentrations may begin in 1 to 3 days; in most patients this increase occurs in 3 to 5 days.[66] Patients on prior digoxin therapy should have a 50% dosage reduction in the digoxin dose when amiodarone is begun, and levels should be obtained every 3 to 5 days for the first 2 weeks of therapy.[64] Monthly levels for the first 6 months may be wise, as we have seen patients, previously stabilized on amiodarone and digoxin, become digoxin toxic 3 to 4 months into therapy. In patients who are on amiodarone when digoxin is added, the digoxin dose should be started at one-half the normal dose and followed.

Amiodarone interacts with a number of antiarrhythmics and this interaction is again complicated by both the long half-life of the drug and the slow onset of action. In patients with life-threatening ventricular arrhythmias, it is common to continue treatment with one antiarrhythmic while adding amiodarone.[60] This double antiarrhythmic coverage is continued until it is felt that the therapeutic effects of amiodarone have started (usually 1–3 weeks).[60] Dosage adjustment of the antiarrhythmic and careful monitoring of blood levels are needed during this time.

Flecainide serum levels show a wide variation, with increases from 5 to 190% with wide interindividual variation.[67] This wide range in serum levels must be kept in mind and each patient on flecainide and amiodarone should be followed very closely. The interaction is not yet understood but may involve a change in either the metabolism or the renal elimination of flecainide, or both. Recommendations are to decrease the flecainide dose by 50% when amiodarone is instituted and to follow levels carefully.

Plasma procainamide levels increase an average of 55%, and levels of its metabolite, N-acetylprocainamide (NAPA), increase by an average of 33% when amiodarone is added to therapy. As for flecainide, the exact mechanism of this interaction is unknown but probably involves changes in both renal and hepatic elimination.[64] Procainamide should be decreased by one third to one half when amiodarone is instituted, and serum levels followed closely.

Quinidine levels can increase by one third to one half in patients who are started on amiodarone. This interaction is also thought to be a combination of reductions in renal and nonrenal clearance and displacement from tissue stores.[64] Quinidine toxicity can occur if the quinidine dosage is not decreased by one third to one half following institution of amiodarone therapy.

Serious or fatal hemorrhage is possible in patients treated with warfarin who do not have their doses adjusted after amiodarone therapy is begun. Amiodarone may directly inhibit vitamin K-dependent clotting cofactors, enhancing the anticoagulant effect of warfarin.[68,69] Hepatic clearance of warfarin appears to be decreased mainly by inhibition of the P450/2C9 isoenzyme of P450 primarily responsible for the conversion of (s)-warfarin to its major metabolite, S-7-hydroxywarfarin,[69] and prothrombin times (PTs) can double in patients without a dosage adjustment. Usually, the PT begins to increase in as few as 1 to 3 days, but the full effect may require weeks to be seen.[62,65] Because of the long half-life of amiodarone, the PTs may remain elevated for months after amiodarone is discontinued and the patient remains on warfarin. Warfarin dosages should be decreased by one half when amiodarone is begun, and careful monitoring of the PT is mandatory. Likewise, when warfarin therapy is initiated in a patient who is or was on amiodarone, one-half the usual dose should be used and the PT monitored carefully.[70]

Beta-adrenergic blocking drugs and calcium channel antagonists appear to work synergistically with amiodarone in causing cardiac conduction blocks and bradycardia.[60,64] Dosage adjustments are often needed for the beta blockers and calcium channel antagonists to prevent this adverse effect. In patients for whom therapy with either a beta blocker or a calcium channel antagonist is considered crucial, artificial pacemakers may be needed to maintain the heart rate within physiologic parameters. If possible, the beta blocker or calcium channel blocker should be discontinued or a dose reduction made when amiodarone is started. Decreasing the dose by one third and following electrocardiograms and heart rates constitute a reasonable approach in most clinical situations.

Amiodarone has caused a three- to fourfold increase in phenytoin levels when added to a regimen where patients were already stabilized on phenytoin.[69] The incidence of this interaction is unpredictable and it may not occur until 3 to 4 weeks after amiodarone therapy has begun. It is recommended that patients with an active seizure history who need phenytoin for control be monitored closely for signs and symptoms of phenytoin toxicity, and phenytoin levels evaluated twice weekly for the first 4 to 6 weeks of amiodarone therapy. The mechanism of the amiodarone–phenytoin interaction is probably reduction of the hepatic clearance of phenytoin. In addition, phenytoin may induce amiodarone metabolism, resulting in lower serum levels. The clinical significance of this interaction is, at present, unknown.[72]

Because of the complexity of the amiodarone drug interactions (reductions in renal and hepatic clearance, displacement from tissue stores, competition for protein binding, and alterations in thyroid function), it is recommended that all concurrently administered drugs be monitored for toxicity when amiodarone is instituted. It is quite possible that there exist drugs whose interactions with amiodarone have not yet been appreciated.

Drug interactions of amiodarone are summarized in Table 10–4.

Intravenous Administration

Intravenous amiodarone is currently undergoing a number of investigational trials in the United States. In contrast to oral amiodarone, which may take days to achieve an antiarrhythmic effect, intravenous amiodarone can achieve this effect in less than 2 hours in some patients.[73] It appears

TABLE 10–4. AMIODARONE DRUG INTERACTIONS

Drug	Onset (days)	Interaction	Management
Warfarin	3–4	PT increases[a] INR increases	Decrease warfarin by half; monitor PT and INR
Digoxin	1–5	Digoxin levels increase	Decrease digoxin by half; monitor levels
Quinidine	2–4	Quinidine levels increase	Decrease quinidine by half; monitor quinidine levels
Procainamide	3–7	Procainamide and NAPA levels increase	Decrease procainamide by one third to one half; monitor levels
Phenytoin	Weeks	Phenytoin level increases	Monitor levels twice weekly; adjust dose
Beta blockers Calcium channel blockers		Additive	Monitor clinical condition/ adjust doses of beta or calcium channel blocker

[a]PT, prothrombin time; INR, International Normalized Ratio.

that the electrophysiologic actions of the intravenous form may be different than those of the oral form. These different electrophysiologic effects are seen on the surface electrocardiogram, where oral form prolongs the corrected QT interval whereas the intravenous form does not.[73,74] It appears that one of the main actions of the intravenous form is prolonging the AH interval, indicating prolongation of conduction through the AV node.[74] Intravenous amiodarone apparently blocks the sodium channels in a rate-dependent effect similar to that of lidocaine, which also does not lengthen the corrected QT interval. This is in contrast to the type IA drugs, which do prolong the QT interval and appear to block the sodium channels at both fast and slow rates.[75]

Intravenous amiodarone has proven effective in the treatment of life-threatening ventricular tachycardia and ventricular fibrillation refractory to conventional treatments.[73,74,76–86] It also is effective in the prevention of recurrent atrial fibrillation and flutter and in the termination of supraventricular tachycardias. It is less efficacious in the termination of atrial fibrillation or flutter.[73,76,79,80] The more serious the arrhythmia (ie, ventricular tachycardia versus ventricular fibrillation) and the more seriously ill the patient (normal versus severe heart failure or shock), the poorer the outcome.[79,81] This, of course, is true with all interventions performed on very ill patients.

Although the onset and mechanism of action may vary between the intravenous and oral forms, the severity of adverse reactions does not. Intravenous amiodarone has been reported to cause serious hypotension during the infusion, which may, in part, be related to the infusion rate or the solvent used (Tween 80).[73,77,78,87,88] Symptomatic bradycardia is also a common adverse effect and may require the use of a pacemaker to restore the cardiac rhythm.[77,80] Acute hepatitis has been reported, with aspartate aminotransferase levels reaching 10 times normal. Liver function tests gradually return to normal on discontinuation of the drug.[89–91] An acute rise in intracranial pressure during the infusion has been reported[92]; no data are available as to whether intracranial pressure changes with long-term administration of the oral form. Intravenous amiodarone is also arrhythmogenic. Multifocal ventricular tachycardia (Torsade de pointes) has been reported to occur during loading with the drug.[93] In addition, the drug has a negative inotropic effect and may worsen heart failure despite its vasodilating properties. It appears that patients with higher ejection fractions (greater than 35%) may be able to compensate for the negative inotropic effects, whereas those with lower ejection fractions may not.[73,87,94]

It must also be noted that although there are no reports of drug interactions with the intravenous form, we should expect many of the same drugs that interact with the oral form also to interact with the intravenous form. These drugs include warfarin, digoxin, quinidine, procainamide, beta-adrenergic blockers, and the calcium channel antagonists.

In addition to using intravenous amiodarone for life-threatening, refractory tachyarrhythmias, it has also been studied as a 24-hour infusion immediately after acute anterior wall myocardial infarction.[94] The major endpoints of death, reinfarction, and sustained ventricular arrhythmias were all less in the amiodarone group, but these differences did not reach statistical significance.

Because of the seriousness of the adverse reactions and the potential for serious drug interactions, intravenous amiodarone should be reserved only for those patients who have life-threatening arrhythmias that are refractory to other treatments and to those patients who cannot take the oral form and who need the drug for prevention of life-threatening arrhythmias.[73,82] Although the doses of intravenous amiodarone varied in the studies, an effective dose for the termination and prevention of tachyarrhythmias was a 5 to 10 mg/kg load over 1 hour, then 20 to 30 mg/kg per 24 hours.[73,74,76,79] In a small group of children with an average age of 6.8 years, the effective intravenous dose was 1 mg/kg over 10 minutes and repeated at 10-minute intervals. Average drug load at the time of therapeutic effect was 4.8 mg/kg. After the bolus doses an intravenous infusion of 10 mg/kg per day was continued for 3 days.[85] Dosing in infants less than 1 year of age should be based on body surface area (mg/m^2) instead of weight (mg/kg).[80]

Intravenous amiodarone is compatible in a number of solutions including Dextrose 5% in Water and Normal Saline. It is also compatible with a number of commonly used drugs and electrolytes including potassium chloride, procainamide, lidocaine, verapamil, and furosemide. Intravenous amiodarone is not compatible with quinidine gluconate.[95]

Adverse Reactions

Amiodarone has a number of potentially serious adverse effects, and up to 85% of the patients taking the drug 4 years or longer experience at least one side effect.[44]

Cardiovascular side effects of long-term therapy include symptomatic bradycardia and conduction defects through the atrioventricular node, which may require placement of a permanent pacemaker.[96–98] Amiodarone may worsen serious ventricular arrhythmias such as ventricular tachycardia, fibrillation, and polymorphous ventricular tachycardia. These rhythms could also be due to a lack of adequate drug effect or predisposing factors such as hypokalemia.[98–100]

The most serious extracardiac side effect would be pulmonary toxicity. This toxic effect appears to be dose related and is usually reversible on discontinuation of the drug.[54–57,101,102] The patient presents with symptoms of a nonproductive cough, weight loss, and exertional dyspnea. The symptoms gradually resolve once the drug is withdrawn, with or without corticosteroid therapy.[54]

A 2 to 4% incidence of both hypo- and hyperthyroidism has been reported. Hypothyroidism responds to either drug discontinuation or thyroid supplementation. Hyperthyroidism resolves on discontinuation of the drug.[98,103–105]

Gastrointestinal side effects consisting of nausea, vomiting, and loss of appetite may occur in up to 50% of patients during the oral loading phase.[50] For this reason it is advisable to give the drug in three to four divided doses, with food, throughout the day when giving oral loading doses.

Hepatic enzyme elevation may occur in as many as 40% of patients taking the drug.[106] Although these enzyme levels will return to normal whether or not the drug is discontinued,[107] there have been cases of fatal hepatic cirrhosis with long-term therapy.[108,109]

Corneal microdeposits occur in up to 90% of patients on chronic oral therapy. These microdeposits can be observed by slit-light examination.[110] The microdeposits do not appear to have an effect on vision and resolve when the drug is discontinued. A second type of ocular effect is the observance of halos of light around objects during acute therapy with high doses. This effect appears to be dose-related and resolves with dose reductions or discontinuation of therapy.[110] There have been no reports of permanent ocular toxicity with amiodarone.[110]

Blue-gray skin discoloration has been reported in less than 1% of the patients receiving amiodarone. This discoloration is due to lipofuscin deposits in the skin and gradually disappears once amiodarone is discontinued.[111–113]

Photosensitivity can occur in 3 to 10% of patients.[110] Patients should be advised to use sunscreens to protect against sunburn whenever exposed to sunlight.[114]

Other less common adverse reactions reported include gynecomastia,[115] sterile epididymitis,[116] and toxic epidermal necrolysis.[117]

In conclusion, amiodarone is a therapeutic agent that is often effective in the treatment of life-threatening arrhythmias when all other agents have failed. This drug, however, does have many serious side effects and potentially serious drug interactions and should be reserved for use only in those cases where other therapies have failed. Proper education on the risks and benefits of this agent is essential if the patient is to make an informed decision as to whether the benefits of the drug are worth the added risks associated with such therapy.

PROCAINAMIDE

Clinical Pharmacology and Therapeutics

Procainamide is a type IA antiarrhythmic that has shown efficacy in the treatment of ventricular as well as supraventricular arrhythmias.[118] Procainamide, as a type IA antiarrhythmic, slows impulse conduction through the atrioventricular node by depressing the flow of sodium ions into cells during phase 0 of the action potential.[119]

In a comparison of the various type I antiarrhythmics, differences exist between each group relative to rate of depolarization and effects on the refractory period. As a type IA antiarrhythmic, procainamide moderately reduces the depolarization rate and prolongs repolarization, or the refractory period. This is in contrast to type IB antiarrhythmics, which shorten repolarization, or the refractory period, and weakly affect the repolarization rate. Type IC antiarrhythmic agents strongly depress depolarization, but have negligible effects on the duration of repolarization, or the refractory period.

Additionally, procainamide has been shown to possess peripheral ganglionic blockade activity, which may result in a significant reduction in systemic blood pressure; it also possesses a weak anticholinergic action, which is of concern in patients being treated for supraventricular tachyarrhythmias. In the setting of a supraventricular tachyarrhythmia, the intrinsic anticholinergic effects of procainamide can result in an increase in electrical conduction through the atrioventricular node into the ventricles.[119]

Clinical Pharmacokinetics

Absorption

The literature reports that approximately 75 to 95% (range 66–113%) of an oral dose of procainamide is readily absorbed from the gastrointestinal tract. The data available represent the use of the rapid-acting form of procainamide in capsules[120]; however, during the last 10 years, with the introduction of sustained-release dosing forms (Procan SR, Pronestyl-SR), comparative data and time to peak serum levels have come into question.

Recent studies have shown that the oral absorption for sustained-release procainamide approximates 68% and that the degree of absorption is similar with each product.[121,122] Of added interest is the potential differences that exist with respect to times to peak absorption for the two dosing forms, which for Procan SR and Pronestyl-SR were shown to be 2.2 and 3.8 hours, respectively.[122] Though fundamentally this may not pose a major problem clinically, concern regarding these differences may play an important factor if one anticipates changing from one sustained-release product to another.

One area that has sparked interest since the initial release of Procan SR is the identification of what appears to be an intact wax matrix in the feces of patients taking the product. This was first thought to be the result of an absorption problem, and alarmed the patients who initially received the product; however, as the manufacturer has acknowledged, this matrix tablet represents the remnants of the total dosage form referred to as a "ghost tablet," the ingredients of which were sieved out during passage through the gastrointestinal tract.

Distribution

Procainamide has been described as an antiarrhythmic that distributes into two compartments: a rather small central compartment (0.1–0.9 L/kg) and a larger peripheral compartment, which represents rather extensive distribution into tissues at steady state. Procainamide does not appear to distribute into fat tissues to any significant degree. This becomes a factor when calculating doses for patients; ideal body weight rather than actual body weight will more closely reflect the distribution of the drug throughout the body.

The distribution of procainamide has been reported to be 2.0 L/kg in patients with normal renal function and normal cardiac output. In circumstances such as prerenal azotemia and congestive heart failure, the volume of distribution has been reported to decrease to about 1.5 L/k, which would necessitate a reduction in doses in such patients.[118]

Additionally, procainamide and N-acetylprocainamide (NAPA) have both been shown to appear in breast milk; consequently, close measurements of procainamide and NAPA levels should be carried out on the neonate.[123]

Procainamide demonstrates a minimal amount of plasma protein binding, about 15%[118];

thus, situations such as hypoalbuminemia and nephrotic syndrome that cause a reduction in available binding sites have little effect on the total disposition of the drug.

Metabolism

The discussion of the metabolism of procainamide is somewhat complicated because the drug is eliminated about equally by hepatic and renal routes. Approximately 50% of the parent compound is excreted in the urine, with the remainder being products of metabolism. This has created a rather significant amount of interest during the last 10 to 15 years because of the identification of at least one metabolite that possesses antiarrhythmic activity (NAPA).

Such formation from the parent compound takes place via acetylation, which is additionally compounded by a genetically determined rate for such acetylation. This difference in the rate of transformation shows a bimodal distribution, with patients falling into either slow or fast acetylator groups, similar to the situation for isoniazid and hydralazine.[118] It has also been shown that approximately 2 to 3% of the NAPA formed through acetylation is deacetylated back to procainamide. The remaining NAPA that is formed in the liver is extensively dependent on the kidney for its final elimination.

A drug–food interaction has been reported to occur in patients after the acute ingestion of ethanol.[124] The mechanism for such an interaction involves an increase in the rate of acetylation of procainamide, resulting in higher concentrations of NAPA. One can speculate that after such acute ingestion, NAPA may accumulate at a higher rate because of its longer half-life; consequently, both procainamide and NAPA levels should be more closely monitored.

Additionally, the process of dealkylation has been identified as a metabolic pathway involved in the production of a second metabolite, desethyl-N-acetylprocainamide (NAPADE), which is formed after the initial dealkylation of para-amino-N-2-(ethylamino)ethylbenzamide (PADE). Neither of these products has been shown to offer any antiarrhythmic activity.[125]

Of additional concern regarding the metabolism of procainamide is the production of an additional compound that has been speculated to be responsible for the development of the procainamide-associated lupus erythematosus syndrome. Such a compound, as in the case of isoniazid and hydralazine, has been speculated to be a hydroxylamine intermediate formed from procainamide. Studies to date reveal that the slow acetylator, besides demonstrating a smaller NAPA/procainamide ratio of about 0.6 as compared with the rapid acetylator ratio of 1–1.2, may have a higher incidence of the described lupus reaction.[126]

One would suspect that dosing adjustments would be required in patients suffering from hepatic disease based on the acetylation of procainamide by the liver; however, the current lack of concrete data requires the clinician to monitor procainamide levels closely in such patients where a prolongation in dosing interval may be required.

Elimination

Approximately 40 to 60% of a procainamide dose is excreted unchanged in the urine (average 50%). Consequently, the half-life for procainamide as the parent compound has been reported to be approximately 3.5 hours without renal impairment and 5 to 20 hours (average 10 hours) in the anephric patient.[127–130]

The prolongation of procainamide half-life with declining renal status has provided several recommendations for dose adjustments in patients with renal impairment.[131] Patients with mild renal failure (glomerular filtration rate [GFR] > 50 mL/min) should be dosed every 6 to 12 hours, and patients with severe renal failure (GFR < 10 mL/min) should be dosed every 8 to 24 hours.

As has been described in the literature, the elimination of NAPA is much more dependent on renal function (up to 85%); therefore, the accumulation of NAPA with declining renal function must be taken into consideration when designing dosing regimens for procainamide. In patients with normal renal function, half-life has ranged between 4 and 15 hours, whereas in the anephric patient the half-life has been reported to be as long as 40 hours.[127–130]

Unlike other agents whose elimination has paralleled the glomerular filtration for any given patient, the elimination of procainamide and NAPA is dependent on proximal renal secretion as well. Consequently, the development of simple nomograms to correct for altered GFRs does not suffice for procainamide. Therefore, the use of procainamide in patients with significant renal impairment is best avoided if possible, but if not, it is best achieved with careful monitoring of both procainamide and NAPA levels as well as a clinical assessment for efficacy and toxicity.

The pharmacokinetic parameters for procainamide are summarized in Table 10–5.

TABLE 10–5. SUMMARY OF PHARMACOKINETIC PARAMETERS FOR PROCAINAMIDE (PA)

Pharmacokinetic Parameter	Value		Comments
Bioavailability	100% (IV)		87% PA[a]
	83% (conventional capsules)		$F' = 0.72$
	80% (sustained-release tablets)		$F' = 0.69$
$t_{1/2,\alpha}$	6 min		
$t_{1/2}$ (h)	Normal	Anuria	
PA	2.5–4.7	5.3–20.7	
NAPA	4.3–15.1	>40	
V_d	2.0 L/kg		Reduced to 1.5 L/kg in congestive heart failure
Protein bound	15%		
Acetylator status:			
bimodal distribution in humans			Slow acetylators show
Slow acetylators	NAPA/PA = 0.60		higher rates of systemic
Fast acetylators	NAPA/PA = 1–1.20		lupus erythematosus
Absorption lag time	PO: 20–30 min		
	IM: 2 min		
Time to peak	PO: 1.5 h		
	IM: 25 min		
Renal excretion	50% PA		
	85% NAPA		
Active metabolites	NAPA		Controversy as to role in treatment of arrhythmias
Serum levels	Variable		See text

[a] 87% of dosage form is procainamide.

Pharmacodynamics

Drug–Drug Interactions

Most drug–drug interactions of significance have centered around altered renal clearance. The H_2 receptor antagonists cimetidine and ranitidine have both been reported to compete for active tubular secretion via the kidney and, thus, necessitate a reduction of procainamide dose in patients receiving these agents (Table 10–6). One such report revealed a decrease in renal clearance from 258 to 197 mL/min when cimetidine was given to patients receiving procainamide.[132]

Though the mechanism has not been completely identified at this time, amiodarone usage has been shown to increase serum procainamide levels by 50% and NAPA levels by 30%. Consequently, as suggested in the literature, use of amiodarone with procainamide may result in elevated levels of procainamide unless reductions in doses occur at the time of initiation of amiodarone therapy.

Therapeutic Efficacy

Few antiarrhythmics currently available for clinical use have had greater documentation of the relationship between antiarrhythmic effects and plasma levels than has procainamide. Initial data presented on a group of patients treated for various arrhythmias revealed a desirable therapeutic range of 4 to 8 µg/mL.[120] The authors also report that at such desired concentrations, therapeutic efficacy was appreciated in 90% of patients, whereas toxic effects occurred in less than 10% of patients evaluated.[120] Additional studies have since been conducted that have revealed slight alterations in the initial therapeutic range as reported above.[120,133–139] Table 10–7 lists the studies that have evaluated the therapeutic and toxic ranges for procainamide and includes brief descriptions of the study methods.

As can be appreciated from Table 10–7, most of the early work done with procainamide centered around a therapeutic range of 4 to 8 µg/mL. This range was to reflect a positive effect of procainamide on arrhythmia suppression, but recently, investigators have begun to suggest that higher serum levels are required to more effectively treat patients with procainamide.

TABLE 10–6. PROCAINAMIDE DRUG INTERACTIONS

Drug	Mechanism	Comments
Cimetidine Ranitidine	Reduced tubular secretion and prolongation of $t_{1/2}$	Reduce PA dose
Amiodarone	Unknown, but increase by 50% PA level and 30% NAPA level	Reduce PA dose to prevent accumulation of PA and NAPA
Ethanol	Acute ingestion reported to increase PA acetylation	Closely monitor PA and NAPA levels for accumulation of NAPA; may need to prolong dosing interval
Trimethoprim	Increased plasma concentration and $t_{1/2}$ for both PA and NAPA	Closely monitor PA and NAPA levels and clinical effects

TABLE 10–7. SUMMARY OF STUDIES EVALUATING PROCAINAMIDE SERUM LEVELS

Investigator	Sample Size	Therapeutic Range (μg/mL)	Comments
Koch-Weser and Klein[120]	142	4–8 PA	Various arrhythmias, no details documenting arrhythmias, frequency of ectopic beats, and duration of observation
Giardina et al[133] PVCs VT	20	4–10 PA 6.3 PA 8.2 PA	Patients with VT[a] required higher PA levels than patients with PVCs along Levels may have been drawn too early after injection for full appreciation of entire clinical effect
Giardina et al[134] Therapeutic Toxic	33	6.8 PA 8.7 NAPA 13.7 PA 17.1 NAPA	Patients with PVCs monitored with Holter monitors Results reported reflect those of 22 patients who responded to therapy
Lima et al[135]	7	> 10.00	Little toxicity when PA levels reached 10 mg/mL
Greenspan et al[136]	16	13.6 PA	All but one patient required levels > 9 for suppression of recurrent VT induced through electrical stimulation
Myerburg et al[137]	6	5.0 + 0.5 PA	Patients with acute MI-induced PVCs
	6	9.3 + 0.7 PA	Patients with recurrent VT to reduce PVCs
Roden et al[138] Therapeutic Toxic	23	9.4–19.5 NAPA (mean trough: 14.3) 10.6–37.9 NAPA (mean trough: 22.5)	
Winkle et al[139] Therapeutic Toxic	11	— 6.9–25.6 NAPA	
Lima et al[135] Conclusions		25–30 PA + NAPA PA: 6–14 NAPA: Evaluate only for toxicity	

[a]VT, ventricular tachycardia.

An additional area of controversy centers on the active metabolite NAPA and its contributions to the antiarrhythmic effects of procainamide. Prior to the availability of NAPA assays and the identification of NAPA as an antiarrhythmic, monitoring of procainamide therapy centered around therapeutic ranges established for procainamide alone. Recently, however, the use of procainamide levels alone or in combination with NAPA has provided much controversy as to the correct method for evaluating a patient's therapy.

Today's dilemma concerns the relationship between procainamide and NAPA and the therapeutic and toxic responses to the substances. Roden et al compared the responses to procainamide and NAPA of 23 patients suffering from premature ventricular contractions (PVCs) and ventricular tachycardia.[138] In the study, 63% of patients receiving procainamide responded favorably as compared with only 30% of the patients who had received NAPA. These findings are consistent with those of others who believe that the differing electrophysiologic activities of the two substances should result in differing response rates.[139]

It has been suggested that the therapeutic concentration range for procainamide should now be regarded as 6 to 14 μg/mL, which represents a 50 to 75% increase over the previously described ranges set by Koch-Weser and Klein.[120] At the same time, it appears that the active metabolite NAPA may not significantly contribute to the antiarrhythmic efficacy but may serve to augment the adverse effects associated with such therapy.[140]

Much work continues to be reported regarding the relationship between procainamide and NAPA with respect to the efficacy and toxicity associated with their use. In the clinical setting, much confusion still arises when procainamide and NAPA serum levels are obtained concomitantly on patients receiving procainamide therapy. It has been suggested that the sum of the two serum levels may be the greatest aid in guiding future adjustments to therapy.[135] In the group evaluated by Lima et al, it was concluded that the sums of procainamide and NAPA levels between 25 and 30 μg/mL were associated with therapeutic efficacy, and that adverse effects became more likely when the combined levels exceeded 30 μg/mL.

In conclusion, routine monitoring of procainamide serum levels has been shown to directly reflect the therapeutic efficacy and toxicity associated with the parent drug. Because as much as 50% of procainamide may be converted to the active metabolite NAPA, concern must exist with respect to the therapeutic levels of this metabolite and their impact on efficacy and toxicity. Questions remain as to the electrophysiologic effects of NAPA, reduced potency of NAPA as compared with procainamide, and controversial nature of NAPA as an antiarrhythmic agent; therefore, routine monitoring does not seem cost-effective at this time. Currently, the routine monitoring of procainamide therapy for serum concentrations between 6 and 14 μg/mL as suggested in the literature suffices in most clinical situations.

There may exist subsets of patients who require routine monitoring of both procainamide and NAPA. The elimination of NAPA via the kidneys may be compromised in patients with declining renal status and may provide a basis for such monitoring. There have been reports of toxic effects in patients with declining renal status because of the accumulation of NAPA.[141]

Of major concern when evaluating serum procainamide levels is timing. As discussed previously, steady-state levels are interpretable and have been shown to correlate well with end-organ tissue concentrations. Consequently, a patient receiving a bolus dose followed by a continuous infusion will attain steady state shortly after receiving the loading dose (approximately 2 hours).[142] Additional levels at 12 hours and then 24 hours would be appropriate when monitoring short-term therapy. Once the desired concentration has been achieved and the patient has responded favorably, levels can be obtained at greater intervals based on the patient setting.

Regardless of the underlying disease process, many clinicians still prefer the active role that the electrocardiogram plays in the monitoring of procainamide therapy. As a type IA antiarrhythmic, the greatest effect of procainamide occurs on the QRS complex (ventricular depolarization). Baseline evaluations of the QT interval aid in the monitoring of pharmacologic as well as toxic effects. The QT interval increases with increasing serum levels of procainamide; however, as the interval approaches 25% of baseline, the clinician exercises extreme caution on increasing doses because of the potential to induce toxicity. Fifty percent prolongation of the QT interval signifies the need to reduce doses, and even abandon therapy.

Myasthenia gravis is a disease involving the cholinergic nervous system in which the lack of acetylcholine activity results in fatigue, muscle weakness, respiratory paralysis, and even death. This disease process becomes of concern pharmacodynamically in patients receiving procainamide, who may experience a potentiation of the drug's anticholinergic properties. Consequently, procainamide is relatively contraindicated in patients with myasthenia gravis. Additionally, patients receiving procainamide should be monitored closely for anticholinergic effects when other anticholinergic agents (propantheline, atropine, etc) are added to therapy.

Adverse Reactions

We have already discussed the relationship between serum procainamide levels and therapeutic effect. Of additional concern are those side effects that are directly related to serum procainamide concentrations. Koch-Weser and Klein were able to identify minor and major side effects that developed as serum procainamide levels approached the upper limits of their initially described therapeutic range of 4 to 8 µg/mL.[120] Minor side effects, including nausea and vomiting, fatigue, weakness, and reduced arterial blood pressure, have been reported with serum levels above 8.0 µg/mL. Major side effects, including significant prolongation of PR, QRS, and QT intervals, development of new arrhythmias, and even cardiac arrest, have been attributed to serum levels in excess of 12.0 µg/mL.[120]

Additional side effects reported in the literature include dizziness, lightheadedness, skin rash, sore throat, and agranulocytosis.

The literature has also described the development of clinically significant hypotension and bradycardia when procainamide is given intravenously at a rapid rate. Consequently, current recommendations include the intravenous administration of procainamide at a rate not to exceed 25 to 50 mg/min.

Much attention has been given in the literature to the development of a drug-induced lupus erythematosus syndrome, which includes antinuclear antibodies (ANA), positive lupus erythematosus preparations, arthralgias, myalgias, and fever. This syndrome has not been directly related to serum procainamide levels, but is a consequence of continuous therapy. Approximately 50 to 80% of patients taking procainamide develop positive ANA, and the full-blown syndrome has been reported to occur in 30 to 50% of these patients. Drug-induced systemic lupus erythematosus is usually not life threatening, but does usually require the cessation of therapy.[126]

Most patients respond favorably within 2 weeks of discontinuing procainamide; however, it may take up to a year for ANA titers to return to normal.

Therapeutic Regimen Design

Several methods have been presented in the literature for the effective dosing of procainamide. As discussed earlier in the chapter, the steady-state concentrations required to treat patients effectively are still undergoing evaluation. For the purposes of this discussion, 8 µg/mL (8 mg/L), representing the upper limit of Koch-Weser and Klein's range, will be used to calculate the dosing requirements for procainamide.[120] The clinician must appreciate that the individual patient, therapeutic indications, clinical experience, and clinical setting dictate the serum level goal.

Calculation of Loading Doses

Using a more traditional dosing regimen based on the available pharmacokinetic parameters one is able to calculate the following dosing regimen for a 70-kg patient suffering from a ventricular arrhythmia in whom congestive heart failure or renal dysfunction is not present.

1. Dose $= C_{av}V_d/F$, where $F = 0.87$ for procainamide HCl.
2. Dose $= (6.0 \text{ mg/L} \times 2 \text{ L/kg})/0.87$.
3. Dose $= 13.80$ mg/kg as a loading dose to obtain procainamide serum levels of 6.0 mg/L.
4. Literature recommendations for 17 mg/kg IBW as a loading dose will result in initial serum levels of 17 mg/kg $= (C_{av} \times 2 \text{ L/kg})/0.87 = 7.4$ mg/L for C_{av}.

Of critical importance in this situation are the parameters used in calculating the volume of distribution (V_d). As discussed previously, the volume of distribution is decreased in patients with congestive heart failure or renal dysfunction to about 1.5 L/kg, which should result in the following change in the preceding calculation.

1. Dose $= (C_{av} \times 1.5 \text{ L/kg})/0.87$.
2. Dose $= (6.0 \text{ mg/L} \times 1.5 \text{ L/kg})/0.87$.
3. Dose $= 10.3$ mg/kg in patients with congestive heart failure.
4. A loading dose of 12 mg/kg IBW, as suggested by several sources, results in initial procainamide concentrations of 12 mg/kg $= (C_{av} \times 1.5 \text{ L/kg})/0.87$.
5. $C_{av} = 6.96$ mg/L.

In the clinical setting, due to the potential acuteness of any arrhythmia, the use of a parenteral loading dose at a rate not to exceed 25 to 50 mg/min has been shown effective. For the above-mentioned patients this would translate to the following orders:

1. No predisposing factors in a 70-kg patient: 13.8 mg/kg $\times$ 70 kg $= 966$ mg, or 1000 mg given over 30–60 minutes.
2. A 70-kg patient with coexisting CHF: 10.3 mg/kg $\times$ 70 kg $= 721$ mg, or 725 mg given over 20–40 minutes.

Calculation of Maintenance Doses

Using the equation for calculating infusion doses below, one is able to calculate the required maintenance infusion rate (K_o) to provide therapeutic levels as the loading dose is eliminated. In a patient with no predisposing factors:

$$C_{ss} = \frac{1.44 \times K_o \times f \times t_{1/2}}{V_d}$$

$$6.0 \text{ mg/L} = \frac{1.44 \times K_o \times 0.87 \times 3.5}{2.0 \text{ L/kg}}$$

$$K_o = 2.74 \text{ mg/kg/h, or } 3.20 \text{ mg/min}$$

In the patient with predisposing factors such as renal dysfunction the infusion rate is altered to reflect the reduction in volume of distribution as well as a prolongation in half-life:

$$C_{av} = \frac{1.44 \times K_o \times f \times t_{1/2}}{1.5 \text{ L/kg}}$$

$$6.00 \text{ mg/L} = \frac{1.44 \times K_o \times 0.87 \times 10}{1.5 \text{ L/kg}}$$

$$K_o = 0.72 \text{ mg/kg/h, or } 0.84 \text{ mg/min}$$

Conversion from Intravenous to Oral Maintenance Therapy

Using the principles described by Lima et al,[135] the following equations can be used to convert a patient successfully treated with intravenous therapy who now requires long-term chronic therapy. In this situation, however, one must take into account the F value of 0.87 when using procainamide HCl, and then calculate actual bioavailability by assuming approximately 83% absorption, or $87 \times 0.83 = F' = 0.72$.

$$\text{daily dose} = \frac{C_{ss}(\text{des}) \times K_o \times 24/ F'}{C_{ss}}$$

where $C_{ss}(\text{des})$ = desired average steady-state concentration, C_{ss} = observed steady-state concentration during intravenous dosing, K_o = maintenance intravenous infusion rate (as mg/h), and F' = bioavailability from oral dose.

In the preceding examples this would translate to the following: The author has chosen to use a steady-state serum concentration of 4.0 mg/L as described by Koch-Weser and Klein when using the range of 4 to 8 mg/L.

In the 70-kg patient discussed above with no renal dysfunction or reduction in cardiac output:

$$\text{daily dose} = \frac{4 \text{ mg/L} \times 3.2 \text{ mg/min} \times 60 \text{ min/h} \times 24 \text{ h}/0.72}{6 \text{ mg/L}}$$

$$4300 \text{ mg} = 4.3 \text{ g in 6–8 doses of a conventional procainamide capsule}$$

If a sustained-release tablet is used, $F' = 0.70$ because the dosage contains 87% procainamide and 80% of the dosage is bioavailable (ie, $0.87 \times 0.80 = 0.70$).

Therefore, 4.5 g would be needed over 24 hours, in 6-hour intervals (1 g q6h).

In the 70-kg patient with either renal or cardiac output reduction:

$$\text{daily dose} = \frac{4 \text{ mg/L} \times 0.84 \text{ mg/min} \times 60 \text{ min/h} \times 24 \text{ h}/0.72}{6 \text{ mg/L}}$$

$$= 1120 \text{ mg} = 1.0 \text{ g in 6–8 doses of a conventional procainamide capsule}$$

If a sustained-release tablet is used, the daily needs would be calculated as 1.7 g over 24 hours, in 6-hour intervals (425 mg q6h).

Sustained-release products should not routinely be used to load patients during initiation of therapy; however, the convenience of a three- or four-times-daily regimen should not be overlooked when designing long-term maintenance therapy.

QUINIDINE

Clinical Pharmacology and Therapeutics

Quinidine, a type IA antiarrhythmic agent, works by inhibiting the fast inward sodium current and, thus, decreasing the maximum rate of rise and amplitude of the cardiac action potential.[143] Studies to date have shown that quinidine causes electrocardiogram changes that include prolongation of the QT interval and, to a lesser degree, the QRS complex duration, which is observed with increasing plasma quinidine concentrations. The effects of quinidine on the QRS complex have proven useful when monitoring for therapeutic as well as toxic effects of the drug.

Additionally, quinidine has been shown to possess a significant atropine-like effect and peripheral alpha-adrenergic blockade, and has been shown capable of increasing atrial conduction into the ventricles.[144] As a type IA antiarrhythmic agent used in the treatment and prevention of both atrial and ventricular tachyarrhythmias, this atropine-like effect may be detrimental in patients being treated with quinidine for such tachyarrhythmias. Atrioventricular (AV) conduction may be increased reflexly through peripheral vasodilation caused either by the alpha-adrenergic blockade or a vagolytic effect induced by quinidine at the atrioventricular node.

The antiarrhythmic efficacy and toxicity of quinidine usually have been shown to correlate with serum concentration of the drug. As mentioned previously, the assay techniques employed have created variations in therapeutic ranges. As the assay techniques have become more specific for quinidine, reports have shown that the effective serum quinidine level for reducing premature ventricular contractions (PVCs) may be as low as 1.0 µg/mL or less.[145] Despite these findings, the authors stated that a satisfactory therapeutic effect did occur in 12 of 14 study subjects whose plasma concentrations ranged from 0.72 to 5.92 µg/mL.[145] In that study, the assay method did not report metabolite concentrations, and this may explain why the lower quinidine concentrations were shown to be efficacious.

Several other studies, using various assay techniques, have shown that therapeutic quinidine levels overlap in the range 2.0–6.0 µg/mL. A previous study defined 3.0 to 6.0 µg/mL as the optimum quinidine concentration range required to convert patients satisfactorily from atrial fibrillation.[146] Though this study is still frequently cited today as a reference for the therapeutic concentration range for quinidine, it is important to appreciate that quinidine was measured along with its metabolites, and the concentration of unchanged drug may have been overestimated. As suggested by one researcher, toxic effects are observed when the serum quinidine level exceeds 6.0 µg/mL.

Consequently, though the literature does suggest a therapeutic serum range for efficacy of quinidine therapy, variations in the manner in which the drug is analyzed have provided controversial ranges for its antiarrhythmic effects.

As mentioned previously, the activity of the quinidine metabolites, specifically 3-hydroxyquinidine and 2'-oxoquinidione, has provided more questions than answers in monitoring quinidine therapy. Though we have provided the reader with a therapeutic range for quinidine, 2.0 to

6.0 µg/mL, methodologic inconsistencies in most of the earlier studies make it impossible to make definite statements regarding optimal serum quinidine levels.[140] Until such controversies are resolved in the literature the following guidelines for using serum drug concentrations for quinidine are recommended:

1. Obtain baseline electrocardiograms on specific patients prior to quinidine therapy to determine the width of the QT interval and QRS complex.
2. Use routine electrocardiogram tracings during the initiation of quinidine to evaluate a therapeutic prolongation of the QT interval and QRS complex, while at the same time monitoring for resolution of the indicated arrhythmia.
3. As the QT interval or QRS complex begins to approach 25% prolongation of the respective baseline measurement, obtain serum quinidine concentrations to ensure attainment of therapeutic levels.
4. If therapeutic concentrations are obtained and the QT interval or QRS complex has been prolonged by 25% of the baseline measurement, begin thinking about an alternate antiarrhythmic.
5. If one of the more specific assays for measuring quinidine are used, mentally reduce the therapeutic quinidine concentration to the lower end of the serum range of 2.0 to 6.0 µg/mL. This will compensate for the potential antiarrhythmic effects of quinidine metabolites not measured in the more specific assays.

Clinical Pharmacokinetics

Absorption

Quinidine is currently available in the form of several salts, each of which possesses specific characteristics associated with absorption, onset of action, and duration of effect. Overall, studies conducted to date reveal quinidine bioavailability of 70 to 80% with significant first-pass elimination.[147] Quinidine sulfate in a conventional dosage form has been shown to be completely absorbed after oral administration from the gastrointestinal tract, and has been detected in the serum within 15 minutes of an oral dose.[148]

Peak levels have been reported within 1 hour of oral administration of conventional quinidine sulfate tablets as compared with the sustained-release form and the gluconate form, which are absorbed more slowly.[149] This change in rate of absorption for the various salts may lend itself to differing uses for each salt based on individual patient requirements.

The gluconate form of quinidine has been reported to produce peak serum levels at 3.6 hours after administration, whereas the polygalacturonate salt of quinidine has been reported to elicit peak serum levels 6 hours after administration.[150,151] Based on the available information in the literature, one would expect that both the gluconate and polygalacturonate salts, as well as the sustained-release sulfate product, would be appropriate for regimens providing less frequent (every 8 to 12 hours) dosing, as compared with conventional dosage form sulfate (every 6 to 8 hours).[152]

Additional claims have been made that the sustained-release salt forms have less potential to produce gastrointestinal intolerance, a common concern for patients receiving the drug orally.

The absorption characteristics of the various salts of quinidine take on added importance when prescribing the various preparations. It is fundamental for the clinician to remember that each salt form contains different amounts of the quinidine base. The sulfate contains 83%, the gluconate contains 62%, and the polygalacturonate contains 60% of the base.[152] Consequently, a 275-mg quinidine polygalacturonate product is equivalent to a 200-mg quinidine sulfate tablet, and a 324-mg quinidine gluconate tablet is equivalent to a 240-mg quinidine sulfate product.[152]

$$324 \text{ mg quinidine gluconate} = 240 \text{ mg quinidine sulfate}$$

$$\cdot = 200 \text{ mg of quinidine base}$$

$$275 \text{ mg quinidine polygalacturonate} = 200 \text{ mg quinidine sulfate}$$

$$= 165 \text{ mg of quinidine base}$$

Quinidine has been given via the intramuscular route with conflicting results regarding the systemic availability.[152,153] An initial report showed that intramuscular administration of quinidine gluconate produces higher peak quinidine concentrations than comparable doses of oral quinidine sulfate.[153] A later report, however, showed rather erratic and incomplete absorption rates with the intramuscular route as compared with the oral route.[152]

Distribution

The distribution kinetics have been described using a two-compartment model consisting of a small central compartment ($V_{d,c} = 0.91$ L/kg) and a larger peripheral compartment ($V_{d,ss} = 3.03$ L/kg).[154] The reported $V_{d,ss}$ is consistent with the range previously reported by others.[147,152] Additionally, the two-compartment model has also been used to determine the short half-life within the central compartment of approximately 7 minutes ($t_{1/2,\alpha}$) for distribution, and the longer half-life within the peripheral compartment of 6 to 8 hours ($t_{1/2,\beta}$) for elimination.

Congestive heart failure has been shown to reduce the normal $V_{d,ss}$ for quinidine from 3.0 to 1.3–2.3 L/kg.[155] One would speculate that this would result in a decrease in the half-life; however, a subsequent reduction in plasma clearance results in only small insignificant differences in serum half-life.[155]

Quinidine has also been shown to be highly protein bound (80–90%), but this may be dependent on pH and/or α_1-acid glycoprotein levels for disease state fluctuations.[156,157] Studies have shown that binding of quinidine to the α_1-acid glycoprotein may help explain the increased amount of free quinidine reported in patients after acute myocardial infarction and in mothers just prior to delivery. In both situations, it is believed that initial α_1-glycoprotein levels are low and increase significantly over time.[158] Consequently, the pharmacologic effect associated with the free quinidine concentrations may be directly related to the amount of circulating α_1-acid glycoprotein.

Though the levels may start off low during various acute diseases (resulting in more free quinidine), a gradual increase in α_1-acid glycoprotein as the illness progresses may result in an eventual reduction in free quinidine levels. It has been suggested that the binding of quinidine to α_1-acid glycoprotein may be more significant than its binding to albumin.[157]

Quinidine has been shown to have little dependence on liver blood flow or low hepatic extractability, which suggests little bioavailability variations with route of administration.[154]

Metabolism

Quinidine is eliminated from the body primarily by metabolism, which represents approximately 83% of any given dose.[159] Quinidine is metabolized in the liver through hydroxylation to

3-hydroxyquinidine and through oxidation to 2-quinolone.[160,161] Much controversy has arisen as to the activity of the various metabolites of quinidine. Recent studies suggest that the 3-hydroxy-quinidine metabolite does possess antiarrhythmic effects similar to those of quinidine, through such effects may be less potent than those of the parent compound.[162] More recently, the contributions of several quinidine metabolites were reported.[163] Of the three metabolites tested, 3-hydroxyquinidine, 2'-oroquinidione, and quinidine N-oxide, the authors concluded that the data indicate that the metabolites accumulate during quinidine infusions, and that the metabolites may have different electrophysiologic effects on the heart and may contribute to the overall antiarrhythmic effects of the parent drug.[163]

Controversy still exists today as to the respective contributions of the quinidine metabolites to the parent drug's pharmacologic activity. This becomes crucial for the clinician who is monitoring quinidine serum levels in the patient being treated for an arrhythmia. Initially quinidine therapy monitoring employed a nonspecific assay that measured both quinidine and its metabolites[164]; however, newer assay techniques have since been developed that measure primarily active quinidine concentrations.

It therefore becomes important for the clinician to identify from the laboratory the assay technique used. Today, most laboratories use a version of the double-extraction technique to measure only the active quinidine concentration. Of concern in many of these laboratories, however, is the measurement of a cardiac contaminant, dihydroquinidine, which has no significant antiarrhythmic activity. As the assay methods continue to be refined, through the use of immunoassays, fluorescence polarization immunoassay, and high-pressure liquid chromatography, the clinician will need to keep abreast of the changes that may be occurring in the specific laboratory employed in his or her practice.[165]

Elimination

The amount of quinidine excreted unchanged in the urine is approximately 17%.[159] Quinidine is a weak base ($pK_a = 8.34$) and its excretion by the kidney is pH dependent. By increasing the urinary pH with antacids, acetazolamide, or sodium bicarbonate, a greater percentage of renal quinidine is in the unionized form, resulting in increased renal tubular reabsorption.

One report showed that average quinidine renal clearance decreased by up to 50% during alkaluria and that such clearance was inversely proportional to urine pH.[166] In the same report, urinary alkalinization resulted in increased serum quinidine concentrations as well as an intensification of electrocardiographic effects.[166]

Pharmacokinetic parameters for quinidine are summarized in Table 10–8.

Pharmacodynamics

Special Populations

Several patient populations have been identified whose pharmacokinetic/pharmacodynamic effects may be altered when quinidine is administered (Tables 10–9 and 10–10).

The liver serves as the major route of inactivation for quinidine. Studies to date, however, do not suggest major dosing alterations for quinidine with reduced liver function.[167] With severe hepatic dysfunction as a result of end-stage liver disease, total body quinidine clearance has been reported to decrease and may require a reduction in dosing regimen.[168]

TABLE 10–8. SUMMARY OF PHARMACOKINETIC PARAMETERS FOR QUINIDINE

V_d (central)	0.9 L/kg
V_d (apparent)	2–3 L/kg (reduced in congestive heart failure to 1.3–2.3 L/kg)
$t_{1/2,\alpha}$	7 min
$t_{1/2,\beta}$	6–8 h (increased to 8–10 h in cirrhosis)
F	0.75 (range, 0.70–0.80)
F'	
Sulfate	0.83
Gluconate	0.62
Polygalacturonate	0.60
Serum levels	2–6 mg/L (depending on assay used)

TABLE 10–9. DRUG–DISEASE ALTERATIONS IN PHARMACOKINETICS AND/OR PHARMACODYNAMICS

Patient Population	Alteration	Cause
Congestive heart failure[172,173]	Negligible	Reduced $V_{d,ss}$ and prolongation of body clearance negate each other.
End-stage liver disease[168]	Quinidine accumulation	$t_{1/2}$ and V_d increase with a decrease in total body accumulation.
Post-myocardial infarction[157,158]	Increased pharmacologic effect, which decreases during the stress	Reduced α_1-acid glycoprotein results in more "free" quinidine initially, but as AAG increases "free" levels decrease.
Elderly[165]	Negligible	Accumulation of metabolites and quinidine is minimal because of reduced creatinine clearance.
Pediatrics[165]	Reduced pharmacologic effect	Shortened $t_{1/2}$ results in lower serum levels.
Postsurgery (acute stress)[157,158]	Reduced pharmacologic effect	Increased AAG binding to quinidine causes a reduction in free quinidine levels.
Dialysis (hemo-/peritoneal)[159]	Decreased pharmacologic effect	Potential exists for loss of drug through dialysis.

TABLE 10–10. DRUG–DRUG ALTERATIONS IN PHARMACOKINETICS AND PHARMACODYNAMICS

Patient Population	Alteration	Cause
Warfarin[176]	Additive hypoprothrombinemia	Additive depression of vitamin K-dependent clotting factors
Antihypertensives[165]	Hypotension	Peripheral vasodilation by quinidine exacerbates antihypertensive effects
Phenothiazines[180]	Additive myocardial depressant effects	QT interval prolongation by both quinidine and the phenothiazines
Muscle relaxants[178,179]	Additive neuromuscular blocking activity,	Quinidine potentiates all neuromuscular blockers
Enzyme inducers (phenytoin, barbiturates, rifampin)[169–171]	reduced pharmacologic effect	Increased rate of metabolism of quinidine
Digitalis glycosides[177]	Increased digitalis effect	Reduction in renal and nonrenal clearance
Antacids[169,175]	Increased renal tubular reabsorption	Urine pH of 7.0, resulting in increased unionized drug and prolongation of $t_{1/2}$
Acetazolamide Sodium bicarbonate[169,175]	Increased pharmacologic effect	Increased urine pH, resulting in increased tubular reabsorption and prolonged $t_{1/2}$
Cimetidine[169,170]	Increased pharmacologic effect	Reduced metabolic clearance

Additionally, several drugs that act as inducers of metabolizing enzymes have been shown to reduce the elimination half-life of quinidine and, thus, increase quinidine dosing requirements.[169–171]

Patients suffering from congestive heart failure pose a potential dilemma to the clinician treating a patient with quinidine. Though there have been reports of a prolongation of half-life in patients with congestive heart failure, other researchers have suggested no significant changes that would necessitate a dosing adjustment.[172,173] Consequently, it is reasonable to assume that reductions in $V_{d,ss}$ associated with prolongation of total body clearance result in only negligible effects on the half-life:

$$t_{1/2} = \frac{V_d \times 0.693}{\text{clearance}}$$

According to this equation, if V_d decreases at a rate equal to the increase in total body clearance, no significant change in half-life will be observed.[174]

Declining renal function has also been studied for its effects on quinidine elimination. As mentioned previously, renal elimination contributes minimally to the body's ability to remove quinidine.[159] Therefore, accumulation of potentially active metabolites such as 3-hydroxyquinidine and 2'oxoquinidione as well as quinidine would not be expected to cause significant changes in dosing requirements in the patient population.[165]

During recent years, increased attention has been given to the effects of various stressful situations on the plasma protein α_1-acid glycoprotein (AAG).[158] As a key participant in the 80 to 90% binding of quinidine in the plasma, alterations in AAG levels would be expected to impact on quinidine disposition.[157] Various stressful situations such as acute myocardial infarction, surgery, and the predelivery phases of pregnancy have been shown to increase AAG levels to accommodate for stress.[158] As the AAG levels increase in response to such stresses, available free quinidine concentrations in the plasma decrease, resulting in a potential need to increase daily doses of the drug.[158] There have been speculative reports that these types of patients may need to have "free" quinidine serum determinations to aid in the dosing adjustments that may be required.[165]

As can be seen from Table 10–10, numerous drug–disease interactions have been described when quinidine is given to various populations of patients.

Numerous drugs have been reported to interact with quinidine through several key mechanisms:

1. Increase in renal tubular reabsorption with a resultant increase in serum quinidine concentrations[169,175]
2. Stimulation of metabolizing enzymes within the liver with a resultant decrease in serum quinidine concentrations[169–171]
3. Inhibition of metabolizing enzymes within the liver with a resultant increase in serum quinidine concentrations[169,170]

Additionally, quinidine has been shown to alter the pharmacokinetics/pharmacodynamics of other agents through several mechanisms:

1. Depression of vitamin K-dependent clotting factors by quinidine with a resultant additive hypo-prothrombinemic effect when used in combination with warfarin[176]
2. Reduction by quinidine of the volume of distribution as well as the renal and nonrenal clearances of digitalis glycosides, resulting in a two- to threefold increase in the glycoside serum level[177]
3. Potentiation by quinidine of nondepolarizing as well as depolarizing muscle relaxants, resulting in a prolongation of muscle relaxation[178,179]
4. Antiarrhythmic effects of quinidine additive to the effects induced by phenothiazines, with a resultant prolongation of QT interval[180]
5. Peripheral alpha-adrenergic blocking effects by quinidine resulting in peripheral dilation, which may add to the hypotensive effects associated with most antihypertensives and peripheral vasodilators[165]

Crucial to the appropriate therapeutic drug monitoring of quinidine is the ability of the clinician to recognize pharmacokinetic/pharmacodynamic alterations caused by diseases and other therapeutic agents, and to respond appropriately prior to alteration and after the alteration returns to normal. This enables the patient to receive adequate quinidine therapy regardless of alterations. An example of such a scenario would include a patient with congestive heart failure being treated with digoxin who is about to receive quinidine for the acute treatment of atrial fibrillation. Recognizing the drug–drug interaction described for digoxin–quinidine should result in a reduction in the current digoxin dose to about half. If quinidine therapy is to be discontinued, it would be equally important to reinstitute higher doses of digoxin therapy. This ensures the maintenance of appropriate serum levels in treatment of the congestive heart failure.

Adverse Reactions

Though the use of quinidine as an antiarrhythmic has become commonplace for the treatment and prevention of atrial and ventricular tachyarrhythmias, a troublesome side effect profile continues to compromise its long-term use.[165] Anorexia, nausea, vomiting, diarrhea, and colic represent the majority of gastrointestinal effects resulting from local irritation and the most frequently reported side effects associated with the drug's use.[181] Despite local irritation, it has been suggested that the incidence of gastrointestinal complaints is independent of route of administration.[181] This observation has led to the current consensus that a central effect may be responsible for the gastrointestinal symptoms.

Diarrhea has been reported to occur in as many as 30% of all patients receiving quinidine, and may be prevented by using aluminum hydroxide gel or decreased by using the polygalacturonate salt.[182,183]

Quinidine is a representative of the cinchona alkaloid family and, as such, has been associated with cinchonism due to increased serum levels. *Cinchonism* is a syndrome of disturbances that include tinnitus, blurred vision, lightheadedness, tremor activity, giddiness, and altered hearing.[165] Reports to date reveal that the syndrome is reversible with declining levels of quinidine once therapy is discontinued.[165]

Many of the reported side effects of quinidine represent extensions of the drug's cardiac and extracardiac pharmacologic responses. Myocardial depression with increased serum quinidine concentrations would be expected to prolong QT intervals, QRS complexes, and perhaps PR intervals, with a resultant increase in the incidence of reentrant arrhythmias.

A recently published study evaluated, using meta-analysis, six trials published between 1970 and 1984 comparing patients who received quinidine therapy with control patients who received no antiarrhythmic therapy.[184] The therapeutic efficacy of quinidine was assessed during at 3-, 6-, and 12-month follow-up. In each study reviewed, a patient's likelihood of being in sinus rhythm at each time interval was significantly greater in the quinidine group versus the control group.[184] Additionally, the authors concluded that the odds of dying were approximately three times greater for the quinidine group as compared with the control group. Therefore, though the study did show that quinidine treatment is more effective than no antiarrhythmic in suppressing recurrences of atrial fibrillation, the efficacy is compromised because of the increase in total mortality associated with quinidine.[184]

As mentioned previously, routine monitoring of electrocardiogram tracings will aid the clinician in identifying many of the quinidine patients predisposed to quinidine-induced arrhythmias.

Reports in the literature reveal that two very troublesome electrocardiographic effects, quinidine syncope and Torsade de pointes, may occur in 1 to 8% of patients receiving the drug.[185–187] During a quinidine syncope episode, ventricular tachycardia or fibrillation, and possibly prolongation of QT intervals, occur in a non-dose-dependent fashion.[152,188,189] The same findings occur with Torsade de pointes, and it has been described as an idiosyncratic reaction.[165] A retrospective review of 31 patients with documented Torsade de pointes led to the conclusion that (1) patients developing Torsade de pointes while on quinidine generally had heart disease complicated by atrial fibrillation, (2) these patients are receiving digoxin and have been for a short period, (3) 67% of these patients manifest prolonged QT intervals while not receiving quinidine, and may have had hypokalemia secondary to diuretic therapy, which may be a risk factor.[186] Some have speculated that Torsade de pointes may be nothing more than an exaggerated digoxin–quinidine interaction.[165]

Additionally, hypersensitivity reactions to quinidine have been reported and include rashes, drug fever, thrombocytopenia, hemolytic anemia, asthma, respiratory depression, systemic lupus erythematosus, hepatitis, and anaphylactic shock.[181] Though occurrence rates for such reactions are less than for the gastrointestinal and pharmacologic effects of quinidine, the significance of such reactions cannot be overstated.

Therapeutic Regimen Design

At present, unlike numerous other agents requiring therapeutic drug monitoring, dosing nomograms have not been developed to aid in calculating appropriate dosing regimens. Through the use of various pharmacokinetic principles, as in the case for procainamide, dosing regimens can be developed to aid in obtaining desired therapeutic serum levels while minimizing drug toxicity.

Calculation of Loading Dose

$$C_{av} = \frac{D_L \times F}{V_d}$$

$$D_L = \frac{2.0 \text{ mg/L} \times 3 \text{ L/kg}}{0.75} = \quad (C_{av} \text{ of 2.0 mg/L randomly chosen})$$

$$D_L = \frac{6 \text{ mg/kg}}{0.75} = 8.0 \text{ mg/kg quinidine base}$$

A 70-kg patient with no alteration in pharmacokinetic parameters could be given the equivalent of 560 mg (8.0 × 70) of quinidine base in the following fashion, orally. Quinidine base is equivalent to 0.83 of quinidine sulfate, or 560 mg base/0.83 = 675 mg quinidine sulfate. Consequently, 200 mg every 2 hours in three or four doses would be administered to load the patient orally.

Calculation of Maintenance Dose

$$C_{av} = \frac{1.44 \times D \times F \times t_{1/2}}{V_d}$$

$$D = \frac{C_{av} \times V_d}{1.44 \times F \times t_{1/2}}$$

$$D = \frac{2.0 \text{ mg/L} \times 3 \text{ L/kg}}{1.44 \times 0.75 \times 7 \text{ hours}}$$

The dose is 0.79 mg/kg/h quinidine base (1327 mg/24 h). Once again, a 70-kg patient with no alteration in pharmacokinetic parameters could be given the equivalent of 1327 mg of quinidine base orally over 24 hours in one of two ways:

- 1327 mg quinidine base = 1598 mg quinidine sulfate (1327/0.83), or 400 mg (2 tablets) every 6 hours of the rapid-release product, or 660 mg (2 tablets) every 8 hours of the sustained-release tablets.

- 1327 mg. quinidine base = 2140 mg quinidine gluconate (1327/0.62), or 648 mg (2 tablets) every 8 hours of the sustained-release product.

The same type of calculation can be made for the patient receiving quinidine who suffers from congestive heart failure or end-stage liver disease, where alterations in volume of distribution and half-life may require changes in pharmacokinetic parameters as follows.

Calculation of Loading Dose

A. Dose $= \dfrac{2.0 \text{ mg/L} \times 2.0 \text{ L/kg}}{0.75}$ (V_d randomly assigned as 2.0 L/kg in this case, assuming CHF)

B. Dose = 5.3 mg/kg Quinidine base, or 5.3 mg/kg/0.83 = 6.4 mg/kg quinidine sulfate orally as 100 mg. every 2 hours in four or five doses to load the patient rapidly.

Calculation of Loading Dose

A. Dose $= \dfrac{2.0 \text{ mg/L} \times 2.0 \text{ L/kg}}{1.44 \times 0.75 \times 7 \text{ hours}}$

The dose is 0.53 mg/kg/h = 890 mg/d quinidine base, or 890/0.83 = 1072 mg/d quinidine sulfate as 200 mg every 6 hours orally, or 890/0.62 = 1435 mg/d quinidine gluconate as 648 mg every 8 to 12 hours of the sustained-release product.

———— QUESTIONS ————

Lidocaine

B.G. is a 62-year-old white man with a long history of coronary artery disease, congestive heart failure with an ejection fraction of 30%, and adult-onset diabetes.

B.G. presented to the emergency room with complaints of "difficulty breathing."

Physical exam reveals a white man in respiratory distress. Findings of note include a loud S_3 gallop on auscultation, 3+ pitting edema up to the knees, and apparent pulmonary edema.

During the examination, the patient complained of dizziness, nausea, and increased shortness of breath. He became unresponsive. No pulses were present and audible breath sounds were absent. CPR was initiated. EKG revealed ventricular tachycardia. B.G. was countershocked with 200, 300, and 360 J with no success. He was intubated, an IV line was obtained, and 1 mg of epinephrine was given. Subsequent countershock of 360 J transiently converted the ventricular tachycardia to sinus rhythm. It was at this point that the decision was made to administer lidocaine.

1. Using the criteria suggested by the American Heart Association, what would you recommend for the initial and subsequent boluses? (B.G. appears to weigh 80 kg.)

2. A total of three bolus doses were administered and an infusion is desired. What do you recommend for the initial infusion rate?

3. What would the bolus doses and maintenance doses be using population-based parameters?

4. One hour into the infusion at the rate you recommended in question 3, the serum level was 3.2 µg/mL. Eight hours into the infusion the serum level of lidocaine was 2.8 µg/mL. As B.G. was having breakthrough ventricular complexes the physicians desire a blood lidocaine level of approximately 4 µg/mL. What would be your recommendation?

5. What are the signs and symptoms of lidocaine toxicity? What can be done to decrease the chances of a patient becoming lidocaine toxic?

Amiodarone

C.P. is a 48-year-old white man who is currently undergoing a workup for syncope thought to be secondary to frequent episodes of sustained ventricular tachycardia. His medical history is significant for mitral valve replacement with a mechanical valve 3 years prior to the current admission. His present medications are digoxin 0.25 mg daily for treatment of atrial fibrillation and warfarin 3 mg daily for prophylaxis of thromboembolic complications secondary to the mechanical heart valve. His laboratory values of note include a digoxin level of 1.94 ng/mL, PT of 19, and INR of 3.4. All other laboratory values were normal.

During the discussion of proposed treatment, the question arises on the use of amiodarone as a first-line antiarrhythmic in C.P. because of its high success rate in the treatment of ventricular tachycardia.

6. Should amiodarone be used as a first-line agent in this instance?

7. If amiodarone is chosen, what drug interactions should we be concerned about and what steps should be taken to prevent adverse consequences secondary to the interactions?

8. What baseline monitoring parameters should be performed before initiating amiodarone?

9. What would be a reasonable loading regimen for C.P.? Is the use of intravenous amiodarone indicated in this patient?

Procainamide

Patient A.M. is a 65-year-old, 195-pound white man who, after sustaining an acute anterior myocardial infarction, is found to have developed several significant runs of ventricular tachycardia. The patient has had minimal urine output to date, and acute management with procainamide is to be initiated.

10. Calculate an appropriate loading dose for procainamide to obtain therapeutic serum levels.

11. Recommend an intravenous dosing regimen for patient A.M. after the acute treatment of the ventricular tachycardia.

12. Assuming that the patient has responded appropriately to your intravenous recommendations, develop an oral dosing regimen that will ensure maximal patient compliance with minimal toxicity.

13. Describe the applicability of serum drug levels in patients receiving procainamide, and suggest alternative monitoring tools.

Quinidine

Patient P.M. is a 58-year-old, 140-pound man with a strong history of liver disease and congestive heart failure requiring digoxin. The patient is seen in the emergency room suffering from atrial fibrillation symptomatic enough to warrant drug therapy. It is determined that therapy with a type IA antiarrhythmic is warranted, and quinidine is chosen.

14. Design a loading dose regimen for initiation of quinidine in this patient who presents with chronic liver disease due to alcohol abuse.

15. Assuming that the patient responds to the loading doses of quinidine, design a maintenance regimen that will be effective in this noncompliant patient.

16. Describe the dosing adjustments for quinidine that may or may not be required in this patient because of concurrent digoxin therapy.

17. Explain the rationale for acidifying the urine in a patient found to be toxic on quinidine.

18. Explain why serum quinidine levels have continued to be useful to the clinician monitoring a patient receiving the drug.

REFERENCES

1. Southwirth JL, McKusick VA, Pierce EC, et al. Ventricular fibrillation precipitated by cardiac catheterization. *JAMA* 1950;143:717–720.
2. Nattel S, Gagne G, Pineau M. The pharmacokinetics of lignocaine and beta-adrenoreceptor antagonists in patients with acute myocardial infarction. *Clin Pharmacokinet.* 1987;13:293–316.
3. Caruth JE, Silverman MD. Ventricular fibrillation complicating acute myocardial infarction: Reasons against the routine use of lidocaine. *Am Heart J.* 1982;104:545–550.
4. Harrison DC, Berte LE. Should prophylactic drug therapy be used in acute myocardial infarction? *JAMA.* 1982;247:2019–2021.

5. Vaughn Williams EM. A classification of antiarrhythmic actions reassessed after a decade of new drugs. *Clin J Pharmacol.* 1984;24:129–147.

6. Boyles RN, Scott DB, Jebson PJ, et al. Pharmacokinetics of lidocaine in man. *Clin Pharmacol Ther.* 1971;12:105–116.

7. Huet PM, LeLorier J, Pomier G, et al. Bioavailability of lidocaine in normal volunteers and cirrhotic patients. *Gastroenterology.* 1978;75:969–974.

8. Scott DB, Jebson PJ, Villani CW, Julian DG. Plasma lignocaine levels after intravenous and intramuscular injection. *Lancet.* 1970;1:41.

9. Prengel AW, Lindner KH, Hahnel J, Ahnefield FW. Endotracheal and endobronchial lidocaine administration: Effects on plasma lidocaine concentration and blood gases. *Crit Care Med.* 1991; 19(7):911–915.

10. Hahmel JH, Lindner KH, Schurmann C, et al. Plasma lidocaine levels and PaO_2 with endobronchial administration: Dilution with normal saline or water? *Ann Emerg Med.* 1990;19:1314–1317.

11. Scott DB, Littlewood DG, Covino BG, Drummond GB. Plasma lignocaine concentrations following endobronchial spraying with an aerosol. *Br J Anaesth.* 1976;48:899–901.

12. Scavone JM, Greenblatt DJ, Fraser DG. The bioavailability of intranasal lidocaine. *Br J Clin Pharmacol.* 1989;28:722–724.

13. Watson WA, Sands MF, Barlow JC, et al. Lidocaine absorption and metabolism after oropharyngeal application in young and young-elderly adults. *Drug Intell Clin Pharm.* 1991;25:463–465.

14. Lie RL, Vermer BJ, Edelbroek PM. Severe lidocaine intoxication by cutaneous absorption. *J Am Acad Dermatol.* 1990;23:1026–1028

15. LeLorier J, Grenon D, Latour Y, et al. Pharmacokinetics of lidocaine after prolonged intravenous infusions in uncomplicated myocardial infarction. *Ann Intern Med.* 1977;87:700–702.

16. Benowitz NL, Meister W. Clinical pharmacokinetics of lignocaine. *Clin Pharmacokinet.* 1978;3:177–201.

17. Burrows FA, Lerman J, LeDez KM. Pharmacokinetics of lidocaine in children with congenital heart disease. *Can J Anaesth.* 1991;38(2):196–200.

18. Woosley RL. Pharmacokinetics and pharmacodynamics of antiarrhythmic agents in patients with congestive heart failure. *Am Heart J.* 1987;114:1280–1291.

19. Mather LE, Thomas J. Metabolism of lidocaine in man. *Life Sci.* 1972;11:915–919.

20. Benowitz NL, Meister W. Pharmacokinetics in patients with heart failure. *Clin Pharmacokinet.* 1976;1:389–405.

21. Chow MSS, Ronfield RA, Ruffett D, et al. Lidocaine pharmacokinetics during cardiac arrest and external cardiopulmonary resuscitation. *Am Heart J.* 1981;102:799–801.

22. Tucker GT, Boyles RN, Bridenbaugh PO, Moore DC. Binding of anilide type local anesthetics in human plasma. *Anesthesiology.* 1970;33:387–390.

23. Denson DD, Toltzio RS, Ernst TF, et al. Rapid estimation of unbound lidocaine clearance in cardiac patients: Implications for reducing toxicity. *J Clin Pharmacol.* 1988;28:995–1000.

24. Collingsworth KA, Strong JM, Atkinson AJ, et al. Pharmacokinetics and metabolism of lidocaine in patients with renal failure. *Clin Pharmacol Ther.* 1975;18:59–64.

25. Joel SE, Bryson SM, Small M, et al. Kinetic predictive technique applied to lignocaine therapeutic monitoring. *Ther Drug Monit.* 1983;5(3):271–277.

26. Davidson R, Parker M, Atkinson A. Excessive serum lidocaine levels during maintenance infusions: Mechanisms and prevention. *Am Heart J.* 1982;104(2):203–208.

27. Williams RL, Blaschke TF, Miffin PJ, et al. Influence of viral hepatitis on the disposition of two compounds with high hepatic clearance: Lidocaine and indocyanine green. *Clin Pharmacol Ther.* 1976;20:290–299.

28. Estes M, Manolia AS, Greenblatt DJ. Therapeutic serum lidocaine and metabolite concentrations in patients undergoing electrophysiologic study after discontinuation of intravenous lidocaine. *Am Heart J.* 1989;117:1060–1064.

29. Suzuki T, Fujita S, Kawai R. Precursor metabolite interaction in the metabolism of lidocaine. *J. Pharm Sci.* 1987;73:136–138.

30. Erickson E, Granberg PO. Studies on the renal excretion of citanest and xylocaine. *Acta Anaesthesiol Scand.* 1965;16:79–85.

31. Nation RL, Triggs EJ, Selig M. Lignocaine kinetics in cardiac patients and aged subjects. *Br J Clin Pharmacol.* 1977;4:439–448.

32. Lie KI, Wellens HS, Van Capille FJ, Furrer D. Lidocaine in the prevention of primary ventricular fibrillation. *N Engl J Med.* 1974;291:1324–1329.

33. Foldes FF, Malloy R, McNall PG, Kowkal LR. Comparison of toxicity of intravenously given local anesthetic agents in man. *JAMA.* 1960;172:1493–1498.

34. Koppanyi T. The sedative, central analgesic and anticonvulsant actions of local anesthetics. *Am J Med Sci.* 1962;244:646–654.

35. Sinatra ST, Jeresty RM. Enhanced atrioventricular conduction in atrial fibrillation after lidocaine administration. *JAMA.* 1977;237:1356–1357.

36. Marriot HJ, Beza CF. Alarming ventricular acceleration after lidocaine administration. *Chest.* 1972; 61:682–683.

37. Pfeifer HJ, Greenblatt DJ, Kock Weser J. Clinical use and toxicity of intravenous lidocaine. A report from the Boston Collaborative Drug Surveillance Program. *Am Heart J.* 1976;92:168–173.

38. Branch RA, Shand DG, Wilkinson CR, et al. The reduction of lidocaine clearance by *dl*-propranolol: An example of hemodynamic drug interaction. *J Pharmacol Exp Ther.* 1973;184:515–519.

39. Ochs HR, Carstens G, Greenblatt D. Reduction in lidocaine clearance by continuous infusion and by co-administration of propranolol. *N Engl J Med.* 1980;303(7):373–377.

40. Wing LM, Miners JO, Birkett DJ, et al. Lidocaine disposition: Sex differences and effects of cimetidine. *Clin Pharmacol Ther.* 1984;35:695–701.

41. Feely J, Guy E. Lack of effect of ranitidine on the disposition of lidocaine. *Br J Clin Pharmacol.* 1983;15:378–379.

42. Freedman MD, Somberg JC. Pharmacology and pharmacokinetics of amiodarone. *J Clin Pharmacol.* 1991;31:1061–1069.

43. Horowitz LN, Greenspan AM, Spielman SR, et al. Usefulness of electrophysiologic testing in evaluation of amiodarone therapy for sustained ventricular tacharrhythmias associated with coronary heart disease. *Am J Cardiol.* 1985;55:367–371.

44. Herre JM, Sauve MJ, Malone P, et al. Long-term results of amiodarone therapy in patients with recurrent ventricular tachycardia or ventricular fibrillation. *J Am Coll Cardiol.* 1989;13(2):442–449.

45. Sloskey G. Amiodarone: A unique antiarrhythmic agent. *Clin Pharm.* 1983;2:330–340.

46. Riva E, Gena M, Latine R, et al. Pharmacokinetics of amiodarone in man. *J Cardiovasc Pharmacol.* 1982;4:270–275.

47. Andreason F, Agerback H, Byerregarrd P. Pharmacokinetics of amiodarone after intravenous and oral administration. *Eur J Clin Pharmacol.* 1981;19:293–299.

48. Pourbaix S, Berger Y, Desager JP. Absolute bioavailability of amiodarone in normal subjects. *Clin Pharmacol Ther.* 1985;37:118–123.

49. Nolan PE, Mayersohm M, Fenster PE, et al. Single dose pharmacokinetics of amiodarone. *Drug Intell Clin Pharm.* 1985;19:463–466.

50. Zipes DP. Amiodarone: Electrophysiologic action, pharmacokinetics and clinical effects. *J Am Coll Cardiol.* 1984;3:1059–1065.

51. Holt DW, Tucker GT, Jackson PR, et al. Pharmacokinetics of amiodarone in man. *J Cardiovasc Pharmacol.* 1982;4:264–269.

52. Follath F. The utility of serum drug level monitoring during therapy with class III antiarrhythmic agents. *J Cardiovasc Pharmacol.* 1992;35(2):278–280.

53. Kowey PR, Friehling TD, Marinikak RA. Safety and efficacy of amiodarone, a low dose perspective. *Chest.* 1988;93(1):54–59.

54. Rakita L, Sobol S, Mostow N, Vrobel T. Amiodarone pulmonary toxicity. *Am Heart J.* 1983;106:906–914.

55. Marchlinski FE, Gansler TS, Waxman HL, Josephson ME. Amiodarone pulmonary toxicity. *Ann Intern Med.* 1985;145:1016–1019.

56. Giardina EG, Schneider M, Barr ML. Myocardial amiodarone and desethylamiodarone concentrations in patients undergoing cardiac transplantation. *J Am Coll Cardiol.* 1990;16:943–947.

57. Harris L, McKenna WJ, Rowland E, et al. Amiodarone, side effects of long-term therapy. *Circulation.* 1983;67:45–51.

58. Plomp TA, Vulsma T, deVijlder JM. Use of amiodarone during pregnancy. *Eur J Obstet Gynecol Reprod Biol.* 1992;43(3):201–207.

59. Lalloz MR, Beffield CG, Greenwood RM, Himsworth RL. Binding of amiodarone by serum proteins and the effects of drugs, hormones, and other ligands. *J Pharm Pharmacol.* 1984;36:366–372.

60. Mason J. Amiodarone. *N Engl J Med.* 1987;316:455–466.

61. Flanagan RJ, Storey GCA, Holt DW, Farmer PB. Identification and measurement of desethylamiodarone in blood plasma specimens from amiodarone treated patients. *J Pharm Pharmacol.* 1982;34:638–643.

62. Berdeaux A, Roche A, Labaille T, et al. Tissue extraction of amiodarone and *N*-desethylamiodarone in man after a single oral dose. *Br J Clin Pharmacol.* 1984;18:759–763.

63. Latini R, Reginato R, Burlingame AL, et al. High performance liquid chromatographic isolation and fast action atom bombardment mass spectrometic identification of di-*N*-desethyl amiodarone, a new metabolite of amiodarone in the dog. *Biomed Mass Spectrum.* 1984;11:466–471.

64. Marcus F. Drug interactions with amiodarone. *Am Heart J.* 1983;92:924–930.

65. Hawthorne GC, Campbell NP, Geddes JS. Amiodarone induced hypothyroidism. *Arch Intern Med.* 1985;145:1016–1019.

66. Moysey JO, Jaggarao NS, Grundy EN. Amiodarone increases plasma digoxin concentrations. *Br Med J.* 1981;282:272.

67. Shea P, Lal R, Kim SS, et al. Flecainide and amiodarone interaction. *J Am Coll Cardiol.* 1986;7:1127–1130.

68. Hamer A, Peter T, Mandel WJ, et al. The potentiation of warfarin anticoagulation by amiodarone. *Circulation.* 1982;65:1025–1029.

69. McGovern B, Geer V, LaRaia RJ, et al. Possible interaction between amiodarone and phenytoin. *Ann Intern Med.* 1984;101:650–651.

70. Heimark LD, Wienkers L, Kinze K, et al. The mechanism of the interaction between amiodarone and warfarin in humans. *Clin Pharmacol Ther.* 1992;51:398–407.

71. Almong S, Shafran N, Halkin H, et al. Mechanism of warfarin potentiation by amiodarone: Dose and concentration dependent inhibition of warfarin elimination. *Eur J Clin Pharmacol.* 1985;28:257–261.

72. Nolan PE, Marcus FI, Karol MD, et al. Effect of phenytoin on the clinical pharmacokinetics of amiodarone. *J Clin Pharmacol.* 1990;30:1112–1119.

73. Kadish A, Morady F. The use of intravenous amiodarone in the acute therapy of life threatening tachyarrhythmias. *Prog Cardiovasc Dis.* 1989;31:281–294.

74. Ikeda N, Koonlawee N, Kannan R, et al. Electrophysiologic effects of amiodarone: Experimental and clinical observation relative to serum and tissue drug concentrations. *Am Heart J.* 1984;108:890–898.

75. Morady F, DiCarlo L, Baerman J, et al. Rate-dependent effects of intravenous lidocaine, procainamide, and amiodarone on intraventricular conduction. *J Am Coll Cardiol.* 1985;6:179–185.

76. Hohnloser S, Meinertz T, Dammbacher T, et al. Electrocardiographic and antiarrhythmic effects of intravenous amiodarone: Results of a prospective, placebo-controlled study. *Am Heart J.* 1991;121:89–95.

77. Mooss A, Mohiuddin S, Hee T, et al. Efficacy and tolerance of high-dose intravenous amiodarone for recurrent, refractory ventricular tachycardia. *Am J Cardiol.* 1990;65:609–614.

78. Nalos P, Ismail Y, Pappas J, et al. Intravenous amiodarone for short-term treatment of refractory ventricular tachycardia or fibrillation. *Am Heart J.* 1991;122:1629–1632.

79. Schmidt A, Konig W, Binner L, et al. Efficacy and safety of intravenous amiodarone in acute refractory arrhythmias. *Clin Cardiol.* 1988;11:485–486.

80. Bucknall C, Keeton B, Curry P, et al. Intravenous and oral amiodarone for arrhythmias in children. *Br Heart J.* 1986;56:278–284.

81. Williams M, Woelfel A, Cascio W, et al. Intravenous amiodarone during prolonged resuscitation from cardiac arrest. *Ann Intern Med.* 1989;110:839–842.

82. Ochi R, Goldenberg I, Almquist A, et al. Intravenous amiodarone for the rapid treatment of life-threatening ventricular arrhythmias in critically ill patients with coronary disease. *Am J Cardiol.* 1989;64:599–603.

83. Leak D. Intravenous amiodarone in the treatment of refractory life-threatening cardiac arrhythmias in the critically ill patient. *Am Heart J.* 1986;111:456–462.

84. Schutzenberger W, Leisch F, Kerschner K, et al. Clinical efficacy of intravenous amiodarone in the short-term treatment of recurrent sustained ventricular tachycardia and ventricular fibrillation. *Br Heart J.* 1989;62:367–371.

85. Remme W, Kruyssen C, Look M, et al. Hemodynamic effects and tolerability of intravenous amiodarone in patients with impaired left ventricular function. *Am Heart J.* 1991;122:96–103.

86. Perry JC, Knilans TK, Marlow D. Intravenous amiodarone for life threatening tachyarrhythmias in children and young adults. *J Am Coll Cardiol.* 1993;22:95–98.

87. Munoz A, Karilla P, Gallay P, et al. A randomized hemodynamic comparison of intravenous amiodarone with and without Tween 80. *Eur Heart J.* 1988;9:142–148.

88. Pye M, Northcote S, Cobbe S. Acute hepatitis after parenteral amiodarone administration. *Br Heart J.* 1988;59:690–691.

89. Morelli S, Guido V, De Marzio P, et al. Early hepatitis during intravenous amiodarone administration. *Cardiology.* 1991;78:291–294.

90. Stevenson R, Nayani T, Davies. Acute hepatic dysfunction following parenteral amiodarone administration. *Postgrad Med.* 1989;65:707–708.

91. Lopez A, Lopez A, Jimenez S, De Elvira M. Acute intracranial hypertension during amiodarone infusion. *Crit Care Med.* 1985;13:688–689.

92. LeRoy G, Haiat R, Barthelemy M, Lionnet F. Torsades de Pointes during loading with amiodarone. *Eur Heart J.* 1987;8:541–542.

93. Bopp P, Rasoamanambelo L, Crevoisier L, et al. Acute hemodynamic effects of intravenous amiodarone in patients with coronary artery disease. *J Cardiovasc Pharmacol.* 1985;7:286–289.

94. Greco R, D'Alterio D, Schiattarella M, et al. Intravenous amiodarone in acute anterior myocardial infarction: A controlled study. *Cardiovasc Drugs Ther.* 1989;2:791–794.

95. Campbell S, Nolan P, Bliss M, et al. Stability of amiodarone hydrochloride in admixtures with other injectable drugs. *Am J Hosp Pharm.* 1986;43:917–921.

96. Lynch JJ, DiCarlo LA, Lucchesi BR. New antiarrhythmic agents: Part VI—The pharmacology and practical use of amiodarone. *Pract Cardiol.* 1985;11:139–167.

97. Fogoros RN, Anderson KP, Winkle RA, et al. Amiodarone: Clinical efficacy and toxicity in 96 patients with recurrent refractory arrhythmias. *Circulation.* 1983;68:88–94.

98. Raeder EA, Podrid PJ, Locun B. Side effects and complications of amiodarone therapy. *Am Heart J.* 1985;109:975–983.

99. Moro C, Romero J, PeireHi MAC. Amiodarone and hypokalemia, a dangerous combination. *Int J Cardiol.* 1986;13:365–368.

100. Gallastegui JL, Bauman JL, Anderson JL, et al. Worsening of ventricular tachycardia by amiodarone. *J Clin Pharmacol.* 1988;28:406–411.

101. Myers JL, Kennedy JI, Plumb VJ. Amiodarone lung: Pathologic findings in clinically toxic patients. *Hum Pathol.* 1987;18:349–354.

102. Adams PC, Gibson GJ, Morley AR et al. Amiodarone pulmonary toxicity: Clinical and subclinical features. *Q J Med.* 1986;229:449–471.

103. Martino E, Aghini-Lombardi F, Mariotti S et al. Amiodarone: A common source of iodine-induced thyrotoxicosis. *Hormone Res.* 1987;26:158–171.

104. Martino E, Aghini-Lombardi F, Mariotti S, et al. Amiodarone iodine-induced hypothyroidism: Risk factors and follow-up in 28 cases. *Clin Endocrinol.* 1987;26:227–237.

105. Martino E, Safran M, Aghini-Lombardi F, et al. Environmental iodine intake and thyroid dysfunction during chronic amiodarone therapy. *Ann Intern Med.* 1984;101:28–34.

106. McGovern B, Garan H, Kelly E, et al. Adverse reactions during treatment with amiodarone hydrochloride. *Br Med J.* 1983;287:175–179.

107. Lewis HJ, Ranard RC, Caruso A, et al. Amiodarone hepatotoxicity: Prevalence and clinicopathologic correlations among 104 patients. *Hepatology.* 1989;9:679–685.

108. Rinder HM, Love JC, Wexler R. Amiodarone hepatotoxicity. *N Engl J Med.* 1986;314:318–319. Letter.

109. Gilinsky NH, Briscoe GW, Kuo CS. Fatal amiodarone hepatotoxicity. *Am J Gastroenterol.* 1988;83:161–163.

110. Marcus FI, Fontaine GH, Frank R, et al. Clinical pharmacology and therapeutic applications of the antiarrhythmic agent, amiodarone. *Am Heart J.* 1981;101:480–493.

111. Heger JJ, Prystowsky EN, Jackman WM, et al. Amiodarone: Clinical efficacy and electrophysiology during long-term therapy for recurrent ventricular tachycardia or ventricular fibrillation. *N Engl J Med.* 1981;305:539–545.

112. Trimble JW, Mendelson DS, Fetter BF, et al. Cutaneous pigmentation secondary to amiodarone therapy. *Arch Dermatol.* 1983;119:914–918.

113. Vos AK. A peculiar cutaneous pigmentation from Cordarone(R). *Dermatologica.* 1972;145:297–303.

114. Ferguson J, DeVane PJ, Wirth M. Prevention of amiodarone-induced photosensitivity. *Lancet.* 1984;2:414. Letter.

115. Antonelli D, Luboshitsky R, Gelbendorf A. Amiodarone-induced gynecomastia. *N Engl J Med.* 1986;315:1553. Letter.

116. Gasparich JP, Mason JT, Greene HL, et al. Amiodarone-associated epididymitis: Drug-related epididymitis in the absence of infection. *J Urology.* 1985;133:971–972.

117. Benini PL, Crosti C, Sala F, et al. Toxic epidermal necrolysis and amiodarone treatment. *Arch Dermatol.* 1985;121:838. Letter.

118. Anderson, JL, Harrison DC, Meffin PJ, et al. Antiarrhythmic drugs: Clinical pharmacology and therapeutic uses. *Drugs.* 1978;15:271–309.

119. Hoffman BF, Rosen MR, Wit AL. Electrophysiology and pharmacology of cardiac arrhythmias. VII. Cardiac effects of quinidine and procaine amide. *Am Heart J.* 1975;90:117–122.

120. Koch-Weser J, Klein SW. Procainamide dosage schedules, plasma concentrations, and clinical effects. *JAMA.* 1971;215:1454–1460.

121. Grasela TH, Sheiner LB. Population pharmacokinetics of procainamide from routine clinical data. *Clin Pharmacokinet.* 1984;9:545–554.

122. Baker BA, Reynolds JR, Gleckel L, et al. Comparative bioavailability of two oral sustained–release procainamide products. *Clin Pharm.* 1988;7:135–138.

123. Pittard WB, Glazier H. Procainamide excretion in human milk. *J Pediatrics.* 1983;102:631–633.

124. Olsen H, Morland J. Ethanol-induced increase in procainamide acetylation in man. *Br J Clin Pharmacol.* 1982;13:203–208.

125. Ruo TI, Morita Y, Atkinson AJ Jr, et al. Identification of desethyl procainamide in patients: A new metabolite of procainamide. *J Pharmacol Exp Ther.* 1981;216:357–362.

126. Henningsen NC, Cederberg A, Hanson A, et al. Effects of long-term treatment with procaine amide: A prospective study with special regard to ANF and SLE in fast and slow acetylators. *Acta Med Scand.* 1975;198:475–482.

127. Koch-Weser J. Pharmacokinetics of procainamide in man. *Ann NY Acad Sci.* 1971;179:370–382.

128. Gibson TP, Atkinson AJ, Matusik E, et al. Kinetics of procainamide and *N*-acetylprocainamide in renal failure. *Kidney Int.* 1977;12:422–429.

129. Connolly SJ, Kates RE. Clinical pharmacokinetics of *N*-acetylprocainamide. *Clin Pharmacokinet.* 1982;7:206–220.

130. Drayer DE, Lowenthal DT, Woosley RL, et al. Cumulation of *N*-acetylprocainamide, an active metabolite of procainamide, in patients with impaired renal function. *Clin Pharmacol Ther.* 1977;22:63–69.

131. Bennett WM, Aronoff GR, Morrison G, et al. Drug prescribing in renal failure: Dosing guidelines for adults. *Am J Kidney Dis.* 1983;3:155–193.

132. Somogyi A, McLean A, Heinzow, B. Cimetidine–procainamide pharmacokinetic interaction in man: Evidence of competition for tubular secretion of basic drugs. *Eur J Clin Pharmacol.* 1983;25: 339–345.

133. Giardina EG, Heissenbuttel RH, Bigger JT. Intermittent intravenous procaineamide to treat ventricular arrhythmias: Correlation of plasma concentration with effect on arrhythmia, electrocardiogram, and blood pressure. *Ann Intern Med.* 1973;78:183–193.

134. Giardina EG, Fenster PE, Bigger JT, et al. Efficacy, plasma concentrations and adverse effects of a new sustained release procainamide preparation. *Am J Cardiol.* 1980;46:855–862.

135. Lima JJ, Goldfarb AL, Conti DR, et al. Safety and efficacy of procainamide infusion. *Am J Cardiol.* 1979;43:98–106.

136. Greenspan AM, Horowitz LN, Spielman SR, et al. Large dose procainamide therapy for ventricular tachyarrhythmia. *Am J Cardiol.* 1980;46:453–462.

137. Myerburg RJ, Kessler KM, Kiem I, et al. Relationship between plasma levels of procainamide, suppression of premature ventricular complexes and prevention of recurrent ventricular tachycardia. *Circulation.* 1981;64:280–289.

138. Roden DM, Reele SB, Higgins SB, et al. Antiarrhythmic efficacy, pharmacokinetics and safety of *N*-acetylprocainamide in human subjects: *Am J Cardiol.* 1980;46:463–468.

139. Winkle RA, Jaillon P, Kates RE, et al. Clinical pharmacology and antiarrhythmic efficacy of *N*-acetyl-procainamide. *Am J Cardiol.* 1981;47:123–130.

140. Follath F, Ganzinger U, Schuetz E. Reliability of antiarrhythmic drug plasma concentration monitoring. *Clin Pharmacokinet.* 1983;8:63–82.

141. Vlasses PH, Ferguson RK, Rocci ML Jr, et al. Lethal accumulation of procainamide metabolite in renal insufficiency. *N Engl J Med.* 1981;305:231.

142. Coyle JD, Lima JL. Procainamide. In: Robinson JD, Charache P, eds. *A Textbook for the Clinical Application of Therapeutic Drug Monitoring.* Chicago: Abbott Labs; 1986:137–148.

143. Kim SY, Benowitz NL. Poisoning due to class IA antiarrhythmic drugs. Quinidine, procainamide and disopyramide. Drug Saf. 1990;5(6):393–420.

144. Bigger JT, Hoffman BF. Antiarrhythmic Drugs. In: Gilman AG, Rall TW, Nies AS, Taylor P, eds. *Goodman and Gilman's The Pharmacological Basis of Therapeutics.* 8th ed. New York: Pergamon Press; 1990:848–857.

145. Carliner NH, Fisher ML, Crouthamel WG, et al. Relation of ventricular premature beat suppression to serum quinidine concentration determined by a new and specific assay. *Am Heart J.* 1980;100: 483–489.

146. Sokolow M, Ball RE. Factors influencing conversion of chronic atrial fibrillation with special reference to serum quinidine concentration. *Circulation.* 1956;14:568–583.

147. Ochs HR, Greenblatt DL, Woo E. Clinical pharmacokinetics of quinidine. *Clin Pharmacokinet.* 1980;5:150–168.

148. Sokolow M, Perloff DB. The clinical pharmacology and use of quinidine in heart disease. *Prog Cardiovasc Dis.* 1961;3:316.

149. Crevasse, L. Quinidine: An update on therapeutics, pharmacokinetics, and serum concentration monitoring. *Am J Cardiol.* 1983;62(14):22I–23I.

150. *Product Information: Quinaglute Dura-Tabs® (quinidine gluconate).* Berlex Labs; 1985.

151. Goldberg WM, Chakrabarti SG. The relationship of dosage schedule to the blood level of quinidine using all available quinidine preparations. *Can Med Assoc J.* 1964;91:991.

152. Greenblatt DL, Pfeifer HJ, Ochs HR, et al. Pharmacokinetics of quinidine in humans after intravenous, intramuscular, and oral administration. *J Pharmacol Exp Ther.* 1977;202:365–378.

153. Mason WD, Covinsky JO. Comparative plasma concentration of quinidine following administration of one intramuscular and three oral formulations to 13 subjects. *J Pharmacol Sci.* 1976;65:1325–1329.

154. Ueda CT, Williamson BJ, Dzindzio BD. Absolute quinidine bioavailability. *Clin Pharmacol Ther.* 1976;20:260–265.

155. Ueda CT, Dzindzio BS. Quinidine kinetics in congestive heart failure. *Clin Pharmacol Ther.* 1978;23:158–164.

156. Chen BH, Taylor EH, Ackerman BH, et al. Effect of pH on free quinidine. *Drug Intell Clin Pharm.* 1988;22:826.

157. Mihaly GW, Cheng MS, Klein MB, et al. Difference in the binding of quinine and quinidine to plasma proteins. *Br J Clin Pharm.* 1987;24:769–774.

158. Kessler KM, Lisker B, Cande C, et al. Abnormal quinidine binding in survivors of prehospital cardiac arrest. *Am Heart J.* 1984;107:665–669.

159. Ueda CT, Hirschfeld DJ, Schermman MM, et al. Disposition kinetics of quinidine. *Clin Pharmacol Ther.* 1976;19:30–36.

160. Palmer K, Martin B, Baggett B, et al. The metabolic fate of orally administered quinidine gluconate in humans. *Biochem Pharmacol.* 1969;18:1845–1860.

161. Brodie BB, Baer JE, Craig LC. Metabolic products of the cinchona alkaloids in human urine. *J Biol Chem.* 1951;188:567–581.

162. Vozeh S, Vematsu T, Guentert TW, et al. Kinetics and electrocardiographic changes after oral 3-OH quinidine in healthy subjects. *Clin Pharmacol Ther.* 1985;37:575–581.

163. Kavanagh KM, Wyse DG, Mitchell LB, et al. Contribution of quinidine metabolites to electrophysiologic responses in human subjects. *Clin Pharmacol Ther.* 1989;46(3):352–358.

164. Hartel G, Harjanne A. Comparison of two methods for quinidine determination and chromatographic analysis of the difference. *Clin Chem Acta.* 1969;23:289–294.

165. Covinsky, JO: Quinidine. In: Robinson JD, Charache P, eds. *A Textbook for the Clinical Application of Therapeutic Drug Monitoring.* Chicago: Abbott Laboratories; 1986:161–171.

166. Gerhardt RE, Knouss RF, Thyrum PT, et al. Quinidine excretion in aciduria and alkaluria. *Ann Int Med.* 1969;71:927–933.

167. Bigger JT Jr. Arrhythmias and antiarrhythmic drugs. *Adv Intern Med.* 1972;18:251.

168. Powell JR, Okada R, Conrad KA, et al. Altered quinidine disposition in a patient with chronic active hepatitis. *Postgrad Med J.* 1982;58:82–84.

169. Hansten PD, Horn JR. *Drug Interact Newslett.* 1991;11:483–490.

170. Mangini RJ, ed. *Drug Interaction Facts.* St Louis: JB Lippincott; 1986.

171. Twum-Baruma Y, Carruthers SG. Evaluation of rifampin–quinidine interaction. *Clin Pharmacol Ther.* 1980;27:290.

172. Carliner NH, Crouthamel WG, et al. Quinidine therapy in hospitalized patients with ventricular arrhythmias. *Am Heart J.* 1979;98:708.

173. Hirschfield DJ, Ueda CT, Rowland M, et al. Clinical and electrophysiological effects of intravenous quinidine in man. *Br Heart J.* 1977;39:309–316.

174. Woosley RL, Shand DG. Pharmacokinetics of antiarrhythmic drugs. *Am J Cardiol.* 1978;41:986–994.

175. Olin B, ed. *Facts and Comparisons.* St Louis: JB Lippincott; 1990.

176. Koch-Weser J. Quinidine-induced hypoprothrombinemic hemorrhage on patients on chronic warfarin therapy. *Ann Intern Med.* 1968;68:511.

177. Hooymans PM, Merkus FW. Current status of cardiac glycoside drug interactions. *Clin Pharm.* 1985;4:404–410.

178. Way WI, Katzung GB, Larson CP Jr. Recurarization with quinidine. *JAMA.* 1967;200:153–154.

179. Schmidt JL, Vick NA, Sadove MS. The effect of quinidine on the action of muscle relaxants. *JAMA.* 1963;183:669–671.

180. Shinn AF, ed. *Evaluations of Drug Interactions.* New York: Macmillan; 1989.

181. Cohen IS, Jick H, Cohen SI. Adverse reactions to quinidine in hospitalized patients: Findings from the Boston Collaborative Drug Surveillance Program. *Prog Cardiovasc Dis.* 1977;20:151–163.

182. Romankiewicz JA, Reidenberg M, Drayer D, et al. The non-interference of aluminum hydroxide gel with quinidine sulfate absorption: An approach to control quinidine-induced diarrhea. *Am Heart J.* 1978;96:518–520.

183. Gerstenblith T, Katabi G, Stein I, et al. Quinidine utilization in cardiac arrhythmias: Report of study involving sulfate and polygalacturonate salts. *NY State J Med.* 1966;66:701–706.

184. Coplen SE, Antman EM, Berlin JA, et al. Efficacy and safety of quinidine therapy for maintenance of sinus rhythm after cardioversion. A meta-analysis of randomized control trials. *Circulation.* 1990;82(4):1106–1116.

185. Reynolds EW, Vander Ark CR. Quinidine syncope and the delayed repolarization syndromes. *Mod Concepts Cardiovasc Dis.* 1976;45:117–122.

186. Bauman JL, Bauernfeind RA, Hoff JV, et al. Torsade de pointes due to quinidine: Observations in 31 patients. *Am Heart J.* 1984;107:425–430.

187. Roden DM, Woosley RL, Primm RK. Incidence and clinical features of the quinidine-associated long QT syndrome: Implications for patient care. *Am Heart J.* 1986;111:1088–1093.

188. Selzer A, Wray HW. Quinidine syncope. *Circulation.* 1964;30:17.

189. Koster RH, Wellens HJ. Quinidine-induced ventricular flutter and fibrillation without digitalis therapy. *Am J Cardiol.* 1976;38:519.

Chapter 11

Antiepileptics

William R. Garnett

Keep in Mind

- Ensure that the patient actually needs an antiepileptic drug.
- Ensure that the antiepileptic drug selected is appropriate for the seizure type.
- Know the pharmacokinetic parameters for the antiepileptic drugs and the factors that may alter them.
- Know the therapeutic ranges of the antiepileptic drugs but do not consider them dogma.
- Monitor antiepileptic drug concentrations.
- Obtain trough antiepileptic drug concentration samples.
- Know when to obtain "free" or unbound concentrations of the antiepileptic drugs.
- Always know the relationship between the time of the last dose and the time of collection of the drug concentration sample.
- Anticipate dosage adjustments.
- Know the dosage form of the drug being used and relate it to the needs of the patient.
- Set specific endpoints for therapy.
- Know the role of the metabolites of the antiepileptic drugs.
- Monitor patient compliance.
- Assess changes in the patient and in the patient's drug therapy.
- Consider the side effect potential in selecting antiepileptic drugs.
- Periodically reassess the need for antiepileptic drug therapy.
- Evaluate new antiepileptic drugs for a better risk-to-benefit ratio for a given drug.

The antiepileptic drugs are drugs with narrow, well-defined therapeutic ranges. Patient outcome management is enhanced by incorporating the preceding principles into a therapeutic drug monitoring plan.[1]

BACKGROUND

Antiepileptic drugs are used to treat epilepsy, which represents the chronic occurrence of paroxysmal firing of neurons that result in seizures. Seizures may be convulsive or nonconvulsive. A single seizure does not represent epilepsy and a single seizure is not treated immediately with anticonvulsants. Therapy is not instituted until remedial causes are excluded. If the seizure is idiopathic, a second seizure is usually required before the initiation of antiepileptic drug therapy.[2] Some patients may have psychogenic seizures and do not need antiepileptic drug therapy at all.[2]

Seizures may be classified as partial or generalized depending on whether they occur in one hemisphere of the brain (partial) or in both (generalized). A partial seizure may spread to both hemispheres and become generalized.[3] Partial and generalized seizures may be differentiated and further classified by signs and symptoms, observation, and an EEG.[4] Seizure classification allows the clinician to select a drug of choice for a given seizure type. For example, carbamazepine is considered the drug of choice for simple and complex partial seizures.[5,6] Valproic acid is accepted as the drug of choice for most generalized seizures except typical absence. Ethosuximide is the drug of choice for this seizure type and is used only for absence seizures. A further classification of multiple seizure types into seizure syndromes will further help in defining drugs of choice.[7]

The dosing interval, the interval between changes in dose, the time to steady state, the estimate of a loading dose, an estimation of a maintenance dose, anticipation of drug interactions, and the pharmacodynamic response all require an understanding of pharmacokinetic principles. The pharmacokinetics may be altered by age, renal failure, liver dysfunction, other drugs, low albumin and other factors. These variables should be taken into consideration in the therapeutic drug monitoring (TDM) of antiepileptic drugs.[8]

The therapeutic ranges are population estimates that predict when the clinician is most likely to observe the desired response and is least likely to observe toxicity. Clinicians should not treat numbers, however, and the therapeutic range should be defined for each patient.[9]

Antiepileptic drug concentrations can be used to assess patient compliance, predict the relative safety of a dosage change, assess the potential for side effects to be related to the antiepileptic drug, identify patients with unusual antiepileptic drug clearances or protein binding, and identify refractory patients who do not respond to therapy. As stated, the concentration should be individualized for each patient and should reflect a concentration that prevents the occurrence of seizures with a minimum of side effects.[10]

In general, trough levels are observed just prior to the next dose of an antiepileptic drug. Enteric-coated sodium divalproex is an exception. Trough levels may be used to define a minimum drug concentration below which the concentration should not fall. Peak concentrations may be obtained when the patient is experiencing intermittent side effects.[9]

The free or unbound drug exists in an equilibrium with the bound drug but it is the free drug that is capable of diffusing across the blood–brain barrier and inducing the pharmacodynamic effect. If protein binding exceeds 90% of the total drug, small changes in the free fraction may have significant clinical consequences. It is the free drug that is metabolized. Therefore, an increase in free drug increases drug clearance, causing the total drug concentration to fall. If the total drug concentration is monitored and adjusted without considering an alteration in the free fraction, the patient may have a toxic reaction despite having a "therapeutic" concentration. Thus for some drugs the free fraction is an important TDM variable.[11]

Phenytoin and valproic acid are highly protein bound. Phenytoin is linearly bound within the therapeutic range; however, renal failure, low albumin, the extremes of age, and other drugs are some of the variables that may alter the protein binding of phenytoin. The protein binding of valproic acid saturates within the therapeutic range. Also, other drugs may displace valproic acid from its binding sites. The other major antiepileptic drugs are not extensively protein bound. Thus the clinician should know when to measure the free fraction of the antiepileptic drugs in addition to, or in lieu of, the total concentration.[8]

Drugs with short half lives, for example, carbamazepine and valproic acid, in patients with rapid clearances may have high peaks and low trough concentrations. The only way that a given concentration may be correctly interpreted is to know the relationship of the time of the collection of the sample to the time of the patient's last dose. If a peak is mistaken for a trough or if the sample is random and has no relationship to either a peak or a trough, the concentration may be meaningless. If the relationship of the timing of the sample to the time of the last dose is not known, the sample may have to be repeated, which increases the cost to the patient. The timing of sample collection is more critical for short-half-life drugs like carbamazepine and valproic acid than it is for drugs with long half-lives like phenobarbital.[8,9]

Many early side effects, especially central nervous system effects, may be minimized by dosage titration. Also, clinicians should anticipate large interpatient variability in pharmacokinetic variables which alters the maintenance dose. Because of the intersubject pharmacokinetic variability and the need to define the desired drug concentration for a given patient, the dose should be titrated. Autoinduction and drug interactions are further reasons for dosage adjustments.[10]

The dosage form, for example, suspension, tablet, capsule, parenteral, may affect the achieved serum concentration, the rate of absorption, the peak-to-trough fluctuation, the maximum concentration, the minimum concentration, or the exact time of the trough. Thus, the clinician must consider the effect of each dosage form. Also, the clinician should know if the patient is receiving a generic formulation. Some epileptic patients may be very sensitive to small changes in the fraction of the drug that is bioavailable. In general, a patient should be maintained on the brand of antiepileptic drug on which he or she is initially titrated. The indiscriminate switching of generic brands is to be discouraged.

The dosage form may also affect the patient's ability to comply with the medication. For example some pediatric and some elderly patients may have difficulty swallowing a solid dosage form. For these patients a liquid would be more appropriate. Rectal administration may be useful for early treatment of emergent conditions, such as acute repetitive seizures and status epilepticus. Rectal dosage forms may have to be extemporaneously compounded using a suspension or parenteral dosage form.[12]

Monotherapy is the preferred approach for antiepileptic drug therapy. The ideal response is control of seizures with no side effects; however, this may not occur in all patients. Therefore, when an antiepileptic drug is started an endpoint should be set. If the patient achieves cessation of his or her seizures with no or tolerable side effects, the therapeutic goal has been reached. If, however, the patient has no or partial response, a second drug should be added and the first drug discontinued. Polytherapy is indicated only if the patient has failed two or more drugs as single agents. Patients on polytherapy may be converted to monotherapy. Complete control of seizures may not be achievable in all patients. Some patients may have to accommodate to some side effects. An assessment for a given patient should be made between the number of acceptable seizures and the degree of acceptable side effects. Also, antiepileptic drug therapy may be discontinued in many patients after a sustained period of no seizures. This is a long-term goal, as there should be at least two to four seizure-free years before the antiepileptic drug is discontinued; however, antiepileptic drugs do not necessarily have to be given for life.[1]

The antiepileptic drugs are extensively metabolized. Some of these metabolites contribute to the efficacy, toxicity, and drug interaction potential of the antiepileptic drugs. The 10,11-diepoxide metabolite of carbamazepine has antiepileptic and central nervous system activity. This metabolite is further metabolized and the concentrations may be altered by other drugs, for example, valproic acid, independent of interactions with the parent drug. Because the diepoxide carbamazepine is active, the patient may demonstrate signs of toxicity when the concentration of parent drug is in the "therapeutic" range. Valproic acid has multiple routes of metabolism. In some patients an alternative metabolic route may result in a metabolite that is potentially liver toxic. Monitoring of parent drug in this situation would not be helpful.[13]

Drug concentrations are meaningless without a knowledge of the patient's compliance. Dosage increases are frequently made if drug concentrations are low and the patient is not having the desired response. If the low concentration is due to poor compliance rather than variability in pharmacokinetic parameters and the patient suddenly starts taking his or her medication, the patient may have a toxic reaction. Alternatively, some patients may take extra doses of their antiepileptic drug because they are coming to the seizure clinic or because they have had a seizure. This may give the false impression of elevated concentrations and may result in dosage lowering or the patient may be judged refractory. It should be remembered that prescribing antiepileptic drugs does not prevent seizures. The patient must ingest the drug to get a response.[8,9]

Antiepileptic drugs may be given for long periods. Physiologic functions may change with time, especially in the neonate, infant, and child.[14] Females may reach childbearing potential or wish to conceive. Other diseases may occur in addition to epilepsy. All of these factors may alter pharmacokinetic parameters and in some cases, for example, pregnancy, the decision to continue therapy with a given antiepileptic drug.[15]

Some side effects of the antiepileptic drugs take time before they are manifested. For example, gingival hyperplasia secondary to phenytoin may not be seen for months after the initiation of the drug. Therefore, new complaints and new observations in a patient on chronic antiepileptic drug therapy should not be dismissed as unrelated to drug therapy without a careful review.[16]

The antiepileptic drugs have pharmacokinetic parameters that make them highly susceptible to drug interactions. The narrow therapeutic ranges make the drug interactions very clinically significant. Therefore, the addition or removal of any drug from the therapeutic regimen of a given patient should be monitored very carefully.[1]

A therapeutic goal in the treatment of epilepsy is to control the seizures with no or minimal side effects. The antiepileptic drugs have differing side effect profiles and this should be considered when selecting the initial drug of choice. The side effect profile explains why carbamazepine and valproic acid have been used with increasing frequency.[17]

Some patients may be at increased risks of developing side effects. For example, patients less than 2 years of age with inborn errors of metabolism who receive multiple drugs are at an increased risk of developing fatal hepatitis secondary to valproic acid therapy. When an antiepileptic drug is started, the side effects should be reviewed and the patient monitored to determine the occurrence and the severity of the side effects.[1]

As discussed, some patients may have their antiepileptic drug therapy discontinued after a sufficiently long seizure-free interval. Also, new data alter the opinion about the need to treat certain seizure types. For example, prophylaxis for febrile seizures with phenobarbital has

TABLE 11–1. PHARMACOKINETIC SUMMARY OF COMMONLY USED ANTIEPILEPTIC DRUGS

		$t_{1/2}$ (h)	Time to C_{ss} (d)	V_d (L/kg)	Bioavailability (%)	Active Metabolite	Protein Bound (%)	Dialysis (% H)[a]	%UC[b]
Phenytoin	A	10–34[c]	7–28	0.6–0.8	90–95	No	90	4	<5%
	C	5–14							
Phenobarbital	A	46–136	14–21	0.6	90–100	No	50	30	20–40
	C	37–73							
Primidone	A	3.3–19	1–4	0.43–1.1	90–100	PB,[e] PEMA	80	30	40
	C	4.5–11							
Carbamazepine		36[e]	21–28[e]	1–2	>75	10,11-CBZ	40–90	20	<1
		8–14[e]							
Valproic acid	A	8–20	1–3	0.1–0.5	100	Yes[f]	90–95[g]	—	<5
Ethosuximide	A	60	6–12	0.67	100	No	0	~50	10–20
Felbamate		22	5	0.73–0.82	>90	No	~25	?	0
Gabapentin		5.3	25	58L	60[h]	No	<3	Yes	100
Lamotrigine		22	5	1.28	>98	No	40–50	?	0

[a] Percent hemodialyzed.

[b] Percent excreted unchanged in the urine.

[c] Because of the Michaelis–Menten kinetics of phenytoin, half-life and time to steady state are inappropriate terms.

[d] Carbamazepine undergoes autoinduction. The half-life is longer after one dose than after repeated dosing. The time to steady state must reflect the time for the autoinduction to be completed.

[e] PB, phenobarbital; PEMA, phenylethylmalonamide; 10,11-CBZ, carbamazepine 10,11-epoxide.

[f] One of the metabolites of valproic acid may be hepatotoxic.

[g] The protein binding of valproic acid saturates within the therapeutic range.

[h] The bioavailability of gabapentin is dose dependent. The bioavailability of the most frequently used doses is 60%.

Abbreviations: A, adult; C, child.

often been recommended; however, recent data indicate that phenobarbital may significantly impair cognition without preventing the recurrence of febrile seizures.[18] This puts the use of chronic phenobarbital for febrile seizure prophylaxis into question. Perhaps a better choice is the use of rectal valproic acid at the first sign of an increased temperature. Another example of the need to reassess drug therapy is found in the results of a prospective study of the prophylactic effects of phenytoin in head trauma. The study showed that phenytoin prevented seizures in the first 7 days but was not different than placebo in preventing the occurrence of late epilepsy.[19]

After a period of little drug development in the area of antiepileptic drug therapy, there are now a number of drugs that are in the later stages of clinical development.[20] New Drug Applications (NDAs) have been approved for felbamate, lamotrigine, and gabapentin. Several other NDAs may be submitted soon. Therefore, the clinician will have new drugs to consider in the treatment of epilepsy. For a given patient some of these new drugs may offer the opportunity to improve seizure control or to maintain seizure control but decrease the side effects. Individual patients should be carefully evaluated to determine if the risk/benefit ratio justifies a change to a new drug.

Table 11–1 provides a summary of the pharmacokinetics of the major antiepileptic drugs. Table 11–2 gives generally accepted therapeutic ranges for the major antiepileptic drugs. At this time no therapeutic range has been defined for the new antiepileptic drugs felbamate, gabapentin, and lamotrigine. Drug interactions are common with the antiepileptic drugs. It is beyond the scope of this chapter to discuss every drug interaction that has been reported with the antiepileptic drugs. Table 11–3 provides a summary of the drug interaction potential of the common antiepileptic drugs. Clinicians should always anticipate drug interactions when any change is made to the therapeutic regimen of a patient taking an antiepileptic drug. The following narrative examines each of the major antiepileptic drugs in detail. Patients who do not respond to these drugs are not likely to respond to the other less effective and more toxic antiepileptic drugs.

TABLE 11–2. THERAPEUTIC RANGES (µg/mL) FOR COMMONLY USED ANTIEPILEPTIC DRUGS

Phenytoin	
Total drug	10–20
Free drug	1–2
Phenobarbital	15–40
Primidone	6–12
Carbamazepine	4–12
Valproic acid	50–150
Ethosuximide	50–100
Felbamate	undefined
Gabapentin	undefined
Lamotrigine	undefined

TABLE 11–3. DRUG INTERACTION POTENTIAL OF COMMON ANTIEPILEPTIC DRUGS

Phenytoin	Enzyme inducer
	Highly protein bound
	Metabolism may be induced or inhibited
Phenobarbital	Enzyme inducer
Primidone	Enzyme inducer
Carbamazepine	Enzyme inducer
	Metabolism may be induced or inhibited
Valproic acid	Enzyme inhibitor
	Highly protein bound
	Metabolism may be induced or inhibited
Ethosuximide	No significant interactions
Felbamate	Enzyme inhibitor (reported interactions with
	phenytoin, carbamazepine, and valproic acid)
	Metabolism may be induced
Gabapentin	No significant interaction
Lamotrigine	Metabolism may be induced or inhibited

MAJOR ANTIEPILEPTIC DRUGS

Carbamazepine

Clinical Pharmacology and Therapeutics

Carbamazepine is structurally related to the tricyclic antidepressants. It is believed either to act on the neuronal sodium channel to reduce sustained, high-frequency repetitive firing of action potentials or to act on synaptic transmission. The epoxide metabolite of carbamazepine is active in animals and is believed to contribute to the efficacy and side effects of carbamazepine in humans.[21]

Carbamazepine was originally approved for the treatment of trigeminal neuralgia and was later found to be effective as an antiepileptic drug.[22] It was approved for use as an antiepileptic drug in 1974. More recently, carbamazepine has been shown to be effective in patients with bipolar depression who are not responsive to lithium.[23]

Carbamazepine is considered the drug of choice for simple and complex partial seizures.[1] It may also be used for some types of generalized seizures such as tonic–clonic and secondarily generalized seizures. It is ineffective in absence seizures.

Clinical Pharmacokinetics

Absorption. Carbamazepine has a slow rate of dissolution, which is believed to result in slow, erratic, and unpredictable absorption in humans.[24] Peak levels are usually seen between 3 and 8 hours after ingestion; however, there is considerable intra- and intersubject variability and peak levels have been reported to occur much later after dosing. The absorption of carbamazepine does not follow a simple first-order process. Absorption may be prolonged in the upper and lower parts of the intestine, resulting in several secondary and tertiary peaks of absorption.[24] Carbamazepine does not undergo first-pass metabolism. Absorption of carbamazepine may be slower following the evening dose.[25]

No intravenous form of carbamazepine is available for human trials. Therefore, the absolute bioavailability of carbamazepine is not known. A 2% oral solution has been reported to be 100% bioavailable.[26] The absorption from oral tablets is estimated to be about 85 to 90%.[27] The chewable tablets and the immediate-release tablets are equivalent in bioavailability and may be interchanged without a change in dose or dosing interval.[28,29] The bioavailability of the suspension is equal to the bioavailability of the immediate-release tablets; however, the suspension is absorbed at a faster rate. Therefore, the total daily dose of carbamazepine is the same using either immediate release or suspension formulations; however, to avoid wide fluctuations in peak to trough concentrations with possible side effects or breakthrough seizures, the suspension should be given in smaller doses at more frequent intervals.[30] The sustained-release formulation is bioequivalent to the immediate-release formulation but may provide a more even serum concentration curve.[31] Total absorption from an enema made by diluting the suspension is comparable to that of the oral formulations, but time to peak concentration may be longer than with the suspension given orally.[32] The FDA recently reported that moisture may decrease the potency of carbamazepine tablets by up to 30%; therefore, it is essential that carbamazepine be stored in a cool, dry place.[33]

Distribution. Animal studies indicate that carbamazepine distributes rapidly and uniformly to various organs and tissues achieving higher concentrations in organs of high blood flow such as the liver, kidney, and brain.[24]

Carbamazepine binds to albumin and to α_1-acid glycoprotein (AAG). AAG may vary with the presence of inflammation, trauma, concurrent antiepileptic drug therapy, and age.[34] Therefore, there are varying reports about the amount of free or unbound drug available in the plasma and the need for free drug monitoring. The free fraction of carbamazepine is estimated at 25%, but reports in epileptic patients have ranged from 10 to 50%. There is a small decrease in the protein binding of carbamazepine in neonates, but binding rates in all other age groups are comparable.[24] Monitoring of the free fraction may be indicated when the clinical presentation of the patient, for example, the presence of side effects or the lack of response, does not coincide with the plasma concentration.[35]

Carbamazepine crosses the placenta, achieving a concentration in the fetus equal to the concentration in the plasma of the mother. The concentration of carbamazepine in breast milk is about 60% of the concentration in the mother's plasma. The concentration of carbamazepine in the saliva and tears approximates the unbound concentration.[24]

Metabolism and Elimination. Carbamazepine is about 99% metabolized before the metabolites are excreted in the urine. The metabolism of carbamazepine follows four major pathways: oxidation, hydroxylation, direct conjugation with glucuronic acid, and sulfur conjugation. The oxidation and hydroxylation pathways account for about 65% of the metabolism of carbamazepine.[36] The most important of the carbamazepine metabolites is the 10,11-epoxide because it is felt to be active and may contribute to the efficacy and toxicity of carbamazepine.[37] In a recent study carbamazepine was replaced by the 10,11-epoxide metabolite without a loss of efficacy.[38] Drug interactions may alter the formation of the 10,11-epoxide metabolite without altering the concentration of the parent drug.[39] The 10,11-epoxide metabolite is further metabolized to a diol metabolite. Clearance of the 10,11-epoxide metabolite is higher than that of the parent drug.[40]

The metabolism of carbamazepine may be altered by other drugs and by itself. Carbamazepine is unique in that it can induce its own metabolism. Clearance of carbamazepine increases with continued dosing.[41] The autoinduction with carbamazepine begins 3 to 5 days into continued therapy; full induction takes 2 to 4 weeks.[41,42] It is mainly the 10,11-epoxide diol pathway that is induced. The autoinduction occurs after each dosage increase.[42] Because of the autoinduction, the concentrations achieved initially can be expected to fall and this should be remembered when evaluating patient compliance. A drop in carbamazepine may reflect autoinduction rather than noncompliance. Autoinduction must be remembered during dosage titration. The potential for other drugs to enhance or inhibit the metabolism of carbamazepine makes drug–drug interactions very likely and significant.[1]

Special Populations. Clearance of carbamazepine may be altered by age.[43] The clearance in children up to age 15 years appears to be higher and more variable than in adults.[44] A higher mg/kg/d dose is likely to be required in children. Older patients have a decreased clearance, suggesting a lower dose. There do not appear to be any age-related changes in absorption, protein binding, and distribution between infants and adults in otherwise healthy patients.[44] Malnutrition has been reported to decrease the bioavailability of carbamazepine in children to about one third of that seen in a normal control group.[45] Females may have a lower clearance than males.[46] The achieved serum concentration is the best guide to dosage regulation.[47]

Chronic renal failure should not affect the clearance of carbamazepine because only 1% of the drug is excreted unchanged.[24] There is no indication that renal disease affects any of the other pharmacokinetic parameters of carbamazepine. Replacement doses are not indicated in patients requiring hemodialysis.[48] The antidiuretic effect of carbamazepine should be remembered in patients with chronic renal failure. Chronic severe liver disease may alter the metabolism of carbamazepine and result in higher blood concentrations.[24]

The apparent clearance of carbamazepine increases in the third trimester of pregnancy and returns to baseline soon after delivery.[49] Carbamazepine diffuses into breast milk.

Pharmacodynamics

Therapeutic Endpoints. The desired therapeutic endpoint for carbamazepine is the abolition of seizures. As carbamazepine is the drug of choice for partial seizures and may be used in some types of generalized seizures, assessment of therapeutic outcome may require both a careful patient history and an EEG.[1] Carbamazepine may control seizures as monotherapy in about 75% of patients.[5]

Carbamazepine has been reported to be more effective in girls than boys and more effective in older patients than in children.[22]

Adverse Reactions. Neurologic side effects are the most commonly reported side effects associated with carbamazepine. These central nervous system effects include lethargy, dizziness, drowsiness, headache, blurred vision, diplopia, ataxia, and incoordination.[50] They are more common at serum concentrations greater than 8 to 12 μg/mL, but each patient seems to have a threshold below which the side effects do not occur. The neurologic side effects may be eliminated or reduced by dosage manipulation. A slow dosage titration will allow the patient time to develop some tolerance to these effects. A reduction in dose will reduce side effects in some patients without a loss in seizure control. These side effects may be controlled in other patients by giving larger dose of carbamazepine in the evening hours and smaller doses in the daytime hours.[1] If unequal doses are given, this should be considered when trough concentrations are measured. Other side effects that are possibly related to serum concentrations are nausea and vomiting, syndrome of inappropriate antidiuretic hormone (SIADH), cardiac disturbances, and osteomalacia which are more common in patients with high serum concentrations.[50] Side effects may occur at concentrations considered to be in the therapeutic range.

In a study of 40 patients, carbamazepine was found to induce the clearance of thyroid hormones. Carbamazepine may also have an inhibitory effect at the hypothalamic level. There was no correlation between serum carbamazepine and thyroid hormone concentration.[51]

There are also idiosyncratic reactions that occur with carbamazepine that cannot be detected nor minimized by concentration monitoring.[50] These include the bone marrow suppression that occurs infrequently with carbamazepine. Frequent CBC monitoring is not indicated for chronic carbamazepine monitoring. A baseline CBC is useful but is not required at every patient visit.[52] It should be remembered that carbamazepine can cause a leukopenia that is not considered dangerous or a harbinger of agranulocytosis or aplastic anemia. A rough guideline is that carbamazepine does not need to be discontinued unless the absolute neutrophil count drops below 1000 cells/mL.

Recent case reports of rare side effects associated with carbamazepine include intractable diarrhea,[53] eosinophilic colitis,[54] encephalopathy,[55] weight gain and increased appetite,[56] positive antinuclear antibodies and systemic lupus erythematosus-like syndrome,[57] hepatotoxicity,[58] bradyarrhythmias,[59] and atrioventricular block.[60] Sinus tachycardia, external ophthalmoplegia and asterixis, and central nervous system dysfunction (coma, seizures, combativeness, drowsiness, ataxia) were associated with carbamazepine overdose cases.[61,62] The half-life of carbamazepine is prolonged in cases of overdose and there is an elevation of the carbamazepine-epoxide/carbamazepine ratio. There is an estimated 1% incidence of spina bifida in children born to women taking carbamazepine.[63]

Patients on monotherapy have fewer side effects and tolerate higher concentrations of carbamazepine than patients on polytherapy.

Drug–Drug Interactions. Carbamazepine is an enzyme inducer and may enhance the metabolism of many drugs undergoing phase I metabolism. Because carbamazepine is extensively metabolized by the liver, its metabolism may be affected by other drugs that induce or inhibit liver microsomal enzymes.[64–66]

A possible synergistic effect is seen with lithium when carbamazepine is used in patients with bipolar depression.

Significant amounts of carbamazepine are lost if undiluted carbamazepine suspension is administered through polyvinyl chloride nasogastric feeding tubes. The dilution with an equal volume of diluent and flushing minimize the adsorption.[67] Enteral feedings do not appear to alter significantly the absorption of carbamazepine.[68]

Disease–Drug Interactions. There is very little information concerning the interaction between carbamazepine and disease states other than epilepsy. Because carbamazepine is extensively metabolized by the liver, it can be postulated that the clearance of carbamazepine would be decreased in patients with significant liver disease. Because almost no drug is excreted unchanged in the urine, significant renal impairment would not be expected to alter the clearance of carbamazepine.[24] Hemodialysis has been shown not to affect the clearance of carbamazepine.[48] Congestive heart failure that causes gut edema may contribute to the variable absorption of carbamazepine. Carbamazepine may cause sodium and water retention, aggravating congestive heart failure. Fever (increased metabolism) and pulmonary disease (decreased metabolism) have been associated with alterations of antiepileptic drug clearance. Protein binding may be altered postoperatively.[24] The change in protein binding and altered metabolism were felt to be responsible for the carbamazepine toxicity that followed cardiothoracic surgery and myocardial infarction.[69]

Clearance of antiepileptic drugs increases during the third trimester of pregnancy and the concentration of carbamazepine should be closely monitored during this period. An increase in dose can be expected. Following delivery the clearance returns to normal and the dose should be reduced.[49]

Therapeutic Regimen Design

Initial Dose. Although a rapid loading dose sequence has been described using 10 mg/kg suspension for children less than age 12 years and 8 mg/kg suspension for patients older than 12 years, a loading dose of carbamazepine is rarely needed. It is preferable to begin therapy with one fourth to one third of the anticipated maintenance dose and to titrate the dose to the individual patient's response. Doses may be increased by one fourth to one third at weekly intervals until the patient becomes seizure free or side effects are intolerable. This allows tolerance to the central nervous system side effects to develop and allows for the anticipation of autoinduction.

Maintenance Dose. Because of autoinduction the serum concentrations of carbamazepine and the patient's seizure frequency should be monitored for at least 1 to 2 months after the achievement of a therapeutic dose and adequate serum concentrations. The presence of other enzyme-inhibiting or -inducing drugs should be considered in titrating the dose of carbamazepine.

Although the manufacturer cautions that doses greater than 1200 mg per day are excessive, the maximal dose of carbamazepine should be determined by the achieved serum concentration, the seizure frequency, and the occurrence of side effects. The usual maintenance doses are 7 to 15 mg/kg/d for patients older than 15 years and 11 to 40 mg/kg/d for patients less than 15 years.

Dosing Interval. Based on the half-life carbamazepine may be dosed twice a day and many patients will tolerate this dosing frequency. This gives higher peaks, however, and in some patients this peak may exceed the threshold for side effects. Therefore, some patients may need a three- or four-times-a-day dosing schedule with conventional immediate-release tablets. The suspension, which is absorbed more quickly, should be given at least three or four times a day.[30] The sustained-release formulation of carbamazepine may be given twice a day.[31]

Dosage Prediction and Adjustment. The variability in the pharmacokinetics of carbamazepine has made dosage prediction difficult. Statistical models and population methods are not generally useful for clinical use.[70,71] A bayesian nonlinear method was clinically acceptable but needed three or four data points for acceptability.[72]

Blood Sampling for Carbamazepine Concentrations. The sampling time for carbamazepine depends on the duration of treatment and whether the clinician is evaluating efficacy or side effects. There is no indication to obtain a blood sample for carbamazepine concentration determination after the first dose unless a rapid loading dose has been given in an emergency situation. Although concentrations should be determined during the course of dosage titration to evaluate endpoints, the concentration may be expected to fall following the full effect of autoinduction. Also, the effect of autoinduction must be remembered if doses are changed during chronic therapy.

Numerous side effects associated with carbamazepine, such as blurred vision, lethargy, and drowsiness, are serum concentration related.[50] Each patient appears to have a threshold for the occurrence of side effects. Therefore, for some patients it may be appropriate to obtain the serum sample between dosing intervals when the side effects are occurring. Given the variability of absorption it is difficult to predict when the peak concentration of carbamazepine will occur.

A trough level, that is, one drawn just before the morning dose, is most appropriate for the evaluation of efficacy. A trough level is particularly important if seizures are not controlled or if there appears to be an increase in seizure activity at the end of a dosing interval.

In addition to the use of serum concentration monitoring in the initial dosage titration, the sudden occurrence of side effects or change in seizure frequency is an indication to monitor carbamazepine concentrations. The serum concentrations of carbamazepine should be closely monitored during the third trimester in pregnant patients. Serum concentrations should be monitored every 6 to 12 months in stable adults and every 4 to 6 months in stable children.

The 10,11-diepoxide metabolite is active but an assay is not routinely available. It may be assayed at research centers.

Therapeutic Range. The reported therapeutic range of carbamazepine is 4 to 12 μg/mL for the treatment of seizures. The exact concentration that will be therapeutic for a given patient must be individually determined. The final target concentration is a balance between seizure control and intolerable side effects. There is a poor correlation between carbamazepine dose and serum concentration.[47]

Dosage Forms. Carbamazepine is available as a 100-mg chewable table and as a 200-mg immediate-release tablet. A suspension is also available. The immediate-release tablet is available from several generic manufacturers. Concern about the generic equivalency of antiepileptic drugs has been raised. A sustained-release formulation (OROS) of carbamazepine is being reviewed by the FDA. A rectal enema has been made by diluting the suspension 1:1 with water.[12] There is no intravenous formulation of carbamazepine.

Valproic Acid

Clinical Pharmacology and Therapeutics

Valproic acid is a unique antiepileptic drug in that it is effective in absence seizures as well as other generalized and partial seizures. It is structurally related to free fatty acids and is the first antiepileptic drug to deviate from the traditional heterocyclic ring structure. It was used for more than 80 years as an organic solvent before it was found to have antiepileptic properties. It was approved as an antiepileptic drug in 1978. Valproic acid has become the drug of choice for primary generalized seizures.[73] More recently it has been used in the treatment of bipolar depression, especially in patients refractory to lithium.[74]

Valproic acid inhibits epileptiform activity at several levels but the exact mechanism is unknown.[75] Originally, valproic acid was thought to act by increasing γ-aminobutyric acid (GABA), which is a neuroinhibitor; however, the concentrations required and the onset of effect are different clinically than in the laboratory model. It has also been postulated that valproic acid potentiates postsynaptic GABA response, but again the clinical concentrations are much less than in the laboratory model. More recently it has been postulated that valproic acid has a direct cellular membrane effect. It is possible that valproic acid works by all or a combination of these mechanisms.[76]

Clinical Pharmacokinetics

Absorption. Valproic acid is rapidly absorbed when given orally.[77] The absorption rate of valproic acid depends on the formulation used. Absorption is fastest from the valproic acid syrup followed by the gelatin capsule, the enteric-coated tablet, and the sprinkle formulations. The time to peak concentration with the syrup and gelatin capsule is between 1 and 3 hours. The enteric-coated tablet and the sprinkle formulations were formulated to delay absorption and to minimize the gastrointestinal irritation associated with valproic acid. Absorption from the enteric-coated tablet does not begin for 2 to 4 hours after administration, but once absorption begins valproic acid reaches the systemic circulation very quickly at a rate similar to that of rapid-release formulations. Peak concentrations with the enteric coated tablets are not seen for 4 to 8 hours. The enteric-coated tablet is not a sustained-release formulation. Recently a circadian effect on the absorption of valproic acid from enteric coated tablets has been reported. Although not designed to be a controlled release formulation, the sprinkle formulation results in a prolonged absorption that approaches a zero order input.[78] The absorption of valproic acid given as a rectal solution, prepared by mixing the syrup and water in a 1:1 ratio, is comparable to that of oral formulations; however, the maximum concentration is lower and the time to peak is longer. The rectal route may be used for maintenance therapy, but the slow absorption precludes its use in emergency situations. After absorption begins the pharmacokinetics of all of the valproic acid formulations are similar.

The bioavailability of all of the valproic acid formulations is believed to be about 100%. Food may delay the rate of drug absorption but does not affect the extent of absorption.[79] There is no first-pass metabolism of valproic acid.[80]

Distribution. More than 90% of valproic acid is ionized at physiologic pH. Therefore, the drug is highly bound to plasma proteins relative to tissue proteins. The volume of distribution of the unbound drug is higher than the volume of distribution for the total drug. At concentrations up to 80 to 100 μg/mL, valproic acid is 90 to 95% bound to plasma proteins, mainly albumin.[81] At higher concentrations, however, the protein binding saturates and the free fraction increases in a percentage that is disproportionate to the amount of dosage increase. The protein binding may be altered in disease states in which the synthesis of albumin may be altered, for example, cirrhosis, chronic renal failure, extremes of age. The diurnal fluctuation seen with valproic acid concentrations is greater with the unbound than with the total concentration.[82] Free fatty acids may compete with valproic acid for binding sites on the albumin molecule.

Valproic acid enters the brain and cerebrospinal fluid (CSF) very rapidly. An equilibrium develops between the CSF and plasma concentrations of valproic acid, and a ratio of about 0.1 to 0.15 is established for the total valproic acid concentration. CSF concentrations have been reported to equal the serum unbound concentrations. Valproic acid also distributes to a variety of other tissues that include the liver, kidney, breast milk, growing bones, intestines, and the developing fetus. Some valproic acid may bind to red blood cells. When given intravenously, valproic acid seems to follow a two-compartment model.[77]

Metabolism and Elimination. Valproic acid is a low extraction drug and is extensively metabolized by the liver. Only 3 to 7% is excreted in the urine as unchanged drug. It is the unbound fraction that is metabolized. Therefore, when protein binding saturates and there is an increase in the percentage of free drug, the metabolism of valproic acid increases. Thus, there is an increase in clearance at higher serum concentrations. With an increase in clearance, the concentration of total drug increases less than the percentage increase in dose. There is significant intersubject variability in the metabolism of valproic acid. The average half-life of valproic acid has been reported to be 12 to 16 hours in adult volunteers[80]; however, the half-life may be affected by the presence of other enzyme-inducing or -inhibiting drugs and is highly variable in a patient population.[83,84]

Valproic acid may be metabolized by conjugation, beta oxidation, and alpha hydroxylation. More than 10 metabolites have been identified. Some of these metabolites may have antiepileptic activity, and one of these, 4-en-valproic acid, has been associated with valproic acid-induced hepatotoxicity. The 4-en-valproic acid metabolite may reflect an abnormal pathway that is used in the presence of other drugs or congenital abnormalities.[85]

Renal elimination does not contribute significantly to the clearance of valproic acid.

Special Populations. Children have a higher clearance of valproic acid than do adults.[86] This may necessitate more frequent dosing in children. The elderly have an increase in the free fraction and a decrease in the clearance of unbound drug. Interestingly, the clearance of total drug is not changed in the elderly.[87]

Liver disease may decrease the protein binding of valproic acid and hence the clearance of unbound drug. Protein binding and, hence, clearance of unbound drug may also be altered in patients with chronic renal failure. Negligible amounts of valproic acid are removed by dialysis. Clearance of valproic acid increases in the third trimester of pregnancy and decreases postpartum.[88]

Pharmacodynamics

Therapeutic Endpoints. Valproic acid is the drug of choice for all types of generalized seizures except classic absence seizures, although it can be used for this seizure type.[1] Valproic acid is also useful in patients with partial seizures.[89] The therapeutic endpoint for valproic acid is the abolition of seizures. The upper end of the therapeutic range for valproic acid remains to be defined, so the dose may continue to be increased in patients who do not experience side effects. The initial drowsiness, sedation, and lethargy associated with valproic acid may be minimized if the dose is titrated properly.[90] The major dose-limiting side effect is gastrointestinal discomfort, which may be minimized by the enteric coated tablet dosage form.[91] Some patients may experience tremor with concentrations greater than 100 μg/mL.

Adverse Reactions. The adverse reactions associated with valproic acid may be divided into physiologic reactions, concentration-dependent reactions, and idiosyncratic reactions. Gastrointestinal complaints constitute the most frequently reported physiologic adverse reactions. Nausea, vomiting, and anorexia were frequently reported with the liquid capsule.[91] These reactions may be significantly reduced with the enteric-coated tablet. The administration of valproic acid is associated with an increase in liver function tests and serum ammonia.[92] Other physiologic side effects associated with valproic acid include alopecia and excessive weight gain.

Central nervous system depression manifested by ataxia, sedation, lethargy, and tiredness are associated with early high concentrations of valproic acid and may be minimized by dosage titration. An adrenergic or essential tremor has been reported in patients with valproic acid concentrations greater than 100 μg/mL. Thrombocytopenia may occur in 6 to 40% of patients exposed to valproic acid, but is responsive to a decrease in dose. The increase in liver function tests may be dose related. Stupor and coma may be seen in patients receiving very high concentrations of valproic acid (175 μg/mL or greater). The primary side effect seen in massive overdoses (up to 20 times therapeutic blood levels) is cerebral edema, but even these concentrations are usually not associated with long term sequelae.[93]

A number of rare and idiosyncratic reactions have been associated with valproic acid. The most significant is a fatal hepatotoxicity. Two recent retrospective reviews of the reported cases of valproic acid-induced hepatotoxicity identified that this reaction is most likely to occur in children less than 2 years of age who are being treated with enzyme-inducing agents or who have inborn errors of metabolism.[94,95] The formation of the 4-en-valproic acid metabolite may represent an alternate pathway of metabolism that is increased in this population and results in hepatotoxicity. Although the exposure of patients to valproic acid has increased significantly, the number of reported cases of valproic acid-induced hepatotoxicity has remained the same or decreased. It has not been possible to anticipate the occurrence of fatal hepatotoxicity by laboratory monitoring. Other idiosyncratic reactions to valproic acid include pancreatitis,[96] pitting edema,[97] and drug-induced systemic lupus erythematosus.[98] Cases of leukopenia with transient neutropenia, transient erythroblastopenia, and bone marrow changes have been reported.[99] Valproic acid has been reported to induce von Willebrand disease type I.[100]

Valproic acid will cross the placenta and into breast milk. Because it can cross the placenta, valproic acid has the potential to cause teratogenicity. Although cases similar to the "hydantoin syndrome" have been reported, the most significant result of valproic acid administration to pregnant females is the occurrence of spina bifida, which may occur in 1% of the off-spring of pregnant patients exposed to valproic acid. The concentration present in breast milk is not high enough to cause side effects.[77]

Valproic acid has been shown to decrease serum carnitine levels, which is a cofactor for mitochondrial metabolism.[101] Carnitine is necessary for the transport of medium- and long-chain fatty acids across mitochondrial membranes and for the regulation of the ratio of free coenzyme A to acylcoenzyme A in the mitochondrion.[102] It has been suggested that patients treated with valproic acid should receive carnitine supplements.[103] Some clinicians have observed that some side effects such as tremor may be decreased by carnitine supplementation; the evidence is main-ly anecdotal. Carnitine has also been suggested as an antidote for valproic acid-induced hepato-toxicity. There have been no controlled trials to determine if carnitine can reduce any of the adverse effects associated with valproic acid. Although its administration cannot be recom-mended for routine supplementation, it may be tried in an individual patient in whom the seizures have been well controlled but who is bothered by side effects.

Valproic acid is remarkably free of cognitive impairment and behavioral side effects.[104]

Drug–Drug Interactions. Valproic acid is an enzyme inhibitor. Most significantly it inhibits the metabolism of phenobarbital and may increase phenobarbital concentrations by as much as 125%.[105] More recently, valproic acid has been reported to inhibit the formation of the 10,11-diepoxide metabolite of carbamazepine without altering the concentration of the parent drug. Because this metabolite of carbamazepine is active and contributes to the side effects associated with carbamazepine, a patient may exhibit signs of carbamazepine toxicity without a change in the serum concentration of parent drug after the addition of valproic acid.[106] Valproic acid is highly protein bound and may displace phenytoin from its binding sites, increasing the free frac-tion and clearance of phenytoin.

Because valproic acid is highly metabolized, its clearance may be altered by other drugs.[107] When other enzyme-inducing antiepileptic drugs are discontinued, clearance of valproic acid decreases and a lower dose is needed to maintain the same serum concentration.[108] Enzyme-inhibiting drugs should decrease the clearance of valproic acid. Valproic acid may also be dis-placed from its binding sites by other highly protein-bound drugs such as aspirin and free fatty acids.[109] It appears that drugs must be present in concentrations similar to that of valproic acid to displace it from its binding sites.

The rate but not the extent of absorption of valproic acid has been shown to be decreased by the concurrent administration with antacids.

Pharmacodynamic interactions have been suggested when valproic acid is given with other drugs such as alcohol and other central nervous system depressants. Absence status developed in 5 of 12 patients on clonazepam when valproic acid was added.[107]

Disease–Drug Interactions. The major effect of disease states on valproic acid is an alteration in protein binding. Liver disease, chronic renal failure, burns, and protein loss result in an increased free fraction of valproic acid. Liver disease does not affect the clearance of valproic acid.

The clearance of valproic acid is not significantly affected by dialysis.[77]

Therapeutic Regimen Design

Initial Dose. Because an intravenous dosage form is not currently available, there is generally no need to give a large loading dose of valproic acid. The product information indicates that the initial dose of valproic acid is 15 mg/kg/d given in divided doses; however, because age and comedication have a significant effect on dose, a more rational approach is to incorporate these variables into the dosing design. Adults clear valproic acid more slowly and may be started on 7.5 mg/kg/d as monotherapy and on 15 mg/kg/d if they are receiving an enzyme-inducing drug. Children may be started on 10 mg/kg/d as monotherapy and on 20 mg/kg/d if they are receiving polytherapy. The dose is then titrated to tolerance and response.[110]

Maintenance Dose. Dosage adjustments may be made every 2 to 3 days until the desired concentration is reached or side effects become intolerable. Because of their higher clearance rates, neonates and children often require larger doses than adults.[111] Doses of 100 mg/kg/d have been used in children. Some types of childhood epilepsy, for example, infantile spasms and West syndrome, may require very large doses of valproic acid.[112,113]

Dosing Interval. Antiepileptic drugs are normally dosed on the half-life of the drug. There is significant variation in the half-life of valproic acid. Some patients may have a half-life that would allow once-daily dosing, whereas others may require four-times-a-day dosing. In general, in children and patients taking enzyme-inducing drugs, valproic acid has a short half-life and more frequent dosing is required.

Dosing Prediction and Adjustment. If a loading dose (LD) is needed, it may be estimated by the following equations:

children $LD = (0.20 \text{ L/kg}) \times (\text{desired } C_{serum}) \times BW \text{ in kg}$

adults $LD = (0.15 \text{ L/kg}) \times (\text{desired } C_{serum}) \times BW \text{ in kg}$

The maintenance dose of valproic acid was successfully predicted in normal volunteers using the Slattery equation. This prediction works provided there is good patient compliance and the binding of valproic acid remains constant. If the binding saturates, the clearance is no longer linear and the dosage prediction using the one-point method of Slattery would not be appropriate.[114]

Attempts to predict the unbound fraction have been unsuccessful.[115]

Dose adjustment may be made as frequently as every 2 to 3 days. A slower titration may be desirable to allow the patient to develop tolerance to the central nervous system side effects.

Blood Sampling for Valproic Acid. The blood sampling of valproic acid should take into account the diurnal variation in the clearance and the dosage form of valproic acid used.[116] Because there is diurnal variation in the pharmacokinetics of valproic acid, a trough level in the morning will not necessarily be the same as a trough level in the evening. To direct therapy appropriately, the level should be obtained at the same time each day.

The trough level of the enteric-coated tablet does not occur immediately prior to the next dose of medication as it does with the syrup and the gelatin capsule. The enteric coating delays the absorption and the trough may not occur for 2 to 4 hours after dosing.

Peak levels may be useful if the patient is having transient side effects.

The type of vacutainer that valproic acid is collected in has been shown to affect concentration. Vacutainer tubes containing sodium citrate in solution resulted in concentrations that were lower for total and free valproic acid, compared with vacutainer tubes containing heparin, EDTA, or nothing. The volume of sodium citrate was believed to dilute the sample, resulting in a falsely low concentration. There does not appear to be a difference in serum and plasma for total or free concentrations.[117]

Samples should be obtained following each dosage increase until the therapeutic concentration for that patient has been determined. After seizure control has been established, concentrations may be monitored every 6 to 12 months.

The unbound fraction of valproic acid should be measured in patients with risk factors for altered protein binding. Also, at higher concentrations where the binding is likely to saturate, the unbound fraction should be measured. The unbound fraction should also be measured in patients who are experiencing side effects at concentrations that are not thought to produce side effects.

Therapeutic Range. A minimal, but not maximal, concentration for valproic acid has been defined.[110] The minimal concentration that is thought to control seizures effectively is 50 μg/mL. The maximal concentration was initially stated to be 100 μg/mL; however, some clinicians have recently advocated pushing the concentration to 150 or 175 μg/mL. Doses required to achieve these concentrations should be carefully monitored for increased seizure control and for concentration-dependent side effects.

Dosage Forms. Valproic acid is available as a syrup (250 mg/5 mL), a gelatin capsule (250 mg), an enteric-coated tablet (125, 250, and 500 mg), and a "sprinkle" (125 mg). The sprinkle may be particularly useful in a pediatric population. A recent study demonstrated that patients prefer it because of its ease of administration, increased palatability, and twice-a-day dosing schedule. These features may enhance compliance in a pediatric population. It may be substituted for the syrup without changing the dose. Because of its prolonged absorption, the "sprinkle" may also be useful in patients with very rapid clearances that result in dramatic peak to trough concentrations.[78] The enteric-coated preparation has significantly less gastrointestinal toxicity associated with it. A rectal enema may be compounded using the oral liquid in a 1:1 ratio with water. An intravenous formulation is under development.

Phenobarbital and Primidone

Clinical Pharmacology and Therapeutics

Phenobarbital and primidone can be considered together because primidone is metabolized to phenobarbital. Phenobarbital was introduced in 1912 and is the oldest antiepileptic drug that is still commonly used.[118] Although its use in the United States has diminished in recent years because of the availability of more effective and less toxic drugs, it is still frequently used; in economically deprived populations it is commonly used because of its low price. Primidone was first commercially available in 1954. Although primidone has inherent antiepileptic activity, it is dosed to achieve a serum phenobarbital concentration consistent with phenobarbital administered alone. In selected patients primidone may have some therapeutic benefit over phenobarbital because of the antiepileptic effect of the parent drug and possible antiepileptic effects of phenylethylmalonamide (PEMA), its other metabolite.[119] Phenobarbital and primidone have been frequently used in partial seizures but the VA Epilepsy Cooperative Study demonstrated that both carbamazepine and phenytoin were more effective and less toxic than either phenobarbital or primidone.[5] Both of these agents may have some use in patients with refractory generalized seizures (except absence). Phenobarbital and primidone may exacerbate absence seizures. Although phenobarbital has been widely used for the prophylaxis of febrile seizures, a recent study indicated that its efficacy is not different from that of placebo and it may diminish cognitive abilities.[18] The availability of an intravenous dosage formulation of phenobarbital makes it a second-line agent for the treatment of status epilepticus.

Although these are old drugs a complete understanding of their mechanism of action is lacking. Though the mechanisms of action of the barbiturates are often considered together, there does appear to be selectivity for antiepileptic activity among them. Phenobarbital raises the seizure threshold by decreasing postsynaptic excitation, possibly by stimulating postsynaptic GABA-ergic inhibitor responses. Phenobarbital may have some effect on reducing sodium uptake but is less potent than phenytoin. Phenobarbital may exert more of its antiepileptic action on abnormal neurons rather than normal neurons, as does phenytoin.[120] Although it has been argued that all of the effects of primidone may be explained by the conversion to phenobarbital, animal models indicate a separate antiepileptic effect of primidone and PEMA. There are no data on the biochemical mechanisms of primidone and PEMA.[121]

Clinical Pharmacokinetics

Phenobarbital and primidone were introduced before extensive pharmacokinetic testing was required and the pharmacokinetics of these drugs are not completely understood.

Absorption. Phenobarbital is absorbed primarily from the small intestine and is rapidly and completely absorbed from oral dosage forms. Bioavailability approaches 100% in children and adults.[122] Newborns may have delayed or incomplete absorption of oral products. Absorption is more rapid from solutions than from tablets. Intramuscular administration may result in a small decrease in bioavailability, although this may be explained by individual variations in clearance. Peak concentrations are reached in 0.5 to 4.0 hours with both oral and intramuscular dosage forms.[123]

There is no intravenous dosage form of primidone so the absolute bioavailability is not known. Bioavailability is comparable between tablet and syrup and has been estimated at about 92%.[124] Although a report of generic inequivalency with primidone has been published, the FDA concluded that it was a therapeutic failure, resulting from patient idiosyncrasy rather than bioequivalency problems.[125]

Distribution. Initially, phenobarbital distributes to highly perfused organs and concentrations may be found in the brain 3 to 20 minutes following intravenous administration.[123] EEG effects document rapid penetration into the central nervous system.[126] Phenobarbital has a bimodal distribution so it then redistributes to all body tissues including fat. A recent report of a morbidly obese patient indicates that the loading dose of phenobarbital should be calculated on total body weight.[127] The volume of distribution of phenobarbital is between 0.6 and 1.0 L/kg for children and adults. Neonates may have a larger volume of distribution. Because phenobarbital is only about 50% protein bound, protein binding is not felt to contribute significantly to the pharmacokinetics. Protein binding may be somewhat lower in neonates. An acidic systemic pH drives phenobarbital into tissues. Phenobarbital crosses the placenta and is secreted into breast milk.[123] Primidone distributes throughout the body in a manner similar to phenobarbital. It does not significantly bind to plasma proteins.[124]

Metabolism and Elimination. Phenobarbital is eliminated by liver metabolism and by renal excretion. Phenobarbital is a low-extraction drug and is eliminated by a first-order process.[128] The half-life of phenobarbital is very long and averages around 70 hours. There is significant variability in the elimination of phenobarbital. Neonates have the longest half-life and infants have the shortest. Although phenobarbital is a potent enzyme inducer, there is no evidence that it may induce its own metabolism. About 20 to 40% of phenobarbital is eliminated unchanged in the urine. The renal clearance of phenobarbital is less than the glomerular filtration rate because there is extensive tubular reabsorption. Renal elimination may be increased by forced diuresis and urinary alkalinization.[129]

Primidone is metabolized to phenobarbital and PEMA. The primidone-to-phenobarbital ratio is highly variable.[130] The parent drug and its metabolites are also eliminated by renal excretion. About 40 to 60% of an administered dose of primidone is eliminated unchanged in the urine. The half-life of primidone is independent of dose or plasma concentration and is consistent with a first-order, linear pharmacokinetic model. The half-life of primidone following a single dose of monotherapy ranges between 8 and 22 hours. Because phenobarbital is an enzyme inducer, the half-life of primidone is believed to decrease with continued dosing. The half-life of primidone following multiple dosing is reported to be between 5 and 19 hours. The longer half-life of phenobarbital allows for greater accumulation, and the shorter half-life of primidone requires more frequent dosing. There is poor correlation between the dose of primidone and its clearance.[120]

Special Populations. The pharmacokinetics of phenobarbital and primidone are affected by age. Neonates have a longer half-life and a larger volume of distribution of phenobarbital than children or adults. There is a significant relationship between age and phenobarbital dose ratio for monotherapy patients.[131] The dose ratio declines in the first year of life, but the dose ratio increases after age 1. A prolonged half-life for patients over age 70 has been reported. Protein malnutrition increases phenobarbital clearance and asphyxia reduces it. Patients with renal or hepatic impairment would be expected to have a decreased clearance of phenobarbital and primidone.[121] One burn patient with uremia was reported to have a free fraction of phenobarbital of 93%.[132] A 4-hour hemodialysis removes about 30% of the phenobarbital in the body and about 32% of a primidone dose. Peritoneal dialysis is about one fourth as efficient as hemodialysis. The clearance of phenobarbital and primidone can be altered by the coadministration of other drugs. Pregnancy may decrease the clearance of primidone and increase the clearance of phenobarbital.[133]

Pharmacodynamics

Therapeutic Endpoints. The desired therapeutic endpoint for phenobarbital and primidone is the abolition of seizures. For patients with mixed seizure disorders, it should be remembered that these drugs can exacerbate absence seizures. The efficacy of phenobarbital and primidone should be carefully balanced against the high rate of adverse reactions that these drugs can cause. They should be used as adjunctive therapy for patients refractory to other antiepileptic drugs.

Adverse Reactions. The VA Epilepsy Cooperative Study helped to define the side effects associated with phenobarbital and primidone.[5] Continued use of phenobarbital and primidone, even at doses that result in serum concentrations considered to be in the therapeutic range, results in significant changes in affect, behavior, and cognitive function. Tolerance may develop to the initial reports of sedation, tiredness, and lethargy; however, although the complaints of these side effects decrease, patients often describe feeling more alert when phenobarbital is discontinued. Long-term administration results in depression and impairment of cognitive functioning. In children a paradoxical hyperactivity may occur. Elderly patients may also become agitated rather than sedated with phenobarbital.[134] A recent case of dystonia occurring at a concentration within the therapeutic range was reported.[135]

Chronic administration of phenobarbital may also result in hematologic side effects manifested by megaloblastic anemia, folate deficiency, decreased production of vitamin K-dependent clotting factors, decreased vitamin D and osteomalacia, and porphyria. Impotence and decreased libido may occur. Gastrointestinal complaints are less common than with other antiepileptic drugs. Skin rashes and other hypersensitivity reactions may occur. Teratogenicity has been associated with phenobarbital.[134]

Primidone shares the adverse reactions of its major metabolite. Initial complaints of weakness, dizziness, and drowsiness occurring with the initiation of therapy may be attributed to the parent drug, but chronic toxicity from the parent drug alone has been difficult to separate from the effects of phenobarbital.[136] Tolerance to the central nervous system side effects of primidone may develop.[137]

Drug–Drug Interactions. Phenobarbital is a potent enzyme inducer of the mixed-function oxidative system. Although cytochrome P450 is the primary enzyme system affected, other enzymes such as NADPH–cytochrome c reductase, UDP-glucuronyl transferase, and the enzymes involved in glucuronic acid synthesis may be induced also. Phenobarbital appears to increase production and to decrease degradation of these enzymes. Therefore, phenobarbital is the prototype drug used to assess drug interactions of these enzyme systems. Phenobarbital has the potential to interact with any drug that is metabolized by the mixed-function oxidative system. Phenobarbital may also increase the clearance of endogenous substances such as vitamin D.[138]

Phenobarbital may compete for the same substrate for metabolism as other drugs such as phenytoin and thus inhibit metabolism.

A significant decrease in phenobarbital clearance occurs when valproic acid is administered concurrently. Increases in phenobarbital concentrations have also been reported with dextropropoxyphene and chloramphenicol. Chlorpromazine, prochlorperazine, and thioridazine may lower phenobarbital concentrations.

A pharmacodynamic interaction may occur if phenobarbital is given with other central nervous system-depressant drugs such as alcohol.

Primidone has a drug interaction profile similar to that of phenobarbital.[139]

Disease–Drug Interactions. The clearance of phenobarbital and primidone may be decreased in patients with liver disease or chronic renal impairment. Patients receiving hemodialysis may need supplemental doses.

Therapeutic Regimen Design

Initial Dose. Phenobarbital is used in the treatment of status epilepticus if the seizures are not controlled by intravenous benzodiazepines and phenytoin. In this emergency situation the loading dose is 20 mg/kg, which should be adequate to achieve serum concentrations within the therapeutic range. In nonemergency conditions, phenobarbital should be started at lower does and titrated to the desired response.

There is no clinically accepted indication for a loading dose of primidone.

Maintenance Dose. The average maintenance dose of phenobarbital needed to achieve a concentration between 15 and 40 µg/mL is 1.5 to 2 mg/kg/d.[119] In children less than 10 years of age the range is 3.0 to 4.5 mg/kg/d, and in neonates the range varies from 2.5 to 5.0 mg/kg/d. The average maintenance dose of primidone in adults averages between 10 and 25 mg/kg/d. In children less than 15 years of age, the maintenance dose has varied between 12 and 23 mg/kg/d. Recent data suggest that children may require larger doses.[140] Limited data in neonates indicate a maintenance dosage range of 12 to 20 mg/kg/d. The maintenance dose will be affected by interindividual variability and by the presence or absence of other drugs. The serum concentration and patient response are the preferred guidelines.

Dosing Interval. The very long half-life of phenobarbital allows for drug accumulation and once-a-day dosing. Patients in a nursing home were switched from multiple daily dosing to once-a-day dosing without a change in their serum concentration.[141] If transient drowsiness, sedation, or lethargy occurs with phenobarbital, the dose may be given at bedtime so that the central nervous system depression may occur during sleep. The short half life of primidone necessitates a three- or four-times-per-day dosing interval.

Dosage Prediction and Adjustment. Phenobarbital is a linear drug and follows a first-order process. Therefore, a maintenance dose may be calculated after an initial dose.[128] The intersubject variability in the primidone-to-phenobarbital conversion precludes dosage prediction with primidone.

Dosage adjustment with phenobarbital must consider the very long half-life of the drug. Steady-state concentrations may not occur for 2 to 3 weeks after initiation of or change in dosing. Only in emergency situations should dose changes be made more frequently than every 2 weeks. The dosage adjustment of primidone will be directed by the kinetics of phenobarbital.

Blood Sampling of Phenobarbital and Primidone. A therapeutic range has been defined for phenobarbital and primidone. Trough level assessment is preferred; however, with a long half-life drug such as phenobarbital, there is minimal peak to trough variability and the timing of sample collection is not as important. The shorter half-life of primidone results in greater peak to trough variability. In nonemergency situations, the assessment of drug concentrations should wait until steady state has been achieved. In emergency situations, concentrations may be assessed to determine the need for another loading dose. Once the therapeutic concentration has been defined for a given patient, serum concentration monitoring may be done every 6 to 12 months.

Except in very unusual cases there is no indication to measure the unbound fraction of either phenobarbital or primidone. Serum and plasma give the same result.

Therapeutic Range. The therapeutic range that has been defined for phenobarbital is 15 to 40 μg/mL. There appears to be little clinical benefit gained by increasing the concentration above 40 μg/mL. The therapeutic range of primidone is 6 to 12 μg/mL. Generally, if the serum concentration of primidone is within the therapeutic range, the serum concentration of phenobarbital is also within the therapeutic range.

Dosage Forms. Phenobarbital is available as an oral tablet (15, 30, 65, and 100 mg), as an elixir (20 mg/5 mL), and as a parenteral formulation (30, 60, and 130 mg/mL) that can be given either intramuscularly or intravenously. Primidone is available as a tablet (50 and 250 mg) and a suspension (250 mg/5 mL).

Phenytoin

Clinical Pharmacology and Therapeutics
Phenytoin was first introduced for clinical use in 1938 and is still widely used as an antiepileptic drug for the suppression of generalized and partial seizures.[142] In the VA Epilepsy Cooperative Study phenytoin was equally efficacious to carbamazepine in the treatment of partial seizures[5]; however, phenytoin was associated with a greater incidence of cognitive and behavioral side effects than carbamazepine.[143] Phenytoin is the antiepileptic drug that is given after an intravenous benzodiazepine in status epilepticus. It is effective in a variety of primary and secondary generalized seizures with the exception of absence seizures. Phenytoin may exacerbate absence seizures.[144] Although phenytoin is still widely used, it has the potential for inducing significant side effects. The appropriate use of phenytoin requires a thorough understanding of its pharmacokinetics and individualization of dosing strategies.

Phenytoin suppresses seizures by blocking posttetanic potentiation by influencing synaptic transmission. The mechanisms postulated for this effect include altering ion fluxes associated with depolarization, repolarization, and membrane stability; altering calcium uptake in presynaptic terminals; influencing calcium-dependent synaptic protein phosphorylation and transmitter release; altering the sodium–potassium ATP-dependent ionic membrane pump; and preventing cyclic nucleotide buildup and cerebellar stimulation. There is disagreement about whether phenytoin interacts with numerous biochemical processes or whether it interacts with a few major regulatory systems in the nervous system that regulate other systems. It has been suggested that phenytoin exerts its greatest effect on normal neuronal cells.[145]

Clinical Pharmacokinetics

Absorption. Phenytoin is a weak organic acid with a high pK_a and is poorly soluble in water. Dissolution is the rate-limiting step to phenytoin's absorption. Anything that affects the dissolution or solubility of phenytoin will affect absorption.[146] Phenytoin toxicity occurred in Australia several years ago when an excipient in a capsule formulation was changed. Following oral administration little absorption occurs in the stomach, where the pH is acidic. Absorption does not begin until the drug enters the duodenum, where the pH is more alkaline. The absorption of phenytoin slows down when the drug enters the jejunum and the ileum. Phenytoin is poorly absorbed from the rectum. Changes in gastrointestinal motility may alter the absorption of orally administered phenytoin. The rate and extent of oral absorption of phenytoin may be affected by particle size. There is evidence suggesting that the rate and amount of oral absorption may be dose dependent and that the absorption of phenytoin may saturate. Absorption may be prolonged and secondary peaks may be seen. Thus, absorption is not first order and is nonlinear. Enterohepatic cycling of phenytoin occurs but there is no first-pass metabolism.[147] The rate and extent of phenytoin absorption may be affected by food and antacids.[148]

The absorption rate varies for different generic formulations of phenytoin. The innovator product (Dilantin) and some generic formulations are extended-release preparations. Other generic formulations are absorbed more rapidly and are termed *prompt-release preparations.* Extended-release and prompt-release preparations should not be interchanged. Only the extended-release preparations should be used for once-a-day therapy. Dilantin suspension has an absorption profile similar to that of Dilantin capsules if the difference in salt content is considered.[146]

When phenytoin is given intramuscularly, it will crystalize in muscle tissues which may be seen on biopsy. These crystals provide a depot of drug. Initially absorption is decreased, but drug continues to be absorbed from the injection site for a prolonged period after the injections are stopped. Thus, intramuscular injection results in erratic and prolonged absorption. The unpredictable absorption plus the pain caused by the injection make the intramuscular injection of phenytoin undesirable.[146] Fosphenytoin is a new water-soluble prodrug of phenytoin and may be given intramuscularly without pain and with rapid attainment of serum phenytoin concentrations.

Distribution. Following absorption phenytoin distributes widely throughout the body. It rapidly enters the brain and is redistributed to other body tissues. Phenytoin is about 90 to 95% bound to plasma proteins. The free fraction distributes into all transcellular fluids including saliva, breast milk, bile, semen, and gastrointestinal fluids. Phenytoin crosses the placental barrier. The volume of distribution of phenytoin is about 0.6 to 0.8 L/kg, which is similar to that of total body water. Obesity may increase the volume of distribution.[146,147]

As phenytoin is highly protein bound and it is the free fraction that is pharmacologically active and is available for metabolism, the protein binding of phenytoin is clinically significant. For most patients the protein binding is predictable and linear throughout the concentrations normally seen clinically; however, the protein binding may be altered by liver disease, chronic renal failure, and other drugs and in very young and old patients. If the free fraction increases, there is an increase in the clearance of phenytoin and the total concentration may decrease. A new equilibrium will be reached. Attempts to increase the total concentration without first evaluating the free fraction may result in phenytoin toxicity. The equations that have been used to normalize phenytoin concentrations in patients with hypoalbuminemia and chronic renal failure have been shown to be unreliable. The equations underpredicted the phenytoin concentration in patients with hypoalbuminemia, and over- and underprediction occurred in patients with renal failure. A better clinical guide is to measure the free fraction.[146,147]

Metabolism and Elimination. Less than 5% of a dose of phenytoin is excreted unchanged in the urine. It is first metabolized to an arene oxide via the cytochrome oxidase system enzyme arene oxidase. Arene oxide is converted spontaneously to 5-(p-hydroxyphenyl)-5-phenylhydantoin (HPPH) and is converted by the enzyme epoxide hydrolase to dihydrodiol. HPPH accounts for 67 to 88% and dihydrodiol accounts for 7 to 11% of the phenytoin metabolites recovered in the urine.[149] The concentration of HPPH in the urine may be used to evaluate malabsorption versus increased capacity for metabolism for patients with low phenytoin serum concentrations who are receiving large doses of phenytoin. A low percentage of HPPH in the urine would suggest malabsorption, whereas the concentration of HPPH would be high in patients with increased metabolic capacity. Phenytoin is a low-extraction drug and its metabolism is not altered by changes in hepatic blood flow. The enzymes that metabolize phenytoin, however, are subject to induction and inhibition.[146]

Michaelis and Menten demonstrated in the early 1900s that enzyme systems have a finite capacity to metabolize substrate. Although their work was with enzyme systems, the Michaelis–Menten principles apply to phenytoin. The metabolism of phenytoin occurs with doses given clinically. When saturation occurs, the metabolism of phenytoin changes from a first-order (linear) process to a zero-order (nonlinear) process. When the metabolizing enzymes saturate, no additional drug can be metabolized. Any additional increase in dose results in a significantly disproportional increase in serum concentration. Small changes in phenytoin dose may result in large increases in serum concentrations.[146] It is clinically unfortunate that this saturation may occur at concentrations that are considered therapeutic. The saturable metabolism of phenytoin means that there is no one dose for every patient. Although 300 mg is frequently given as "the maintenance dose," this will not be adequate for every patient. If 300 mg is given as a maintenance dose, about 55% of the patients will have a steady-state concentration less than 10 μg/mL, about 30% will achieve a concentration of 10 to 20 μg/mL, and about 15% will have concentrations above 20 μg/mL. Therefore, the dose of phenytoin must be individualized to the given patient (see Dosing Prediction and Adjustment).

The metabolism of phenytoin can be described by the Michaelis–Menten equation

$$D = \frac{V_{max} \times C_p}{K_m + C_p}$$

where D is the dose (mg/d), V_{max} is the maximum rate of metabolism (mg/d), K_m is the serum concentration at which the rate of metabolism is half-maximal (μg/mL), and C_p is the serum concentration (μg/mL).

The published ranges for V_{max} and K_m are 100 to 1000 mg/d and 1 to 15 μg/mL, respectively. Because of the large and independent variability in these values, the metabolism of phenytoin may saturate at any concentration.[150] The V_{max} has been shown to decline with age and the K_m may be affected by concurrent drug therapy. Some patients may saturate at low serum concentrations of phenytoin, and other patients may not display any evidence of saturation at all.[151]

It is not possible to predict prospectively the concentration at which a given patient will saturate. Any change in dose should be accompanied by careful patient monitoring[152] (see Dosing Prediction and Adjustment).

Because phenytoin displays Michaelis–Menten kinetics, elimination is not linear and half-life is an inappropriate term. Half-life assumes concentration-independent elimination. Therefore, for phenytoin it is better to refer to the time required to eliminate 50% ($t_{50\%}$). The average $t_{50\%}$ is 22 hours but may range from 7 to 42 hours. As half-life is an inappropriate term, it cannot be used to determine when phenytoin may reach steady state. The time to reach 90% of steady state ($t_{90\%}$) may be as long as 50 days for a patient with a V_{max} of 425 mg/d and a low K_m of 1 μg/mL and as short as 8 days for a patient with a V_{max} of 700 mg/d and a K_m of 12 μg/mL. The unknown time to steady state should be considered whenever dosage adjustments are made.[146]

Special Populations. Age may affect the metabolism of phenytoin.[153] Premature and term newborn infants may not have a mature hydroxylation enzyme system. Therefore, clearance may be reduced in this population. Children have higher clearances of phenytoin and usually require larger doses and more frequent dosing intervals than adults. The elderly may have a lower clearance. The Michaelis–Menten kinetics of phenytoin make it difficult to evaluate metabolism across age groups.[146,149]

The protein binding of phenytoin may be altered by a number of mechanisms. Patients with chronic renal failure may have hypoalbuminemia, which would reduce phenytoin binding. In addition, patients with chronic renal failure retain some high-molecular-weight molecule that is capable of displacing phenytoin from its binding sites on albumin. The very young, the elderly, and patients with liver disease may have low albumins and decreased protein binding of phenytoin. Burn patients may also have decreased phenytoin binding because of lost fluids and low albumin.[146,149]

The clearance of phenytoin increases in the third trimester of pregnancy. Clearance returns to normal postpartum.[154]

The clearance of phenytoin is not altered by hemo- or peritoneal dialysis. Plasmapheresis removes clinically insignificant amounts of phenytoin.[155]

Pharmacodynamics

Therapeutic Endpoints. The desired therapeutic endpoint for phenytoin therapy is the suppression of seizures. Phenytoin has been used in partial seizures and in generalized seizures with the exception of absence. It is a first-line agent in the treatment of generalized tonic–clonic status epilepticus.[144] Recently, its prophylactic use for head trauma-induced seizures has been questioned. In a prospective controlled trial phenytoin was effective in preventing seizures for 7 days following head trauma, but was no different than placebo in preventing late seizures.[19] The suppression of seizures must be balanced against the phenytoin-induced side effects.

Adverse Reactions. Phenytoin may cause acute and chronic side effects. The most often described acute toxic effect is a disturbance of the vestibuloocular system. This is generally considered to be concentration related, with nystagmus occurring at concentrations greater than 20 μg/mL, ataxia occurring at concentrations greater than 30 μg/mL, and lethargy occurring at concentrations greater than 40 μg/mL. This relationship should not be relied on exclusively. Many patients will have these side effects at lesser concentrations and many will not demonstrate them at higher concentrations. Also, some patients may develop ataxia or lethargy without having other symptoms. Other symptoms of acute toxicity include involuntary movements, exacerbation of seizures, and severe mental depression manifested by delirium, psychosis, encephalopathy, or coma.[156]

It is difficult to determine if the chronic side effects associated with phenytoin are concentration or duration dependent.[156] The cognitive and behavioral side effects appear to be more pronounced at higher concentrations. The severity of gingival hyperplasia, which is the most frequently encountered chronic side effect, ranges from mildly disfiguring to requiring oral surgery.[157] Patients should be encouraged to practice good oral hygiene, which may minimize the gum hypertrophy.[158] Phenytoin may cause other cosmetic side effects, including hirsutism and coarsening of facial features. Phenytoin decreases folic acid, which may result in a megaloblastic anemia.[159] Phenytoin also decreases vitamin D, which may result in osteomalacia. Chronic administration of phenytoin has been associated with cardiac arrhythmias, peripheral neuropathy, carbohydrate intolerance, decreased concentrations of total thyroxine and free thyroxine, interference with pituitary–adrenal function, and immunologic disturbances. Idiosyncratic reactions associated with phenytoin include skin rashes, Stevens–Johnson syndrome, pseudolymphoma, bone marrow suppression, lupuslike reactions, and hepatitis. Phenytoin has been reported to cause teratogenicity.[160] The incidence of "fetal hydantoin syndrome" versus the malformations that occur in epileptic mothers without antiepileptic drugs has not been determined.[161]

Drug–Drug Interactions. Phenytoin is highly protein bound and is metabolized by enzymes that are subject to induction and inhibition. Also, phenytoin is an enzyme inducer. Therefore, phenytoin is associated with numerous drug–drug interactions. Because phenytoin has a very narrow therapeutic range, these interactions are usually clinically significant.[162,163]

In addition to the numerous drug–drug interactions, phenytoin may also interact with nutritional factors. Although the mechanism is undefined, the administration of continuous enteral nutrient tube feedings is reported to decrease the absorption of phenytoin.[164] Whereas phenytoin decreases folic acid concentrations, the supplementation of folic acid increases the clearance of phenytoin and may induce breakthrough seizures.[165]

Influenza vaccine has been reported to increase the clearance of phenytoin.[166]

Disease–Drug Interactions. As previously discussed patients with chronic renal failure have a decreased protein binding of phenytoin and an increased free fraction.[67] Other diseases that reduce albumin, such as liver disease, burns, and protein malnutrition, will alter protein binding. Fever has resulted in a decrease in phenytoin concentrations, presumably because of enzyme induction.[168] Patients with head trauma may have a more rapid clearance of phenytoin for the first 7 to 14 days after the trauma.[169]

Therapeutic Regimen Design

Initial Dose. In acute situations such as status epilepticus a loading dose of 18 to 20 mg/kg phenytoin may be given by intravenous infusion.[170] Because phenytoin contains propylene glycol as a solvent, the rate of infusion should not exceed 50 mg/min and should be slower for geriatric patients. The phenytoin should be mixed with normal saline to a concentration of 10 mg/mL or less. The admixture may be infused through a 0.22-nm millimicron inline filter. The tubing should be flushed before and after the phenytoin infusion.[1]

Oral loading doses may also be given in less critical situations. Because of the saturation of absorption, divided doses seem to be better absorbed and better tolerated. Although loading doses of 1000 mg have been cited, a mg/kg load is more appropriate. The total dose is divided and given at 2- to 6-hour intervals until the load is completed.

Serum concentrations should be drawn to confirm the adequacy of the loading dose.

Maintenance Dose. Because phenytoin displays Michaelis–Menten kinetics, the maintenance dose must be individualized. The standard practice of giving patients 300 mg/d will result in subtherapeutic or toxic levels in many patients. Following a loading dose patients may be started on 5 to 6 mg/kg/d. Concentrations should be measured after 4 to 7 days to ensure that appropriate concentrations are being achieved. Dosage adjustments must be made cautiously because of the indeterminate amount of time it may take to attain steady state or $t_{90\%}$ and because the concentration at which metabolism saturates cannot be prospectively predicted. General ranges of maintenance doses are for adults, 3 to 7 mg/kg/d; for children, 5 to 15 mg/kg/d; and for neonates, 3 to 5 mg/kg/d. The 30-mg capsule, 50-mg tablet, and 100-mg capsule can all be used to individualize the dosing of phenytoin (see Dosage Prediction and Adjustment). The adequacy of the maintenance dose should be confirmed with serum concentration monitoring.[171]

Dosing Interval. It is usually desirable to dose the antiepileptic drugs based on their pharmacokinetic half-life, but half-life is an inappropriate term when applied to phenytoin. Many adult patients will have a $t_{50\%}$ of about 22 hours. This allows once-a-day dosing in these patients. Neonates and children have faster clearances and may require more frequent dosing.

The absorption of phenytoin may saturate. Therefore, larger doses may be less well absorbed if given as a single dose. It is recommended that larger doses be divided to facilitate absorption.[146]

Dosage Prediction and Adjustment. The nonlinear Michaelis–Menten kinetics of phenytoin make dosage prediction very difficult; however, because of the protracted time it can take to achieve $t_{90\%}$, it would be clinically desirable to be able to predict phenytoin dosing. Several methods have been proposed for predicting phenytoin dosing. All of these methods have inherent problems that require clinical judgment for appropriate use.[172] None of these methods replaces careful patient monitoring.

In reviewing the Michaelis–Menten equation, $D = (V_{max} \times C_p)/(K_m + C_p)$, one could calculate a new dose for a desired concentration, for example, 15 µg/mL, if one knew both V_{max} and K_m; however both of these values are unknown at the time of dosage initiation. An estimate of drug dosing can be made by assigning a value to either V_{max} or K_m and using the dose and serum concentration achieved at the first steady state to calculate the other Michaelis–Menten parameter. K_m is assumed to have the least variability and an average value of 4 µg/mL can be assigned. After the V_{max} is calculated, the equation could be solved for the desired concentration. Nomograms have been developed to obviate the need for mathematical calculations. The obvious limitation to this technique is that K_m fluctuates widely and the dose calculated may be more or less than the real dose. This method is not useful in acute care situations because a steady-state concentration is needed.

Nomograms requiring two different steady-state concentrations that result from two different doses have been developed. These nomograms are more accurate because they allow for the calculation of both V_{max} and K_m. Their use is limited because of the requirement for steady-state concentrations with two different doses.[173] An example is shown in Figure 2–5.

A population clearance method has been described by Graves et al.[174] This method requires one steady-state concentration with one dose. This method uses the equation

$$D_n = (D_o/SC_o) \times SC_d^{0.199} \times SC_o^{0.804}$$

where D_n = new dose, D_o = original dose, SC_o = original steady-state concentration, and SC_d = desired steady-state concentration. This method has been shown to be more reliable than the one-point nomograms or methods that fix V_{max} or K_m. It is particularly useful in an ambulatory setting. It is limited by the need to have a steady-state concentration.[175]

Bayesian forecasting has the greatest potential for predicting phenytoin dosing in an acute situation. This method can use concentrations after the first dose and before steady state is achieved; however, sophisticated computer support is required.

An empiric method of dosing phenytoin is to give a loading dose and obtain a trough concentration 24 hours before the first maintenance dose. The patient is started on 5 mg/kg/d and the concentration determined after 5 days. An adjustment is made depending on the trend of the concentration. A recently published guideline suggests that if the phenytoin is less than 7 µg/mL, the dose can safely be increased by not more than 100 mg/d; if the phenytoin concentration is between 7 and 12 µg/mL, the dose should not be increased by more than 50 mg/d; and if the phenytoin concentration is greater than 12 µg/mL, the dose should not be increased by more than 30 mg/d.[176] Phenytoin is available in dosage strengths that allow this type of individualized patient dosing.

Any method of predicting or adjusting phenytoin should be accompanied by careful patient monitoring for side effects, efficacy, and serum concentration.[171]

Blood Sampling for Phenytoin. Because of the intervariability in Michaelis–Menten kinetics, the narrow therapeutic range, and the potential for a myriad of drug interactions, it is essential that the serum concentration of the total and, in selected patients, the free fraction be monitored. The efficacy of a loading dose should be assessed after 24 hours to ensure the adequacy of the load and the necessity for another loading dose prior to maintenance therapy. In the hospital setting there is no need for daily phenytoin concentrations, however. The effect of a change in dose will not be seen for a prolonged period. Concentration determination every 2 to 5 days should be adequate unless the patient is continuing to seize or has side effects.

In the ambulatory setting concentrations can be monitored 7 days after a dosage change and then every 2 to 4 weeks until steady state is confirmed. The patient should be instructed to call the clinician if he or she experiences nystagmus, ataxia, or lethargy. The possibility of a protracted time to reach steady state should be remembered.

For patients with normal albumin, no other diseases, and no other drugs, monitoring the total serum concentration should be adequate; however, the free fraction should be measured if patients have side effects with concentrations in the "therapeutic range." For patients with chronic renal failure, liver disease, low albumin, and drugs highly bound to albumin, the free fraction may be a better guide to therapy than the total concentration. Equations to predict free levels have not resulted in uniformly accurate predictions.[176]

There is no indication that there is a difference between the serum and plasma concentrations. The wax matrix in Tiger Top or Speckled Top serum collection containers has been shown to bind free drug. Although the binding is not necessarily clinically significant, it may be significant for pharmacokinetic or drug interaction studies.[177]

Therapeutic Range. The therapeutic range for phenytoin is defined as 10 to 20 μg/mL for total drug concentration. Although the incidence of side effects increases at concentrations above 20 μg/mL, many patients will tolerate higher concentrations without visible side effects. Also, some patients may have an adequate response at concentrations below 10 μg/mL. Patients with very low concentrations, for example, less than 5 μg/mL, should have the need for continued therapy reevaluated.

Because phenytoin is about 90% protein bound, the free fraction is about 10%. Therefore, the therapeutic range of the free fraction is 1 to 2 μg/mL.[171]

Dosage Forms. Phenytoin is available as a chewable tablet (50 mg), capsules (30 and 100 mg), suspension (30 mg/5 mL and 125 mg/5 mL), and parenteral formulation (50 mg/mL). Phenytoin is also available in a fixed combination with phenobarbital (100 mg of phenytoin with 16 or 32 mg of phenobarbital). Phenytoin chewable tablets and suspension are composed of phenytoin acid, whereas phenytoin capsules and phenytoin parenteral are composed of phenytoin sodium. The phenytoin sodium is 92% phenytoin acid. For patients at the Michaelis–Menten saturation point this difference could be clinically important. Therefore, when formulations are changed, the difference in salt form should be considered.[146] The prompt-release and the extended-release capsules are not interchangeable.[178] Phenytoin suspension will settle, resulting in a difference in concentration between the top and bottom of the bottle. If the suspension is not resuspended, this can result in variable doses being given. A recent study demonstrated that phenytoin resuspends readily with minimal shaking and stays in suspension for periods of up to five weeks. When the suspension is used, it should be shaken well and a calibrated measuring device used to measure the dose.[179]

A prodrug formulation of phenytoin has been developed by adding a phosphate group to the phenytoin structure. When the prodrug reaches the systemic circulation, the phosphate group is rapidly cleaved off, leaving phenytoin. Addition of the phosphate group results in enhanced solubility in water, negating the need for propylene glycol as a solvent.[180] Preliminary data indicate that there is less pain associated with the intramuscular use of the prodrug and that the prodrug may be given by rapid intravenous infusion.

Ethosuximide

Clinical Pharmacology and Therapeutics
Ethosuximide is a highly specific antiepileptic drug. It is very effective in reducing the frequency of absence seizures but is not effective in suppressing other types of generalized seizures or in suppressing either simple or complex partial seizures. It is believed that ethosuximide exerts its

antiepileptic effect by either a direct modification of membrane function in excitable cells or an alteration of chemically mediated neurotransmission, or both.[181]

Ethosuximide is indicated only for the prevention of absence seizures, which are seen primarily in children. An adult with a diagnosis of absence seizures should be carefully evaluated by EEG to differentiate absence from simple or complex partial seizures. Therefore, the use of ethosuximide in adults should be questioned. Consequently, most of the data concerning ethosuximide are derived from studies in children or from healthy adult volunteers.[182]

Clinical Pharmacokinetics

The pharmacokinetics of ethosuximide are poorly understood despite the fact that ethosuximide is an old antiepileptic drug and there is a sensitive and specific assay for the drug. Ethosuximide has been described as following a one-compartment model with first-order input.[183]

Absorption. In humans ethosuximide is rapidly absorbed and peak concentrations are achieved in 3 to 7 hours. The time to peak concentration is somewhat faster with a single dose than after repeated dosing.

The lack of an intravenous dosage form for humans prevents the determination of absolute bioavailability in humans. In monkeys, absolute bioavailability was 93 to 97.5%, and in dogs, oral bioavailability was 88 to 95%. The bioavailability of ethosuximide in humans is assumed to be complete. Although the syrup and capsule are equal in bioavailability, absorption is faster from the syrup.[183]

Distribution. Ethosuximide does not bind to plasma proteins. A cerebrospinal fluid-to-plasma-to-saliva ratio of 1.0 indicates that most of the drug in the plasma is in the unbound form. Ethosuximide is uniformly distributed throughout the body except for body fat. Ethosuximide does not distribute into body fat. Thus, the apparent volume of distribution of ethosuximide is approximately 70% of body weight, which is equivalent to that of total body water. The apparent volume of distribution V_d is 0.69 L/kg in children less than 10 years of age and 0.62 to 0.67 L/kg in adults. Ethosuximide crosses the placenta and passes into breast milk, achieving concentrations similar to the concentration in the mother's plasma.[183]

Metabolism and Elimination. Ethosuximide is poorly extracted by the liver and therefore does not undergo first-pass metabolism. Ethosuximide is first hydroxylated and then conjugated to inactive metabolites before being excreted into the urine.[184] The apparent clearance of ethosuximide in normal adults has been estimated at 10 ± 4 mL/h/kg, which is less than hepatic blood flow and demonstrates that the elimination of ethosuximide is not flow dependent. The half-life of ethosuximide is shorter in children than adults. The half-life in children has been reported to be 30 hours versus 60 hours in adults. Data in neonates are derived from case reports and indicate that the half-life in neonates is between 32 and 41 hours. The total body clearance of ethosuximide is reported to be 16 mL/h/kg in children and 10 to 13 mL/h/kg in adults. The half-life of ethosuximide has been reported to be unaffected by dose size and to be constant with repeated dosing; however, a 15% decrease in total body clearance that was attributed to a decrease in the nonrenal clearance has also been described.[182] Two studies have suggested that ethosuximide may display nonlinear kinetics at the upper end of the therapeutic range. Smith et al reported that in individual patients, successive dose increments of equal size produced disproportionately greater increases in steady-state concentrations.[185] An evaluation by Bauer et al indicated that 7 of 10 patients demonstrated evidence of nonlinearity.[186] Therefore, there may be significant variability in the dose and steady-state concentration relationship of ethosuximide, especially at the upper end of the therapeutic range. The asymmetric center in ethosuximide is quartenary, making racemization unlikely.[187] There does not appear to be any stereoselectivity in the metabolism of ethosuximide. The measurement of total ethosuximide is adequate for therapeutic monitoring.[2]

Special Populations. Younger patients seem to require larger doses of ethosuximide to achieve similar serum concentrations.[188] Smith et al indicated that females achieve a higher serum concentration from a given dose than do males.[185] The serum concentration of ethosuximide has been reported to increase postpartum.[189] Ethosuximide is significantly removed by hemodialysis and patients on hemodialysis may need supplemental doses of ethosuximide.[190] Based on the known pharmacokinetics of ethosuximide, one could postulate that the dose of ethosuximide should be reduced in patients with liver disease and possibly should be reduced in patients with chronic renal failure. There are, however, no studies to document these postulates.[183]

Pharmacodynamics

Therapeutic Endpoints. The desired therapeutic endpoint for ethosuximide is the abolition of absence seizures. In some cases this may require EEG monitoring to evaluate. Ethosuximide is indicated only for the treatment of absence seizures and may exacerbate other seizure types. Ethosuximide is very effective as monotherapy for absence seizures. In refractory patients, the combination of ethosuximide and valproic acid may be more effective than either drug alone.[181]

Adverse Reactions. Patients should also be monitored for ethosuximide side effects. The most frequent side effects of ethosuximide are nausea and vomiting, which may be related to the size of the dose. Other side effects that may be concentration related are abdominal discomfort, anorexia, drowsiness, fatigue, lethargy, dizziness, hiccups, and headache. Headaches may persist after a dosage reduction. The behavioral and cognitive side effects of ethosuximide have not been well documented. Rare side effects associated with ethosuximide include skin rashes, systemic lupus erythematosus, blood dyscrasias, and changes in liver function tests.[191]

Drug–Drug Interactions. Reports of drug interactions with ethosuximide are rare and often poorly documented. The ratio of ethosuximide serum concentrations to dose was significantly higher when ethosuximide was given alone than when it was given with carbamazepine, primidone, or valproic acid.[188] Other studies have reported an increase in ethosuximide concentrations when given with valproic acid.[192,193] The interaction with valproic acid may be complex and may require the presence of other concurrent antiepileptic drugs or high concentrations of valproic acid.[194] Isoniazid has been reported to increase ethosuximide concentrations,[195] and ethosuximide has been reported to increase the concentration of phenytoin in single case reports.[196]

Disease–Drug Interactions. Patients on hemodialysis lose about 50% of their ethosuximide stores in a 6-hour dialysis. Therefore, they require increased monitoring pre- and postdialysis and may require supplemental dosing.[190]

Patients with impaired liver and renal function may require lower doses.

Therapeutic Regimen Design

Initial Dose. Absence seizures are not life threatening and therefore a loading dose of ethosuximide is not indicated. As with most antiepileptic drugs, it is better to initiate therapy with a low dose and titrate the dose upward until a desired therapeutic dose is achieved or intolerable side effects occur.[181] The data from Chang indicate that there is a significant difference in the dose–concentration relationship between children 3 to 10 years of age and children older than 11 years of age.[183] Battino et al had similar results.[188] This is at variance with the data from Smith et al, who did not find a significant difference in the ethosuximide concentration-versus-dose relationship between patients under 10 years of age and those over 15 years of age.[185] An initial dose of 20 mg/kg/d in children less than 11 years old will result in a mean plasma concentration of 50 μg/mL. In older patients an initial dose of 15 mg/kg/d will result in a similar mean concentration.[2]

Maintenance Dose. The dose of ethosuximide may be increased until the desired serum concentration is achieved. The generally accepted maximum dose is 30 mg/kg/d in adults and 40 mg/kg/d in children; however, the resulting serum concentration and response versus tolerance should be the ultimate determinants of maximum dose.[182]

Dosing Interval. Based on the half-life of ethosuximide, the dose could be given once a day.[197] This regimen has been used successfully. In some patients, however, the incidence of gastrointestinal side effects increases with the dose. Therefore, the dose may need to be given twice a day to minimize the gastrointestinal side effects.[191]

Dosage Prediction and Adjustment. The attempts to predict doses of ethosuximide based on previous serum concentrations or the serum concentration that will result from a given increase in dose of ethosuximide have universally been unsuccessful. Therefore, dosage adjustment of ethosuximide must be done by titration and clinical monitoring. At the low end of the dosing range, a first-order process may be assumed. A time to steady state of 6 days in children and 12 days in adults can be assumed and used to plan changes in doses and monitoring of serum concentrations. Doses at the upper end of the therapeutic range should be adjusted more cautiously because of the possible nonlinear kinetics.[182]

Blood Sampling for Ethosuximide Concentration. The indications for monitoring ethosuximide concentrations include a poor response to therapy, questionable compliance, low doses, and maintenance of optimal concentrations.

Ethosuximide has a long half-life. This should be taken into consideration in determining when to collect blood samples after the initial dose and after a dosage change. The initial sample or the sample after a change in dose should not be drawn for at least 6 days in children and

12 days in adults, which would allow the patient to reach steady state. Samples may be drawn earlier if the patient is experiencing unexpected side effects.[182]

The long half-life of ethosuximide would suggest minimal changes in the peak-to-trough ratio; however, trough concentrations are recommended. The trough concentration would be more important if the patient were on a once-a-day regimen.[181]

There is no indication that serum concentrations are different than plasma concentrations.

Because of the negligible protein binding of ethosuximide, there is no indication for determining unbound ethosuximide. The evaluation of ethosuximide in saliva or in tears is predictive of serum concentration and may be used in some patients if intravenous sampling is not possible.[182]

Once the desired therapeutic response has been achieved, serum samples can be monitored every 4 to 6 months. A change in response or the onset of unusual side effects indicates a need to monitor serum concentrations.

Therapeutic Range. The therapeutic range of ethosuximide is described as 40 to 100 μg/mL. Within this range 80% of patients achieve partial control and 60% become seizure free. In a small number of patients concentrations up to 150 μg/mL may be needed to achieve complete seizure control.[181]

Dosage Forms. Ethosuximide is available as a 250-mg capsule and as an oral solution that contains 250 mg of ethosuximide per 5 mL. There is no parenteral form of ethosuximide available for human use.

INVESTIGATIONAL ANTIEPILEPTIC DRUGS

The last major antiepileptic drug approved by the FDA was valproic acid in 1978. To rectify this the Epilepsy Branch of the National Institute of Neuromuscular Disorders and Stroke collaborated with the pharmaceutical industry and clinicians to screen and clinically test new compounds for possible efficacy as antiepileptic drugs.[198] This effort has resulted in three drugs that have been approved or are in the final stages of approval by the FDA. These drugs are felbamate, gabapentin, and lamotrigine. These drugs have all demonstrated efficacy in patients who have been refractory to or unable to tolerate available antiepileptic drugs. Several more drugs may be submitted for New Drug Applications soon.[199]

Felbamate (Approved 1993)

Clinical Pharmacology and Therapeutics

Felbamate is structurally related to meprobamate; however, it has been shown not to have the tolerance and dependency that have been associated with meprobamate. In preclinical tests it had a broader spectrum of antiepileptic activity than phenytoin or carbamazepine.[200] Felbamate appears to act as an antagonist of the glycine receptor site on the N-methyl-D-aspartate (NMDA) receptor. This action inhibits the initiation and propagation of seizures. Felbamate increases seizure threshold and prevents seizure spread.[201] The clinical trials with felbamate have used innovative designs that include active controls, patients who have been removed from all antiepileptic drugs for evaluation of seizure surgery, and patients with Lennox–Gastaut syndrome.[202,203] Felbamate has been approved for use in adults 14 years and older as monotherapy and adjunctive therapy in partial seizures with and without secondary generalization and for children 2 years and older as adjunctive therapy for the Lennox–Gastaut syndrome.[204] The drug is recommended for patients not responding satisfactorily to other antiepileptics.

Clinical Pharmacokinetics

Absorption. Felbamate is rapidly and well absorbed orally with a T_{max} of 1 to 4 hours and an apparent oral bioavailability exceeding 90%. The absorption is unaffected by food or antacids.[205]

Distribution. There is negligible protein binding (20–25%) with felbamate. The binding is dependent on the concentration of albumin. Felbamate has a volume of distribution of 0.7 L/kg.[205]

Metabolism and Elimination. Felbamate is metabolized to three inactive metabolites and has a half life of 14 to 20 hours in healthy volunteers. The half-life is shorter in patients comedicated with other antiepileptic drugs which may induce its metabolism.[205] About 40 to 50% of the drug is eliminated unchanged in the urine.[206] Felbamate displays linear pharmacokinetics and the concentrations are dose proportional.

Special Populations. The effects of age, gender, pregnancy, renal failure, and hepatic impairment on the pharmacokinetics of felbamate have not been reported.

Pharmacodynamics

Therapeutic Endpoints. No therapeutic range has been established.[207] Felbamate is dosed to patient response using seizure frequency and side effects as therapeutic endpoints.

Adverse Reactions. Felbamate has been well tolerated in clinical trials. Postmarketing surveillance, however, has recommended restricting the drug to patients refractory to other antiepileptics. The two most serious adverse reactions observed during postmarketing surveillance have been aplastic anemia and liver failure. There has been no evidence of tolerance or physical dependence. The reported central nervous system side effects (diplopia, dizziness, blurred vision, headache, ataxia) may have been related to interactions with concurrent antiepileptic drugs. Other side effects include gastrointestinal distress, nausea, vomiting, anorexia, weight loss, and insomnia. Side effects have been more common in polytherapy.[207] The dose of concurrent antiepileptic drugs should be reduced when felbamate is initiated to reduce the incidence of side effects.

Drug–Drug Interactions. Felbamate has been shown to inhibit the clearance of phenytoin, valproic acid, and the 10,11 diepoxide metabolite of carbamazepine.[208–210] The dose of these drugs should be reduced by about 30% when felbamate is initiated. The drug interactions with felbamate are dose proportional and the clinician should reduce the dose of concurrent antiepileptic drugs each time the dose of felbamate is increased. Interactions other than phenytoin, carbamazepine, and valproic acid have not been studied.

Therapeutic Regimen Design

Initial Dose. If felbamate is used as monotherapy, the dose is initiated at 1200 mg/d (15 mg/kg in children).[204]

Maintenance Dose. Felbamate is increased by 600 mg every 2 weeks up to a maximum dose of 3600 mg (45 mg/kg in children). When felbamate is used in combination with other antiepileptic drugs, the dose of the concurrent antiepileptic drug should be reduced by 30 to 50% at the initiation of felbamate, and further reductions should occur as the dose is increased. Doses higher than 3600 mg have been tolerated in clinical trials.[204]

Dosing Interval. Felbamate is dosed three times a day.[204]

Dosage Prediction and Adjustment. The dose of felbamate is based on clinical response.

Blood Sampling for Felbamate. At this time no therapeutic range has been defined for felbamate and routine blood sampling is not recommended.[204]

Dosage Forms. Felbamate is available as 400- and 600-mg tablets and as a 600 mg/5 mL suspension.[204]

Gabapentin (Approved 1993)

Clinical Pharmacology and Therapeutics

Gabapentin is a structural analog of GABA and was synthesized as a GABA agonist; however, it does not interact with $GABA_A$ or $GABA_B$ and has no direct GABA-mimetic action or no effect on GABA metabolism and causes no increase in GABA concentrations. Although its mechanism of action is independent of GABA, its spectrum of antiepileptic activity is similar to those of other GABA-mimetic drugs.[211,212] Gabapentin appears to bind to a systemic amino acid carrier protein.[213] Gabapentin is approved for adjunctive therapy for partial seizures with or without secondary generalization in adults with epilepsy.[214]

Clinical Pharmacokinetics

Absorption. Gabapentin is absorbed by an active process and the bioavailability decreases with an increase in dose. The bioavailability of a 400-mg dose is about 25% less than that of a 100-mg dose. The bioavailability of doses that are likely to be used clinically (300–600 mg) is about 60%. Gabapentin is rapidly absorbed, with a T_{max} between 2 and 4 hours. The absorption of gabapentin is unaffected by food.[215]

Distribution. Gabapentin appears to follow a three-compartment model. There is no protein binding of the drug and it has a volume of distribution of 50 L/kg.[215]

Metabolism and Elimination. There is no metabolism of gabapentin. About 77% of a given dose is excreted unchanged in the urine, with the rest being excreted in the feces. The renal clearance of gabapentin equals the total drug clearance. The half life is about 5.3 hours.[215]

Special Populations. Gabapentin is eliminated exclusively by renal elimination and dosage adjustments will be necessary in patients with significantly impaired renal function.[215] For patients with a creatinine clearance greater than 60 mL/min the dose is 1200 mg/d, for patients with a creatinine clearance between 30 and 60 mL/min the dose is 600 mg/d, for patients with a creatinine clearance of 15 to 30 mL/min the dose is 300 mg/d, and for patients with a creatinine less than 15 mL/min the dose is 150 mg per day (300 mg every other day).[214] The Cockroft and Gault equation may be used to estimate creatinine clearance in the elderly and in patients with chronic renal failure.

The pharmacokinetics of gabapentin in the elderly, children less than 12 years of age, and pregnant females have not been reported. No dosage alteration in patients with hepatic impairment would be anticipated based on the renal elimination.

Pharmacodynamics

Therapeutic Endpoints. The dose of gabapentin is adjusted based on clinical response and side effects. A therapeutic range has not been defined.[216–218]

Adverse Reactions. Central nervous system side effects are the most frequently reported side effects with gabapentin. Fatigue, somnolence, dizziness, and ataxia are the most frequently reported side effects. Other side effects reported more frequently than placebo-induced effects include nystagmus, tremor, and diplopia. The central nervous system effects of gabapentin are less than or equal to those of traditional antiepileptic drugs.[216–218]

Drug–Drug Interactions. There have been no reported drug interactions. Based on the lack of liver metabolism and protein binding, drug interactions are not anticipated. It is possible that drugs could compete for renal elimination.

Disease–Drug Interactions. The dose of gabapentin should be reduced in patients with renal impairment.[214]

Therapeutic Regimen Design

Initial Dose. The dosing of gabapentin is initiated at 300 mg at bedtime on the first day. The dose is increased to 300 mg twice a day on the second day and 300 mg three times a day on the third day.[214]

Maintenance Dose. The dose is then titrated as needed up to 1800 mg per day. Doses up to 2400 or 3600 mg per day have been used safely.[218]

Dosing Interval. Gabapentin is dosed three times a day. The package insert indicates that the dosing interval should not exceed 12 hours, except in patients with significant renal impairment.[214]

Dosage Prediction and Adjustment. Doses of gabapentin are adjusted based on clinical response.

Blood Sampling. At this time no therapeutic range has been defined for gabapentin and routine blood sampling is not recommended.

Dosage Forms. Gabapentin is available as 100-, 300-, and 400-mg capsules.[214]

Lamotrigine (Approved 1994)

Clinical Pharmacology and Therapeutics
Lamotrigine is structurally related to antifolate drugs. It was developed for its antifolate activity but has been found to have only weak antifolate activity.[219] It is believed to inhibit the release of glutamate and aspartate and possibly to interact with the sodium channel. The drug is being studied primarily in patients with partial seizures.[220]

Clinical Pharmacokinetics

Absorption. The drug is rapidly and well absorbed, reaching peaks in 1 to 3 hours. It follows a one-compartment model and has first-order absorption and elimination. The drug is linear and dose proportional.[221]

Distribution. The drug is about 55% protein bound and has a volume of distribution of about 1.1 L/kg.[221]

Metabolism and Elimination. About 70% of a dose of lamotrigine is metabolized in the liver by glucuronide conjugation. The glucuronide conjugate accounts for about 90% of the total drug recovery. Less than 1% of the drug is excreted renally. The half-life of lamotrigine is about 20 to 24 hours in drug-naive subjects. The half-life is about 14.3 hours in patients receiving enzyme-inducing drugs concurrently and about 24 hours in drug-naive patients.[222] The half-life is prolonged in patients taking valproic acid. There is no first-pass metabolism and there is no evidence of saturable pharmacokinetics.[223] One report suggests that there may be some autoinduction.[224] There is considerable intersubject variability in pharmacokinetics but very little intrasubject variability in the elimination of lamotrigine. The metabolism may be moderately reduced in Gilbert's syndrome.[225]

Special Populations. The pharmacokinetics in special populations have not been reported.

Pharmacodynamics

Therapeutic Endpoints. The dose of lamotrigine is adjusted based on clinical response and side effects. A therapeutic range has not been defined.

Adverse Reactions. The drug has a wide margin of safety and a low potential for toxicity.[225] The primary side effects of lamotrigine involve the central nervous system. Diplopia, drowsiness, ataxia, and headache are the most frequently reported side effects.[226] Lamotrigine may cause several types of skin rash. Some of these rashes may necessitate the withdrawal of lamotrigine. The incidence of skin rash appears to be increased in patients who are also receiving valproic acid.

Drug–Drug Interactions. Phenytoin and carbamazepine decrease the half-life of lamotrigine.[223] Valproic acid causes a dramatic increase in the half-life of lamotrigine. Lamotrigine does not interfere with the clearance of phenytoin or carbamazepine.

Therapeutic Regimen Design

Initial Dose. In patients who are taking enzyme-inducing drugs, lamotrigine should be started at a dose of 100 mg/d, and in patients taking valproic acid and enzyme inhibitors, the dose should be started at 50 mg/d.

Maintenance Dose. In patients taking enzyme-inducing drugs lamotrigine should be increased by 100 mg/d per week up to a total dose of 500 mg/d, and in patients taking valproic acid and enzyme inhibitors, the dose should be increased by 50 mg/d every 2 weeks.

Dosing Interval. Lamotrigine is dosed every 12 hours.

Dosing Prediction and Adjustment. Doses of lamotrigine are adjusted based on clinical response.

Blood Sampling. At this time there is no defined therapeutic range for lamotrigine and routine concentration monitoring is not recommended.

Dosage Forms. The dose will be between 50 and 300 mg/d.[224] Availability of dosage terms is expected to be 100-, 150-, and 200-mg scored tablets.

ANTIEPILEPTICS UNDERGOING PHASE III TRIALS

Vigabatrin

Vigabatrin is a synthetic derivative of GABA. It inactivates GABA-T which is the enzyme that metabolizes GABA. Thus, vigabatrin prevents the breakdown of GABA and increases the functional pool of GABA. Vigabatrin substitutes for a natural substrate and thus demonstrates stereospecificity. There is a lag time between the administration of vigabatrin and the onset of effect. There is also a persistence of effect for about 6 days after the drug is removed.[227] Vigabatrin is being studied primarily in patients with partial epilepsy.[228,229]

The drug reaches maximal concentration in 1 to 2 hours. It has a half-life of 4.2 to 5.6 hours; the half-life may be prolonged in the elderly. There is zero protein binding and the volume of distribution is 0.8 L/kg, which may be larger in children. Vigabatrin is linear over doses currently being used. Renal elimination accounts for about 70% of the elimination.[230] Vigabatrin may interact with phenytoin and carbamazepine but the interaction may not be seen for 4 to 6 weeks. The drug is given in doses of 1000 to 3000 mg/d. It is dosed twice a day because of its pharmacodynamic effects.[231]

Clinical trials with vigabatrin were stopped several years ago because of the reports of "intramyelinic edema," or vacuoles in the brains of animals in preclinical trials. This has never been shown in humans who seem to tolerate the drug well and clinical trials have resumed. The side effects reported with initial administration of vigabatrin include drowsiness, fatigue, dizziness, and behavioral changes. Side effects seen with chronic dosing are drowsiness, ataxia, and weight gain.[232]

Flunarizine

Flunarizine is a calcium channel blocker that has been widely used in Europe for the treatment of migraine headaches. It appears to reduce excessive transmembrane influx of calcium ions but does not appear to interfere with normal calcium ion exchange. The drug has a very long half-life and a very large volume of distribution, is highly protein bound, and displays significant intersubject variability. It is metabolized mainly by the liver, with minimal amounts being excreted unchanged in the urine. There is no evidence of drug interactions and it is generally well tolerated. The most common side effects are altered central nervous system functioning, weight gain, and extrapyramidal symptoms.[233]

CONCLUSIONS

Patients are therapeutic failures with the antiepileptic drugs because of inappropriate drug selection, inappropriate dose, poor compliance, and refractoriness. The applications of the principles discussed in this chapter will facilitate the selection, dosing, and monitoring of the antiepileptic drugs. Clinicians should continually work with patients to reinforce the appropriate use of the antiepileptic drugs. The new antiepileptic drugs that may soon be available may potentially offer seizure control for some patients who are not currently controlled or who are currently experiencing side effects with their antiepileptic drugs.

———— QUESTIONS ————

1. A patient is diagnosed as having complex partial epilepsy and is started on carbamazepine 100 mg tid (1-week interval). He has the following doses and plasma level responses:

Dose	CBZ Level (μg/mL)
100–100–100	2.4
100–100–200	3.1

200–100–200	4.8
200–200–200	6.2
200–200–200	4.0
200–200–200	3.1

Explain this patient's response. What would you recommend?

2. L.B. is an adult woman who weighs 65 kg. She is having two to three seizures per day for which carbamazepine is indicated. Knowing that the average apparent clearance of carbamazepine is 75 mL/h/kg in adults, the physician predicts a daily dosage of 700 mg for this woman to attain a steady-state concentration of 6 μg/mL. After 1 day of therapy at this daily dose, the patient complains of blurred vision, nausea, and dizziness. A blood sample is taken and reveals a carbamazepine plasma concentration of 10 μg/mL. How should this adverse reaction be handled?

3. R.D. is a 43-year-old man who continues to have seizures despite phenytoin doses of 600 mg each morning. He takes the drug orally and is very compliant. He is on no other medicine. His neurologic examination was normal and there are no signs of drug toxicity. The steady-state phenytoin trough level is 13 μg/mL. The phenytoin dose was increased to 700 mg/d. On this dose the patient stopped having seizures but after 3 weeks he was found to have a lateral gaze nystagmus. The serum phenytoin concentration was found to be 26 μg/mL. What would you recommend for this patient?

4. A 31-year-old epileptic woman has been well controlled on 300 mg of phenytoin per day for more than 3 years. Her serum concentration has been 15 μg/mL. During the third trimester of her pregnancy, however, she has been having frequent seizures. The serum concentration is reported to be 7 μg/mL. How would you manage this case?

5. A 12-year-old girl has been diagnosed as having primary generalized seizures. She is started on valproic acid 250 mg qid. She achieves an initial decrease in seizure frequency and has a serum concentration of 60 μg/mL; however, she complains of abdominal pain and gastrointestinal distress. What would you recommend in this case?

6. W.S. has been receiving valproic acid for 2 years for control of his generalized seizures. He has been controlled and without side effects, with a trough serum concentration of around 125 μg/mL. Following a recent sprained ankle, he began taking aspirin. His parents noticed that he had become lethargic. On neurologic examination he was found to have a tremor. His serum valproic acid concentration was 110 μg/mL. How would you assess this patient?

7. A.W. is a 10-year-old boy with partial seizures. He has been well stabilized on carbamazepine with good control of his seizures and no side effects. He has been seen every 3 months for the last year with serum concentrations of 8 μg/mL. His mother calls to complain of the sudden onset of lethargy and blurred vision. A history reveals

that the patient had developed an ear infection 7 days ago and that the pediatrician had started him on erythromycin. How do you assess this patient?

8. A 6-year-old girl has difficult-to-control generalized seizures. She is started on valproic acid. She is receiving 750 mg every 8 hours and achieves a trough concentration of only 35 μg/mL. What would you assess in this patient?

9. A 31-year-old woman patient who weighs 60 kg has been taking 300 mg of phenytoin per day for 2 months for primary generalized tonic–clonic seizures. She has had one seizure in the last 2 weeks and her phenytoin concentration is 8 μg/mL. Calculate a new dose for this patient.

10. C.G.S. is a 35-year-old man who has complex partial seizures that occasionally are secondarily generalized. He is taking 300 mg of carbamazepine four times a day but continues to have two or three complex partial seizures per month and a secondarily generalized tonic–clonic convulsion every 5 or 6 months. He developed gingival hyperplasia on phenytoin and was very tired on phenobarbital. It is decided that this patient may benefit from a trial of felbamate. How would you manage this patient?

REFERENCES

1. Garnett WR. Epilepsy. In: DiPiro JT, Talbert RL, Hayes PE, et al, eds. *Pharmacotherapy: A Pathophysiologic Approach.* Norwalk, CT: Appleton & Lange; 1993:879–903.
2. Shinnar S. Treatment decisions in childhood seizures. In: Dodson WE, Pellock JM, eds. *Pediatric Epilepsy.* New York: Demos; 1993:215–221.
3. Dreifuss FE. The epilepsies: Clinical implications of the international classification. *Epilepsia.* 1990;31(suppl. 3):S3–S10.
4. Manford M, Hart YM, Sander AS, et al. The National General Practice Study of Epilepsy: The syndromic classification of the International League Against Epilepsy applied to epilepsy in a general population. *Arch Neurol.* 1992;49:801–808.
5. Mattson RH, Cramer JA, Collins JF, et al. Comparison of carbamazepine, phenobarbital, phenytoin, and primidone in partial and secondarily generalized tonic–clonic seizures. *N Engl J Med.* 1985;313:145–151.
6. Mattson RH, Cramer JA, Collins JF, et al. A comparison of valproate with carbamazepine for the treatment of complex partial seizures and secondarily generalized tonic–clonic seizures in adults. *N Engl J Med.* 1992;327:765–771.
7. Mattson RH. Selection of drugs for the treatment of epilepsy. *Semin Neurol.* 1990;10:406–413.
8. Thompson AH, Brodie MJ. Pharmacokinetic optimization of anticonvulsant therapy. *Clin Pharmacokinet.* 1992;23:216–230.
9. Choonara IA, Rane A. Therapeutic drug monitoring of anticonvulsants: State of the art. *Clin Pharmacokinet.* 1990;18:318–328.
10. Pugh CB, Garnett WR. Current issues in the treatment of epilepsy. *Clin Pharm.* 1991;10:335–358.
11. Lenn NJ, Robertson M. Clinical utility of unbound antiepileptic drug blood levels in the management of epilepsy. *Neurology.* 1992; 42:988–990.

12. Garnett WR, Cloyd JC. Dosage form considerations in the treatment of pediatric epilepsy. In: Dodson WE, Pellock JM, eds. *Pediatric Epilepsy.* New York: Demos; 1993:241–252.
13. Eadie MJ. Formation of active metabolites of anticonvulsant drugs: A review of their pharmacokinetic and therapeutic significance. *Clin Pharmacokinet.* 1991;21:27–41.
14. Dodson WE. Pharmacokinetic principles of antiepileptic therapy. In: Dodson WE, Pellock JM, eds. *Pediatric Epilepsy.* New York: Demos; 1993:2231–2240.
15. Yerby Mark S. Teratogenicity of anticonvulsant medications. In: Dodson WE, Pellock JM, eds. *Pediatric Epilepsy.* New York: Demos; 1993:265–279.
16. Pellock JM. Efficacy and adverse effects of antiepileptic drugs. *Pediatr Clin North Amer.* 1989; 36:435–448.
17. Scheuer ML, Pedley TA. The evaluation and treatment of seizures. *N Engl J Med.* 1990;323:1468–1474.
18. Farwell JR, Lee YJ, Hirtz D, et al. Phenobarbital for febrile seizures–Effects on intelligence and on seizure recurrence. *N Engl J Med.* 1990;322:364–369.
19. Temkin NR, Dikmen SS, Wilensky AJ, et al. A randomized, double-blind study of phenytoin for the prevention of post-traumatic seizures. *N Engl J Med.* 1990;323:497–502.
20. Rogawshi, Porter RJ. Antiepileptic drugs: Pharmacological mechanisms and clinical efficacy with consideration of promising developmental stage compounds. *Pharmacol Rev.* 1990;42:223–286.
21. Loiseau P, Buche B. Carbamazepine—Clinical use. In: Levy R, Mattson B, Meldrum B, et al, eds. *Antiepileptic Drugs.* 3rd ed. New York: Raven Press; 1989:533–554.
22. Dodson WE. Carbamazepine and oxycarbamazepine. In: Dodson WE, Pellock JM, eds. *Pediatric Epilepsy.* New York: Demos; 1993:303–314.
23. Ketter TA, Pazzaglia PJ, Post RM. Synergy of carbamazepine and valproic acid in affective illness: Case report and review of the literature. *J Clin Psychopharmacol.* 1992;12:276–281.
24. Morselli PL. Carbamazepine—Absorption, distribution and excretion. In: Levy R, Mattson R, Meldrum B, et al, eds. *Antiepileptic Drugs.* 3rd ed. New York: Raven Press; 1989:473–490.
25. Hartley R, Forsythe WJ, McLain B, et al. Daily variations in steady-state plasma concentrations of carbamazepine and its metabolites in epileptic children. *Clin Pharmacokinet.* 1991;20:237–244.
26. Gerardin A, Dobois JP, Moppert J, et al. Absolute bioavailability of carbamazepine after oral administration of a 2% syrup. *Epilepsia.* 1990;31:334–338.
27. Sanchez A, Duran JA, Serrano JS. Steady-state carbamazepine plasma concentration–dose ratios in epileptic patients. *Clin Pharmacokinet.* 1986;11:411–414.
28. Maas B, Garnett WR, Pellock JM, et al. A comparative bioavailability study of carbamazepine tablets and a chewable tablet formulation. *Ther Drug Monit.* 1987;9:28–33.
29. Patsalos PN. A comparative pharmacokinetic study of conventional and chewable carbamazepine in epileptic patients. *Br J Clin Pharmacol.* 1990;29:574–577.
30. Garnett WR, Carson SP, Pellock JM, et al. Comparison of carbamazepine and 10,11–diepoxide levels in children following chronic dosing with Tegretol suspension and Tegretol tablets. *Neurology.* 1987;37(suppl 1):93–94. Abstract.
31. Thakker KM, Mangat S, Garnett WR, et al. Comparative bioavailability and steady state fluctuations of Tegretol commercial and carbamazepine OROS tablets in adult and pediatric epileptic patients. *Biopharm Drug Dispos.* 1992;13:559–569.
32. Neuvonen PJ, Tokola O. Bioavailability of rectally administered carbamazepine mixture. *Br J Clin Pharmacol.* 1987;24:839–841.
33. Carbamazepine and moisture. *Medicom.* 1990;8:442.
34. Baruzzi A, Contin M, Perucca E, et al. Altered serum protein binding of carbamazepine in disease states associated with an increased alpha$_1$–acid glycoprotein concentration. *Eur J Clin Pharmacol.* 1986;31:85–89.
35. Gianelli M, Gentile S, Verze L, et al. Free drug levels monitoring as a detector of false metabolic refractory epilepsy. *Eur Neurol.* 1988;28:349–353.

36. Faigle JW, Feldmann KF. Carbamazepine–Biotransformation. In: Levy R, Mattson R, Meldrum B, et al, eds. *Antiepileptic Drugs.* 3rd ed. New York: Raven Press; 1989:491–504.
37. Sumi M, Watari N, Umezawa O, et al. Pharmacokinetic study of carbamazepine and its epoxide metabolite in humans. *J Pharmacobiodyn.* 1987;10:652–661.
38. Tomson T, Almkvist O, Nilsson BY, et al. Carbamazepine-10,11-epoxide in epilepsy: A pilot study. *Arch Neurol.* 1990;47:888–892.
39. Kerr BM, Levy RH. Carbamazepine—Carbamazepine epoxide. In: Levy R, Mattson R, Meldrum B, et al, eds. *Antiepileptic Drugs.* 3rd ed. New York: Raven Press; 1989:505–520.
40. Robbins DK, Wedlund PJ, Baumann RJ, et al. Inhibition of epoxide hydrolase by valproic acid in epileptic patients receiving carbamazepine. *Br J Clin Pharmacol.* 1990;29:759–762.
41. Mikati MA, Browne TR, Collins JG, et al. Time course of carbamazepine autoinduction. *Neurology.* 1989;39:592–594.
42. Bertilsson L, Tomson T, Tybring G. Pharmacokinetics: Time-dependent changes—Autoinduction of carbamazepine epoxidation. *J Clin Pharmacol.* 1986;26:459–462.
43. Levy RH, Kerr BM. Clinical pharmacokinetics of carbamazepine. *J Clin Psychiatry.* 1988;49(suppl):58–61.
44. Hockings N, Pall A, Moody J, et al. The effects of age on carbamazepine pharmacokinetics and adverse effects. *Br J Clin Pharmacol.* 1986;22:725–728.
45. Bano G, Raina RK, Sharma DB. Pharmacokinetics of carbamazepine in protein energy malnutrition. *Pharmacology.* 1986;32:232–236.
46. Summers B, Summers RS. Carbamazepine clearance in paediatric epilepsy patients: Influence of body mass, dose, sex and co-medication. *Clin Pharmacokinet.* 1989;17:208–216.
47. Gilman JT. Carbamazepine dosing for pediatric seizure disorders: The highs and lows. *Drug Intell Clin Pharm Ann Pharmacother.* 1991;25:1109–1112.
48. Kandrotas RJ, Oles KS, Gal P, et al. Carbamazepine clearance in hemodialysis and hemoperfusion. *Drug Intell Clin Pharm Ann Pharmacother.* 1989;23:137–140.
49. Dam M, Christiansen J, Munck O, et al. Antiepileptic drugs: Metabolism in pregnancy. *Clin Pharmacokinet.* 1979;4:53–62.
50. Gram L, Jensen PK. Carbamazepine—Toxicity. In: Levy R, Mattson R, Meldrum B, et al, eds. *Antiepileptic Drugs.* 3rd ed. New York: Raven Press; 1989:555–565.
51. Isojarvi JIT, Pakarinen AJ, Myllyla VV. Thyroid function in epileptic patients treated with carbamazepine. *Arch Neurol.* 1989;46:1175–1178.
52. Pellock JM, Willmore LJ. A rational guide to routine blood monitoring in patients receiving antiepileptic drugs. *Neurology.* 1991;41:961–964.
53. Iyer V, Holmes JW, Richardson RL. Intractable diarrhea from carbamazepine. *Epilepsia.* 1992;33:185–187.
54. Anttila V-J, Valtonen M. Carbamazepine-induced eosinophilic colitis. *Epilepsia.* 1992;33:119–121.
55. Stommel EW. Carbamazepine encephalopathy. *Neurology.* 1992;42:705.
56. Lampl Y, Eshel Y, Rapaport A, et al. Weight gain, increased appetite, and excessive food intake induced by carbamazepine. *Clin Neuropharmacol.* 1991;14:251–255.
57. De Giorgio CM, Rabinowicz AL, Olivas RD. Carbamazepine-induced antinuclear antibodies and systemic lupus erythematosus-like syndrome. *Epilepsia.* 1991;21:128–129.
58. Forbes GM, Jeffrey GP, Shilkin KB, et al. Carbamazepine hepatotoxicity: Another cause of the vanishing bile duct syndrome. *Gastroenterology.* 1992;102:1385–1388.
59. Labrecque J, Cote M-A, Vincent P. Carbamazepine-induced atrioventricular block. *Am J Psychiatry.* 1992;149:572–573.
60. Kasarskis EJ, Kuo C-S, Berger R, et al. Carbamazepine-induced cardiac dysfunction: Characterization of two distinct clinical syndromes. *Arch Intern Med.* 1992;152:186–191.
61. Weaver DF, Camfield P, Fraser A. Massive carbamazepine overdose: Clinical and pharmacologic observations of five episodes. *Neurology.* 1988;38:755–759.

62. Ng K, Silbert PL, Edis RH. Complete external ophthalmoplegia and asterixis with carbamazepine toxicity. *Aust NZ J Med.* 1991;21:886–887.
63. Jones KL, Lacro RV, Johnson KA, et al. Pattern of malformations in the children of women treated with carbamazepine during pregnancy. *N Engl J Med.* 1989;320:1661–1666.
64. Ketter TA, Post RM, Worthington K. Principles of clinically important drug interactions with carbamazepine. Part I. *J Clin Psychopharmacol.* 1991;11:198–203.
65. Ketter TA, Post RM, Worthington K. Principles of clinically important drug interactions with carbamazepine. Part II. *J Clin Psychopharmacol.* 1991;11:306–313.
66. Pitlick WH, Levy RH. Carbamazepine—Interactions with other drugs. In: Levy R, Mattson R, Meldrum B, et al, eds. *Antiepileptic Drugs.* 3rd ed. New York: Raven Press; 1989:521–531.
67. Clark-Schmidt AL, Garnett WR, Lowe DR, et al. Loss of carbamazepine suspension through nasogastric feeding tubes. *Am J Hosp Pharm.* 1990;47:2034–2037.
68. Bass J, Miles MV, Tennison MB, et al. Effects of enteral tube feeding on the absorption and pharmacokinetic profile of carbamazepine suspension. *Epilepsia.* 1989;30:364–369.
69. Wright PS, Seifert CF, Hampton EM. Toxic carbamazepine concentrations following cardiothoracic surgery and myocardial infarction. *Drug Intell Clin Pharm Ann Pharmacother.* 1990;24:822–826.
70. Racine-Poon A, Dubois JP. Predicting the range of plasma carbamazepine concentrations in patients with epilepsy. *Stat Med.* 1989;8:1327–1337.
71. Gonzalez ACA, Sanchez MJG, Hurle AD-G. Contribution of serum level monitoring in the individualization of carbamazepine dosage regimens. *Int J Clin Pharmacol Ther Toxicol.* 1988;26:409–412.
72. Garcia MJ, Alonso AC, Maza A, et al. Comparison of methods of carbamazepine dosage, individualization in epileptic patients. *J Clin Pharm Ther.* 1988;13:375–380.
73. Bourgeois BFD. Valproate: Clinical use. In: Levy R, Mattson R, Meldrum B, et al, eds. *Antiepileptic Drugs.* 3rd ed. New York: Raven Press; 1989:633–651.
74. McElroy SL, Keck PE, Pope HG, et al. Valproate in the treatment of bipolar disorder: Literature review and clinical guidelines. *J Clin Psychopharmacol.* 1992;12:42S–52S.
75. Faingold CL, Browning RA. Mechanisms of anticonvulsant drug action. II. Drugs primarily used for absence epilepsy. *Eur J Pediatr.* 1987;146:8–14.
76. Fariello R and Smith MC. Valproate: Mechanism of action. In: Levy R, Mattson R, Meldrum B, et al, eds. *Antiepileptic Drugs.* 3rd ed. New York: Raven Press; 1989:567–575.
77. Levey RH, Shen DD. Valproate: Absorption, distribution, and excretion. In: Levy R, Mattson R, Meldrum B, et al, eds. *Antiepileptic Drugs.* 3rd ed. New York: Raven Press; 1989:583–599.
78. Cloyd JC, Kriel RL, Jones-Saete CM, et al. Comparison of sprinkle versus syrup formulations of valproate for bioavailability, tolerance, and preference. *J Pediatr.* 1992;120:634–638.
79. Ohdo S, Nakano S, Ogawa N. Circadian changes of valproate kinetics depending on meal condition in humans. *J Clin Pharmacol.* 1992;32:822–826.
80. Zaccara G, Messori A, Moroni F. Clinical pharmacokinetics of valproic acid—1988. *Clin Pharmacokinet.* 1988;15:367–389.
81. Kodama Y, Koike Y, Kimoto H, et al. Binding parameters of valproic acid to serum protein in healthy adults at steady state. *Ther Drug Monitor.* 1992;14:55–60.
82. Bauer LA, Davis R, Wilensky A, et al. Valproic acid clearance: Unbound fraction and diurnal variation in young and elderly adults. *Clin Pharmacol Ther.* 1985;37:697–700.
83. Chiba K, Suganuma T, Ishizaki T, et al. Comparison of steady-state pharmacokinetics of valproic acid in children between monotherapy and multiple antiepileptic drug treatment. *J Pediatr.* 1985;106:653–658.
84. Cloyd JC, Kriel RL, Fischer JH. Valproic acid pharmacokinetics in children. II. Discontinuation of concomitant antiepileptic drug therapy. *Neurology.* 1985;35:1623–1627.
85. Kondo T, Ishida M, Kaneko S, et al. Is 2-propyl-4-pentenoic acid, a hepatotoxic metabolite of valproate, responsible for valproate-induced hyperammmonemia? *Epilepsia.* 1992;33:550–554.

86. Kall K, Otten N, Johnston B, et al. A multivariable analysis of factors governing the steady-state pharmacokinetics of valproic acid in 52 young epileptics. *J Clin Pharmacol.* 1985;25:261–268.

87. Zaccara G, Messori A, Moroni F. Clinical pharmacokinetics of valproic acid. *Clin Pharmacokinet.* 1988;15:367–389.

88. Omtzigt JGC, Nau H, Los FJ, et al. The disposition of valproate and its metabolites in the late first trimester and early second trimester of pregnancy in maternal serum, urine, and amniotic fluid: Effect of dose, co-mediation, and the presence of spina bifida. *Eur J Clin Pharmacol.* 1992;43:381–388.

89. Dean JC, Penry JK. Valproate monotherapy in 30 patients with partial seizures. *Epilepsia.* 1988;29:140–144.

90. Wilder BJ, Karas BJ, Hammond EJ, et al. Twice daily dosing of valproate with divalproex. *Clin Pharmacol Ther.* 1983;34:501–504.

91. Rimmer EM, Richens A. An update on sodium valproate. *Pharmacotherapy.* 1985;5:171–184.

92. Zaxxara G, Paganini M, Campostrini R, et al. Effect of associated antiepileptic treatment on valproate-induced hyperammonemia. *Ther Drug Monitor.* 1985;7:185–190.

93. Driefuss FE. Valproate: Toxicity. In: Levy R, Mattson R, Meldrum B, et al, eds. *Antiepileptic Drugs.* 3rd ed. New York: Raven Press; 1989:643–651.

94. Dreifuss FE, Santilli N, Langer DH, et al. Valproic acid hepatic fatalities: A retrospective review. *Neurology.* 1987;37:379–385.

95. Dreifuss FE, Langer DH, Moline KA, et al. Valproic acid hepatic fatalities. II. US experience since 1984. *Neurology.* 1989;39:201–207.

96. Binek J, Hany A, Heer M. Valproic-acid-induced pancreatitis: Case report and review of the literature. *J Clin Gastroenterol.* 1991;13:690–693.

97. Ettinger A, Moshe S, Shinnar S. Edema associated with long-term valproate therapy. *Epilepsia.* 1990;31:211–213.

98. Bleck TP, Smith MC. Possible induction of systemic lupus erythematosus by valproate. *Epilepsia.* 1990;31:343–345.

99. Ganick DJ, Sunder T, Finley JL. Severe hematologic toxicity of valproic acid: A report of four patients. *Am J Pediatr Hematol/Oncol.* 1990;12:80–85.

100. Kreuz W, Lide R, Funk M, et al. Valproate therapy induces von Willebrand disease type I. *Epilepsia.* 1992;33:178–184.

101. Opala G, Winter S, Vance C, et al. The effect of valproic acid on plasma carnitine levels. *Am J Dis Child.* 1991;145:999–1001.

102. Willmore LJ, Pellock JM. Valproate toxicity: Risk-screening strategies. *J Child Neurol.* 1991;6:3–6.

103. De Vivo DC, Tein I. Primary and secondary disorders of carnitine metbolism. *Int Pediatr.* 1990;5:134–141.

104. Trimble MR. Antiepileptic drugs, cognitive function, and behavior in children: Evidence from recent studies. *Epilepsia.* 1990;31(suppl 4):S26–S29.

105. Vourgeois BFD. Pharmacologic interactions between valproate and other drugs. *Am J Med.* 1988; 84(suppl 1A):29–33.

106. Duncan JS, Patsalos PN, Shorvon SD. Effects of discontinuation of phenytoin, carbamazepine, and valproate on concomitant antiepileptic medication. *Epilepsia.* 1991;32:101–115.

107. Mattson RH, Cramer JA. Valproate—Interactions with other drugs. In: Levy R, Mattson R, Meldrum B, et al, eds. *Antiepileptic Drugs.* 3rd ed. New York: Raven Press; 1989:621–632.

108. Jann MW, Fidone GS, Israel MK, et al. Increased valproate serum concentrations upon carbamazepine cessation. *Epilepsia.* 1988;29:578–581.

109. Goulden KJ, Dooley JM, Camfield PR, et al. Clinical valproate toxicity induced by acetylsalicylic acid. *Neurology.* 1987;37:1392–1394.

110. Chadwick DW. Concentration–effect relationships of valproic acid. *Clin Pharmacokinet.* 1985;10:155–165.

111. Gal P, Oles KS, Gilman JT, et al. Valproic acid efficacy, toxicity, and pharmacokinetics in neonates with intractable seizures. *Neurology.* 1988;38:467–471.

112. Prats JM, Garaizar C, Ruka MJ, et al. Infantile spasms treated with high doses of sodium valproate: Initial response and follow-up. *Dev Med Child Neurol.* 1991;33:617–625.

113. Ohtsuka Y, Amano R, Mizukawa M, et al. Treatment of intractable childhood epilepsy with high-dose valproate. *Epilepsia.* 1992;33:158–164.

114. May CA, Garnett WR. Prediction of steady state levels of valproic acid as determined from single plasma concentrations after the first dose. *Clin Pharmacol.* 1983;2:143–147.

115. Miles MV, Snead OC, Thorn MD. Predictability of unbound antiepileptic drug concentrations in children treated with valproic acid and phenytoin. *Clin Pharm.* 1988;7:688–693.

116. Bauer LA, Davis R, Wilensky A, et al. Diurnal variation in valproic acid clearance. *Clin Pharmacol Ther.* 1984;35:505–509.

117. Tarasidis CG, Garnett WR, Kline BJ, et al. Influence of tube type, storage time, and temperature on the total and free concentration of valproic acid. *Ther Drug Monit.* 1986;8:373–376.

118. Painter MJ. Phenobarbital: Clinical use. In: Levy R, Mattson R, Meldrum B, et al, eds. *Antiepileptic Drugs.* 3rd ed. New York: Raven Press; 1989:329–340.

119. Smith DB. Primidone: Clinical use. In: Levy R, Mattson R, Meldrum B, et al, eds. *Antiepileptic Drugs.* 3rd ed. New York: Raven Press; 1989:423–438.

120. Prichard JW, Ransom BR. Phenobarbital: Mechanism of action. In: Levy R, Mattson R, Meldrum B, et al, eds. *Antiepileptic Drugs.* 3rd ed. New York: Raven Press; 1989:267–282.

121. Bourgeois BFD. Primidone: Biotransformation and mechanism of action. In: Levy R, Mattson R, Meldrum B, et al, eds. *Antiepileptic Drugs.* 3rd ed. New York: Raven Press; 1989:401–412.

122. Meyer MC, Straughn AB, Raghow G. Absorption of phenobarbital from tablets and elixir. *J Pharm Sci.* 1984;73:485–488.

123. Rust RS, Dodson WE. Phenobarbital: Absorption, distribution, and excretion. In: Levy R, Mattson R, Meldrum B, et al, eds. *Antiepileptic Drugs.* 3rd ed. New York: Raven Press; 1989:293–304.

124. Cloyd JC, Leppik IE. Primidone: Absorption, distribution, and excretion. In: Levy R, Mattson R, Meldrum B, et al, eds. *Antiepileptic Drugs.* 3rd ed. New York: Raven Press; 1989:391–400.

125. Wyllie E, Pippenger CE, Rothner AD. Increased seizure frequency with generic primidone. *JAMA.* 1987;258:1216–1217.

126. Sannita WG, Balbi A, Giscchino F, et al. Quantitiative EEG effects and drug plasma concentration of phenobarbital, 50 and 100 mg single-dose oral administration to healthy volunteers: Evidence of early CNS bioavailability. *Neuropsychobiology.* 1990–1991;23:205–212.

127. Wilkes L, Danziger LH, Rodvold KA. Phenobarbital pharmacokinetics in obesity: A case report. *Clin Pharmacokinet.* 1992;22:481–484.

128. Browne TR, Evans JE, Szabo GK, et al. Studies with stable isotopes. II. Phenobarbital pharmacokinetics during monotherapy. *J Clin Pharmacol.* 1985;25:51–58.

129. Anderson GD. Phenobarbital: Biotransformation. In: Levy R, Mattson R, Meldrum B, et al, eds. *Antiepileptic Drugs.* 3rd ed. New York: Raven Press; 1989:305–312.

130. Streete JM, Berry DJ, Pettit LI, et al. Phenylethylmalonamide serum levels in patients treated with primidone and the effects of other antiepileptic drugs. *Ther Drug Monit.* 1986;8:161–165.

131. Painter MJ. Benzodiazepines and the barbiturates in the treatment of childhood epilepsy. In: Dodson WE, Pellock JM, eds. *Pediatric Epilepsy: Diagnosis and Therapy.* New York: Demos; 1993:281–289.

132. Pugh CB. Phenytoin and phenobarbital protein binding alterations in a uremic burn patient. *Drug Intell Clin Pharm.* 1987;21:264–267.

133. Abattino D, Sinelli S, Bossi L, et al. Changes in primidone/phenobarbitone ratio during pregnancy and the puerperium. *Clin Pharmacokinet.* 1984;9:252–260.

134. Mattson RH, Cramer JA. Phenobarbital: Toxicity. In: Levy R, Mattson R, Meldrum B, et al, eds. *Antiepileptic Drugs.* 3rd ed. New York: Raven Press; 1989:341–355.

135. Lacayo Alvaro, Mitra N. Report of a case of phenobarbital-induced dystonia. *Clin Pediatr.* 1992;31:252.
136. Leppik IE, Cloyd JC. Primidone: Toxicity. In: Levy R, Mattson R, Meldrum B, et al, eds. *Antiepileptic Drugs.* 3rd ed. New York: Raven Press; 1989:439–445.
137. Leppik IE, Cloyd JC, Miller K. Development of tolerance to the side effects of primidone. *Ther Drug Monit.* 1984;6:189–191.
138. Kutt H. Phenobarbital: Interactions with other drugs. In: Levy R, Mattson R, Meldrum B, et al, eds. *Antiepileptic Drugs.* 3rd ed. New York: Raven Press; 1989:313–327.
139. Fincham RW, Schottelius DD. Primidone: Interactions with other drugs. In: Levy R, Mattson R, Meldrum B, et al, eds. *Antiepileptic Drugs.* 3rd ed. New York: Raven Press; 1989:413–422.
140. Suzuki Y, Cox S, Hayes J, et al. Phenobarbital doses necessary to achieve "therapeutic" concentrations in children. *Dev Pharmacol Ther.* 1991;17:79–87.
141. Wroblewski BA, Garvin WH. Once-daily administration of phenobarbital in adults: Clinical efficacy and benefit. *Arch Neurol.* 1985;42:699–700.
142. Friedlander WJ. Putnam, Merritt, and the discovery of Dilantin. *Epilepsia.* 1986;27(suppl 3): S1–S21.
143. Smith DB, Mattson RH, Cramer JA, et al. Results of a nationwide Veterans Administration Cooperative Study comparing the efficacy and toxicity of carbamazepine, phenobarbital, phenytoin, and primidone. *Epilepsia.* 1987;28(suppl 3):S50–S58.
144. Willder BJ, Rangel RJ. Phenytoin: Clinical use. In: Levy R, Mattson R, Meldrum B, et al, eds. *Antiepileptic Drugs.* 3rd ed. New York: Raven Press; 1989:233–239.
145. DeLorenzo RJ. Phenytoin: Mechanism of action. In: Levy R, Mattson R, Meldrum B, et al, eds. *Antiepileptic Drugs.* 3rd ed. New York: Raven Press; 1989:143–158.
146. Tozer T, Winter M. Phenytoin. In: Evans W, Schentag J. Jusko W, eds. *Applied Pharmacokinetics: Principles of Therapeutic Drug Monitoring.* 3rd ed. Vancouver, WA: Applied Therapeutics, Inc; 1992:26-1–26-29.
147. Woodberry DM. Phenytoin: Absorption, distribution, excretion. In: Levy R, Mattson R, Meldrum B, et al, eds. *Antiepileptic Drugs.* 3rd ed. New York: Raven Press; 1989:177–195.
148. Cacek AT. Review of alterations in oral phenytoin bioavailability associated with formulation, antacids, and food. *Ther Druk Monit.* 1986;8:166–171.
149. Browne TR and Chang T. Phenytoin: Biotransformation. In: Levy R, Mattson R, Meldrum B, et al, eds. *Antiepileptic Drugs.* 3rd ed. New York: Raven Press; 1989:197–213.
150. Grasela TH, Sheiner LB, Rambeck B, et al. Steady-state pharmacokineitcs of phenytoin from routinely collected patient data. *Clin Pharmacokinet.* 1983;8:355–364.
151. Bauer LA, Blouin RA. Phenytoin Michaelis–Menten pharmacokinetics in Caucasian paediatric patients. *Clin Pharmcokinet.* 1983;8:545–549.
152. Costeff H, Groswasser Z, Soroker N, et al. Covariance analysis of laboratory variance in steady-state phenytoin concentrations. *Clin Pharmacokinet.* 1991;20:331–335.
153. Bauer LA, Blouin RA. Age and phenytoin kinetics in adult epileptics. *Clin Pharmacol Ther.* 1982;31:301–304.
154. Eadie MJ, McKinnon GE, Dickinson RG, et al. Phenytoin metabolism during pregnancy. *Eur J Clin Pharmacol.* 1992;43:389–392.
155. White RL, Garnett WR, Kline BJ, et al. Removal of phenytoin during plasma exchange. *J Clin Aperosis.* 1987;3:147–150.
156. Reynolds EH. Phenytoin: Toxicity. In: Levy R, Mattson R, Meldrum B, et al, eds. *Antiepileptic Drugs.* 3rd ed. New York: Raven Press; 1989:241–255.
157. Brown RS, Beaver WT, Bottomley WK. On the mechanism of drug-induced gingival hyperplasia. *J Oral Pathol Med.* 191;20:201–209.
158. Pihlstrom BL, Carlson JF, Smith QT, et al. Prevention of phenytoin associated gingival enlargement—A 15-month longitudinal study. *J Peridontol.* 1980;51:311–317.

159. Berg MJ, Rincham RW, Ebert BE, et al. Decrease of serum folates in healthy male volunteers taking phenytoin. *Epilepsia.* 1988;29:67–73.

160. Dodson WE. Phenytoin and related drugs. In: Dodson WE, Pellock JM, eds. *Pediatric Epilepsy: Diagnosis and Therapy.* New York: Demos; 1993:291–302.

161. Yerby MS. Teratogenicity of anticonvulsant medication. In: Dodson WE, Pellock JM, eds. *Pediatric Epilepsy: Diagnosis and Therapy.* New York: Demos; 1993:265–279.

162. Nation RL, Evans AM, Milne RW. Pharmacokinetic drug interactions with phenytoin (Part I). *Clin Pharmcokinet.* 1990;18:37–60.

163. Nation RL, Evans AM, Milne RW. Pharmacokinetic drug interactions with phenytoin (Part II). *Clin Pharmcokinet.* 1990;18:131–150.

164. Saklad JJ, Graves RH, Sharp WP. Interaction of oral phenytoin with enteral feedings. *J Parenteral Enteral Nutr.* 1986:10:322–323.

165. Berg MJ, Fincham RW, Ebert BE, et al. Phenytoin pharmacokinetics: Before and after folic acid administration. *Epilepsia.* 1992;33:712–720.

166. Smith CD, Bledsoe MA, Curran R, et al. Effect of influenza vaccine on serum concentrations of total and free phenytoin. *Clin Pharm.* 1988;7:828–832.

167. Krumlovsky FA. Phenytoin in end-stage renal disease. *Int J Artifical Organs.* 1992;15:69–70.

168. Fleppik IE, Fischer J, Kriel, et al. Altered phenytoin clearance with febrile illness. *Neurology.* 1986;36:1367–1370.

169. Boucher BA, Rodman JH, Jaresko GS, et al. Phenytoin pharmacokinetics in critically ill trauma patients. *Clin Pharmacol Ther.* 1988;44:675–683.

170. Vozeh S, Uematsu T, Aarons L, et al. Intravenous phenytoin loading in patients after neurosurgery and in status epilepticus: A population pharmacokinetic study. *Clin Pharmacokinet.* 1988;14:122–128.

171. Levine M, Chang T. Therapeutic drug monitoring of phenytoin: Rationale and current status. *Clin Pharmacokinet.* 1990;19:341–358.

172. Pryka RD, Rodvold KA, Erdman SM. An updated comparison of drug dosing methods. Part I: Phenytoin. *Clin Pharmacokinet.* 1991;20:209–217.

173. Welty TE, Robinson FC, Mayer PR. A comparison of phenytoin dosing methods in private practice seizure patients. *Epilepsia.* 1986;27:76–80.

174. Graves N, Cloyd J, Leppik I, et al. Phenytoin dosage predictions using population clearances. *Drug Intell Clin Pharm.* 1982;16:473.

175. Toscan JP, Jameson JP. Comparison of four single-point phenytoin dosage prediction techniques using computer-simulated pharmacokinetic values. *Clin Pharm.* 1986;5:396–402.

176. Mauro LS, Mauro VF, Bachmann KA, et al. Accuracy of two equations in determining normalized phenytoin concentrations. *Drug Intell Clin Pharm Ann Pharmacother.* 1989;23:64–68.

177. Fitzsimmons WE, Garnett WR. Effect of serum separator tubes on phenytoin concentration. *Clin Pharmacol.* 1986;5:923–925.

178. Mikati M, Basset N, Schacter S. Double-blind randomized study comparing brand-name and generic phenytoin monotherapy. *Epilepsia.* 1992;33:359–365.

179. Sakaar M, Karnes HT, Garnett WR. Effects of storage and shaking on the settling properties of phenytoin suspension. *Neurology.* 1989;39:202–209.

180. Jamerson BD, Donn KH, Dukes GE, et al. Absolute bioavailability of phenytoin after 3-phosphorloxymethyl phenytoin disodium (ACC-9653) administration to humans. *Epilepsia.* 1990;31:592–597.

181. Sherwin AL. Ethosuximide—Clinical use. In: Levy R, Mattson R, Meldrum B, et al, eds. *Antiepileptic Drugs.* 3rd ed. New York: Raven Press; 1989:685–698.

182. Garnett WR. Ethosuximide. In: Taylor WJ, Caviness MHD, eds. *A Textbook for the Clinical Application of Therapeutic Drug Monitoring.* Irving, TX: Abbott Laboratories; Diagnostics Division. 1986:225–235.

183. Chang T. Ethosuximide—Absorption, distribution, and excretion. In: Levy R, Mattson R, Meldrum B, et al, eds. *Antiepileptic Drugs.* 3rd ed. New York: Raven Press; 1989:671–678.

184. Chang T. Ethosuximide–Biotransformation. In: Levy R, Mattson R, Meldrum B, et al, eds. *Antiepileptic Drugs*. 3rd ed. New York: Raven Press; 1989:679–683.

185. Smith GA, McKauge L, Dubetz D, et al. Factors influencing plasma concentrations of ethosuximide. *Clin Pharmacokinet*. 1979;4:38–52.

186. Bauer LA, Harris C, Wilensky AJ, et al. Ethosuximide kinetics: Possible interaction with valproic acid. *Clin Pharm Ther*. 1982;31:741–745.

187. Villen T, Bertilsson L, Sjoqvist F. Nonstereoselective disposition of ethosuximide in humans. *Ther Drug Monit*. 1990;12:514–516.

188. Battino D, Cusi C, Franceschetti S, et al. Ethosuximide plasma concentrations: Influence of age and associated concomitant therapy. *Clin Pharmacokinet*. 1982;7:176–180.

189. Koup JR, Rose JQ, Cohen ME. Ethosuximide pharmacokinetics in a pregnant patient and her newborn. *Epilepsia*. 1978;19:535–539.

190. Marbury TC, Lee CC, Perchalski RJ et al. Hemodialysis clearance of ethosuximide in patients with chronic renal failure. *Am J Hosp Pharm*. 1981;38:1757–1760.

191. Dreifuss FE. Ethosuximide—Toxicity. In: Levy R, Mattson R, Meldrum B, et al, eds. *Antiepileptic Drugs*. 3rd ed. New York: Raven Press; 1989:699–705.

192. Mattson RH, Cramer JA. Valproic acid and ethosuximide interaction. *Ann Neurol*. 1980;7:583–584.

193. Bourgeois BFD. Combination of valproate and ethosuximide: Antiepileptic and neurotoxic interaction. *J Pharmacol Exp Ther*. 1988;247:1128–1132.

194. Pisani F, Nurbone MC, Trunfio C, et al. Valproic acid–ethosuximide interaction: A pharmacokinetic study. *Epilepsia*. 1984;25:229–233.

195. Van Wieringen A, Vriglandt CM. Ethosuximide intoxication caused by interaction with isoniazid. *Neurology*. 1983;33:1227–1228.

196. Dawson GW, Brown HW, Clark BG. Serum phenytoin after ethosuximide. *Ann Neurol*. 1978;4:583–584.

197. Bachmann K, Schwartz J, Sullivan T, et al. Single sample estimate of ethosuximide clearance. *Int J Clin Pharmacol Ther Toxicol*. 1986;24:546–550.

198. Porter RJ, Rogawski MA. New antiepileptic drugs: From serendipity to rational discovery. *Epilepsia*. 1992;33(suppl. 1):S1–S6.

199. Graves NM, Leppik IE. Antiepileptic medications in development. *Drug Intell Clin Pharm. Ann Pharmacother*. 1991;25:978–986.

200. White HS, Wolf HH, Swinyard EA, et al. A neuropharmacological evaluation of felbamate as a novel anticonvulsant. *Epilepsia*. 1992;33:564–572.

201. Leppik IE, Graves NM. Potential antiepileptic drugs: Felbamate. In: Levy R, Mattson R, Meldrum B, et al, eds. *Antiepileptic Drugs*. 3rd ed. New York: Raven Press; 1989:983–990.

202. Sachdeo R, Kramer LD, Rosenberg A, et al. Felbamate monotherapy: Controlled trial in patients with partial onset seizures. *Ann Neurol*. 1992;32:386–392.

203. Efficacy of felbamate in childhood epileptic encephalopathy (Lennox–Gastaut syndrome). *N Engl J Med*. 1993;328:29–33.

204. Felbamate package insert, 1993.

205. Graves NM. Felbamate. *Ann Pharmacother*. 1993;27:1073–1081.

206. Graves NM, Ludden TM, Holmes GB, et al. Pharmacokinetics of felbamate, a novel antiepileptic drug: Application of mixed-effect modeling to clinical trials. *Pharmacotherapy*. 1989;9:372–376.

207. Sofia RD, Kramer L, Perhach JL, et al. Felbamate. In: Pisani F, Perucca E, Avanzini G, et al, eds. *New Antiepileptic Drugs (Epilepsy Research Supplement 3)*. New York: Elsevier; 1991:103–108.

208. Fuerst RH, Graves NM, Leppik IE, et al. Felbamate increases phenytoin but decreases carbamazepine concentration. *Epilepsia*. 1988;29:488–491.

209. Graves NM, Holmes GB, Fuerst RH, et al. Effect of felbamate on phenytoin and carbamazepine serum concentrations. *Epilepsia*. 1989;30:225–229.

210. Albani F, Theodore WH, Washington P, et al. Effect of felbamate on plasma levels of carbamazepine and its metabolites. *Epilepsia.* 1991;32:130–132.
211. Schmidt B. Potential antiepileptic drugs: Gabapentin. In: Levy R, Mattson R, Meldrum B, et al, eds. *Antiepileptic Drugs.* 3rd ed. New York: Raven Press; 1989:925–935.
212. Sivenius J, Kalviainen R, Ylinen A, et al. Double-blind study of gabapentin in the treatment of partial seizures. *Epilepsia.* 1991;32:539–542.
213. Goa KL, Sorkin EM. Gabapentin—A review of its pharmacological properties and clinical potential in epilepsy. *Drugs.* 1993;46:409–427.
214. Neurontin® (gabapentin) package insert, Parke-Davis, Morris Plains, NJ: January 1994.
215. Richens A. Clinical pharmacokinetics of gabapentin. In: Chadwick D, ed. *New Trends in Epilepsy Management: The Role of Gabapentin.* International Congress and Symposium Series No. 198. London: Royal Society of Medicine Services; 1993:41–46.
216. Browne TR. Efficacy and safety of gabapentin. In: Chadwick D, ed. *New Trends in Epilepsy Management: The Role of Gabapentin.* International Congress and Symposium Series No. 198. London: Royal Society of Medicine Services; 1993:47–57.
217. Foot M, Wallace J. Gabapentin. In: Pisani F, Perucca E, Avanzini G, et al, eds. *New Antiepileptic Drugs (Epilepsy Research Supplement 3).* New York: Elsevier; 1991:109–114.
218. Chadwick D. The role of gabapentin in epilepsy management. In: Chadwick D, ed. *New Trends in Epilepsy Management: The Role of Gabapentin.* International Congress and Symposium Series No. 198. London: Royal Society of Medicine Services, 1993:59–65.
219. Gram L. Potential antiepileptic drugs: Lamotrigine. In: Levy R, Mattson R, Meldrum B, et al, eds. *Antiepileptic Drugs.* 3rd ed. New York: Raven Press; 1989:947–953.
220. Richens A, Yuen AWC. Overview of the clinical efficacy of lamotrigine. *Epilepsia.* 1991;32(suppl 2):S13–S16.
221. Rambeck B, Wolf P. Lamotrigine clinical pharmacokinetics. *Clin Pharmacokinet.* 1993;25:433–443.
222. Ramsay RE, Pellock JM, Garnett WR, et al. *Epilepsy Rev.* 1991;10:191–200.
223. Peck AW. Clinical pharmacology of lamotrigine. *Epilepsia.* 1991;suppl 2:S9–S12.
224. Yau MK, Adams MA, Wargin MM, et al. A single-dose and steady-state pharmacokinetic study of lamotrigine in healthy male volunteers. Presented at the Third International Cleveland Clinic-Bethel Epilepsy Symposium on Antiepileptic Drug Pharmacology. Cleveland, June 16–20, 1992.
225. Yuen AWC. Lamotrigine. In: Pisani F, Perucca E, Avanzini G, et al, eds. *New Antiepileptic Drugs (Epilepsy Research Supplement 3).* New York: Elsevier; 1991:115–123.
226. Betts T, Goodwin G, Withers RM, et al. Human safety of lamotrigine. *Epilepsia.* 1991;32(suppl 2):S17–S21.
227. Sabers A, Gram L. Pharmacology of vigabatrin. *Pharmacol Toxicol.* 1992;70:237–243.
228. Dam M. Long-term evaluation of vigabatrin (gamma vinyl GABA) in epilepsy. *Epilepsia.* 1989;30(suppl 3):S26–S30.
229. Reynolds EH, Ring HA, Farr IN, et al. Open, double-blind and long-term study of vigabatrin in chronic epilepsy. *Epilepsia.* 1991;32:530–538.
230. Rey E, Pons G, Olive G. Vigabatrin: Clinical pharmacokinetics. *Clin Pharmacokinet.* 1992;23:267–278.
231. Richens A. Potential antiepileptic drugs: Vigabatrin. In: Levy R, Mattson R, Meldrum B, et al, eds. *Antiepileptic Drugs.* 3rd ed. New York: Raven Press; 1989:937–946.
232. Michelucci R, Tassinari CA. Vigabatrin. In: Pisani F, Perucca E, Avanzini G, et al, eds. *New Antiepileptic Drugs (Epilepsy Research Supplement 3).* New York: Elsevier; 1991:193–196.
233. Binnie CD. Potential antiepileptic drugs: Flunarizine and other calcium entry blockers. In: Levy R, Mattson R, Meldrum B, et al, eds. *Antiepileptic Drugs.* 3rd ed. New York: Raven Press; 1989:971–982.

Chapter 12

Chloramphenicol

Milap C. Nahata

Keep in Mind

- Chloramphenicol has a broad spectrum of antimicrobial activity. It is generally bacteriostatic, but has been shown to be bactericidal against *Streptococcus pneumoniae* and *Haemophilus influenzae.*

- Initial dose should be 25 mg/kg/day in premature and full-term infants less than 2 weeks of age; and 50 mg/kg/day in divided doses for older infants (2 weeks–1 year), children, adolescents, adults and geriatric patients.

- Infuse intravenous chloramphenicol succinate over a 20- to 60-minute period.

- Measure peak blood concentrations about 1 hour after administration of chloramphenicol capsules; 1.5 to 3 hours after chloramphenicol palmitate suspension; and 0.5 to 1.5 hours after a 20- to 60-minute infusion of chloramphenicol succinate.

- Use a rapid enzyme immunoassay (EMIT) to measure chloramphenicol; use high-performance liquid chromatography (HPLC) to measure both chloramphenicol and succinate ester.

- Chloramphenicol causes two types of adverse effects: dose independent (idiosyncratic) and dose dependent.

- Monitor chloramphenicol serum concentrations early in therapy, for example, 24 hours after initiation of therapy, to ensure optimal doses in patients with proven infection who are likely to receive chloramphenicol for 7 days or longer. It is not necessary to measure chloramphenicol concentration in patients with presumed infection, who may receive chloramphenicol for 3 or 4 days, pending microbial sensitivity results, unless there is renal or hepatic dysfunction or subtherapeutic or toxic drug concentrations are suspected.

- Monitor hematologic function at the start of therapy, at the end of 1 week, and every 3 days thereafter to minimize toxicity.

- Phenobarbital, phenytoin, and rifampin may decrease the serum concentration of chloramphenicol by inducing its metabolism. On the other hand, chloramphenicol may increase the serum concentration of chlorpropamide, phenytoin, and tolbutamide by decreasing their metabolism.

- Repeat measurement of chloramphenicol serum concentration may be needed if liver or kidney function changes markedly; initial concentrations are outside the therapeutic range; an interacting drug is added or discontinued; or the patient does not respond clinically or experiences toxic effects.

Chloramphenicol was discovered in 1947. It quickly became one of the commonly used antibiotics because of its (1) broad spectrum of antimicrobial activity; (2) efficacy in the treatment of a variety of infections, including those involving the central nervous system; and (3) worldwide availability. Reports of idiosyncratic and dose-related toxicity, however, led to a decline in the use of chloramphenicol. In the 1970s and early 1980s, chloramphenicol once again became the drug of choice for the treatment of presumed or proven systemic infections caused by ampicillin-resistant *Haemophilus influenzae* type b, the most common pathogen causing bacterial meningitis in infants and children. These patients are now treated with a third-generation cephalosporin at most institutions in developed countries. Chloramphenicol, however, is still a useful drug in the treatment of central nervous system infections, typhoid fever, rickettsial disease, anaerobic infections, and certain infections of the eye.[1] This is particularly true when drugs of first choice cannot be used. It should be noted that in much of the developing world, chloramphenicol continues to be used widely for treating a variety of infections.

The major concern about chloramphenicol use is its toxicity. Fortunately, some of the dose-related adverse effects can be prevented by therapeutic drug monitoring. The goal of this chapter is to provide an overview of the pharmacokinetics, pharmacodynamics, dosage regimens, adverse effects, drug–drug interactions, and monitoring guidelines of chloramphenicol, so that it can be used optimally in pediatric and adult patients.

CLINICAL PHARMACOLOGY AND THERAPEUTICS

The antimicrobial action of chloramphenicol depends on its binding to 50 S subunit of bacterial ribosomes. This binding inhibits the formation of peptide bonds.

Chloramphenicol has a broad spectrum of antimicrobial activity. It is active in vitro against many Gram-positive aerobic bacteria, including *Streptococcus pneumoniae* and other streptococci, and many Gram-negative microorganisms, including *Haemophilus influenzae*, *Neisseria meningitidis*, *Shigella*, and *Salmonella*. It is also active against many anaerobic microorganisms, including *Bacteroides fragilis*, *Bacteriodes melaninogenicus*, *Clostridium*, *Fusobacterium*, and *Veillonella*. Other organisms inhibited by chloramphenicol include *Rickettsia*, *Chlamydia*, and *Mycoplasma*.[2]

Although chloramphenicol is generally considered bacteriostatic, it is bactericidal to *H. influenzae* and *S. pneumoniae*. Susceptible aerobic microorganisms such as *H. influenzae*, *S. pneumonia*, *Neisseria*, and *Salmonella* are inhibited at chloramphenicol concentrations of 0.1 to 5.0 μg/mL, whereas anaerobes may be inhibited at about 8.0 μg/mL. Ampicillin and chloramphenicol have synergistic in vitro antimicrobial activity.[2,3]

Chloramphenicol resistance is usually plasmid mediated, and occurs as a result of the production of chloramphenicol acetyltransferase. Strains of *H. influenzae* resistant to chloramphenicol have rarely been reported. Some strains of *Salmonella*, staphylococci, *Shigella*, and *Escherichia coli* may also be resistant.[3]

Chloramphenicol is effective in the treatment of a variety of infections, particularly when potentially less toxic drugs are contraindicated or ineffective. Therapy should be initiated empirically, pending the results of susceptibility tests. Chloramphenicol should be discontinued if the organism is sensitive to a less toxic antibiotic or resistant to chloramphenicol.[2]

Typhoid fever

Ampicillin and amoxicillin are considered the drugs of choice in the treatment of typhoid fever (enteric fever) caused by *Salmonella typhi*, except in severe cases, for which chloramphenicol is recommended. There are two concerns: (1) a few strains of *Salmonella* may be resistant to chloramphenicol; (2) in about 10% of patients, chloramphenicol may not eradicate the organism, leading to a temporary or permanent carrier state.[2,3]

Infections caused by *Haemophilus influenzae*

Haemophilus influenzae type b may cause serious systemic infections including bacterial meningitis, osteomyelitis, septic arthritis, cellulitis, epiglottitis, and septicemia. Although cephalosporins are commonly used, chloramphenicol may be considered if cephalosporins are contraindicated or ineffective.[2,3]

Rickettsial Infections

Tetracycline is the drug of choice in the treatment of Rocky Mountain spotted fever and other infections caused by *Rickettsia*. Chloramphenicol, however, is considered the drug of choice when tetracyclines are contraindicated, for example, in children younger than 8 years of age or in pregnant women.[2] It should be noted that the safety of chloramphenicol during pregnancy has not been established, as it crosses the placenta and appears in breast milk. It should be used with extreme caution in pregnant women at term or during labor and in nursing women because of potential toxic effects on the fetus or child.[2,3]

Other Infections

Because of the toxicity asssociated with chloramphenicol, it is considered an alternative antibiotic when first-line drugs are ineffective or contraindicated in a variety of other infections. These may include meningitis caused by susceptible pathogens, such as *S. pneumoniae* and *N. meningitidis*; cerebral abscess or intraabdominal infections caused by anaerobes; in conjunction with tetracycline for melioidosis caused by *Pseudomonas pseudomallei*; and as one of the antibiotics in patients with cystic fibrosis who frequently develop resistance to antimicrobial agents.[3]

CLINICAL PHARMACOKINETICS

Dosage Forms

For the treatment of systemic infections, chloramphenicol is available in three dosage forms:
- Chloramphenicol sodium succinate is indicated for parenteral use. When reconstituted, each 1-g vial contains the equivalent of 100 mg of chloramphenicol per milliliter. This inactive prodrug must be hydrolyzed by esterases, primarily in the liver, to active chloramphenicol. It is administered routinely by the intravenous route, although limited data

indicate the intramuscular route may be used. Caution should be used if the drug is administered intramuscularly as therapeutic failures have been reported.

- Chloramphenicol palmitate suspension is administered orally. Each 5 mL contains 150 mg of chloramphenicol. This inactive prodrug must be hydrolyzed in the gut by pancreatic enzymes to active chloramphenicol.
- Each chloramphenicol capsule for oral use contains 250 mg of chloramphenicol base.

Chloramphenicol is also available as 0.16%, 0.25%, and 0.5% ophthalmic solutions; a 1% ophthalmic ointment; a 0.5% otic solution; and a 1% topical cream.

Absorption

In adults receiving chloramphenicol capsules, 50 mg/kg/d in four doses or 1 g every 6 hours, the C_{max} and T_{max} have averaged 8 to 14 µg/mL and 1.0 hour, respectively.[4] The mean C_{max} and T_{max} ranged from 19 to 28 µg/mL and from 1.5 to 3.0 hours, respectively, after administration of chloramphenicol palmitate 19 to 27 mg/kg every 6 hours to pediatric patients.[3] Absorption of chloramphenicol from chloramphenicol palmitate is incomplete, delayed, and erratic in premature infants.[5]

Absorption of chloramphenicol after intramuscular administration of chloramphenicol succinate was reported to be lower than that achieved after intravenous or oral administration.[6] A recent study, however, has demonstrated comparable C_{max} and area-under-curve (AUC) values after intramuscular and intravenous doses of chloramphenicol succinate in infants and children (1 month to 6 years).[7] Further studies are needed before intramuscular administration can be recommended for routine clinical use.

Comparative studies have shown higher AUC values after oral palmitate than intravenous succinate,[8] except in newborn infants[5] and patients with cystic fibrosis who may lack pancreatic enzymes.[9]

The mean bioavailability of chloramphenicol from intravenous succinate ranges from 0.64 to 0.93, depending on the patient's age (Table 12–1). Bioavailability is highest in premature infants because of their decreased ability to eliminate unchanged chloramphenicol succinate by the kidney; thus, a larger fraction of dose is available for hydrolysis to chloramphenicol.[10]

In patients with cystic fibrosis receiving pancreatic supplementation, the mean relative bioavailability of chloramphenicol was 0.69 after intravenous succinate and 0.64 after oral palmitate compared with chloramphenicol base; the bioavailability was substantially lower (0.42) after oral palmitate in patients not receiving pancreatic enzymes.[9]

In premature infants, the bioavailability of chloramphenicol from oral palmitate is not known; however, dosage increases from 25 to 50 mg/kg were necessary to achieve therapeutic serum concentrations of chloramphenicol.[5]

Distribution

Chloramphenicol penetrates into various body organs and fluids including liver, kidney, placenta, cerebrospinal fluid, aqueous and vitreous humor of the eye, ascitic fluid, and breast milk. Unlike penicillins and cephalosporins, penetration into the cerebrospinal fluid is independent of meningeal inflammation.[3]

TABLE 12–1. SUMMARY OF CHLORAMPHENICOL PHARMACOKINETICS

Common dosage forms	Chloramphenicol palmitate PO
	Chloramphenicol succinate IV
Active moiety	Chloramphenicol
Effective peak concentration	10–20 µg/mL
Time to peak concentration	1.0–3.0 h
Potentially toxic concentration	>30 µg/mL
Bioavailable fraction	0.64–0.93
Bioavailability	Higher from PO palmitate than from IV succinate, except in
	newborn infants and in those with cystic fibrosis
Bioavalability from IV chloramphenicol succinate	Highest in newborn infants
Distribution	Liver, kidney, placenta, cerebrospinal fluid, aqueous and
	vitreous humor of the eye, ascitic fluid, and breast milk
Plasma protein binding	30–50%
Apparent distribution volume	
Adults	0.55–0.98 L/kg
Infants and children	0.63–1.55 L/kg
Major metabolite	Chloramphenicol monoglucuronide
Total body clearance (Cl)	
Adults	1.3–3.6 mL/min/kg
Infants and children	1.5–4.7 mL/min/kg
Nonrenal clearance	90% of Cl in adults and 70–80% of Cl in infants and children
Renal elimination	Glomerular filtration, tubular secretion, and reabsorption
Elimination half-life	
Adults	2.3–5.1 h
Infants and children	3.5–10 h
Time to steady state	12–50 h

The average plasma protein binding of chloramphenicol was about 50% in normal adults, 40% in adult patients with cirrhosis, and 30% in premature infants.[3] The mean apparent volume of distribution has ranged from 0.55 to 0.98 L/kg in adults and from 0.63 to 1.55 L/kg in pediatric patients (Table 12–2).

Metabolism

Chloramphenicol palmitate must be hydrolyzed by pancreatic lipases in the gut, and chloramphenicol succinate primarily by esterases in the liver, to active chloramphenicol. Chloramphenicol is metabolized in the liver by glucuronyl transferases to inactive glucuronide metabolites.[3]

The mean total clearance of chloramphenicol has ranged from 1.3 to 3.6 mL/min/kg in adults and from 1.5 to 4.7 mL/min/kg in pediatric patients. The nonrenal clearance of chloram-

TABLE 12-2. PHARMACOKINETIC DATA OBTAINED AFTER INTRAVENOUS ADMINISTRATION OF CHLORAMPHENICOL SUCCINATE

Age	Mean f	Mean Cl (mL/min/kg)	Mean Cl_r (mL/min/kg)	Mean V_d, (L/kg)	Mean $t_{1/2}$ (h)	Reference
31.8 ± 3.4 wk[a]	0.93	1.73	0.36	1.55	10.1	10
8.4 ± 3.4 wk[b]						
0.64 ± 0.3 y	0.71	2.54	0.43	0.76	3.5	15
10.7 ± 7.5 y	0.64	1.59	0.44	0.63	4.8	15
0.4-84 mo	ND[c]	1.50	ND	0.64	4.6	16
3-18 mo	ND	2.11[d]	ND	ND	ND	17
4-72 mo	ND	4.68[d]	ND	1.39[d]	3.9	18
19-64 y	ND	3.21	0.33	0.81	3.2	19
43-72 y	ND	1.29	0.14	0.55	5.1	12
Adults						
Normal	ND	3.57[d]	ND	0.92[d]	2.3	11
Cirrhosis	ND	1.99[d]	ND	0.98[d]	3.9	11

[a] Gestational age.
[b] Postnatal age.
[c] Not determined.
[d] Because these studies assumed complete hydrolysis of chloramphenicol succinate to chloramphenicol, the Cl and V_d are likely to be overestimated.

phenicol accounts for 90% of its total clearance in adults and 70 to 80% of total clearance in infants and children (Table 12–2).

Elimination

Chloramphenicol undergoes glomerular filtration as well as tubular secretion and reabsorption. The mean elimination half-life of chloramphenicol is 2.3 to 5.1 hours in adults, 3.5 to 4.8 hours in children and infants older than a mean age of 2 weeks, and 10.1 hours in infants born prematurely with mean postnatal age of about 2 months (Table 12–2).

About 5 to 30% of a chloramphenicol succinate dose may be excreted unchanged in the urine. Newborn infants may accumulate chloramphenicol succinate because of underdeveloped kidney function, leading to increased serum concentration and bioavailability of chloramphenicol.[3,10]

Special Populations

Clearance of chloramphenicol is decreased in patients with severe liver disease. The mean total clearance of chloramphenicol was about 3.6 mL/min/kg in normal adults compared with 2.0 mL/min/kg in adult patients with cirrhosis of the liver.[11] Elevated serum concentrations of chloramphenicol have also been reported in anephric patients (40 to 160 µg/mL),[12,13] and those with acidosis (30–84 µg/mL).[14]

PHARMACODYNAMICS

Research studies and clinical experience have shown that chloramphenicol is effective when the C_{max} is between 10 and 20 µg/mL. These concentrations exceed the minimum inhibitory concentration (MIC) of most common susceptible pathogens by severalfold in blood and cerebrospinal fluid. Thus, C_{max} should be monitored to ensure efficacy.

Chloramphenicol may cause two types of adverse effects: idiosyncratic (dose independent) and dose dependent. Aplastic anemia, the most serious idiosyncratic reaction, occurs in about one of every 40,000 people treated with chloramphenicol; this is not preventable, as it may occur at any dose or concentration and with any dosage form of chloramphenicol. Dose-dependent adverse effects, however, can be identified and minimized by monitoring chloramphenicol serum concentration (Table 12–3).

Gray baby syndrome has been most commonly reported in infants who received chloramphenicol doses of 100 to 300 mg/kg/d. Serum concentrations of chloramphenicol in two infants immediately before death were found to be 75 and 180 µg/mL.[20] This syndrome is characterized by vomiting, abdominal distension, anorexia, and respiratory distress after 3 to 4 days of therapy. After the initial symptoms, hypotension, gray color, greenish diarrhea, and progressive shock occur. The mortality of gray baby syndrome is approximately 40%; the remaining 60% recover completely after stopping chloramphenicol therapy.[3]

Acidosis has been reported in four infants and children after chloramphenicol succinate 100 mg/kg/d. The C_{max} of chloramphenicol was 30 µg/mL in one and between 62 and 84 µg/mL in

TABLE 12–3. ADVERSE DRUG REACTIONS OF CHLORAMPHENICOL

Adverse Effect	Frequency[a]	Clinical Comments
Increase in serum iron	1	Usually mild; reversible; dose related; may continue therapy
Reticulocytopenia	1	Usually mild; reversible; dose related; may continue therapy
Decrease in hemoglobin	1	Usually mild; reversible; dose related; may continue therapy
Thrombocytopenia	2	Usually mild; reversible; dose related; may continue therapy
Leukopenia	3	May be severe; reversible; dose related; may need to discontinue therapy in severe cases
Neutropenia	4	May be severe; reversible; dose related; may need to discontinue therapy in severe cases
Gray baby syndrome	5	May be fatal; related to concentration above 75 μg/mL; must discontinue therapy
Acidosis	5	May be severe; related to concentration above 30 μg/mL; may need to discontinue therapy in severe cases
Aplastic anemia	6	Often fatal; irreversible; not related to dose, route, and duration of therapy

[a] Frequency scale of 1 (most common) to 6 (least common) at usual dose.

the remaining three patients.[14] Cardiovascular collapse occurred in an anephric patient who received chloramphenicol succinate (0.8 g followed by 0.5 g every 6 hours). The serum concentration of chloramphenicol was 161 μg/mL 1 hour after the dose.[13]

The most common adverse effects of chloramphenicol after administration of recommended doses are leukopenia and anemia; some patients also develop thrombocytopenia, eosinophilia, and neutropenia. Recent studies have shown a lack of correlation between serum concentration and occurrence of these adverse effects.[7,21,22] There was a trend toward a higher cumulative dose in pediatric patients who developed toxic effects (1.2–1.8 g/kg) versus those who did not (0.9–1.1 g/kg), but the difference was not statistically significant.[21] Additional unknown factors (eg, concentration in the marrow or genetic factors) may predispose patients to these adverse effects.

THERAPEUTIC REGIMEN DESIGN

The role of therapeutic drug monitoring should be broader than monitoring serum concentration. It should include confirmation of appropriate drug, dose, dosage regimen, and method of drug administration and establishment of guidelines for monitoring serum drug concentrations, laboratory parameters, efficacy, adverse effects, drug–drug interactions, and cost of therapy (Table 12–4).

Chloramphenicol is effective when its C_{max} is between 10 and 20 μg/mL. Toxicity rarely occurs at a C_{max} below 30 μg/mL. Thus, an attempt should be made to keep C_{max} between 10 and 20 μg/mL, not to exceed 30 μg/mL. Although some have suggested that trough serum concentrations should be between 5 and 10 μg/mL,[23] no studies have found a correlation between

TABLE 12–4. DOSAGE REGIMENS OF CHLORAMPHENICOL

Type of Patients[a]	Dose[b]
Premature infants or newborn infants <2 wk of age	25 mg/kg/d
Infants (>2 wk–1 y), children, adolescents,[c] adults, elderly[c]	50 mg/kg/d

[a] The dose should be reduced in severe liver and kidney disease; cystic fibrosis patients with low pancreatic enzymes may require higher doses of chloramphenicol palmitate; maintenance doses should be individualized based on the serum concentration of chloramphenicol.
[b] Dose divided in four parts.
[c] Limited data exist about dose requirements.

trough concentration and efficacy or adverse effects. Little is known about the relationship between efficacy or adverse effects and AUC or about the length of time the serum concentration must exceed the MIC of chloramphenicol.

Sampling Times

As the efficacy and certain adverse effects of chloramphenicol are associated with its C_{max}, blood samples should be obtained at T_{max}. C_{max} appears to occur about 1 hour after oral chloramphenicol capsules, 1.5 to 3.0 hours after oral chloramphenicol palmitate suspension, and 0.5 to 1.5 hours after completion of a 20- to 30-minute intravenous infusion of chloramphenicol succinate.[3] Trough concentrations should be obtained at the end of the dosage interval, that is, just prior to the next dose.

Influence of Infusion Method on Drug Concentration

Studies have shown that the method of intravenous drug infusion can markedly influence the serum concentrations of chloramphenicol (Table 12–5). For example, injection of a dose into an intravenous tubing port closer to the patient and infusion at a faster rate of delivery lead to high serum concentrations of chloramphenicol.[24] This may result in unpredictable serum concentrations, particularly in infants and children who typically are infused at low flow rates to maintain a delicate fluid balance. Inaccurate serum concentrations may result in inappropriate pharmacokinetic calculations and, consequently, incorrect dosage recommendations.

Methods to Measure Serum Concentration

Although a variety of analytic methods have been used to measure chloramphenicol serum concentrations, two types of methods are used most frequently in clinical settings. The enzyme-mediated immunoassay technique (EMIT, Syva Company) is most suitable for routine measurement of chloramphenicol. It is rapid, reproducible, specific, and easy to use for the quantitation of chloramphenicol. It cannot, however, be used to measure the prodrug, chlorampheni-

TABLE 12–5. SIGNIFICANT DRUG INTERACTIONS WITH CHLORAMPHENICOL

Drug	Mechanism	Clinical Comment
Tolbutamide	Inhibition of tolbutamide metabolism by chloramphenicol	May need to decrease the dose of tolbutamide
Chlorpropamide	Inhibition of chlorpropamide metabolism by chloramphenicol	May need to decrease the dose of chlorpropamide
Warfarin	Inhibition of warfarin metabolism by chloramphenicol	May need to decrease the dose of warfarin
Phenobarbital	Stimulation of chloramphenicol metabolism by phenobartital	Monitor serum concentration of chloramphenicol; may need to increase the dose of chloramphenicol
Phenytoin	Stimulation of chloramphenicol metabolism by phenytoin, inhibition of phenytoin metabolism by chloramphenicol, or both	Monitor serum concentration of chloramphenicol and phenytoin; may need to adjust the dose of both
Rifampin	Stimulation of chloramphenicol metabolism by rifampin	Monitor serum concentration of chloramphenicol; may need to increase the dose of chloramphenicol

col succinate, or the metabolites of chloramphenicol. In such special situations or for research purposes, high-performance liquid chromatography (HPLC) should be used.[3]

Monitoring Hematologic Function

A complete blood count including differential and platelet count should be monitored at the start of therapy, after 1 week of therapy, and every 3 days thereafter during therapy to identify and prevent further toxicity.[3]

Repeat Measurement of Serum Concentration

Chloramphenicol serum concentration should be measured again if (1) liver or kidney (and gastrointestinal for oral therapy) function changes markedly; (2) the initial serum concentration is outside the therapeutic range; (3) the patient does not respond clinically or has a toxic reaction; and (4) interacting drugs such as phenobarbital, phenytoin, and rifampin are added to or eliminated from the regimen.

If the serum concentration is uninterpretable, measurement of chloramphenicol succinate concentrations can identify patients with abnormal hydrolysis to chloramphenicol. In some patients receiving the typical 10 to 14 days of therapy, the serum concentration of chloramphenicol may decline without alteration in dose.[25] Patients with extremely high serum concentrations can be treated with hemodialysis, charcoal column perfusion, or whole blood exchange transfusion.[3,26]

Estimation of Dosage Requirement

A method for estimating dosage requirements from a single serum concentration obtained 6 hours (C_{min}) after the initial intravenous dose has been proposed.[27] This approach has not, however, been tested in subsequent studies and requires exclusion of patients with low or changing clearance and those who are severely ill, for example, patients who are in shock or receiving vasoactive or interacting drugs. This can exclude a large number of patients.

Clearance is estimated by using the equation

$$\log Cl = -0.17 - 0.066\, C_{min} \tag{12-1}$$

where C_{min} is chloramphenicol serum concentration 6 hours after the initial intravenous dose. The dose is estimated as

$$\text{dose (mg/kg/d)} = C_{av,ss} \text{ (mg/L)} \times Cl \text{ (L/kg/h)} \times 24\text{ h} \tag{12-2}$$

where $C_{av,ss}$ is the desired mean steady-state serum concentration (15 µg/mL in most cases) and Cl is clearance.

Assuming a C_{min} of 5 µg/mL, Equation 12–1 will yield

$$\log Cl = -0.17 - 0.066 \times 5$$
$$\log Cl = -0.50$$
$$Cl = 0.316$$

Substituting this value of clearance in Equation 12–2 and assuming $C_{av,ss}$ is 15 µg/mL yields

$$\text{dose} = 15 \times 0.316 \times 24$$
$$= 113\text{ mg/kg/d}$$

In this example, the one-point method appears to suggest nearly twice the normally recommended doses for initial therapy. This method should be used with caution because it has not been validated following the original report in 20 infants and children.

────── QUESTIONS ──────────────────────────────

1. A 6-month-old infant is diagnosed with bacterial meningitis caused by *Haemophilus influenzae* type b. The patient has a documented history of severe allergic reactions to penicillin and cephalosporin. What should be recommended, and how should therapy be monitored?

2. A seriously ill patient is receiving chloramphenicol succinate by infusion. Blood samples are obtained 1 hour after infusion and at the end of the dosage interval. C_{max} and C_{min} are 15 and 10 µg/mL, respectively. No liver or renal disease is present. What can explain the small decline in serum concentration over a 6-hour period?

3. A decision is made to add chloramphenicol to the antibiotic regimen in an adult patient with cystic fibrosis. What should be recommended?

4. A patient with brain abscess is being treated with chloramphenicol succinate. Phenobarbital is added to the regimen for seizure control. What would be its effect on chloramphenicol serum concentrations, and how should the therapy be monitored?

REFERENCES

1. Feigin RD, Cherry JD. *Textbook of Pediatric Infectious Diseases*. Philadelphia: WB Saunders; 1981.
2. Chloramphenicol. In: *AHFS Drug Information*. Bethesda, MD: American Society of Hospital Pharmacists; 1991:191–194.
3. Nahata MC. Chloramphenicol. In Evans WE, Schentag JJ, Jusko WJ, eds. *Applied Pharmacokinetics*. 3rd ed. Spokane, WA: Applied Therapeutics: 1991.
4. Chloromycetin Kapscals. In: *Physicians' Desk Reference*. 45th cd. Oradcll, NJ: Mcdical Economics Company; 1991:1627–1628.
5. Shankaran S, Kauffman RE. Use of chloramphenicol palmitate in neonates. *J Pediatr.* 1984;105:113–116.
6. Glazko AJ, Bill WA, Kinke AW, et al. Absorption and excretion of parenteral doses of chloramphenicol sodium succinate (CMS) in comparison with peroral doses of chloramphenicol (CM). *Clin Pharmacol Ther.* 1977;21:104. Abstract.
7. Roy TE, Krieger E, Craig G et al. Studies on the absorption of chloramphenicol in normal children in relation to the treatment of meningitis. *Antibiot Chemother.* 1952;11:505–516.
8. Kauffman RE, Thirumoorthi MC, Buckley JA, et al. Relative bioavailability of intravenous chloramphenicol succinate and oral chloramphenicol palmitate in infants and children. *J Pediatr.* 1981;99:963–967.
9. Dickinson CJ, Reed MD, Stern RC, et al. The effect of exocrine pancreatic function on chloramphenicol pharmacokinetics in patients with cystic fibrosis. *Pediatr Res.* 1988;23:388–392.
10. Nahata MC, Powell DA. Comparative bioavailability and pharmacokinetics of chloramphenicol after intravenous chloramphenicol succinate in premature infants and older patients. *Dev Pharmacol Ther.* 1983;6:23–32.
11. Koup JR, Lau AH, Bodsky B, et al. Chloramphenicol pharmacokinetics in hospitalized patients. *Antimicrob Agents Chemother.* 1979;15:651–657.
12. Slaughter RL, Pieper JA, Cerra FB, et al. Chloramphenicol succinate kinetics in critically ill patients. *Clin Pharmacol Ther.* 1980;28:69–77.
13. Phelps SJ, Tsiu W, Barrett FF, et al. Chloramphenicol-induced cardiovascular collapse in an anephric patient. *Pediatr Infect Dis J.* 1987;6:285–288.
14. Evans LS, Kleiman MB. Acidosis as a presenting feature of chloramphenicol toxicity. *J Pediatr.* 1986;108:475–477.
15. Nahata MC, Powell DA. Bioavailability and clearance of chloramphenicol after intravenous chloramphenicol succinate. *Clin Pharmacol Ther.* 1981;30:368–372.
16. Sack CM, Koup JR, Opheim KE, et al. Chloramphenicol succinate kinetics in infants and young children. *Pediatr Pharmacol.* 1982;2:93.
17. Burckart GJ, Barrett FF, Straugh AB, et al. Chloramphenicol clearance in infants. *J Clin Pharmacol.* 1982;22:49–52.
18. Sack CM, Koup JR, Smith AL. Chloramphenicol pharmacokinetics in infants and young children. *Pediatrics.* 1980;66:579–584.
19. Burke JT, Wargin WA, Sherertz RJ, et al. Pharmacokinetics of intravenous chloramphenicol sodium

succinate in adult patients with normal renal and hepatic function. *J Pharmacokinet Biopharm.* 1982;10:601–614.

20. Burns LE, Hodgman JE, Cass AB. Fatal circulatory collapse in premature infants receiving chloramphenicol. *N Engl J Med.* 1959;261:1318–1321.

21. Nahata MC. Lack of predictability of chloramphenicol toxicity in pediatric patients. *J Clin Pharm Ther.* 1989;14:297–303.

22. Sherry B, Smith AL, Kronmal RA. Anemia during *Haemophilus influenzae* type b meningitis: Lack of an effect of chloramphenicol. *Dev Pharmacol Ther.* 1989;12:188–189.

23. Ristuccia AM. Chloramphenicol: Clinical pharmacology in pediatrics. *Ther Drug Monit.* 1985;7:159–167.

24. Nahata MC, Powell DA, Glazer JP, Hilty M. Effect of intravenous flow rate and injection site on *in vitro* delivery of chloramphenicol succinate and in vivo kinetics. *J Pediatr.* 1981;99:463–466.

25. Nahata MC, Powell DA. Chloramphenicol serum concentration falls during chloramphenicol succinate dosing. *Clin Pharmacol Ther.* 1983;33:308–313.

26. Slaughter RL, Cerra FB, Koup JR. Effect of hemodialysis on total body clearance of chloramphenicol. *Am J Hosp Pharm.* 1980;37:1083–1086.

27. Koup JR, Sack CM, Smith AL, et al. Rapid estimation of chloramphenicol clearance in infants and children. *Clin Pharmacokinet.* 1981;6:83–88.

Chapter 13

Cyclic Antidepressants

Gregory B. Toney
Larry Ereshefsky

Keep in Mind

- Imipramine, desipramine, nortriptyline, and perhaps amitriptyline have well-established therapeutic ranges. Additionally, evidence for plasma concentration-versus-response relationships for clomipramine and bupropion appears clinically useful. Obtaining plasma concentrations of other antidepressants has little to no value for therapeutic drug monitoring at this time.

- To judge the effectiveness of an antidepressant in an individual patient, the patient must receive adequate doses (or therapeutic plasma concentrations) for a minimum of 2 to 4 weeks. The most common reason for failure of antidepressant therapy is inadequate dose or inadequate length of clinical trial.

- If a dosage formulation is switched in a stabilized patient (ie, brand to generic), obtain a plasma concentration prior to the switch. This would be helpful for dose adjustment, if necessary, because of possible differences in bioavailability (useful for any of the cyclic depressants).

- Oral and systemic clearance of cyclic antidepressants may be decreased in the elderly, who may be more sensitive to adverse effects and, thus, may require lower than usual dose ranges.

- Children have increased metabolic rates, leading to shorter elimination half-lives. Children require divided daily doses rather than once-daily dosing. Once adolescence is reached, the pharmacokinetic profile begins to resemble that seen in adults.

- Dose ranges for cyclic antidepressants should be reduced in hepatic impairment, although dose adjustments are not routinely required in renal impairment.

- In cardiac disease, decreases in cardiac output may require decreased doses of many cyclic antidepressants. Tricyclic antidepressants are not recommended in patients with baseline corrected QT intervals greater than 450 milliseconds.

- Demethylated active metabolites are routinely monitored along with the parent compound. Monitoring of hydroxymetabolites adds little value to therapeutic drug monitoring at this time.

- Drugs that inhibit or induce the cytochrome P450 system, particularly the P450IID6 isozyme system, are the most common drugs that interact significantly with cyclic antidepressants. Displacement from protein binding sites rarely causes significant interactions in the majority of patients.

- Approximately 5 to 10% of the population have the slow hydroxylater phenotype and may show increased plasma concentrations and longer elimination half-lives of tertiary and secondary amines; however, rapid hydroxylators may be more likely to exhibit nonlinear kinetics with these cyclic antidepressants. Patients with the most rapid clearance at lower doses may be the most likely to show nonlinear kinetics.

- Prospective dosing techniques are best used in medically compromised patients, in whom an extremely long elimination half-life might be expected, or in other metabolically distinct populations such as the elderly, children, and slow hydroxylators.

- Standardized collection techniques will yield the most consistent and valid therapeutic drug monitoring results. Radioimmunoassay and enzyme immunoassay are adequate for clinical application but more sophisticated chromatographic techniques are required for research. HPLC represents the best compromise between the two situations.

Methods for analytic measurement of cyclic antidepressants (CADs) have been developed since the early 1960s. Today, therapeutic drug monitoring (TDM) programs are an important part of the clinical management of antidepressant therapy. For TDM programs for CADs to be optimally designed and executed, a basic knowledge of the pharmacokinetic characteristics of CADs is necessary. Policies and procedures used for plasma sample timing, handling, storage, and assay should be designed with the pharmacokinetic characteristics of CADs in mind to increase the accuracy, validity, and clinical utility of TDM results.

The clinical utility of TDM for CADs is well documented. The American Psychiatric Association Task Force on the Use of Laboratory Tests in Psychiatry[1] recommended the clinical use of antidepressant plasma concentrations (C_p) for imipramine (IMI), desipramine (DMI), and nortriptyline (NT), all of which have well-established therapeutic ranges. Plasma CAD concentrations are particularly useful in certain clinical situations such as the nonresponding patient, where noncompliance is suspected, in patients with cardiovascular disease, where significant drug interactions may occur, when significant side effects occur, in overdose situations, and for special populations such as the elderly or children and adolescents. Monitoring of plasma CAD concentrations is also important in research attempting to establish plasma concentration–therapeutic response relationships for various CADs, that is, establishing a therapeutic range for an antidepressant.

CLINICAL PHARMACOLOGY AND THERAPEUTICS

Cyclic antidepressants are used to treat several psychiatric disorders including major depression, panic disorder, generalized anxiety disorder, obsessive–compulsive disorder (OCD), eating disorders, attention deficit hyperactivity disorder (ADHD), and enuresis in children. The pharmacologic action of CADs and the observed latency of response for specific psychiatric disorders provide clues to the underlying therapeutic actions of CADs.

The primary pharmacologic effect of CADs is blockade of high-affinity reuptake mechanisms in norepinephrine (NE), serotonin (5HT), and dopamine (DA) neurons. The degree of specificity for one neurotransmitter system over another varies for each CAD (Table 13–1). In general, effects of tertiary amine tricyclic antidepressants (TCAs) are more balanced between

TABLE 13–1. RELATIVE EFFECTS ON NEUROTRANSMITTER REUPTAKE BLOCKADE

Antidepressants	Reuptake Inhibition		
	NE	5HT	DA
Tricyclic Agents			
Tertiary Amines			
Doxepin	+	++	−
Amitriptyline	++	++	−
Imipramine	+++	++	−
Trimipramine	++	+	−
Clomipramine	++	++++	−
Secondary Amines			
Protriptyline	+++	++	−
Nortriptyline	+++	++	−
Desipramine	++++	+	−
Other Cyclic Agents			
Amoxapine	+++	++	−
Bupropion	+	−	+
Maprotiline	+++	+	−
Trazodone	−	++	−
Venlafaxine	+++	++++	+
Selective Serotonin Reuptake Inhibitors			
Fluoxetine	−	++++	−
Sertraline	−	+++++	−
Fluvoxamine	−	++++	−
Paroxetine	−	+++++	−

Adapted from Bryant SG, Brown CS. Major depression. In: Young LY, Koda-Kimble MA, eds. Applied Therapeutics: The Clinical Use of Drugs. *4th ed. Spokane, WA: Applied Therapeutics; 1988:1231—1254, with permission.*

NE and 5HT, with the exception of clomipramine (CMI), which predominantly blocks 5HT reuptake compared with NE. The secondary amines tend to be more specific for NE than 5HT. The exact mechanism of action of bupropion is unclear, although it is thought to be linked to its weak reuptake blocking activity in NE and DA neurons. A relatively new class of antidepressants, the selective serotonin reuptake inhibitors (SSRIs), have high affinity for blockade of 5HT reuptake sites, with little or no effect on NE or DA reuptake. Recently, venlafaxine, a non-TCA antidepressant with potent 5HT and NE reuptake blocking activity, has become available.

Acute administration of CADs results in increased concentrations of NE, 5HT, and DA in the neuronal synapse. This effect was once believed to be responsible for the antidepressant activity of CADs and resulted in the monoamine deficiency hypothesis of depression; however, neurotransmitter concentrations are increased immediately and resolution of depressive symptoms requires 4 to 6 weeks of chronic dosing. Subsequent neuropharmacologic studies have shown delayed effects of CADs on receptor binding and second messenger systems. The time course of these changes corresponds much more closely to the latency of response seen in depression.

Chronic CAD administration has generally been associated with a decrease in beta-adrenergic receptor density[2,3] although not all CADs have been associated with beta-adrenergic receptor downregulation.[2,4–6] A decrease in serotonin type 2 (5HT-2) receptor density also appears to be a consistent finding following chronic CAD dosing.[7] Consistent changes in alpha-1- or alpha-2-adrenergic receptors have not been observed across studies.[2,8–11] Chronic CAD administration does lead to functional changes in neuronal second messenger systems, specifically a decrease in NE-stimulated cAMP production.[2–4] Functional changes in second messenger systems are not always correlated with changes in receptor density. Mianserin, an atypical antidepressant, decreases NE-stimulated cAMP production without decreasing beta-adrenergic receptor density.[2,4,12] This suggests that the ultimate therapeutic effect of antidepressants is decreased sensitivity of the beta-adrenergic system. CADs may restore the efficiency of neurotransmission in the noradrenergic system and thereby restabilize the noradrenergic system within its normal homeostatic range. This view is currently the most accepted hypothesis of depression, called the *dysregulation hypothesis.*[13] This hypothesis may be useful in explaining the underlying neural mechanisms in other psychiatric illness as well. The dysregulation hypothesis states that neuronal regulatory mechanisms normally act to maintain homeostasis of CNS functioning. If these regulatory mechanisms are impaired, CNS functioning can occasionally fall outside the normal homeostatic range and normal functioning cannot be reestablished. The end result of this malfunctioning is seen as symptoms of psychiatric illness. The specific neuronal pathways or areas of the brain that are affected determine the specific symptoms exhibited and, therefore, the type of psychiatric illness.

In addition to depression, CADs are useful in other psychiatric disorders. In some disorders the response latency is much shorter and suggests a different underlying therapeutic effect. For example, response latency to CADs in ADHD is much shorter, occurring in hours to days. This suggests that the therapeutic effect of CADs in ADHD is related to increased neurotransmitter concentrations in DA and NE pathways after acute dosing, rather than receptor changes induced by chronic dosing. OCD has been shown to respond to antidepressant agents with potent 5HT reuptake blockade, such as CMI, fluoxetine (FLX), and other SSRIs. The latency to maximum therapeutic response is delayed compared with major depression; usually approximately 8 to 12 weeks of treatment is required for maximal effect. This suggests a different mechanism of therapeutic effect, which has not been determined at this time.

The pharmacologic effects of binding to receptor systems other than NE, 5HT, and DA reuptake sites are primarily adverse effects rather than therapeutic effects. Newer CADs, such as the selective 5HT reuptake blockers, exhibit limited binding to other receptor systems compared with TCAs and, therefore, exhibit an improved adverse effect profile. TCAs possess clinically significant binding to cholinergic, histaminic, and alpha-1-adrenergic receptors. Anticholinergic activity of TCAs produces dry mouth, blurring of vision, constipation, urinary retention, and decreased sweating. At higher TCA concentrations, anticholinergic delirium can occur (see Concentration and Toxicity). TCAs bind to both H_1 and H_2 histamine receptors. Binding to the H_1 receptor is more clinically important, associated with sedation produced by TCAs. TCAs can also bind to alpha-1-adrenergic receptors and produce cardiovascular effects such as postural hypotension, which can lead to dizziness and reflex tachycardia.

TCAs and their metabolites can also produce adverse effects by acting directly on cardiac tissue. TCAs produce cardiac effects similar to those elicited by class IA antiarrhythmics. The most common effect is prolongation of cardiac conduction. TCAs, at or just above therapeutic plasma concentrations, can prolong PR and QRS intervals above baseline values. Patients with preexisting cardiac conduction abnormalities may be at increased risk of developing atrioventricular (AV) heart block with TCA treatment.[14] Also, prolongation of QRS or corrected QT (QT_c) interval can cause ventricular arrhythmias including Torsade de pointes. It is generally recommended that use of TCAs be avoided in patients with baseline QT_c intervals greater than approximately 450 milliseconds. TCAs may occasionally be used in nondepressed cardiac patients. IMI and NT have been shown to suppress premature ventricular contractions (PVCs) and complex features, such as bigeminy, trigeminy, and ventricular tachycardia.

Tricyclic antidepressants do not appear to affect cardiac output significantly in patients with moderate to severe impairment of left ventricular function.[15-18] Some TCAs may be less likely to produce clinically observable effects in this population. NT appears to produce a lower incidence of intolerable orthostatic hypotension in patients with moderate to severe left ventricular impairment compared to IMI.[16,18,19]

CLINICAL PHARMACOKINETICS

The pharmacokinetic parameters of CADs are summarized in Table 13–2.

Dosage Forms

All CADs are available in solid oral dosage forms, either tablets or capsules. Doxepin (DOX), NT, and FLX are also available in oral solution form. Parenteral dosage forms are available for amitriptyline (AMI) and IMI.

There is some evidence suggesting that significant intraindividual differences in bioavailability (*F*) and absorption rate may occur in some individuals between generic and brand name drug formulations.[20] Significant differences in bioavailability between formulations could translate clinically into loss of therapeutic effect, through decreases in plasma CAD concentration, or toxic effects, through increases in plasma CAD concentration. Changes in therapeutic effect or adverse effects have been reported when changing from brand to generic dosage forms of DMI.[21,22] Obtaining plasma CAD concentrations may be prudent when making dosage form changes, so that if significant changes in plasma CAD concentration do occur, the oral dose can be adjusted to attain the previous plasma CAD concentration. This may be especially important in patients in whom therapeutic effect is difficult to attain or in populations at risk for adverse effects.

TABLE 13–2. PHARMACOKINETIC PROPERTIES OF CYCLIC ANTIDEPRESSANTS

Antidepressant	Bioavailability (%)	Unbound Fraction (%)	Volume of Distribution[a] (L/kg)	Clearance[b]	Half-life[c] (h)
Amitriptyline	30–60	3–15	6.4–36	19–72	9–46
Bupropion	>90	20	27–63	126–140	9.6–20.9
Clomipramine	36–62	2–10	9–25	23–122	15–62
Desipramine	33–51	8–27	24–60	78–168	12–28
Doxepin	13–45	15–32	9–33	41–61	8–25
Fluoxetine	70–80	6	12–42	5.6–42	26–220
Fluvoxamine	NA[d]	23	>5	NA	13–19
Imipramine	22–77	4–37	9.3–23	32–102	6–28
Maprotiline	79–87	12	16–32	17–34	27–50
Nortriptyline	46–70	7–13	15–23	17–79	18–56
Paroxetine	~50	5	3–28	15–92	10–16
Protriptyline	75–90	6–10	15–31	8.4–23.4	54–118
Sertraline	≥44	>3	25[d]	96	26
Trimipramine	18–63	3–7	17–48	40–105	16–40
Venlafaxine	NA	71–75	4–11	58–112	3–7

[a] In steady state or in slowest phase of elimination.
[b] Plasma clearance.
[c] Biologic half-life in slowest phase of elimination.
[d] Not available.
[e] Data from animal studies.

Adapted from DeVane CL. Cyclic antidepressants. In: Evans WE, Schentag JJ, Jusko WJ, eds. Applied Pharmacokinetics: Principles of Therapeutic Drug Monitoring 2nd ed. Spokane, WA: Applied Therapeutics; 1986:852–907, with permission.

Absorption

The CADs are basic lipophilic compounds that are mostly ionized in the acidic medium of the stomach. Because of this, very little absorption occurs until the drug enters the more basic environment of the small intestine. Once in the intestines, absorption is almost complete for all CADs except maprotiline.[23] The absorption rate of most TCAs is relatively rapid, with maximum plasma concentration (C_{max}) occurring 2 to 8 hours after single or multiple dosing.[24,25] Bupropion, trazodone, and venlafaxine are rapidly absorbed, with C_{max} occurring within 1 to 4 hours.[26–28] Other CADs are more slowly absorbed. Maprotiline, a strong base with a pK_a of 10.5, is almost completely protonated at physiologic pH and crosses lipophilic membranes relatively slowly, C_{max} occurring at approximately 8 hours.[29] Protriptyline is also slowly absorbed, with C_{max} occurring between 6 and 12 hours (mean, 8.5 hours).[30] All SSRIs have similar absorption rates, with average C_{max} occurring at approximately 5 to 8 hours.[31–33]

It is believed that food has little effect on absorption of most CADs. Food does not change the bioavailability, C_{max}, or T_{max} of IMI.[34] Food can delay the absorption of trazodone, with decreased C_{max} but no effect on area under curve (AUC).[27] Food delays the absorption of FLX by approximately 3.5 hours but has no effect on AUC.[31] Increased bioavailability has been observed when sertraline is given with food, with a 32% increase in C_{max} and 39% increase in AUC.[32]

As absorption is considered to be complete for the CADs, the "first-pass" effect is responsible for most of the drug that does not reach systemic circulation.[35] The large first-pass effect results in a low systemic F for most CADs, with values ranging from 0.20 to 0.70. Exceptions to the characteristic low F are maprotiline, protriptyline, and FLX, with F values of 0.70 to 0.90, and bupropion, with F greater than 0.90.[36] Because a large proportion of an administered dose is eliminated during first-pass metabolism for many CADs, changes in the extent or rate of metabolism of CADs can significantly affect the resultant C_{max} and clearance. The extraction ratio (E) of these compounds can be useful in understanding the effects of changes in observed C_{ps} seen during drug–drug interaction or concomitant medical illnesses. E is defined as $1 - F$ and is a measure of the efficiency of drug clearance by the liver. Most CADs have intermediate E values (0.3–0.7). For these drugs, changes in either hepatic blood flow (Q) or intrinsic hepatic clearance (Cl_{int}) may result in alterations in hepatic clearance (Cl_H). For most CADs, concomitant enzyme inducers will lower plasma CAD concentrations and increase dose requirements, whereas concomitant enzyme inhibitors will have the opposite effect. Also important are changes in hepatic blood flow, where decreased cardiac output, with resultant decrease in Q, may increase plasma CAD concentrations and decrease dose requirements. Maprotiline, protriptyline, and bupropion are exceptions because of their high F values of 0.75 to 0.90, with resultant low E values of 0.10 to 0.25. The clearance of these drugs should be affected significantly by hepatic enzyme inducers or inhibitors but very little by alterations in hepatic blood flow.

Distribution

Cyclic antidepressants have high lipid solubility and are extensively distributed in the body tissue. The range of octanol:water partition coefficients for most CADs is approximately 10^3 to 10^5.[36] The volume of distribution (V_d) is relatively large for CADs and exhibits high interindividual variation. Volume of distribution V_d ranges from 3 to 63 L/kg for the various compounds[36] (see Table 13–2). The highest concentrations of IMI are found in lung, kidney, brain, small intestine, liver, skeletal muscle and skin; the lowest concentrations are in plasma and adipose tissue.[37] As there appear to be a relatively low TCA concentrations in adipose tissue, obesity may not result in significant alterations in volume of distribution compared with nonobese patients. All other factors being equal, this means that doses for obese and nonobese patients may not differ significantly.

Metabolism and Excretion

Clearance of CADs is almost entirely by hepatic metabolism, illustrated by less than 5% of an administered dose of IMI being excreted unchanged in the urine.[38] The major metabolic pathways of TCAs are demethylation and hydroxylation with subsequent glucuronide conjugation. Minor pathways include N-oxidation and dealkylation. TCAs are metabolized by ring hydroxylation of the parent compound or N-demethylation of the side chain followed by ring hydroxylation. Following ring hydroxylation, glucuronide conjugation occurs, leading to elimination in the urine or bile. There is some evidence that biliary enterohepatic recirculation occurs with these compounds.[39] The major pathways of IMI, the most extensively studied TCA, are shown in Figure 13–1. Metabolism of IMI involves demethylation to form its active metabolite, DMI, and then hydroxylation to form 2-OH-DMI. Alternatively, IMI can be hydroxylated to 2-OH-IMI. Both 2-OH-IMI and 2-OH-DMI are conjugated and eliminated as the respective glucuronides. Other TCAs are eliminated similarly with some variations.

Non-TCA CADs also undergo extensive hepatic metabolism. Amoxapine is hydroxylated to form 7-OH-amoxapine (with antipsychotic properties) and 8-OH-amoxapine (with antidepressant properties), both of which may be further conjugated and eliminated in the urine.[36] Trazodone undergoes hydroxylation and N-oxidation, with production of an active metabolite, *m*-chlorophenylpiperazine, and an inactive propionic acid derivative, which accounts for approximately 20% of the dose.[36] Bupropion, a monocyclic antidepressant, is metabolized by side-chain oxidation to acidic metabolites or to basic *erythro*-amino alcohol, *threo*-amino alcohol, and an active hydroxy metabolite.[36] Maprotiline is demethylated to its principal desmethyl metabolite. Both this and the parent compound can be further metabolized through multiple minor pathways such as aromatic hydroxylation and oxidation of the side chain.[36] FLX can undergo demethylation to an active metabolite, norfluoxetine. Glucuronide conjugates of both FLX and norfluoxetine are recovered in the urine, as is another metabolite, hippuric acid.[31] Sertraline is also demethylated to a partially active metabolite, desmethylsertraline, possessing 20% of the potency of the parent compound.[32] Appearance of conjugates of sertraline or desmethylsertraline has not been reported. Paroxetine is metabolized to a catachol intermediate and then is in part demethylated and conjugated to a glucuronide or sulfate.[40] Fluvoxamine undergoes primarily oxidative demethylation, producing approximately 65% of metabolites. Lesser proportions of metabolites are produced by degradation at amino or methoxy groups or removal of the entire ethanolamine group.[41] None of the metabolites of paroxetine or fluvoxamine is thought to be active. Venlafaxine is demethylated to form its major active metabolite, *O*-desmethylvenlafaxine, and two minor metabolites, *N*-desmethylvenlafaxine and *N,O*-didesmethylvenlafaxine. A small amount of venlafaxine (1–10%) and all its metabolites are excreted renally.[28]

The cytochrome P450 mixed-function oxidase system catalyzes the major metabolic path-

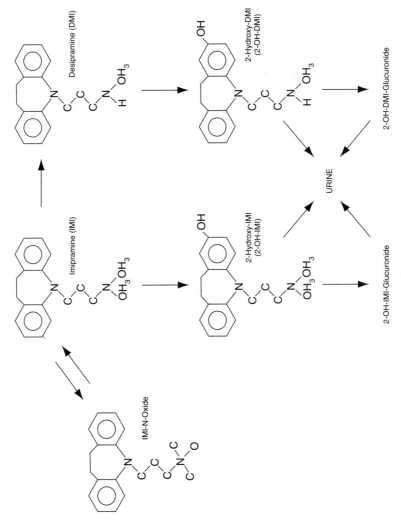

Figure 13–1. Major metabolic pathways of imipramine.

ways of CADs. The P450 system is composed of several distinct isoenzyme subfamilies which are responsible for catalyzing the different metabolic reactions on various substrates. Recent evidence suggests that major demethylation pathways of IMI, and presumably other TCAs, are catalyzed by P450IA and P450IIIA isoenzyme systems.[42] The major hydroxylation pathways of many TCAs are catalyzed by the cytochrome P450IID6 isoenzyme system. The P450IID6 isoenzyme system is the most extensively studied of all the cytochrome P450 subfamilies. Several widely used drugs have been identified as having high affinity for the P450IID6 system and, therefore, can frequently present situations for significant drug interactions (see Drug–Drug Interactions). Additionally, genetic polymorphism is a predominate feature of the P450IID6 system and can therefore be a source of significant interindividual variation in metabolic rates (see Pharmacogenetics). Metabolism through alternative minor pathways may be increased when the major metabolic pathway is compromised, such as with drug–drug interactions or when these enzymes are deficient because of genetic factors.

Special Populations

Geriatrics

Age-related changes in drug metabolism and excretion can be significant, especially for drugs with a low therapeutic index. TDM can be especially important in the elderly because not all patients show the same degree of age-related changes, leading to a high degree of variability in this population.[43] Decreased metabolic capacity of the liver and decreased hepatic blood flow can decrease the clearance of CADs, possibly leading to increased side effects and toxicity. Decreases in renal clearance of unconjugated hydroxy metabolites can lead to their accumulation with chronic dosing. This may be significant, as some of these metabolites are thought to possibly contribute to toxicity.[1]

Not all metabolic pathways for CADs may be equally affected by aging. Several single dose and chronic dosing studies have shown decreased clearance and/or increased plasma concentrations of tertiary amines AMI, IMI, CMI, and DOX in elderly patients.[43–51] Other studies have suggested that other mechanisms, such as changes in the volume of distribution, may be responsible for differences in observed clearance and resultant plasma concentrations.[52] Effects of aging on clearance of secondary amine CADs is less well demonstrated. Some studies on NT and DMI have not found any significant effect of increasing age on clearance,[53–56] whereas fewer have shown a significant decrease in clearance.[48] In one study, the half-life of DMI was found to be slightly decreased in elderly men only and no significant decrease in oral clearance of DMI was observed.[51] The weight of the evidence suggests that demethylation, the primary step in the metabolism of tertiary amines, may be more impaired than hydroxylation, the primary step in the metabolism of secondary amines, with increasing age. This difference is illustrated in a study where IMI, DMI, and their hydroxy metabolites were evaluated following IMI administration. Only IMI:DMI ratios and not IMI:OH-IMI or DMI:OH-DMI ratios differed between young and elderly patients, suggesting an impairment in demethylation and not hydroxylation.[51] As hydroxylation for many TCAs is controlled by the P450IID6 system, this suggests that the P450IID6 system may be less affected by aging. Employing lower target dose ranges may be more important when using tertiary amines, such as IMI, AMI, and DOX, in the elderly compared with secondary amines, such as DMI, NT, and protriptyline.

Decreased renal flow and reduced glomerular filtration with increasing age can result in accumulation of hydroxy metabolites. Elevations of OH-DMI and OH-NT levels following chronic dosing have been observed in elderly patients.[57–60] Although these metabolites do accumulate in elderly patients, the clinical significance is unclear. CAD doses are not adjusted routinely in the elderly because of hydroxy metabolite accumulation unless clinically indicated by occurrence of adverse effects.

Pediatrics

Differences in the pharmacokinetics of CADs in pediatric patients are less well defined because of the small number of studies conducted to date. Drug distribution into deep tissue stores may be altered in children because of a higher proportion of lean body mass to fatty tissue compared with adults.[61] Children also have an increased hepatic surface area-to-body weight ratio. During late infancy and childhood, the hepatic metabolic rate for many drugs is higher than in adults. Clinically, this means that divided daily doses rather than once-daily doses are required in children to minimize peak-to-trough fluctuations in plasma concentration. Because of relatively rapid and individualized rates of somatic maturation, children may display a wider interindividual variation in elimination rate than adults, increasing the need of TDM to optimize dose titration. Extent of protein binding also differs in children. A higher unbound fraction (f_u) of IMI has been observed in neonates compared with adults (26% versus 14%). Seven- to ten-year-olds show values intermediate between those of neonates and adults.[62] A higher f_u may explain why a lower therapeutic range for IMI (125–250 ng/mL) appears sufficient for children.

Hepatic Disease

Surprisingly little literature exists on the effect of hepatic disease on CADs. A significant effect of hepatic disease on the disposition of CADs is expected, as the major route of elimination for CADs is by hepatic metabolism. Hepatic disease has been noted to have an effect on the P450 isoenzyme subfamilies that are implicated in CAD metabolism. P450IA2 enzymes were found to be decreased in cirrhosis but not in hepatocellular carcinoma. Although P450IIIA enzymes have been shown to have only a nonsignificant trend toward diminished levels in cirrhosis, there are reports in patient with cirrhosis of altered clearance of drugs known to be substrates for P450IIIA.[63,64] The effect of cirrhosis on P450IID6 enzymes is not determined at this time.

Alterations in clearance and resultant plasma concentrations may be expected in the clinical setting. The large first-pass effect exhibited by most CADs may be significantly reduced, resulting in increased bioavailability characterized by increased C_{max} and AUC. In addition, the elimination half-life of CADs can be significantly prolonged. Both of these effects indicate that lowering of the usual dose range of CADs is recommended in hepatic dysfunction.

Renal Disease

Studies of CADs in chronic renal failure and hemodialysis patients have shown no effect on disposition of parent compounds and demethylated metabolites, whereas renally eliminated conjugated and unconjugated hydroxy metabolites can be markedly elevated in these patients.[65,66] Although there is limited evidence that hydroxy metabolites contributes to pharmacologic effect or toxicity, most manufacturers recommend starting with lower doses of CADs in individuals with significant renal impairment for general safety reasons. In hemodialysis patients, where renally eliminated metabolites will be removed during the dialysis procedure, additional dose adjustments are not generally needed. An exception to this is venlafaxine, where dose reductions of 25% are recommended for mild to moderate renal impairment and a 50% reduction is recommended in severe renal impairment and in hemodialysis patients.

Cardiovascular Disease

Significant decreases in cardiac output, resulting in decreased hepatic blood flow, can potentially increase the bioavailability of CADs, with intermediate E values of 0.3 to 0.7. In patients with congestive heart failure or other causes of decreased left ventricular function, dose reductions may be required because of increased bioavailability to achieve desired steady state plasma concentrations. Exceptions are maprotiline, protriptyline, and bupropion, which have low E values of 0.1 to 0.25. Decreases in cardiac output should have little effect on the disposition of these CADs. Therefore, dose adjustment for this reason should not be necessary with CADs with low E values.

Nonlinear Pharmacokinetics

Reports of nonlinear pharmacokinetics in some patients have implications for dosing adjustments based on steady-state plasma concentrations (C_{ss}) and for prospective dosing methods. If a nonlinear pharmacokinetic profile occurs in a patient, disproportionately greater increases can be seen in steady-state plasma concentration following a dosage increase. The occurrence of apparent nonlinear kinetics has been best documented with DMI and IMI. In one case, a 300% increase in the DMI C_p value was observed following a 69% increase in dose.[67] In another case, a 14-fold increase in the DMI C_p value following a threefold increase in DMI dose was reported.[68] Nonlinear kinetic behavior has also been observed with desmethyltrimipramine following increasing doses of trimipramine.[69] Although evidence for nonlinear kinetic behavior is more limited for AMI and NT, nonlinearity could also be anticipated for these compounds. FLX has shown limited nonlinear kinetics by an observed increase in elimination half-life from approximately 2 to 4 days following long-term administration.[70]

Nonlinear kinetic behavior of IMI and DMI has been associated with extensive metabolizers of sparteine[71] (see Pharmacogenetics). In this study, one third of subjects showed disproportionate increases in IMI plus DMI C_p values of 50% or greater above predicted values following dose increases. These subjects had the lowest plasma concentrations on an initial low dose of IMI and all of these subjects were rapid metabolizers of sparteine. Similar findings were observed in a study of nonlinearity of DMI.[72] In both of these studies, nonlinear changes occurred at doses of IMI and DMI within the usual dosing range. Other studies have also found nonlinear changes in IMI and DMI within the usual dosing range.[73–75] These data indicate that rapid hydroxylators are more likely to show nonlinear kinetics. It is possible these patients have baseline hydroxylation rates that are already close to capacity, exhibiting relatively low K_m and V_{max}, and thus hydroxylation enzyme systems are easily saturated. This is supported by a study of IMI and DMI metabolism in rats that revealed that 2-hydroxylation of IMI and DMI is mediated by a high-affinity, low-capacity (saturable) enzyme system, whereas N-demethylation of IMI is mediated by a low-affinity, high-capacity (nonsaturable) enzyme system.[76] There is one case report of nonlinear changes in DMI clearance in a slow hydroxylator following overdose.[77] The significance of these data is unclear because possible alterations in clearance have not been systematically studied in overdose. P450IID6 enzymes, which catalyze metabolism of DMI, may be expected to become saturated in overdose situations regardless of hydroxylator status.

It has been estimated that approximately one third of patients may show clinically significant nonlinear increases in plasma DMI concentrations with increasing doses of DMI and IMI.[71,72] Doses within the normal therapeutic dosing range, greater than 150 mg/d for DMI and 125 to 300 mg/day for IMI, have been implicated in nonlinear kinetic behavior. These implicated dose ranges may explain why less evidence exists for nonlinear kinetics with NT, as the upper end of the normal dosing range for NT is 150 mg/d because of its lower therapeutic range.

Identification of predictive factors for patients likely to show nonlinear kinetics would be helpful to limit the potential for producing toxicity. Phenotyping for hydroxylator status (see Pharmacogenetics) may be useful in identifying individuals who are more likely to exhibit nonlinear kinetics. Significant nonlinear kinetics have been observed more commonly in the elderly, in rapid hydroxylators, and with concomitant administration of drugs that undergo hydroxylation. In the clinical setting, careful monitoring of elderly patients, patients with unusually low plasma CAD concentrations at low doses, and patients with drug–drug interactions would be indicated.

Pharmacogenetics

Underlying genetic factors can also result in significant differences in metabolism of CADs between patients. Genetic polymorphism for metabolism of CADs has been characterized by deficiency of specific enzymes in the cytochrome P450 system. Various compounds can be used as probes to detect differences in metabolism under polymorphic genetic control or deficiencies in metabolic enzymes. Debrisoquine, a peripheral-acting monoamine oxidase inhibitor, produces a hydroxylated metabolite via the cytochrome P450IID6 system. With the debrisoquine test, approximately 5 to 10% of the Caucasian population shows an inherited deficiency of oxidative hydroxylation.[78,79] The ratio of debrisoquine to its hydroxylated metabolite concentrations in the urine can be used to characterize a patient's enzyme phenotype. A low debrisoquine:OH-debrisoquine ratio denotes a rapid or extensive hydroxylator, whereas a high debrisoquine:OH-debrisoquine ratio identifies a slow or poor hydroxylator. The distribution of hydroxylator status in the Caucasian population is bimodally distributed, with the division between rapid and slow hydroxylators occurring at approximately 12:1 (debrisoquine:OH-debrisoquine).[80] Other compounds can also be used as probes to phenotype individuals. Hydroxylation of sparteine and O-methylation of dextromethorphan are accomplished through the P450IID6 pathway and can also be used to differentiate poor and rapid hydroxylators.

As many CADs undergo oxidative hydroxylation by the P450IID6 isoenzyme system, the metabolism of these compounds is under the same genetic control. There is a strong relationship between ratios of debrisoquine with DMI and NT with respect to clearance and their resultant plasma concentrations.[81-84] A significant association also exists between the debrisoquine: sparteine ratio and urinary ratio of DMI:OH-DMI.[85-87] A relationship between the ratios of debrisoquine with IMI and AMI has not been demonstrated. This supports the evidence that demethylation of IMI and AMI is catalyzed by another P450 isoenzyme system, probably P450IA or P450IIA.[42]

Differences in hydroxylation rate can be observed as clinically significant differences in oral and systemic clearance and have implications for dosing. First-pass hydroxylation has been shown to become saturated in rapid but not slow hydroxylators.[88] In addition, there appears to be a higher occurrence of nonlinear kinetic behavior in rapid hydroxylators. Rapid hydroxylators may show disproportionately large changes in plasma concentration following dose changes because of enzyme saturation at doses within the usual dosing range.[71,72]

Differential effects of drug–drug interactions have been observed in rapid and slow hydroxylators. Quinidine, a potent inhibitor of DMI hydroxylation, markedly decreases the hydroxylation of DMI in rapid but not slow hydroxylators.[89] Inhibition of hydroxylation by quinidine results in the metabolic status of rapid hydroxylators resembling that of slow hydroxylators. Analogous but less marked effects have been seen with cimetidine and quinine.[89,90] In the clinical setting, when inhibitors of hydroxylation are added to a regimen, dose reductions would likely be required in rapid hydroxylators but would less likely be required in slow hydroxylators. Differential effects of enzyme induction on rapid and slow hydroxylators appear not to have been investigated at this time. Overall, it seems that both slow and rapid hydroxylators may exhibit pharmacokinetic characteristics that can be clinically significant. Higher than usual plasma CAD concentrations for a given dose may occur in slow hydroxlators because of a decreased rate of metabolism. Additionally, a subpopulation of rapid hydroxylators may show nonlinear changes in plasma CAD concentrations following dose increases (see Nonlinear Pharmacokinetics).

There is also some evidence for interethnic differences in CAD metabolism. Studies of hydroxylator status suggest that the frequency of poor metabolizers is much lower in non-Caucasian populations.[91–93] The Asian population appears to have lower clearance rates of TCAs. Asians were found to have higher 24-hour plasma CMI concentrations compared with British subjects.[94] Asians also show a slower rate of DMI metabolism and a higher incidence of anticholinergic side effects compared with Caucasians.[95] Blacks have shown significantly higher plasma NT concentrations following NT administration, although no differences were seen following AMI administration.[55] In another study, no difference in oral clearance of IMI was observed between blacks, Caucasians, and Hispanics.[43] Differences in NT metabolism were also not observed between Caucasian and Hispanics.[96]

Hydroxylator phenotype is not routinely determined in most settings. A debrisoquine or sparteine test is simple and can be instituted in most laboratories. Phenotyping need only be done once in a person's life. It may be clinically useful to consider such a capability if there is a high degree of use of drugs that are metabolized through the P450IID6 system. At present, this applies to tricyclic antidepressants, some antipsychotics (eg, thioridazine and perphenazine), and some antiarrhythmics (eg, propafenone and flecainide).

PHARMACODYNAMICS

Concentration and Response Relationship

For most CADs, the relationship between plasma concentration and clinical response is unclear. The American Psychiatric Association Task Force on the Use of Laboratory Tests in Psychiatry[1] found that only IMI, DMI, and NT have plasma concentration–response relationships established well enough to warrant routine clinical use (Table 13–3). IMI (plus DMI) shows a linear or sigmoidal plasma concentration–response relationship, with a therapeutic threshold of

TABLE 13–3. RECOMMENDED THERAPEUTIC PLASMA CONCENTRATION RANGES FOR TREATMENT WITH ANTIDEPRESSANTS

Antidepressant	Plasma Concentration Range
Routine	
Imipramine (+ desipramine)	180–350 ng/mL
Desipramine	115–250 ng/mL
Amitriptyline (+ nortriptyline)	120–250 ng/mL
Nortriptyline	50–150 ng/mL
Other	
Clomipramine (+ desmethylclomipramine)	150–350 ng/mL (MD)[a]
	100–250 ng/mL (OCD)
Bupropion	<100 ng/mL
Hydroxybupropion	<1200 ng/mL

[a] MD, major depression; OCD, obsessive–compulsive disorder.
Adapted from DeVane CL. Cyclic antidepressants. In: Evans WE, Schentag JJ, Jusko WJ, eds. Applied Pharmacokinetics: Principles of Therapeutic Drug Monitoring. *2nd ed. Spokane, WA: Applied Therapeutics; 1986:852–907, with permission.*

approximately 180 ng/mL. The upper end of the range appears to be determined by increase in adverse effects rather than decrease in therapeutic effect. A practical limit is approximately 350 ng/mL, but this is not absolute and depends on the patient's tolerance. Data on DMI suggest a therapeutic threshold of approximately 115 ng/mL.[97] Earlier studies suggested the possibility of a therapeutic window for DMI.[98–100] More recent studies are equivocal on the existence of a therapeutic window versus a therapeutic range. The upper limit appears to be approximately 250 ng/mL, but again this is not absolute and is based primarily on patient tolerance.

Nortriptyline appears to be the CAD with the best defined plasma concentration–response relationship. Repeated studies have shown a therapeutic window of approximately 50 to 150 ng/mL.[101–105] Therefore, in patients with plasma NT concentrations above 150 ng/mL, chances of response are increased by lowering the dose to achieve a plasma NT concentration less than or equal to 150 ng/mL. Most studies on plasma concentration–response relationship with AMI (plus NT) show either a linear or curvilinear relationship.[106–109] The lower threshold of AMI plus NT for response appears to be approximately 120 ng/mL. Studies that show a curvilinear response suggest an upper limit of approximately 250 ng/mL. One possible explanation for differing results on the shape of the AMI plasma concentration–response curve may be the contribution of NT to overall response. NT has a well-established curvilinear response curve and may be a major contributor to response in many patients treated with AMI. In these patients, if the plasma concentration of NT exceeds its therapeutic window there may be a decrease in response and, therefore, a curvilinear plasma concentration–response curve for AMI plus NT. Two large trials investigating plasma AMI concentration versus response did not find a relationship.[110,111] One of these trials may have included many AMI nonresponders, as only one third of patients in the trial responded and therefore the results may not be valid.[110] Although AMI is not recommended for routine monitoring by the APA Task Force,[1] monitoring of AMI in a TDM system may be justified because NT is a major active metabolite with a well-established therapeutic range and because there are existing data on which to base guidelines for AMI monitoring.

Since the release of the American Psychiatric Association Task Force on the Use of Laboratory Tests in Psychiatry[1] additional information has been obtained on plasma concentration–response relationships for other CADs, particularly CMI and bupropion.

The evidence for a well-defined plasma concentration–response relationship for CMI in the treatment of depression has been controversial. Potential reasons for inconsistent findings include choice of optimal study dose due to high interindividual variability; a principal active metabolite, desmethylclomipramine (DCMI), with a long half-life which accumulates over a 3- to 4-week period and thus results in a continually changing DCMI:CMI ratio during the usual study period; use of different analytic methods resulting in differing degrees of success in detecting any plasma concentration–response relationship; and lack of measurement of other potentially active metabolites.[112] Although studies investigating plasma concentration–response relationships for any drug are associated with these difficulties, analysis of the bulk of data on use of CMI in depression suggests that CMI-plus-DCMI plasma concentrations below 150 ng/mL are usually associated with nonresponse and concentrations above 450 ng/mL are usually associated with toxicity and even nonresponse.[112,113] As higher doses of CMI (> 250 mg/d) have been associated with increased risk of seizures, caution should be taken when approaching the upper end of the estimated therapeutic range. It may be prudent to use a conservative upper limit of approximately 350 ng/mL to reduce the risk of toxicity. In addition to depression, the plasma concentration (C_p)–response relationship of CMI has been investigated in OCD. The same methodologic difficulties noted above also occur in studies on OCD and results have been mixed. Half of the studies support a positive relationship between CMI C_p and OCD response, and a third suggest a tendency toward a negative relationship between plasma DCMI concentration and OCD response.[114–119] A positive relationship between plasma CMI concentration and OCD response would be suspected on a theoretical basis. CMI has a higher 5HT:NE activity ratio compared with DCMI, and it is thought that the therapeutic efficacy of CMI, and the SSRIs, in OCD is related to 5HT reuptake blockade.[120–124] Studies that do support a plasma CMI concentration–response relationship for OCD indicate an effective plasma CMI concentration range of 100 to 250 ng/mL.[114,119] Further investigation is needed to definitively support a plasma CMI concentration–OCD response relationship. Routine monitoring of CMI plus DCMI may be beneficial in depression. Routine monitoring of plasma CMI concentrations in OCD is probably not supported at this time, although occasional monitoring may be useful in special cases, such as when drug–drug interactions are present.

A plasma concentration–response relationship has also been investigated for bupropion.[125–128] From these studies it appears that lower plasma bupropion concentrations are associated with better antidepressant response than the higher concentrations. Antidepressant response is associated with plasma bupropion concentrations less than 100 ng/mL, with the highest likelihood of response at 20 to 50 ng/mL.[128] Measuring the metabolite hydroxybupropion may also be useful. Nonresponse and toxicity have been associated with plasma hydroxybupropion concentrations greater than 1000 to 1200 ng/mL.[128,129]

Concentration and Toxicity

Toxicity of TCAs is manifested primarily as anticholinergic and cardiovascular effects (Table 13–4). TCAs are extremely dangerous in overdose, with death most commonly associated with cardiovascular toxicity. A relationship between plasma TCA concentration and increased incidence of anticholinergic and cardiovascular adverse effects has been observed. Increased incidences of anticholinergic adverse effects are associated with plasma TCA concentrations greater than 500 ng/mL, although some patients may experience common anticholinergic adverse effects at lower plasma TCA concentrations.[130] One study looking at anticholinergic delirium found that six of seven patients with a plasma AMI concentration greater than 450 ng/mL experienced delirium, whereas none of these patients had delirium at 300 to 450 ng/mL.[131] Anticholinergic adverse effects and delirium may be present with lower TCA levels if concomitant drugs with anticholinergic properties are present. A study investigating plasma TCA concentrations in cases of TCA-induced seizures found a mean plasma TCA concentration of 734 ng/mL (range, 438–1200).[132] Severe cardiac toxicity has been associated with plasma TCA concentrations greater than 1000 ng/mL. A QRS interval of greater than 100 milliseconds, which is associated with a lethal TCA overdose, is correlated with plasma TCA concentrations greater than 1000 ng/mL.[133,134]

Central nervous system toxic effects as a result of bupropion administration appear to be associated with high plasma hydroxybupropion concentration, occurring at approximately 1000 ng/mL in some patients, although other individuals may tolerate hydroxybupropion in this range.[128] Seizures are also assumed to occur at high plasma concentrations of bupropion and its metabolites. Exact information is lacking due to inadequate plasma concentration monitoring of bupropion and its metabolites in cases of bupropion-induced seizures.

Factors That May Affect Dose, Concentration, and Response Relationship

In general, plasma CAD concentrations are usually reported to be pharmacokinetically linear within the usual dosing range; however, there are populations that represent exceptions to this rule. Factors that can affect the relationship between dose, plasma concentration, and response include presence of active metabolites, protein binding, significant drug–drug interactions, nonlinear pharmacokinetics, and pharmacogenetics. The following sections detail these factors that may significantly affect the pharmacodynamics of CADs and influence the interpretation of TDM results.

Active Metabolites

Hepatic metabolism of CADs produces metabolites that can be pharmacologically active. Many of the metabolites tend to accumulate with chronic dosing. This suggests they have longer half lives than the parent compound, although the exact half-lives of many of these metabolites are not well characterized because of the lack of studies in which the metabolite is administered as the test drug.

An important question for TDM programs is, Do all active metabolites of an administered drug need to be quantified? The answer is yes, only if inclusion of metabolite concentrations sig-

TABLE 13–4. ADVERSE EFFECTS OF ANTIDEPRESSANT AGENTS

Antidepressant	Anticholinergic Potency	Neurologic		Cardiac	
		Sedation	Seizures	Orthostasis	Arrhythmias
Tricyclic Agents					
Tertiary Amines					
Doxepin	+++	++++	+++	++	++
Amitriptyline	++++	++++	+++	+++	++++
Imipramine	+++	+++	+++	++++	++++
Trimipramine	++++	++++	+++	+++	++++
Clomipramine	++++	++++	++++	+++	++++
Secondary Amines					
Protriptyline	+++	+	++	++	++++
Nortriptyline	+++	+++	++	+	+++
Desipramine	++	++	++	+++	+++
Other Cyclic Agents					
Amoxapine	+++	++	+++	+	++
Bupropion	–	–	+++	–	–
Maprotiline	+++	+++	++++	++	+++
Trazodone	–	+++	++	+++	+
Venlafaxine	–	+	+	–/+	+
Selective Serotonin Reuptake Inhibitors					
Fluoxetine	–	–/+	+	–	–
Sertraline	–	–/+	+	–	–
Paroxetine	–	–/+	–	–/+	–
Fluvoxamine	–	+	+	–/+	–/+

Adapted from Bryant SG, Brown CS. Major depression. In: Young LY, Koda-Kimble MA, eds. Applied Therapeutics: The Clinical Use of Drugs. 4th ed. Spokane, WA: Applied Therapeutics; 1988:1231–1254, with permission.

nificantly increases the strength of the plasma concentration–response relationship compared with measurement of the routinely measured compounds alone. The assessment of a relationship between the clinical effects of CADs and the plasma concentrations of hydroxy metabolites has been attempted, but data are limited because of the lack of clinical studies in which hydroxy metabolites have been administered as the test drug. Inclusion of a measured 2-OH-DMI concentration with DMI concentration does not improve the correlation with observed response compared with measuring DMI alone.[97] Similarly, including plasma 10-OH-NT concentrations with AMI and NT results in only slight improvements in the correlation of plasma concentration with response.[135] 10-OH-AMI and 2-OH-IMI would also be expected to be clinically unimportant for TDM because of low hydroxy metabolite-to-parent compound ratios.[36] In general, the ratio of hydroxy metabolite to parent compound is relatively low, with the exception of 10-OH NT:NT, so that minimal contribution to response or toxicity would be expected. In patients with renal impairment and in the elderly, however, hydroxy metabolites accumulate and can significantly exceed the parent compound or its demethylated metabolites.[135]

When administering tertiary amine parent compounds, routine measurement of secondary amine metabolites should be done, such as measuring DMI when administering IMI or measuring NT when administering AMI. Routine measurement of hydroxy metabolites is probably not justified at this time because of the lack of little clear evidence for relationships with efficacy or adverse effects. Measurement of hydroxy metabolites might be useful in the renally impaired population.

Protein Binding

As CADs are basic compounds, they tend to bind to α_1-acid glycoprotein, lipids, and cholesterol. A negative correlation exists between the unbound fraction of IMI and concentration of α_1-acid glycoprotein, whereas no correlation has been observed between unbound fraction of IMI and albumin concentration.[136] The extent of total protein and lipid binding by CADs can be highly variable (see Table 13–2). Using various ultrafiltration techniques, an approximately twofold difference has been observed in mean unbound fraction for IMI, ranging between 4.2 and 10.9% in healthy subjects.[136–138] This range of difference may be due to the different ultrafiltration techniques used and differences in IMI binding to different polymorphic forms of α_1-acid glycoprotein, proportions of which can vary between individuals.[139] There may also be intraindividual changes in CAD binding over time. Plasma concentrations of α_1-acid glycoprotein are not consistent over time. Inflammation, malignancy, myocardial infarction, "stress," and various hematologic conditions can increase α_1-acid glycoprotein concentrations. Hepatic disease, nephrotic syndrome, pregnancy, malnutrition, and use of oral contraceptives can decrease α_1-acid glycoprotein. The clinical significance of these changes is unknown, although large changes in α_1-acid glycoprotein ($\geq 25\%$) may be necessary to significantly alter unbound fraction. Changes in plasma lipoprotein concentration may also affect unbound fraction, as seen with decreased unbound fraction of IMI with hyperlipoproteinemia.[140]

Would measurement of free drug concentrations (D_f) improve TDM programs? Relatively few studies have looked at free drug concentrations and clinical response. Methodologic issues include the following: (1) ultrafiltration techniques can lose drug as a result of drug binding to filtration devices[36]; (2) equilibrium dialysis can be difficult; (3) free drug concentrations can typically fall below the detection of many conventional assays; and (4) these techniques are not readily available in most laboratories. Protein binding ranges in patients follow a normal distribution.[141–143] For the majority of patients, the degree of protein binding is relatively consistent, although significant differences in unbound fraction can occur in a small proportion of patients that fall in the extremes of the population distribution. Misinterpretation of TDM results and inappropriate adjustments in CAD dosing are possible in these small numbers of patients. In general, changes in protein binding may not produce changes in unbound fraction that are of significant magnitude to justify routine measurement of free drug concentrations for the majority of patients. Free drug concentration monitoring may be appropriate in specific clinical situations where patients are unresponsive throughout the normal therapeutic range or when increased adverse effects at low plasma CAD concentrations are observed.

Drug–Drug Interactions

Drug–drug interactions are the most common reason why standard doses of CADs yield widely divergent plasma concentrations and therapeutic effects. Drug–drug interactions can be either pharmacodynamic or pharmacokinetic in nature. Pharmacodynamically, drugs may interact at the level of the receptor system and alter the neuronal physiologic environment. Pharmacodynamic interactions affect the therapeutic effects of CADs by altering the ability of the target tissue to demonstrate a physiologic response to CADs. Pharmacokinetic interactions can alter absorption, distribution, and metabolic or renal clearance. Pharmacokinetic alterations affect the drug concentration at the site of action and result in changes in the duration or intensity of effect. This chapter focuses on pharmacokinetic drug interactions; information on pharmacodynamic interactions can be found in other sources.

Pharmacokinetic drug–drug interactions generally affect certain hepatic metabolic enzyme systems and result in alterations in the CAD dose–plasma concentration relationship. The hepatic enzyme system usually responsible for pharmacokinetic drug interactions with CADs is the cytochrome P450 microsomal enzyme system. As mentioned above, oxidative demethylation of IMI and AMI, and possibly other CADs, may be catalyzed by the P450IA and P450IIIA isoenzyme systems. The importance of demethylation reactions is that active metabolites of many CADs are produced by demethylation of the parent compound. Oxidative hydroxylation reactions are predominantly catalyzed by the P450IID6 isoenzyme system. These reactions generally change the parent compound or its active metabolites to metabolites with significantly lower activity. Drug interactions that affect these enzyme systems can alter the bioavailabilty or clearance of CADs and significantly alter the resultant drug concentrations from a given dose.

Agents that cause enzyme induction or inhibition alter metabolic clearance of CADs, leading to decreased or increased plasma CAD concentrations, respectively. The magnitude of effect of enzyme inducers versus inhibitors on clearance can be relatively large. A greater than threefold difference between effects of enzyme inducers and inhibitors has been observed for oral clearance of DOX.[43] Increases in plasma concentration following initiation of an enzyme inhibitor or discontinuation of an enzyme inducer can lead to improved response or can precipitate toxic effects. Alternatively, discontinuing an enzyme inhibitor or initiating an enzyme inducer can decrease plasma concentration and reduce response, possibly leading to relapse. Dose adjustments are often necessary to maintain a target steady-state plasma concentration within the therapeutic range when an interacting drug is coadministered.

Hepatic clearance of CADs is most significantly increased by drugs that induce the cytochrome P450 microsomal enzyme system, for example, carbamazepine, phenobarbital, phenytoin, rifampin, and tobacco (cigarette smoking). These agents appear to be general inducers of the P450 microsomal enzyme system, as the clearance of many drugs metabolized by different P450 isoenzyme subfamilies is increased. Some agents can have a very powerful metabolic inducing effect in some patients. Carbamazepine causes up to tenfold increases in clearance of psychotropics in some patients.[144] Time to onset and maximal induction effect is important in optimal timing of monitoring of induction effects. Onset of induction occurs within 2 days for rifampin compared with 1 week for phenobarbital. Enzyme induction with carbamazepine begins after 3 to 5 days and is not complete for approximately 1 month or longer.[145] Maximal metabolic induction can require 2 or more weeks, leading to an extended lag period before maximal effect on steady-state plasma concentrations of CADs is seen.[146] CADs should be monitored for approximately twice the time expected to achieve the maximal induction effect following introduction of an enzyme inducing agent. This should ensure that the maximal enzyme inducing-effect on steady-state plasma CAD concentrations will be observed in the individual and appropriateness of dose adjustments can be assessed.

A possible source of enzyme induction that is often overlooked is cigarette smoking. The enzyme-inducing effect of tobacco smoking has been demonstrated for AMI, NT, IMI, DMI, CMI, and DOX.[43,45,147–149] Cigarette smoking had been thought to induce cytochrome P448 enzymes with little or no effect on cytochrome P450 enzymes[150]; however, recent evidence also implicates cigarette smoking in induction of P450IA isoenzyme system.[151] Induction of P450IA isoenzymes would be thought to increase the rate of demethylation, as this isoenzyme system has been associated with demethylation of IMI. From the data it is unclear whether smoking has a greater inducing effect on demethylation or hydroxylation. Some studies support greater induction of demethylation,[152] whereas others support both pathways being affected.[148,153,154] Onset and peak effects on CAD clearance are not well determined but the magnitude of the inducing effect of cigarette smoking may be substantial in some patients. Almost a twofold increase in DOX oral clearance has been observed in smokers compared with nonsmokers.[43] This degree of enzyme induction could lead to decreased efficacy of CADs at the usual therapeutic doses in some smokers. Also, termination of smoking, including switching to nicotine gum or patches, may lead to increases in plasma CAD concentrations with increase in adverse or toxic effects.

Drugs that inhibit the cytochrome P450 system can decrease the metabolism of many drugs. Enzyme inhibition can occur by competitive or noncompetitive mechanisms. For competitive inhibition, the interacting drug is an alternative substrate for the metabolizing enzymes. In noncompetitive inhibition, the interacting drug binds to a site other than the active site and inactivates the enzyme. Drugs that directly inhibit the metabolic enzymes, through either competitive or noncompetitive mechanisms, will result in clearance changes within 24 to 48 hours of achieving effective concentrations. Drugs that interfere with synthesis of metabolic enzymes take longer to achieve maximal inhibition effect, up to 1 or 2 weeks.[146]

Cimetidine shows a significant inhibitory effect on metabolic clearance of many drugs, including CADs. Cimetidine appears to interact with P450 heme iron complex so that cimetidine is a nonselective inhibitor of many P450 subfamilies. Therefore, cimetidine would be expected to decrease clearance of most CADs, particularly CADs with low bioavailability (high extraction ratio). Cimetidine has been observed to increase the bioavailability of IMI from 40 to 75%, increase the IMI C_{max} from 19.3 to 34.4 ng/mL, and cause twofold increases in the AUCs of IMI and DMI following oral administration of IMI.[155] DOX and AMI have also been reported to interact with cimetidine.[156–158] A 42% decrease in plasma NT concentration has been observed following discontinuation of cimetidine. This interaction was confirmed when plasma NT concentration significantly increased on rechallenge with cimetidine and then decreased again with discontinuation.[159]

Coadministration of several commonly used drugs can inhibit the clearance of CADs. Drug interactions of this nature are most extensively studied with the P450IID6 isoenzyme system. Some drugs that inhibit this pathway may be substrates for the P450IID6 system, such as thioridazine and propafenone,[160,161] whereas others, such as haloperidol and quinidine, apparently are not.[162,163] Table 13–5 lists several drugs that are thought to be substrates for or inhibitors of the P450IID6 isoenzyme system. As demethylation of TCAs appears to be catalyzed by two separate isoenzyme systems, P450IA2 and P450IIIA, inhibition in one pathway can be compensated for by the other. Therefore, inhibitors of demethylation may cause only minor changes in clearance, whereas inhibitors of hydroxylation may have a more significant effect on clearance.

Cyclic antidepressants may commonly be coadministered with other psychotropic drugs that have been reported to increase plasma CAD concentrations, such as alprazolam, methylphenidate, and antipsychotics.[36,164] A twofold increase in mean plasma DMI concentrations has been observed in patients receiving concomitant antipsychotics compared with those

TABLE 13–5. COMMON DRUGS OR METABOLITES THAT INHIBIT P450IID6

Psychotropics	*Antiarrhythmics*
Amitriptyline	Encainide
Chlorpromazine	Flecainide
Clomipramine	Mexiletine
Desipramine	Propafenone
Fluoxetine	Quinidine
Fluphenazine	
Fluvoxamine	*Antihypertensives*
Haloperidol	Alprenolol
Imipramine	Captopril
Levopromazine	Labetalol
Norfluoxetine	Nicardipine
Nortriptyline	Oxprenolol
Paroxetine	Penbutolol
Perphenazine	Propranolol
Sertraline	Timolol
Thioridazine	
	Other Drugs
	Codeine
	Dextromethorphan
	Diphenhydramine

not taking antipsychotics.[165] Also, greater than a twofold decrease in steady-state plasma NT concentration has been observed following discontinuance of perphenazine.[104] Other nonpsychotropic drugs, such as contraceptive steroids and disulfiram, have also been reported to alter plasma TCA concentrations.[166,167] The magnitude and clinical significance of these interactions can vary from individual to individual. Presence of known or potential interactions should alert the clinician that TDM may be useful in these situations.

All current SSRIs have been identified as potential inhibitors of the P450IID6 isoenzyme system. Combined treatment with TCAs and SSRIs may be undertaken in some depressed patients who fail to respond adequately to CAD monotherapy. Numerous case reports have been published of increased plasma TCA concentrations following coadministration of FLX.[168] In a controlled study of effect of FLX on plasma IMI and DMI concentrations, up to a tenfold decrease in clearance and prolonged half-life up to fourfold were observed for both IMI and DMI. Inhibition of hydroxylation of IMI and DMI appeared to be affected without significant effect of demethylation of IMI.[169] This finding is consistent with the inhibitory effect of FLX and norfluoxetine on P450IID6. The duration of FLX interactions are prolonged[170] because of the long half-life of FLX and norfluoxetine. Paroxetine has been noted to decrease clearance of DMI in rapid metabolizers but not poor metabolizers of sparteine[171] (see Pharmacogenetics). Sertraline is observed to be a potent inhibitor of sparteine metabolism, controlled by P450IID6,[172] although sertraline has been observed to only marginally increase DMI concentrations.[173] Contrary to the other SSRIs, fluvoxamine has been found to inhibit N-demethylation, with significantly weaker effects on hydroxylation. Fluvoxamine has been noted to increase plasma concentrations of IMI, AMI, and CMI, with little effect on the concentrations of their demethylated metabolites.[174,175] This is explained by the finding that fluvoxamine is the only SSRI with significant inhibition of demethylation and its relatively low affinity for P450IID6 compared with the other SSRIs.[172,176]

Ethanol ingestion can have differing effects on plasma CAD concentrations. Acutely, ethanol inhibits microsomal oxidation through its metabolite, acetaldehyde, which depletes NADPH. Ethanol, at higher concentrations, has a direct competitive effect on P450 enzymes and can also impede conjugation reactions by inhibiting UPP-glucuronic acid synthesis. Alternatively, chronic ethanol ingestion may be associated with enzyme induction, as long as hepatic cirrhosis is not present. Mixed results on induction effects on demethylation and hydroxylation have been observed. Higher clearance rates and lower plasma concentrations of IMI and DMI have been observed in alcoholic subjects compared with nonalcoholics patients.[177,178] In a study of AMI biotransformation in alcoholics, lower plasma concentrations of NT and AMI plus NT, but not of AMI, were observed in alcoholics versus nonalcoholics, suggesting enhanced hydroxylation in the alcoholic group.[179] Alternatively, during chronic dosing of CMI, a significant lower demethylation clearance but not hydroxylation clearance was observed in recently detoxified alcoholics compared with a nonalcoholic reference group.[180] The mixed results in these studies may be due to varying degrees of hepatic impairment in the study samples. Taken together, chronic ethanol consumption, in the absence of significant liver impairment, can induce the metabolism of CADs and lower resultant plasma CAD concentrations.

Endogenous or exogenous binding compounds, such as α_1-acid glycoprotein or cholesterol, can also be affected by concomitant medications or alcohol. Other weakly basic drugs are most likely to show ability to displace CADs from α_1-acid glycoprotein. Common drugs that have relatively high binding to α_1-acid glycoprotein include alprenolol, disopyramide, erythromycin, lidocaine, meperidine, methadone, and quinidine. Displacement leads to an increase in unbound fraction and typically a corresponding increase in volume of distribution.[181] Depending on the elimination characteristics of the drug, there may or may not be a corresponding change in steady-state plasma concentration. Potentially significant changes in steady-state plasma concentration as a result of alterations in plasma protein binding of CADs are limited because of their large volume of distribution. Looking at a worst case scenario, when a displacer drug is administered along with a CAD, the unbound fraction might increase immediately as a result of displacement from α_1-acid glycoprotein. The increased concentration of unbound drug can equilibrate rapidly with total body tissue because of the large volume of distribution. This would result in a reduction in steady-state plasma concentration with only a modest increase in unbound fraction. Additionally, an increased unbound fraction due to displacement increases the amount of drug available for metabolism, and there is a corresponding increase in clearance. Both of these effects lead to a lower steady-state plasma concentration but no expected significant change in unbound drug concentration. In each of these cases no change in dose would likely be required. In general, drug interactions that affect protein binding of CADs are usually not clinically significant because of the pharmacokinetic characteristics of CADs. Changes in free drug concentration may occasionally be significant enough to alter the usual plasma concentration–response relationships and make TDM results more difficult to interpret correctly. Measurement of free drug concentrations may be indicated in special situations such as when both a protein binding displacer and a enzyme inhibitor are used along with a CAD.

As the CADs are almost exclusively eliminated by metabolism, drugs affecting glomerular filtration or tubular reabsorption do not significantly alter the disposition of the parent compound. Many CADs, however, have hydroxy metabolites that are renally eliminated. Drug interactions or disease states that decrease renal clearance may lead to excessive accumulation of hydroxy metabolites in these patients. As in renal impairment, dose adjustments are not routinely made in these cases.

Therapeutic drug monitoring becomes increasingly important for monitoring changes in steady-state plasma concentrations of CADs when interacting drugs are added or deleted from a regimen. TDM can be used to guide dosage changes to prevent potential toxicity or loss of therapeutic effect for CADs with known therapeutic ranges. When medications that interact with CADs are added or deleted, changes in therapeutic response or side effect profiles should be interpreted within the context of these interactions.

THERAPEUTIC REGIMEN DESIGN

Prospective Dosing

A potential use of TDM programs is prospective dosing based on measuring plasma concentrations following single dose administration of cyclic antidepressants. Traditional TDM requires plasma sampling at steady state; however, individualizing drug dosage regimens at the outset of treatment might reduce the time necessary to achieve a clinical response. The prospective dosing method requires several assumptions: (1) the drug follows a linear, non-dose-dependent pharmacokinetic model; (2) no time-dependent pharmacokinetic changes occur; (3) absorption is rapid and complete; (4) samples are obtained in the postdistribution elimination phase of the plasma concentration–time profile; and (5) the therapeutic range for the drug is established. The cyclic antidepressants meet most of these assumptions for the general population; however, there have been some case reports and studies suggesting nonlinear pharmacokinetics for CADs (see Nonlinear Pharmacokinetics).

More than one method can be used to predict steady-state plasma CAD concentrations. The approach most simple to implement and use clinically is the single-dose, single-point method. This method was originally used for lithium[182] but has been applied to IMI,[183,184] DMI,[185] and NT.[186–191] A single dose of drug is administered and a plasma concentration is obtained 24 to 72 hours postdose. Nomograms were constructed in some of these studies to assist in the estimation of the correct maintenance dose. Using a 24-hour postdose plasma concentration of DMI, a moderately strong relationship was observed ($r^2 = 0.84$) between predicted and observed steady-state plasma concentrations.[184] The predictive power of the method is increased by using a 72-hour sample compared with a 24-hour sample.[188] Studies show that results from the single-point method are comparable to those of more complicated AUC methods. Estimation of a therapeutic maintenance dose with the single-point method is superior to that obtained with the method that calculates the half-life in plasma.[192]

The potential problem with using the single point method is the need to measure low plasma concentrations. This problem is magnified when attempting to use 72-hour samples compared with 24-hour samples. To use a single dose effectively, single-point method access to a sensitive, rigorously maintained assay system is necessary (see Analytic Methods). Other factors that influence the results are possible transient changes in clearance over the test period, such as alcohol consumption within 24 to 48 hours of the test period. All prospective dosing techniques are based on the assumption of a linear pharmacokinetic model. If nonlinearity occurs within the usual dosing range for the patient then the predicted dosage for the target steady-state plasma concentration would be invalid.

Prospective dosing techniques are not often used although they may be very useful in certain situations, such as medically compromised patients, where an extremely long half-life might be expected or in other metabolically distinct populations such as the elderly, children, and slow hydroxylators. This technique can help identify patients with an extremely low rate of clearance. This would reduce the risk of adjusting the dose too rapidly, resulting in a toxic plasma TCA concentration.

Analytic Techniques

For valid and reliable use of TDM results, sampling, storage, and assay of blood samples must be reliable. Rigorous attention to quality control and well trained technicians are important to maintaining internal consistency of results. Periodically it may be necessary to validate a TDM system by correlating results with other reference laboratories. By developing standardized protocols for sampling, storage, and assay of blood samples reliability of TDM is increased. The need for standardization is most important when TDM systems are used for research applications.

Sampling and Storage

Plasma samples are usually obtained at steady state so that plasma concentrations can be accurately interpreted. Although there is a wide range of half-lives across all patients, the mean half-life for most routinely measured CADs is usually in the 24-hour range for most healthy adults. In most cases where plasma CAD concentrations are obtained, the steady-state plasma concentration is achieved after approximately 5 days. Notable exceptions to this rule would be FLX and protriptyline, which are not routinely measured currently.

To implement an effective and efficient TDM program, sampling times should be standardized in relation to dosing schedules to ensure meaningful interpretation of plasma concentrations. For routine monitoring at steady state, samples should be obtained during the terminal elimination phase, usually 8 to 12 hours after the last administered dose. Studies looking at differences in plasma concentrations of NT, AMI, IMI, and DMI as a function of dosing schedule, for example, divided daily doses versus single bedtime dose, have shown relatively consistent postdistribution phase plasma concentrations for these drugs.[101,193] No significant differences have been found between dosing schedule and clinical efficacy or severity of side effects.[194] This means that regardless of dosing schedule of CADs, samples taken 8 or more hours after the last dose should be reliable.

No difference has been demonstrated in analytic determination of CADs between serum and plasma. Either of these media is appropriate for analysis of CADs, although there is a significant increase in red blood cell concentrations compared with plasma or serum concentrations. Cooling of CAD blood samples is not recommended because of possible temperature-induced reequilibration of red blood cell and plasma drug concentrations. Also, plasticizers in rubber stoppers, such as tris(2-butoxyethyl) phosphate, can cause spurious reductions in plasma CAD concentrations as a result of displacement from plasma binding proteins and reequilibration into red blood cells. At one time this was a problem with Vacutainer collection tubes (Becton-Dickinson) but this problem has been corrected.[195–197] Because of these factors, CAD blood samples should be collected in appropriate collection tubes and centrifuged as soon as possible after phlebotomy.

Once centrifuged, TCAs appear to be stable in plasma or serum for at least 1 week at room temperature.[198] For TCAs, samples can be shipped to laboratories unfrozen. Newer CADs may not be as stable as TCAs. Bupropion exhibits a 54-hour half-life in plasma at room temperature[36] and therefore should be frozen if not analyzed immediately. Also, degree of stability when frozen is not well established for newer CADs. IMI and DMI samples appear stable for up to 1 year when frozen.[36] When archiving samples is routine, such as in research studies, or when analyzing CADs without established stability data, sample integrity over time should be supported by stability studies.

Analytic Methods

A variety of analytic methodologies are available for measuring plasma CAD concentrations (see Table 13–6). The gold standard for analysis of CADs is gas chromatography coupled with mass spectrometery (GC–MS). GC–MS is a highly reliable method with high specificity and selectivity. The disadvantage is that the cost of equipment and operation is high. Gas chromatography can be coupled with other types of detectors, such as an alkali flame ionization detector (GC–AFID) or an electron capture detector (GC–EC). GC–AFID retains an adequate degree of sensitivity and selectivity while lowering costs of operation relative to GC–MS. Compared with GC–AFID, GC–EC has a higher degree of sensitivity but lower specificity and a higher difficulty of operation. High performance liquid chromatography (HPLC) is becoming

TABLE 13–6. ANALYTIC METHODOLOGIES FOR CYCLIC ANTIDEPRESSANT PLASMA CONCENTRATIONS

Method[a]	Sample[b] Requirement (mL)	Speed (samples/h)	Sensitivity (ng/mL)	Specificity	Difficulty of Operation	Cost
GC–MS	1–4	15	1.0	Excellent	High	High
GC–AFID	1–2	6–8	5	Good	Moderate	Moderate
GC–EC	1–3	6–8	1.0	Good	Moderate	Moderate
HPLC	1–3	4–6	2–5	Good	Low	Moderate
RIA	< 1.0	> 10	< 1	Low	Low	Low
EMIT	< 1.0	> 10	10[c]–25	Low to good[c]	Low	Low

[a] GC, gas chromatography; MS, mass spectrometry; AFID, alkali flame ionization detector; EC, electron capture detector; HPLC, high-performance liquid chromatography; RIA, radioimmunoassay; EMIT, enzyme immunoassay.

[b] Serum or plasma.

[c] Second generation systems.

Adapted from DeVane CL. Cyclic antidepressants. In: Evans WE, Schentag JJ, Jusko WJ, eds. Applied Pharmacokinetics: Principles of Therapeutic Drug Monitoring. 2nd ed. Spokane, WA: Applied Therapeutics; 1986:852–907, with permission.

more popular for analysis of CADs. Coupled with a fluorescence or electrochemical detector, HPLC can provide adequate sensitivity and selectivity for clinical applications or research. It has an intermediate level of cost and difficulty of operation. Immunoassay methods for CAD measurement are also available. Radioimmunoassay (RIA) and enzyme immunoassay (EMIT) techniques have a low difficulty and cost of operation and require only small sample volumes. These techniques, in general, do not have adequate specificity for research use because of interference by metabolites; however, newly modified EMIT systems from Abbott (TDX) appear to have improved specificity and sensitivity. RIA and older EMIT techniques may be adequate if only clinical application is necessary and available funding and technical support are limited. At this time, HPLC probably provides the best compromise of the chromatographic methods when the instrument can be dedicated to CAD analysis.

CONCLUSION

Use of TDM is warranted for those CADs with established therapeutic plasma concentration ranges. Continuing research needs to be done investigating plasma concentration–response relationships for other CADs, particularly the newer agents. Results of this research may add to the recommended use of TDM in the routine clinical management of patients receiving CADs. Additionally, more complex patients who have a concurrent medical illness, are receiving concomitant medications, or are suspected of having toxic effects; the elderly; and noncompliant patients may warrant TDM even for those CADs for which the therapeutic range is less certain. Pharmacokinetic principles can facilitate more precise dosing of those CADs that are potentially toxic, improving the benefit-to-risk profile for these medications.

_____ QUESTIONS _____

1a. M.S. is a 36-year-old white woman who was recently admitted to your hospital. Her diagnosis is major depression, recurrent episode. She has two prior admissions for major depression and was effectively treated with NT. After 1 week she is on NT 100 mg/d with a C_{ss} of 112 ng/mL. She admits to the psychiatrist that she hears voices telling her that she is "no good and she should die." The psychiatrist starts her on perphenazine 4 mg po bid. One week later, she says that the voices have gone away but she is feeling more "down." A NT C_p is drawn and comes back at 196 ng/mL. Why has M.S.'s NT C_p increased and why has her clinical response deteriorated? What recommendation would you make?

1b. Her psychiatrist stops the perphenazine and M.S. improves. Two weeks later she is discharged from the hospital on NT 100 mg/d. She is to continue her current treatment for at least 3 months and is to be seen by the psychiatrist every month until her drug therapy is discontinued. M.S. misses her first outpatient appointment. Her husband calls in to say that she had been in an automobile accident and is in the hospital. He says that she will come in as soon as she is well. Two weeks later M.S. is able to come in to see the psychiatrist. She reports that she is beginning to feel depressed again. During the automobile accident she hit her head and a neurologist started her on Dilantin while in the hospital. The psychiatrist orders a NT C_p and it comes back at 32 ng/mL. What has happened to cause her NT C_p to decrease? What recommendation would you make?

2. G.R. is admitted to your hospital because he attempted suicide. His diagnosis is major depression. The psychiatrist starts G.R. on DMI 25 mg po tid. One week later, there has been no change in G.R.'s symptoms. A DMI C_p is drawn and comes back at 42 ng/mL. The psychiatrist states that this is a rather low DMI C_p for this dose. Over the next 2 weeks the psychiatrist increases the DMI dose to 200 mg/d. One week later, G.R. complains that he has problems urinating and gets very dizzy when he gets up from sitting. The psychiatrist is concerned, so he orders a DMI C_p drawn and also sends a blood sample to a psychopharmacology research lab to determine the DMI:OH-DMI ratio in plasma. The DMI C_p is 466 mg/mL and the DMI:OH-DMI ratio is 1:3.65. G.R. is classified as a rapid hydroxylator. What has happened to G.R.? Why is he having problems urinating and with dizziness? What is your recommendation?

3. T.P. is a patient at the outpatient psychiatry clinic where you work. She is currently taking NT 125 mg/d, prescribed by the clinic psychiatrist. She informs you that her family practice physician has given her a new drug for hypertension. This drug has only recently been released and you know very little about it. You do some drug information research to find out if this drug will have any interactions with her NT. As this drug is so new, its drug interaction profile is not well established; however, you do learn that the drug is hepatically metabolized through the P450IID6 isozyme subfamily. What effect may this have on NT C_p and what recommendations would you give to the clinic psychiatrist.

REFERENCES

1. Task Force on the Use of Laboratory Tests in Psychiatry. Tricyclic antidepressants—Blood level measurements and clinical outcome: An APA task force report. *Am J Psychiatry.* 1985;142:155–162.
2. Charney DS, Menkes DB, Heninger GR. Receptor sensitivity and the mechanism of action of antidepressant treatment. Implications for the etiology and therapy of depression. *Arch Gen Psychiatry.* 1981;38:1160–1180.
3. Wolfe BB, Harden TK, Sporn JR, et al. Presynaptic modulation of beta adrenergic receptors in rat cerebral cortex after treatment with antidepressants. *J Pharmacol Exp Ther.* 1978;207:446–457.
4. Mishra R, Janowsky A, Sulser F. Action of mianserin and zimelidine on the norepinephrine receptor coupled adenylate cyclase system in brain: Subsensitivity without reduction in beta-adrenergic receptor binding. *Neuropharmacology.* 1980;19:983–987.
5. Manji H, Brown JH. The antidepressant effect of β-adrenoreceptor subsensitivity: A brief review and clinical implications. *Can J Psychiatry.* 1987;32:788–796.

6. Nelson DR, Pratt GD, Palmer KJ, et al. Effect of paroxetine, a selective 5–hydroxytryptamine reuptake inhibitor, and beta-adrenoreceptors in rat brain: Autoradiographic and functional studies. *Neuropharmacology.* 1991;30:607–616.

7. Abel MS, Villegas F, Abreu J, et al. The effect of rapid eye movement sleep deprivation on cortical beta-adrenergic receptors. *Brain Res Bull.* 1983;11:729–734.

8. Cohen RM, Ebstein RP, Daly JW, et al. Chronic effects of a monoamine oxidase-inhibiting antidepressant: Decreases in functional alpha-adrenergic autoreceptors precede the decrease in norepinephrine-stimulated cyclic adenosine 3′: 5′-monophosphate systems in rat brain. *J Neurosci.* 1982;2:1588–1595.

9. Cohen RM, Campbell IC, Dauphin M, et al. Changes in alpha- and beta-receptor densities in rat brain as a result of treatment with monoamine oxidase inhibiting antidepressants. *Neuropharmacology.* 1982;21:293–298.

10. Vetulani J, Antkiewicz-Michaluk L, Rokosz-Pelc A, et al. Chronic electroconvulsive treatment enhances the density of [^{3}H]prazosin binding sites in the central nervous system of the rat. *Brain Res.* 1983;275:392–395.

11. Vetulani J, Antkiewicz-Michaluk L, Rokosz-Pelc A. Chronic administration of antidepressant drugs increases the density of cortical [^{3}H]prazosin binding sites in the rat. *Brain Res.* 1984;310:360–362.

12. Mobley PL, Sulser F. Norepinephrine stimulated cyclic AMP accumulation in rat limbic forebrain slices: Partial mediation by a subpopulation of receptors with neither alpha nor beta characteristics. *Eur J Pharmacol.* 1979;60:221–227.

13. Siever LJ, Davis KL. Overview: Toward a dysregulation hypothesis of depression. *Am J Psychiatry.* 1985;142:1017–1031.

14. Roose SP, Glassman AH, Giardina EG, et al. Tricyclic antidepressants in depressed patients with cardiac conduction disease. *Arch Gen Psychiatry.* 1987;44:273–275.

15. Veith RC, Raskind MA, Caldwell JH, et al. Cardiovascular effects of tricyclic antidepressants in depressed patients with chronic heart disease. *N Engl J Med.* 1982;306:954–959.

16. Glassman AH, Johnson LL, Giardina EG, et al. The use of imipramine in depressed patients with congestive heart failure. *JAMA.* 1983;250:1997–2001.

17. Giardina EG, Bigger JTJ, Glassman AH, et al. Desmethylimipramine and imipramine on left ventricular function and the ECG: A randomized crossover design. *Int J Cardiol.* 1983;2:375–389.

18. Roose SP, Glassman AH, Giardina EG, et al. Cardiovascular effects of imipramine and bupropion in depressed patients with congestive heart failure. *J Clin Psychopharmacol.* 1987;7:247–251.

19. Roose SP, Glassman AH, Giardina EG, et al. Nortriptyline in depressed patients with left ventricular impairment. *JAMA.* 1986;256:3253–3257.

20. Greenblatt DJ, Shader RI. Bioequivalence of generic drugs in clinical psychopharmacology. *J Clin Psychopharmacol.* 1987;7:A21–A22.

21. Rosenbaum JF, Falk WE, Gastfriend DR, et al. Acute distress after switch from Norpramin to generic desipramine. *Am J Psychiatry.* 1989;146:122. Letter

22. Perera CC. Generic vs. brand name: A case history. *Ohio Med.* 1989;85:506. Letter

23. Reiss W, Dubey L, Funfgeld EW, et al. The pharmacokinetic properties of maprotiline in man. *J Int Med Res.* 1975;3:16–41.

24. Gram LF, Sondergaard I, Christiansen J, et al. Steady-state kinetics of imipramine in patients. *Psychopharmacology (Berl).* 1977;154:255–261.

25. Sutfin TA, DeVane CL, Jusko WJ. The analysis and disposition of imipramine and its active metabolites in man. *Psychopharmacology.* 1984;82:310–317.

26. Lai AA, Schroeder DH. Clinical pharmacokinetics of bupropion: A review. *J Clin Psychiatry.* 1983;44:82–84.

27. Bryant SG, Ereshefsky L. Antidepressant properties of trazodone. *Clin Pharm.* 1982;1:406–417.

28. Klamerus KJ, Maloney K, Rudolph RL, et al. Introduction of a composite parameter to the pharma-

cokinetics of venlafaxine and its active metabolite *O*-desmethylvenlafaxine. *J Clin Pharmacol.* 1992; 32:716–724.

29. Alkalay D, Wagner WE, Carlsen S. Bioavailability and kinetics of maprotiline. *Clin Pharmacol Ther.* 1980;27:697–703.

30. Ziegler VE, Biggs JT, Wylie LT, et al. Protriptyline kinetics. *Clin Pharmacol Ther.* 1978;23:580–584.

31. Benfield P, Heel RC, Lewis SP. Fluoxetine: A review of its pharmacodynamic and pharmacokinetic properties and therapeutic efficacy in depressive illness. *Drugs.* 1986;32:481–508.

32. DeVane CL. Pharmacokinetics of the selective serotonin reuptake inhibitors. *J Clin Psychiatry.* 1992; 53:13–20.

33. Van Harten J. Clinical pharmacokinetics of selective serotonin reuptake inhibitors. *Clin Pharmacokinet.* 1993;24:203–220.

34. Abernethy DR, Divoll M, Greenblatt DJ. Absolute bioavailability of imipramine: Influence of food. *Psychopharmacology (Berl).* 1984;83:104–106.

35. Rubin EH, Biggs JT, Preskorn SH. Nortriptyline pharmacokinetics and plasma levels: Implications for clinical practice. *J Clin Psychiatry.* 1985;46:418–424.

36. DeVane CL. Cyclic antidepressants. In: Evans WE, Schentag JJ, Jusko WJ, eds. *Applied Pharmacokinetics: Principles of Therapeutic Drug Monitoring.* 2nd ed. Spokane, WA: Applied Therapeutics; 1986:852–907.

37. Bickel MH, Graber BE, Moor M. Distribution of chlorpromazine and imipramine in adipose and other tissues of rats. *Life Sci.* 1983;33:2025–2031.

38. Gram LF, Kofod B, Christiansen J, et al. Imipramine metabolism: pH dependent distribution and urinary excretion. *Clin Pharmacol Ther.* 1970;12:239–244.

39. Dencker H, Dencker SJ, Green A, et al. Intestinal absorption, demethylation and enterohepatic circulation of imipramine. *Clin Pharmacol Ther.* 1976;19:584–586.

40. Kaye CM, Haddock RE, Langley PF, et al. A review of the metabolism and pharmacokinetics of paroxetine in man. *Acta Psychiatr Scand Suppl.* 1989;350:60–75.

41. Overmars H, Scherpenisse PM, Post LC. Fluvoxamine maleate: Metabolism in man. *Eur J Drug Metab Pharmacokinet.* 1983;8:269–280.

42. Lemoine A, Gautier JC, Azoulay D, et al. Major pathway of imipramine metabolism is catalyzed by cytochromes P-450 1A2 and P-450 3A4 in human liver. *Mol Pharmacol.* 1993;43:827–832.

43. Ereshefsky L, Tran-Johnson T, Davis CM, et al. Pharmacokinetic factors affecting antidepressant drug clearance and clinical effect: Evaluation of doxepin and imipramine—New data and review. *Clin Chem.* 1988;34:863–880.

44. Nies A, Robinson DS, Friedman MJ, et al. Relationship between age and tricyclic antidepressant plasma levels. *Am J Psychiatry.* 1977;134:790–793.

45. John VA, Luscombe DK, Kemp H. Effects of age, cigarette smoking and the oral contraceptive on the pharmacokinetics of clomipramine and its desmethyl metabolite during chronic dosing. *J Int Med Res.* 1980;8 (suppl):88–95.

46. Hrdina PD, Rovei V, Henry JF, et al. Comparison of single dose pharmacokinetics of imipramine and maprotiline in the elderly. *Psychopharmacology (Berl).* 1980;70:29–34.

47. Henry JF, C.Altamura C, Gomeni R, et al. Pharmacokinetics of amitriptyline in the elderly. *Int J Clin Pharmacol Ther. Toxicol.* 1981;19:1–5.

48. Burch JE. The demethylation of amitriptyline: A cross-over study of steady state plasma levels of amitriptyline and nortriptyline in depressed patients. *Psychopharmacology (Berl).* 1983;80: 254–258.

49. Preskorn SH, Mac DS. Plasma levels of amitriptyline: Effect of age and sex. *J Clin Psychiatry.* 1985;46:276–277.

50. Abernethy DR, Greenblatt DJ, Shader RI. Imipramine and desipramine disposition in the elderly. *J Pharmacol Exp Ther.* 1985;232:183–188.

51. Benetello P, Furlanut M, Zara C. Imipramine pharmacokinetics in depressed geriatric patients. *Int J Clin Pharmacol Res.* 1990;13:191–195.
52. Schulz P, Turner-Tarmyasu K, Smith G, et al. Amitriptyline disposition in young and elderly normal men. *Clin Pharmacol Ther.* 1983;33:360–366.
53. Turbott J, Norman TR, Burrows GD, et al. Pharmacokinetics of nortriptyline in elderly volunteers. *Commun Psychopharmacol.* 1980;4:225–231.
54. Cutler NR, Zavadil AP, Eisdorfer C, et al. Concentrations of desipramine in elderly women. *Am J Psychiatry.* 1981;138:1235–1237.
55. Ziegler VE, Biggs JT. Tricyclic plasma levels: Effects of age, race, sex and smoking. *JAMA.* 1977;238:2167–2169.
56. Katz IR, Simpson GM, Jethanandani V, et al. Steady state pharmacokinetics of nortriptyline in the frail elderly. *Neuropsychopharmacology.* 1989;2:229–236.
57. Kitanaka I, Ross RJ, Cutler NR, et al. Altered hydroxydesipramine concentrations in elderly depressed patients. *Clin Pharmacol Ther.* 1982;31:51–55.
58. Young RC, Alexopoulus GS, Shamoian CA, et al. Plasma 10–hydroxynortriptyline concentrations in elderly depressed patients. *Clin Pharmacol Ther.* 1984;35:540–544.
59. Nelson JC, Atillasoy E, Mazure C, et al. Hydroxydesipramine in the elderly. *J Clin Psychopharmacol.* 1988;8:428–433.
60. Schneider LS, Cooper TB, Suckow RF, et al. Relationship of hydroxynortriptyline to nortriptyline concentration and creatinine clearance in the depressed elderly outpatients. *J Clin Psychopharmacol.* 1990;10:333–337.
61. Szefler SJ, Milsap R. Special pharmacokinetic considerations in children. In: Evans WE, Schentag JJ, Jusko WJ, eds. *Applied Pharmacokinetics: Principles of Therapeutic Drug Monitoring.* 2nd ed. Spokane, WA: Applied Therapeutics; 1986:294–306.
62. Winsberg BG, Perel JM, Hurwic MJ, et al. Imipramine protein binding and pharmacokinetics in children. *Adv Biochem Psychopharmacol.* 1974;9:425–431.
63. Guengerich FP, Turvey CG. Comparisons of several cytochrome P-450 enzymes and epoxide hydroxylase in normal and disease states using immunochemical analysis of surgical liver samples. *J Pharmacol Exp Ther.* 1991;256:1189–1191.
64. Ene MD, Roberts CJC. Pharmacokinetics of nifedipine after oral administration in chronic liver disease. *J Clin Pharmacol.* 1987;27:1001–1004.
65. Dawling S, Lynn K, Rosser R, et al. Nortriptyline metabolism in chronic renal failure: Metabolite elimination. *Clin Pharmacol Ther.* 1982;32:322–329.
66. Lieberman JA, Cooper TB, Suckow RF, et al. Tricyclic antidepressant and metabolite levels in chronic renal failure. *Clin Pharmacol Ther.* 1985;37:301–307.
67. Dugas JE, Bishop DS. Nonlinear desipramine pharmacokinetics: A case study. *J Clin Psychopharmacol.* 1985;5:43–45.
68. Amsterdam J, Brunswick D, Mendels J. The clinical application of tricyclic antidepressant pharmacokinetics and plasma levels. *Am J Psychiatry.* 1980;137:653–662.
69. Musa MN. Nonlinear kinetics of trimipramine in depressed patients. *J Clin Pharmacol.* 1989;29:746–747.
70. Bergstrom RF, Lemberger L, Farid NA, et al. Clinical pharmacology and pharmacokinetics of fluoxetine: A review. *Br J Psychiatry.* 1988;153:47–50.
71. Sindrup SH, Borsen K, Gram LF. Nonlinear kinetics of imipramine in low and medium plasma level ranges. *Ther Drug Monit.* 1990;12:445–449.
72. Nelson JC, Jatlow P. Nonlinear desipramine kinetics: Prevalence and importance. *Clin Pharmacol Ther.* 1987;41:666–670.
73. Bjerre M, Gram LF, Kragh-Sorensen P, et al. Dose-dependent kinetics of imipramine in elderly patients. *Psychopharmacology (Berl).* 1981;75:354–357.

74. Cooke RG, Warsh JJ, Stancer HC. The non-linear kinetics of desipramine and 2–hydroxydesipramine in plasma. *Clin Pharmacol Ther.* 1984;36:343–349.

75. Brosen K, Gram LF, Klysner R, et al. Steady-state levels of imipramine and its metabolites: Significance of dose-dependent kinetics. *Eur J Clin Pharmacol.* 1986;30:43–49.

76. Chiba M, Fujita S, Suzuki T. Pharmacokinetic correlation between in vitro hepatic microsomal kinetics and in vivo metabolism of imipramine and desipramine in rats. *J Pharm Sci.* 1989;79:281–287.

77. Spina E, Henthorn T, Eleborg L. Desmethylimipramine overdose: Nonlinear kinetics in a slow hydroxylator. *Ther Drug Monit.* 1985;7:239–241.

78. Clark DWJ. Genetically determined variability in acetylation and oxidation. Therapeutic implications. *Drugs.* 1985;29:342–375.

79. Steiner E, Bertilsson L, Sawe J, et al. Polymorphic debrisoquine hydroxylation in 757 Swedish subjects. *Clin Pharmacol Ther.* 1988;44:431–435.

80. Brosen K. Recent developments in hepatic drug oxidation: Implications for clinical pharmacokinetics. *Clin Pharmacokinet.* 1990;18:220–239.

81. Woolhouse N, Adjepon-Yamoah KK, Mellstrom B, et al. Nortriptyline and debrisoquine hydroxylations in Ghanian and Swedish subjects. *Clin Pharmacol Ther.* 1984;36:374–378.

82. Sjoqvist F, Bertilsson L. Clinical pharmacology of antidepressant drugs. In: Udsin E, Asberg M, Bertilsson L, et al, eds. *Frontiers in Biochemical and Pharmacological Research in Depression. Advances in Biochemical Psychopharmacology.* New York: Raven Press; 1984:359–372.

83. Sjoqvist F, Bertilsson L. Slow hydroxylation of tricyclic antidepressants—Relationship to polymorphic drug oxidation. In: Kalow W, eds. *Ethnic Differences in Reactions to Drugs and Xenobiotics.* New York: Liss; 1986:169–188.

84. Baumann P. New aspects in research on blood levels and bioavailability of antidepressants. *Psychopathology.* 1986;19:79–84.

85. Brosen K, Otton V, Gram LF. Imipramine demethylation and hydroxylation: impact of the sparteine oxidation phenotype. *Clin Pharmacol Ther.* 1986;40:543–549.

86. Brosen K, Klysner R, Gram LF, et al. Steady-state concentrations of imipramine and its metabolites in relation to the sparteine/debrisoquine polymorphism. *Eur J Pharmacol.* 1986;30:679–684.

87. Spina E, Steiner E, Ericsson O, et al. Hydroxylation of desmethylimipramine: Dependence on the debrisoquine hydroxylation phenotype. *Clin Pharmacol Ther.* 1987;41:457–461.

88. Brosen K, Gram LF. First-pass metabolism of imipramine and desipramine: Impact of the sparteine oxidative phenotype. *Clin Pharmacol Ther.* 1988;43:400–406.

89. Steiner E, Dumont E, Spina E, et al. Inhibition of desipramine 2–hydroxylation by quinidine and quinine. *Clin Pharmacol Ther.* 1988;43:577–580.

90. Spina E, Steiner E. Differences in the inhibitory effect of cimetidine on desipramine metabolism between rapid and slow debrisoquine hydroxylators. *Clin Pharmacol Ther.* 1987;42:278–282.

91. Iyun AO, Lennard MS, Tucker GT, et al. Metoprolol and debrisoquine metabolism in Nigerians: Lack of evidence for polymorphic oxidation. *Clin Pharmacol Ther.* 1986;40:387–394.

92. Lou YC, Ying L, Bertilsson L, et al. Low frequency of debrisoquine hydroxylation in a native Chinese population. *Lancet.* 1987;2:852–853.

93. Nakamura K, Goto F, Ray WA, et al. Interethnic differences in genetic polymorphism of debrisoquine and mephenytoin hydroxylation between Japanese and Caucasian populations. *Clin Pharmacol Ther.* 1985;38:402–408.

94. Allen JJ, Rack PH, Vaddadi KS. Differences in the effects of clomipramine on English and Asian volunteers: Preliminary report on a pilot study. *Postgrad Med J.* 1977;53:79–86.

95. Pi EH, Tran-Johnson TK, Walker NR, et al. Pharmacokinetics of desipramine in Asian and Caucasian volunteers. *Psychopharmacol Bull.* 1989;25:483–487.

96. Gaviria M, Gil A, Javaid J. Nortriptyline kinetics in Hispanic and Anglo subjects. *J Clin Psychopharmacol.* 1986;6:227–231.

97. Nelson JC, Jatlow P, Quinlan DM, et al. Desipramine plasma concentration and antidepressant response. *Arch Gen Psychiatry.* 1982;39:1419–1422.

98. Amin MM, Cooper R, Khalid R, et al. A comparison of desipramine and amitriptyline plasma levels and therapeutic response. *Psychopharmacol Bull.* 1978;14:45–46.

99. Khalid R, Amin MM, Ban TA. Desipramine plasma levels and therapeutic response. *Psychopharmacol Bull.* 1978;14:43–44.

100. Friedel RO, Veith RC, Bloom V, et al. Desipramine plasma level and clinical response in depressed outpatients. *Commun Psychopharmacol.* 1979;3:81–87.

101. Kragh-Sorensen P, Eggert-Hansen CE, Larsen NE. Long-term treatment of endogenous depression with nortriptyline with control of plasma levels. *Psychol Med.* 1974;4:174–180.

102. Kragh-Sorensen P, Hansen CE, Baastrup PC, et al. Self-inhibiting action of nortriptyline's antidepressant effect at high plasma levels. *Psychopharmacologia.* 1976;45:305–312.

103. Ziegler VE, Clayton PJ, Taylor JR, et al. Nortriptyline levels and therapeutic response. *Clin Pharmacol Ther.* 1976;20:458–463.

104. Kragh-Sorensen P, Eggert-Hansen CE, Asberg M. Plasma levels of nortriptyline in the treatment of endogenous depression. *Psychol Med.* 1977;49:444–456.

105. Montgomery S, Braithwaite R, Dawling S. High plasma nortriptyline levels in the treatment of depression. *Clin Pharmacol Ther.* 1978;23:309–314.

106. Ziegler VE, Co BT, Taylor JR, et al. Amitriptyline plasma levels and therapeutic response. *Clin Pharmacol Ther.* 1976;19:795–801.

107. Kupfer DJ, Hanin I, Spiker DG, et al. Amitriptyline plasma levels and clinical response in primary depression. *Clin Pharmacol Ther.* 1977;22:904–911.

108. Vandel S, Vandel B, Sandoz M, et al. Clinical response and plasma concentration of amitriptyline and its metabolite nortriptyline. *Eur J Pharmacol.* 1978;14:185–190.

109. Montgomery SA, McAuley R, Rani SJ, et al. Amitriptyline plasma concentration and clinical response. *Br Med J.* 1979;1:230–231.

110. Coppen A, Ghose K, Montgomery S, et al. Amitriptyline plasma concentration and clinical effect (A World Health Organization Collaborative Study). *Lancet.* 1978;1:63–66.

111. Robinson DS, Cooper TB, Ravaris CL, et al. Plasma tricyclic plasma levels in amitriptyline-treated depressed patients. *Psychopharmcology (Berl).* 1979;63:223–231.

112. Balant-Gorgia AE, Gex-Fabry M, Balant LP. Clinical pharmacokinetics of clomipramine. *Clin Pharmacokinet.* 1991;20:447–461.

113. Balant-Gorgia AE, Balant LP, Garrone G. High blood concentrationsof imipramine or clomipramine and the therapeutic failure: A case report study using therapeutic drug monitoring data. *Ther Drug Monit.* 1989;11:415–420.

114. Stern RS, Marks IM, Mawson D, et al. Clomipramine and exposure for compulsive rituals. II. plasma levels, side effects and outcome. *Br J Psychiatry.* 1980;136:161–166.

115. Insel TR, Murphy DL, Cohen RM, et al. Obsessive–compulsive disorder: A double-blind study of clomipramine and clorgyline. *Arch Gen Psychiatry.* 1983;40:605–612.

116. Thoren P, Asberg M, Bertilsson L, et al. Clomipramine treatment of obsessive–compulsive disorder. *Arch Gen Psychiatry.* 1980;37:1289–1294.

117. Flament MF, Rapoport JL, Berg CJ, et al. Clomipramine treatment of childhood obsessive–compulsive disorder. *Arch Gen Psychiatry.* 1985;42:977–983.

118. Kaviskis Y, Marks IM. Clomipramine in obsessive–compulsive disorder ritualizers treated with exposure: Relations between dose, plasma levels, outcome and side effects. *J Clin Psychopharmacol.* 1988;95:113–118.

119. Mavissakalian MR, Jones B, Olson S, et al. Clomipramine in obsessive–compulsive disorder: clinical response and plasma levels. *J Clin Psychopharmacol.* 1990;10:261–268.

120. Zohar J, Intel TR. Drug treatment of obsessive–compulsive disorder. *Affective Disorders.* 1987;13:193–202.

121. Benkelfat C, Murphy DL, Zohar J, et al. Clomipramine in obsessive–compulsive disorder. *Arch Gen Psychiatry.* 1989;46:23–28.

122. Goodman WK, Price LH, Rasmussen SA, et al. Efficacy of fluvoxamine in obsessive–compulsive disorder. *Arch Gen Psychiatry.* 1989;46:36–44.

123. Dominguez RA. Serotonergic antidepressants and their efficacy in obsessive compulsive disorder. *J Clin Psychiatry.* 1992;53:56–59.

124. Riddle MA, Scahill L, King RA, et al. Double-blind, crossover trial of fluoxetine and placebo in children and adolescents with obsessive-compulsive disorder. *J Am Acad Child Adol Psychiatry.* 1992;31:1062–1069.

125. Preskorn SH. Antidepressant response and plasma concentration of bupropion. *J Clin Psychiatry.* 1983;44:137–139.

126. Fogel P, Mamer OA, Chouinard G, et al. Determination of plasma bupropion and its therapeutic effect. *Biomedic Mass Spectrom.* 1984;11:629–632.

127. Goodnick PJ. Wellbutrin blood levels and clinical response. Paper presented at 144th annual meeting of the American Psychiatric Association; 1991; New Orleans, LA.

128. Preskorn SH. Should bupropion dosage be adjusted based upon therapeutic drug monitoring? *Psychopharmacol Bull.* 1992;27:637–643.

129. Golden RN, DeVane CL, Laizure SC, et al. Bupropion in depression: The role of metabolites in clinical outcome. *Arch Gen Psychiatry.* 1985;45:145–149.

130. Crome P, Braithwaite RA. Relationship between clinical features of tricyclic antidepressant poisoning and plasma concentrations in children. *Arch Dis Child.* 1977;53:902–905.

131. Preskorn SH, Simpson S. Tricyclic-antidepressant-induced delirium and plasma concentration. *Am J Psychiatry.* 1982;139:822–823.

132. Preskorn SH, Fast GA. Tricyclic antidepressant-induced seizures and plasma drug concentration. *J Clin Psychiatry.* 1992;53:160–162.

133. Petit JM, Spiker DG, Ruwitch JF, et al. Tricyclic antidepressant plasma levels and adverse effects after overdose. *Clin Pharmacol Ther.* 1977;21:47–51.

134. Bailey DN, Van Dyke C, Langou RA, et al. Tricyclic antidepressant: plasma levels and clinical findings in overdose. *Am J Psychiatry.* 1978;135:1325–1328.

135. Breyer-Pfaff U, Gaertner HJ, Kreuter F, et al. Antidepressive effect and pharmacokinetics of amitriptyline with consideration of unbound drug and 10–hydroxynortriptyline plasma levels. *Psychopharmacology (Berl).* 1982;76:240–244.

136. Piafsky KM, Borga O. Plasma protein binding of basic drugs. II. Importance of alpha-1 acid glycoprotein for interindividual variation. *Clin Pharmacol Ther.* 1977;22:545–549.

137. Borga O, Azarnoff DL, Forshell GP, et al. Plasma protein binding of tricyclic antidepressants in man. *Biochem Pharmacol.* 1969;18:2135–2143.

138. Kristensen CB. Imipramine serum protein binding in healthy subjects. *Clin Pharmacol Ther.* 1983;34:689–694.

139. Tinguely D, Baumann P, Conti M, et al. Interindividual differences in the binding of antidepressives to plasma proteins: The role of the variants of alpha$_1$–acid glyoprotein. *Eur J Pharmacol.* 1985;27:661–666.

140. Krauss RM, Levy RI, Fredrickson DS. Selective measurement of two lipase activities in post heparin plasma from normal subjects and patients with hyperlipoproteinemia. *J Clin Invest.* 1974;54:1107–1124.

141. Glassman AJ, Hurvic MH, Perel JM. Plasma binding of imipramine and clinical outcome. *Am J Psychiatry.* 1973;130:1367–1369.

142. Potter WZ, Muscettola G, Goodwin FK. Binding of imipramine to plasma protein and to brain tissue: Relationship to CSF tricyclic levels in man. *Psychopharmcology (Berl).* 1979;63:187–192.

143. Freilich DI, Giardina EG. Imipramine binding to alpha$_1$-acid glycoprotein in normal subjects and cardiac patients. *Clin Pharmacol Ther.* 1984;35:670–674.

144. Ereshefsky L, Jann MW, Saklad SR, et al. The controversy over the bioavailability of psychotropic drugs: Historical perspective and pharmacokinetic overview. *J Clin Psychiatry.* 1986;47:6–15.

145. Eichelbaum M, Kothe KW, Hoffman F, et al. Use of stable carbamazepine to study its kinetics during chronic carbamazepine treatment. *Eur J Clin Pharmacol.* 1982;23:241–244.

146. Powell JR, Cate EW. Induction and inhibition of drug metabolism. In: Evans WE, Schentag JJ, Jusko WJ, eds. *Applied Pharmacokinetics: Principles of Therapeutic Drug Monitoring.* 2nd ed. Spokane, WA: Applied Therapeutics; 1986:139–186.

147. Perel JM, Irani JM, Hurivic M, et al. Tricyclic antidepressants: relationships among pharmacokinetics, metabolism and clinical outcome. In Garrattini ed. *Depressive Disorders.* Stuttgart: FK Schattauer, 1978:325–336.

148. Linnoila M, George L, Guthrie S, et al. Effect of alcohol consumption and cigarette smoking on antidepressant levels of depressed patients. *Am J Psychiatry.* 1981;138:841.

149. D'Arcy PF. Drug interactions and reactions update. *Drug Intell Clin Pharm.* 1984;18:302–306.

150. Jusko WJ. Influence of cigarette smoking on drug metabolism in man. *Drug Metab Rev.* 1979;9:221–228.

151. Vistisen K, Loft S, Poulsen HE. Cytochrome P450 IA2 activity in man measured by caffeine metabolism: Effect of smoking, broccoli and exercise. *Adv Exp Med Biol.* 1991;283:407–411.

152. Gex-Fabry M, Balant-Gorgia AE, Balant LP, et al. Clomipramine metabolism: Model based analysis of variability factors from drug monitoring data. *Clin Pharmacokinet.* 1990;19:241–255.

153. Vestal RE, Wood AJ. Influence of age and smoking on drug kinetics in man: Studies using model compounds. *Clin Pharmacokinet.* 1980;5:309–319.

154. Sutfin TA, Perini GI, Molnar G, et al. Multiple-dose pharmacokinetics of imipramine and its major active and conjugated metabolites in depressed patients. *J Clin Psychopharmacol.* 1988;8:48–53.

155. Abernethy DR, Greenblatt DJ, Shader RI. Imipramine–cimetidine interaction: Impairment of clearance and enhanced absolute bioavailability. *J Pharmacol Exp Ther.* 1984;229:702–705.

156. Abernethy DR, Todd E. Doxepin–cimetidine interaction: Increased doxepin bioavailability during cimetidine treatment. *J Clin Psychopharmacol.* 1986;6:8–12.

157. Curry SH, DeVane CL, Wolfe MM. Cimetidine interaction with amitriptyline. *Eur J Clin Pharmacol.* 1985;29:429–433.

158. Curry SH, DeVane CL, Wolfe MM. Pharmacology of combined antidepressant/H$_2$-blocking drug therapy. *Psychopharmacol Bull.* 1986;22:220–222.

159. Miller DD, Sawyer JB, Duffy JP. Cimetidine's effect on steady-state serum nortriptyline concentrations. *Drug Intell Clin Pharm.* 1983;17:904–905.

160. Siddoway LA, Thompson KA, McAllister CB, et al. Polymorphism of propafenone metabolism and disposition in man: Clinical and pharmacokinetic consequences. *Circulation.* 1987;75:785–791.

161. von Bahr C, Guengerich FP, Movin G, et al. *The Use of Human Liver Banks in Pharmacogenetic Research.* Heidelberg: Springer Verlag; 1989.

162. Mikus G, Ha HR, Vozeh S, et al. Pharmacokinetics and metabolism of quinidine in extensive and poor metabolizers of sparteine. *Eur J Clin Pharmacol.* 1986;31:69–72.

163. Gram LF, Debruyne D, Caillard V, et al. Substantial rise in sparteine metabolic ratio during haloperidol treatment. *Br J Clin Pharmacol.* 1989;27:272–275.

164. Grasela THJ, Antal EJ, Ereshefsky L, et al. An evaluation of population pharmacokinetics in therapeutic trials. Part II. Detection of a drug–drug interaction. *Clin Pharmacol Ther.* 1987;42:433–441.

165. Nelson JC, Jatlow PI. Neuroleptic effect on desipramine steady-state plasma concentrations. *Am J Psychiatry.* 1980;137:1232–1234.

166. Abernethy DR, Greenblatt DJ, Shader RI. Imipramine disposition in users of oral contraceptives. *Clin Pharmacol Ther.* 1984;6:792.

167. Ciraulo DA, Barnhill J, Boxenbaum H. Pharmacokinetic interaction of disulfiram and antidepressants. *Am J Psychiatry.* 1985;142:1371–1374.

168. Vandel S, Bertschy G, Bonin B, et al. Tricyclic antidepressant plasma levels after fluoxetine addition. *Pharmacopsychiatry.* 1992;25:202–207.

169. Bergstrom RF, Peyton AL, Lemberger L. Quantification and the mechanism of fluoxetine and tricyclic antidepressant interaction. *Clin Pharmacol Ther.* 1992;51:239–248.

170. Westmeyer J. Fluoxetine-induced tricyclic toxicity: Extent and duration. *J Clin Pharmacol.* 1991;31:388–392.

171. Brosen K, Skjelbo E, Rasmussen BB, et al. Fluvoxamine is a potent inhibitor of cytochrome P4501A2. *Biochem Pharmacol.* 1993;45:1211–1214.

172. Skjelbo E, Brosen K. Inhibitors of imipramine metabolism by human liver microsomes. *Br J Clin Pharmacol.* 1992;34:256–261.

173. Preskorn SH, Alderman J, Chung M, et al. Pharmacokinetics of desipramine coadministered with sertraline or fluoxetine. *J Clin Psychopharmacol.* 1994;14:90–98.

174. Bertschy G, Vandel S, Vandel B, et al. Fluvoxamine–tricyclic antidepressant interaction. An accidental finding. *Eur J Clin Pharmacol.* 1991;40:119–120.

175. Spina E, Pollicino AM, Avenoso A, et al. Effect of fluvoxamine on the pharmacokinetics of imipramine and desipramine in healthy subjects. *Ther Drug Monit.* 1993;15:243–246.

176. Crewe HK, Lennard MS, Tucker GT, et al. The effect of selective serotonin re-uptake inhibitors on cytochrome P4502D6 (CYP2D6) activity in human liver microsomes. *Br J Clin Pharmacol.* 1992;34:262–265.

177. Ciraulo DA, Alderson LM, Chapron DJ, et al. Imipramine disposition in alcoholics. *J Clin Psychopharmacol.* 1982;2:2–7.

178. Ciraulo DA, Barnhill JG, Jaffe JH. Clinical pharmacokinetics of imipramine and desipramine in alcoholics and normal volunteers. *Clin Pharmacol Ther.* 1988;43:509–518.

179. Sandoz M, Vandel S, Vandel B, et al. Biotransformation of amitriptyline in alcoholic depressive patients. *Eur J Clin Pharmacol.* 1983;24:615–621.

180. Balant-Gorgia AE, Gay M, Gex-Faby M, et al. Persistent impairment of clomipramine demethylation in recently detoxified alcoholic patients. *Ther Drug Monit.* 1992;14:119–124.

181. Rowland M, Tozer TN. *Clinical Pharmacokinetics.* Philadelphia: Lea & Febiger; 1980.

182. Cooper TB, Bergner P-EE, Simpson GM. The 24–hour serum lithium level as a prognosticator of dosage requirements. *Am J Psychiatry.* 1973;130:601–603.

183. Brunswick DJ, Amsterdam JD, Mendels J, et al. Prediction of steady-state imipramine and desmethylimipramine plasma concentrations from single-dose data. *Clin Pharmacol Ther.* 1979;25:605–610.

184. Potter WZ, Zavadil AP, Kopin IJ, et al. Single-dose kinetics predicts steady-state concentrations of imipramine and desipramine. *Arch Gen Psychiatry.* 1980;37:314–320.

185. Cooper TB, Bark N, Simpson GM. Prediction of steady-state plasma and saliva levels of desmethylimipramine using a single dose, single time point procedure. *Psychopharmacol (Berl).* 1978;74:115–121.

186. Cooper TB, Simpson GM. Prediction of individual dosage of nortriptyline. *Am J Psychiatry.* 1978;135:333–335.

187. Brunswick DJ, Amsterdam J, Schless A, et al. Prediction of steady state plasma concentrations of amitriptyline and nortriptyline from a single dose 24 hour level in depressed patients. *J Clin Psychiatry.* 1980;41:337–340.

188. Dawling S, Crome P, Braithwaite RA. Pharmacokinetics of single oral doses of nortriptyline in depressed elderly hospital patients and young healthy volunteers. *Clin Pharmacokinet.* 1980; 5:394–401.

189. Dawling S, Crome P, Braithwaite RA, et al. Nortriptyline therapy in elderly patients: Dosage prediction after a single dose pharmacokinetic study. *Eur J Pharmacol.* 1980;18:147–150.

190. Redman FC, Bowden CL, Lehmann LS. Single dose prediction of amitriptyline and nortriptyline requirement in unipolar depression. *Curr Ther Res.* 1980;27:635–642.

191. Dawling S, Crome P, Heyer EJ, et al. Nortriptyline therapy in elderly patients: Dosage prediction from plasma concentration at 24 hours after a single 50 mg dose. *Br J Psychiatry.* 1981;139:413–416.
192. Braithwaite RA, Dawling S, Montgomery S. Prediction of steady-state plasma concentrations and individual dosage regimens of tricyclic antidepressants from a single test dose. *Ther Drug Monit.* 1982;4:27–31.
193. Ziegler VE, Biggs JT, Rosen SH, et al. Imipramine and desipramine plasma levels: Relationship to dosage schedule and sampling time. *J Clin Psychiatry.* 1978;39:660–663.
194. Ziegler VE, Knesevich JW, Wylie LT, et al. Sampling time, dosage schedule, and nortriptyline plasma levels. *Arch Gen Psychiatry.* 1977;34:613–615.
195. Borga O, Piafsky KM, Nilsen OG. Plasma protein binding of basic drugs. I. Selective displacement from alpha-1 acid glycoprotein by tris-(2–butoxyethyl) phosphate. *Clin Pharmacol Ther.* 1977;22:539–544.
196. Brunswick DJ, Medels J. Reduced levels of tricyclic antidepressants in plasma from vacutainers. *Commun Psychopharmacol.* 1977;1:131–134.
197. Veith RC, Raisys VA, Perera C. The clinical impact of blood collection methods on tricyclic antidepressants as measured by GC/MS-SIM. *Commun Psychopharmacol.* 1978;2:491–494.
198. Zetin M, Rubin R, Rydzewski R. Tricyclic sample stability and the vacutainer effect. *Am J Psychiatry.* 1981;138:1247–1248.

Chapter 14

Cyclosporine

David I. Min

Keep in Mind

- Monitor renal function, liver function, and electrolytes.
- Review the concurrent medications and check the potential impact on cyclosporine concentrations, when the new drug is added or the existing drug is discontinued.
- Avoid use of nephrotoxic drugs with cyclosporine if possible.
- Use the same assay method and sample matrix for cyclosporine concentration monitoring consistently (ie, same laboratory in case of outpatient monitoring).
- Confirm the timing of blood draw and the last dose (ie, true trough) if the cyclosporine level is unexpectedly high or low.
- In a renal transplant patient, there is no definite indicator to differentiate graft rejection from cyclosporine-induced nephrotoxicity except renal biopsy.
- Identify any risk factors of altered cyclosporine absorption in the gastrointestinal tract.
- Cyclosporine bioavailability is poor and unpredictable just after liver transplantation, and intravenous dosing is needed for adequate immunosuppression.
- Cyclosporine absorption will improve significantly after the T-tube is clamped in liver transplantation and a dosage adjustment will be needed.
- Do not draw a blood sample from the same line used for intravenous cyclosporine administration.
- Identify various factors that may increase or decrease the metabolism of cyclosporine.
- Identify various factors that may enhance cyclosporine toxicity.
- Therapeutic ranges will change according to the assay method and sample matrix.
- The bioavailability of cyclosporine may change as time passes after transplantation.
- Counsel patients on the importance of taking cyclosporine at the same time and under same conditions daily, if possible.
- Maintain adequate cyclosporine concentrations when the doses of concurrent immunosuppressants are reduced or stopped because of their side effects.
- Counsel patients on the signs and symptoms of potential cyclosporine toxicity.
- Counsel patients on the importance of dental hygiene and risk of cyclosporine-induced gingival hyperplasia.

Cyclosporine, a cyclic peptide of 11 amino acids (molecular weight, 1203), was originally extracted from the fungus *Tolipocladium inflatum Gams*.[1] It has potent immunosuppressive activity and a selective ability to inhibit activation of T lymphocytes.[2] Cyclosporine is used to prevent allograft rejection in solid organ transplantation patients and in graft-versus-host disease in bone marrow transplant patients and to prevent or treat various autoimmune diseases. Allograft survival rates for renal, cardiac, hepatic, and pancreatic transplant recipients have significantly improved since cyclosporine was introduced for clinical use in 1978.[3–6] It also appears that cyclosporine is effective in preventing acute graft-versus-host disease in bone marrow transplant recipients.[7] Some patients with autoimmune diseases such as uveitis,[8] diabetes,[9] and myasthenia gravis[10] may benefit from cyclosporine therapy. Although a relationship has been demonstrated between blood or serum cyclosporine concentration and therapeutic effect, the difference between subtherapeutic and toxic concentrations of cyclosporine is narrow. In addition, dosing of cyclosporine is complicated by unpredictable, large intra- and interindividual variability in its pharmacokinetics. Many factors influence the pharmacokinetics of cyclosporine.[11] The therapeutic effect of cyclosporine in organ transplantation cannot be readily assessed and cyclosporine concentrations cannot be predicted on the basis of the dose alone. In considering the serious consequences of subtherapeutic cyclosporine concentrations, such as allograft rejection, and of toxic concentrations, such as renal failure, the careful monitoring of cyclosporine concentrations is essential for optimal care of patients receiving this drug.

CLINICAL PHARMACOLOGY AND THERAPEUTICS

Cyclosporine is a potent immunomodulator that acts selectively at an early stage in the activation of T lymphocytes by inhibiting production of soluble proliferative factors, interleukin-2 (IL-2) and other cytokines.[12] This is an important step for transplanted graft rejection or progress of autoimmune diseases. It does not suppress bone marrow function, which sets it apart from other immunosuppressive agents such as azathioprine.

Mechanism of Action

Cyclosporine does not act on the initial plasma membrane events of signal reception, transduction or calcium influx. The immunosuppressive activity of cyclosporine appears to be mediated by intracellular receptors.[13] At therapeutic concentrations, it enters the cell passively, and binds a cytoplasmic protein termed *cyclophilin,* which is the same enzyme known as peptidyl-prolyl-*cis–trans*-isomerase.[14] This enzyme catalyzes proline peptide bond isomerization, which is a rate-limiting step in protein folding.[14] After cyclosporine forms the cyclosporine–cyclophilin complex, this complex binds to and inhibits the Ca^{2+}-dependent phosphatase calcineurin.[15] Calcineurin is found to be the common molecular target mediating the immunosuppressive actions of cyclosporine and other immunosuppressive agents such as tacrolimus (FK 506).[16] Calcineurin is required for the proper assembly of a transcription factor that then binds to the IL-2 gene and initiates synthesis of IL-2 and other cytokines such as interferon-gamma.[16] IL-2 and other cytokines are necessary for helper and cytotoxic T-cell activation, proliferation, and maturation. A lack of cytokines disrupts the activation and proliferation of the helper and cytotoxic T cells that are essential for the rejection process.[12] Once IL-2 gene activation has expressed on T cells, however, cyclosporine is unable to inhibit IL-2-dependent activation, because it does not block IL-2 receptor expression or binding of IL-2 to its receptor. In addition, there is some evidence that suppressor T cells are relatively spared by cyclosporine therapy, which is important for halting the progress of autoimmune diseases. Cyclosporine is used mainly for prevention of rejection; it is relatively ineffective in reversing the process once rejection develops.

Therapeutic Use

Cyclosporine is used for prophylaxis of allograft rejection in organ transplantation, usually in conjunction with other immunosuppressive agents such as corticosteroids and azathioprine. It has improved allograft survival significantly in most solid organ transplantation. For example, 1-year graft survival for cadaveric renal transplants has improved by approximately 10 to 20% in most cyclosporine-including protocols. Other beneficial effects include reduced incidence of acute rejection or infectious complications compared with azathioprine–prednisone protocols.[17] Cyclosporine's beneficial effects are more significant in other solid organ transplantations such as liver and heart transplants. An improved immunosuppression with cyclosporine-containing protocols has changed liver and heart transplantation from experimental procedures to rapidly growing therapeutic modalities. It has also been used in preventing graft-versus-host disease in bone marrow transplantation and in treating autoimmune diseases.

CLINICAL PHARMACOKINETICS

Pharmacokinetic characteristics of cyclosporine in humans are highly variable in transplant patients as well as healthy volunteers under standardized conditions.[18] Significant factors influencing cyclosporine pharmacokinetics are illustrated in Figure 14–1, and pharmacokinetic parameters are summarized in Table 14–1. In addition, there is some confusion because the pharmacokinetic parameters are different depending on the cyclosporine analytic methods and sample matrix. This section discusses studies using specific analytic methods with whole blood samples, unless otherwise indicated.

Absorption

Cyclosporine is slowly and incompletely absorbed from the gastrointestinal tract after oral or intramuscular administration.[19,20] Intramuscular injection is not used clinically because of poor, unpredictable bioavailability. Absorption of cyclosporine in the gastrointestinal tract is highly variable, with a mean bioavailability of approximately 30% (range, <5 to 92%).[21,22] The absorption process of cyclosporine is best described by a zero-order kinetic model.[23] The zero-order absorption kinetics explain that an absorption window may exist in the upper part of the small intestine and that carrier-mediated transfer of cyclosporine across the intestinal wall may occur.[24] It is also postulated that the decrease in bioavailability with increasing dose is due to limited solubility in the gastrointestinal tract.[24] Cyclosporine appears in the blood after 0 to 0.9 hour, and the absorption half-life ranges from 0.5 to 2 hours.[25] Peak concentration (C_{max}) is usually achieved 2 to 6 hours after administration of the oral solution or soft gelatin capsule.[26] After

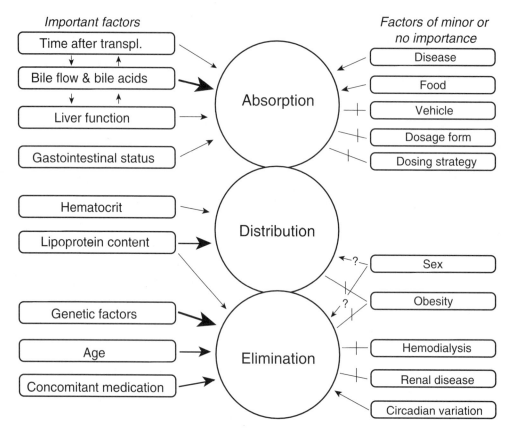

Figure 14–1. Factors with and without effect on the pharmacokinetics of cyclosporine. (*From Lindholm A. Factors influencing the pharmacokinetics of cyclosporine in man.* Ther Drug Monit. *1991;13:473, with permission.*)

single doses of 14 mg/kg given once daily, peak serum concentrations reach 1103 ± 570 ng/mL (SD) in renal transplant patients.[27] The poor bioavailability of cyclosporine appears to be related to the outcomes of renal transplantation. Patients with cyclosporine bioavailability of less than 25% have an increased risk of renal allograft loss (63% versus 83%).[22] The various factors influencing the bioavailability of cyclosporine are summarized in Table 14–2.

Bile acid has been shown to facilitate the bioavailability of many fat-soluble vitamins. It appears to emulsify cyclosporine, which facilitates lipophilic cyclosporine absorption. Liver transplant patients have very poor absorption of oral cyclosporine in the initial posttransplant period, when the bile fluid is drained externally via a T-tube.[11] Cyclosporine concentrations can increase two- to sixfold, when the T-tube is clamped and the bile flow is allowed to flow into the gastrointestinal tract.[11] Because of the variable concentrations of cyclosporine, many centers have used intravenous cyclosporine after liver transplant, gradually reducing the intravenous

TABLE 14–1. SUMMARY OF CYCLOSPORINE PHARMACOKINETICS[a]

Parameter	Average ± SD
Bioavailability (%)	
Renal	30 ± 13
Liver (pediatric)	<5–18[b]
Liver (adult)	27 ± 13
Heart	35 ± 11
Bone marrow	34[c]
First-pass metabolism (%)	10–27[b]
Enterohepatic circulation	Metabolites only
Protein binding (%)	>95
Clearance (mL/min/kg)	
Renal	5.7 ± 1.8
Liver	5.5[c]
Bone marrow	10.1 ± 1
T_{max} (h)	4.0 ± 1.8
C_{max} (ng/mL)[d]	1103 ± 570
V_{ss} (L/kg)	4.5 ± 1.5
Distribution $t_{1/2\alpha}$ (h)	1.1
Elimination $t_{1/2\beta}$ (h)	
Renal	11.4 ± 4.4
Uremic	15.8 ± 8.4
Liver failure	20.4 (10.8–48)
Hepatic metabolism (%)	>99
Biliary excretion (%)	>90
Hemodialysis	No effect
Peritoneal dialysis	No data available
Hemoperfusion	No effect

[a] All parameters based on whole blood samples and HPLC assay method except when indicated otherwise.
[b] Range.
[c] No SD reported; range = 20–50% (serum, RIA).
[d] This C_{max} is based on dose of 10 mg/kg.
Sources. References 18, 20, 21, 27, 38.

dose when the T-tube is clamped and increasing the oral dose to maintain sufficient cyclosporine blood concentrations.

Results on the effect of food on cyclosporine absorption are conflicting,[28–30] although effect appears to be related to the content of the food.[30] Gupta et al showed that the fat content of food is a major determining factor.[30] It was found that there was a significant increase in bioavailability in healthy volunteers (21–53%) when cyclosporine was given with a high-fat breakfast. It was explained that the increased outflow of bile stimulated by fatty meals enhances the absorption of cyclosporine.

TABLE 14–2. VARIOUS FACTORS AFFECTING CYCLOSPORINE BIOAVAILABILITY

Factor	Comments
T-tube (bile flow)	Increase oral cyclosporine dose or use IV before T-tube clamping and reduce dose after T-tube clamping.
Time after transplant	Bioavailability increases by 39% 3 mo after transplantation.
Liver function	Bioavailability is poor (<5%) in poor liver function.
Gastric emptying	Bioavailability increases when gastric emptying is increased by metoclopramide.
High-fat diet	Bioavailability increases.
Length of small bowel	Bioavailability decreases in the patient with short bowel.

Bioavailability gradually improves over several weeks following transplantation. It is observed clinically that patients require lower doses of cyclosporine to maintain the same trough concentrations several weeks after transplantation. This phenomenon can be explained partly by prolonged ileus in the early postoperative period, which attributes to poor absorption; however, in a longitudinal pharmacokinetic study before and after renal transplantation, Odlind et al noted that in the six patients tested 3 months posttransplantation, bioavailability had increased by almost 50% compared with the pretransplantation test.[31] It was not clear whether the change was related to amelioration of the uremic condition or other changes in lipid absorption.

It has been observed that the absorption of cyclosporine is impaired in patients with diarrhea. In bone marrow transplant recipients, orally administered cyclosporine was absorbed poorly or minimally in the presence of clinical intestinal dysfunction of any cause, such as chemoradiation enteritis, acute graft-versus-host disease of the intestine, and candida enteritis.[32] Patients without vomiting or diarrhea consistently showed cyclosporine serum values peaking 3 or 4 hours after an oral dose . It was found that the area under the curve (AUC) of cyclosporine in patients with diarrhea (>500 mL/72 h) was 38% of that in patients without diarrhea (polyclonal radioimmunoassay, serum).[32] Impaired cyclosporine absorption has also been found in pediatric liver transplant patients with diarrhea.[33] In liver transplant patients the hepatic function may be poor immediately after transplantation and bile production and flow may be reduced to one third of the normal production. Burckart et al reported that bioavailability was the least in liver recipients with liver disease and high serum bilirubin levels. These patients absorbed less than 5% of a given dose of cyclosporine.[33]

Any factors influencing gastric emptying and gastrointestinal motility influence the bioavailability of cyclosporine. Drugs increasing gastric emptying such as metoclopramide enhance cyclosporine absorption by 29%.[34] Another factor found to be important in cyclosporine absorption is small bowel length. Whitington et al concluded that the length of the small bowel was the chief determinant of the required dose of orally administered cyclosporine in children after liver transplantation and that the children require larger doses due to the limited absorptive surface of their intestine.[35] Patients with short gut syndrome or extensive intestinal resection also have decreased cyclosporine bioavailability (3% of bioavailability).[36]

Distribution

The distribution of cyclosporine is described by two phases[37]: initial rapid distribution phase with a half-life of 0.1 hour ($t_{1/2,\alpha}$), followed by a slower distribution phase with a half-life of 1.1 hour ($t_{1/2,\beta}$). The volume of distribution is variable, ranging from 2.9 to 4.7 L/kg in renal, liver, and bone marrow transplant patients,[38,39] but from 1.3 to 1.5 L/kg in healthy volunteers and heart transplant patients.[39,40] Cyclosporine is widely distributed into blood cells. In vitro studies with radiolabeled cyclosporine show that in blood, 58% of the circulating cyclosporine is bound to red blood cells, 4% to granulocytes, 5% to lymphocytes, and 33% is in plasma.[41] Binding of cyclosporine to red blood cells appears to be saturable and dependent on temperature and hematocrit, which may be a significant source of variability when serum or plasma samples are used for cyclosporine monitoring.[42,43] Plasma cyclosporine concentrations separated at 37°C were found to be 15% higher that those separated at 36°C.[44] This may imply that during febrile episodes, the distribution of cyclosporine shifts from blood cells to plasma. In plasma, cyclosporine is highly bound to plasma proteins (>95%), mainly lipoproteins, which constitute 10 to 15% of all plasma proteins.[45] Of the lipoproteins, high-density lipoprotein binds 43 to 57% of cyclosporine in plasma, low-density lipoprotein binds 25%, and very low density lipoprotein binds 2%.[46] Measuring the fraction of unbound cyclosporine in plasma is technically difficult because of adsorption of cyclosporine on the ultrafiltration membrane. The fraction of drug unbound in plasma ranges from 1.4 to 12% depending on the different techniques used.[47,48] Lindholm and Henricsson reported a 5-fold intraindividual variability and a 2.3-fold interindividual variability in the mean free fraction of cyclosporine in plasma.[49] They have also observed a significant correlation between the unbound fraction in plasma and the onset of acute rejection in renal transplant recipients.[49] Cyclosporine is distributed widely throughout body tissues, concentrating in organs, such as liver, pancreas, lungs, and kidneys.[50] The highest concentrations, which are found in fat and liver tissues, are up to 10-fold higher than blood concentrations. Despite the high concentrations in fat tissue, obesity was found to have no significant effect on cyclosporine volume of distribution based on serum or blood concentrations.[51] This indicates that the dose of cyclosporine in obese patients should be based on lean body weight rather than actual body weight. Cyclosporine does not readily penetrate the intact blood–brain barrier, and lower concentrations were found in the brain; however, liver transplant patients may have a functional abnormality in the blood–brain barrier because of sustained liver failure. Low serum cholesterol levels as well as prolonged liver disease appear to contribute to an increased risk of serious central nervous system toxic effects, such as mental confusion and seizures.[52] Cyclosporine passes the placenta and measurable concentrations are detected in the amniotic fluid and fetal blood, as well as in maternal breast milk.[53]

Metabolism

Cyclosporine is extensively metabolized by the hepatic cytochrome P450IIIA isoenzymes.[54] These isoenzymes are composed of at least four genes, among which P450IIIA4 (P450NF) is responsible for about 80% of cyclosporine metabolism in the liver.[55] Cyclosporine metabolic pathways in the body involve hydroxylation, N-demethylation, cyclization, and oxidation. Cyclosporine is metabolized to the metabolites M1, M9, M4N, and others.[56] Although cytochrome P450IIIA is located mainly in the liver, there is some evidence that cytochrome P450IIIA enzymes of gastric mucosa enterocytes contribute to presystemic metabolism of cyclosporine in the gastrointestinal tract.[57] More than 30 metabolites have been isolated and their chemical structures characterized, and all metabolites were found to preserve the cyclic oligopeptide structure. High concentrations of the metabolites in the blood raise the question of whether these metabolites contribute to the immunosuppressive activity or toxicity of the parent drug. So far, there is no evidence that the metabolites have significant immunosuppressive activity compared with cyclosporine. Only M1, which is the predominant metabolite in the blood, was found to have about 10% of the immunosuppressive activity of the parent drug.[58] None of the metabolites appears to have significant nephrotoxicity. Cyclosporine is a low- to intermediate-clearance drug, and its clearance is therefore dependent on the intrinsic enzyme activity and the unbound fraction in the blood. Clearance was reported to average 5.7 mL/min/kg in adult kidney recipients, 5.5 mL/min/kg in adult liver recipients, and 10 to 13 mL/min/kg in bone marrow transplant patients.[38,59] In healthy volunteer and heart transplant patients, clearance is slightly lower (about 4 mL/min/kg) than in other patient groups.[38,59]

The mean elimination half life varies from 7 to 24 hours depending on the type of transplant and concurrent disease states.[38,59] In adult renal transplant recipients with near-normal renal function, the mean half-life of cyclosporine is about 10 hours.[38] Because cyclosporine is metabolized in the liver, cyclosporine clearance is significantly reduced and half-life is prolonged in patients with liver diseases, averaging 20 hours (range, 10–48 hours).[38]

In one study with bone marrow recipients,[60] a 23% reduction in clearance of cyclosporine and prolonged half-life (32.1 hours) were observed in patients with hyperbilirubinemia (serum bilirubin > 20 mg/L). The clearance of cyclosporine was also decreased by 30% in renal recipients with impaired hepatic function.[61] Cyclosporine doses should be decreased in most patients with hepatic failure. A few pharmacokinetic studies have reported a second peak, which occurs about 4 to 6 hours after the first peak.[38,62] The reason for the double peak is not clear. One explanation is that undissolved cyclosporine, due to the limited solubility of cyclosporine in the gastrointestinal tract, can be resolubilized and absorbed several hours later by bile acid secretion possibly stimulated by food.[62] The other possible explanation is that the sulfate-conjugated metabolites of cyclosporine excreted through the bile may be degraded by intestinal bacteria into parent cyclosporine, which can then be reabsorbed in the gastrointestinal tract.[11] In usual clinical dosage ranges, cyclosporine appears to be metabolized first-order processes,[63] though some studies suggest nonlinear increases in plasma concentration as cyclosporine dosage was increased.[64] A few case reports of high-dose cyclosporine intoxication, however, did not indicate any nonlinear cyclosporine elimination.[65,66]

The clearance of cyclosporine is clearly dependent on the age of patients. In pediatric patients, cyclosporine clearance is generally twice as fast as in adult liver recipients. For example, Burckart et al reported that cyclosporine clearance in pediatric liver recipients (about 1–5 years) was 9.3 mL/min/kg compared with 5.5 mL/min/kg in adult liver transplant patients.[33] Because of this, some pediatric patients require three-times-daily dosing schedules to maintain adequate trough cyclosporine concentrations compared with twice- or once-a-day dosing schedule in adult patients.

Although circardian variations of cyclosporine clearance are observed, they appear to be clinically insignificant. Canafax et al found that the evening dosing of cyclosporine increases the total AUC of cyclosporine and its metabolites (M1 and M9) compared with morning dosing of cyclosporine in six pancreas transplant patients.[67] On the other hand, Venkataramanan et al found an increased clearance of cyclosporine at nighttime in two liver transplant recipients.[68]

Elimination

In humans, biliary excretion is the major pathway of elimination of cyclosporine. Because of extensive metabolism, most biliary excretion consists of the metabolites and less than 1% of the dose of cyclosporine is detected in the bile.[69] Urinary excretion of cyclosporine is a minor pathway of elimination because cyclosporine is highly lipophilic and extensively metabolized by the liver. According to a study in which radiolabeling was used, only 6% of the radioactivity is excreted in the urine in 96 hours, and most of radioactivity comes from the metabolites M1, M1c, and M9, which are present in higher concentrations than the parent drug in the urine.[70] Renal failure does not appear to impair cyclosporine excretion.[71]

PHARMACODYNAMICS

Drug–Drug Interactions

Numerous interactions between cyclosporine and other drugs can produce troublesome clinical effects.[72-74] The clinically significant drug–drug interactions are summarized in Table 14–3.

It is not known if antacids can decrease cyclosporine absorption, but there appears to be no effect.[75] No effects were seen when cholestyramine was given 1 hour before or 4 hours after the cyclosporine dose.[72,73] Metoclopramide increases cyclosporine levels, and severe diarrhea can decrease cyclosporine levels.[34]

As cyclosporine is extensively metabolized by the hepatic cytochrome P450IIIA enzyme system, various drugs that induce or inhibit these enzymes usually have significant effects on cyclosporine concentrations. Antiepileptic drugs, such as phenytoin, phenobarbital, and carbamazepine, induce these enzymes and decrease the concentration of cyclosporine. Phenytoin effects on cyclosporine metabolism begin as early as 2 days after phenytoin starts, last at least 2 weeks after its discontinuation, and usually necessitate two or three times higher cyclosporine doses.[74] A good alternative antiepileptic drug might be valproic acid, which likely has no effect on cyclosporine concentrations. The antitubercular drugs rifampin and isoniazid are also potent inducers of the P450IIIA enzymes and reduce cyclosporine concentrations.[73,74]

Drugs that inhibit the hepatic microsomal enzymes increase cyclosporine concentrations; for example, ketoconazole has caused a tenfold increase in cyclosporine concentrations with subsequent increases in serum creatinine levels.[75] Fluconazole can increase cyclosporine concentrations slightly after 2 weeks of therapy.[76] Giving erythromycin to a patient on cyclosporine typically causes cyclosporine concentrations to increase up to threefold 2 to 14 days after the initiation of therapy.[77]

Calcium channel blockers, such as diltiazem and nicardipine, can slightly increase cyclosporine concentrations, but nifedipine appears to have no effect.[78] Hormones such as danazol, norethisterone, and methyltestosterone have been reported to increase cyclosporine concentrations, but the clinical significance of this interaction remains unclear. H_2 blockers such as cimetidine, ranitidine, and famotidine appear to have no effect on cyclosporine pharmacokinetics.[74]

TABLE 14–3. CLINICALLY IMPORTANT DRUG INTERACTIONS OF CYCLOSPORINE

Drugs	Mechanism	Effects	Management
Antiepileptic drugs Phenytoin Phenobarbital Carbamazepine	Increased cyclosporine metabolism and reduced bioavailability by induction of cytochrome p450 enzyme	Cyclosporine trough levels drop within 48 h of initiation of these drugs and remain low for at least 2 wk after discontinuation	Increase cyclosporine dose with frequent monitoring of cyclosporine levels or use valproic acid, which has no interaction.
Rifampicin or INH	Same as above	Same as above	Increase cyclosporine dose with frequent monitoring of cyclosporine levels.
Octreotide	Reduced cyclosporine absorption	Cyclosporine levels decrease within 24 to 48 h.	Increase oral cyclosporine dose or use IV cyclosporine; frequent monitoring of cyclosporine levels is required.
Azole antifungal agents Ketoconazole Fluconazole Itraconazole	Inhibition of liver cytochrome P-450 enzyme by these drugs	Cyclosporine levels significantly increase ($\times 2$–10) within 2 d, resulting in nephrotoxicity (ketoconazole > itraconazole > fluconazole)	Reduce cyclosporine dose with frequent monitoring of levels.
Macrolide antibiotics Erythromycin Josamycin	Inhibition of liver and GI cytochrome P450 enzymes	AUC ($\times 2$) and cyclosporine trough levels ($\times 2$–3) increase.	Same as above
Calcium channel blockers Verapamil Diltiazem Nicardipine	Same as above	Same as above	Reduce cyclosporine dose or use nifedipine, isradipine, or nitrendipine.
Oral contraceptives and danazol	Same as above	Same as above	Reduce cyclosporine dose.
Cholesterol-lowering drugs Lovastatin Simvastatin Pravastatin		Incidence of rhabdomyolysis or muscle pain increases.	Switch to non-HMG CoA[a] inhibitors or reduce the dose of these drugs with careful monitoring.

[a] Hydroxymethylglutaryl coenzyme A.

458

TABLE 14–4. SIDE EFFECTS OF CYCLOSPORINE

Side Effects	Incidence	Symptoms	Management
Nephrotoxicity	Most patients	Slowly rising BUN and serum creatinine, decreasing urine output	Monitor blood level; avoid nephrotoxic drugs.
Hypertension	23–100%	Increased blood pressures	Use same measures as for general hypertension.
Hyperkalemia	Uncommon	Elevated serum potassium levels, renal dysfunction is risk factor	Institute diuretic therapy with serum potassium monitoring; use Kayexalate.
Hepatotoxicity	Up to 50%	Hyperbilirubinemia, elevated liver enzymes	Reduce cyclosporine dose; effects are generally mild and no treatment is necessary.
Neurotoxicity	15%	Hand tremors, paresthesis (common), seizure, mental confusion (rare)	Reduce cyclosporine dose; monitor serum magnesium and cholesterol levels.
Hirsutism	30%	Hair growth on the dorsum of the hand, arms, and face	
Gingival hyperplasia	Uncommon	Gum overgrowth	Instruct patient on dental hygiene.

Amphotericin B, aminoglycosides, trimethoprim–sulfamethoxazole, melphalan, furosemide, mannitol, indomethacin, and the cephalosporins increase the incidence of adverse renal effects when given with cyclosporine therapy.[72,73] Drugs that decrease cyclosporine-induced renal effects include spironolactone, enalapril, prazosin, thromboxane synthetase inhibitors, and some prostaglandins.[72,73]

The combination of cyclosporine and lovastatin has been reported to cause a myalgia, rhabdomyolysis syndrome.[79] Patients on cyclosporine are prone to gingival hyperplasia, which can be worsened by other drugs such as phenytoin and nifedipine.

Cyclosporine causes various side effects, of which dose-related nephrotoxicity is the most common and serious. The major side effects of cyclosporine are summarized in Table 14–4.

Adverse Reactions

Nephrotoxic Effects

Almost all patients who receive cyclosporine have some degree of cyclosporine-related renal dysfunction at any dose. Cyclosporine-induced renal dysfunction has been well documented. Cyclosporine-induced nephrotoxicity appears in three basic types[80–82]: first, acute, reversible reduction of glomerular filtration rate; second, tubular toxicity with possible enzymuria and aminoaciduria; and third, irreversible interstitial fibrosis and arteriopathy at a later period, usually 6 months to 12 months after transplantation. The exact mechanism of cyclosporine-induced nephrotoxicity is not completely understood, but cyclosporine appears to disturb the normal activity of various vasoactive substances in the kidney. First, cyclosporine alters the balance of the vasodilator prostacycline and its antagonist thromboxane A_2 in renal cortical tissue.[83] The evidence to support this hypothesis is that prostacycline levels are reduced in cyclosporine-treated patients and the thromboxane A_2 synthesis inhibitor appears to improve renal function. More rare, severe forms of nephrotoxicity manifest as a form of thrombotic microangiopathy which consists of glomerular thrombosis formation and a microangiographic anemia.[84] Cyclosporine appears to reduce prostacycline production, which causes unopposed thromboxane effects. Cyclosporine-induced thrombotic microangiopathy is a serious condition, which may cause graft loss.

Second, it has also been reported that cyclosporine may increase concentrations of the endothelial cell-derived vasoconstrictive peptide endothelin.[85] Cyclosporine added directly to cultured human vascular cells increases the level of endothelin in the culture medium. In the rat model, 20 mg/kg IV cyclosporine caused circulating endothelin levels to increase more than 20 times. Although endothelin appears to affect all vascular vessels, renal vessels are especially susceptible to endothelin's vasoconstrictor effects. These effects produce severe renal vasoconstriction, a decrease in renal blood flow, and a decrease in glomerular filtration rate, usually without morphologic changes, although chronic effects may progress to interstitial fibrosis.

There is controversy over whether cyclosporine increases the incidence of delayed graft function in cadaveric renal transplantation. It may not increase the incidence of delayed graft function per se; however, it appears to enhance ischemic injury of the kidney, require prolonged dialysis support, and delay the recovery from acute tubular necrosis once it occurs.[86] Because of this potential additional insult of cyclosporine on the cadaveric kidney, many transplant centers use sequential initiation of cyclosporine in the immediate posttransplant period by avoiding cyclosporine until diuresis begins.

The possibility of long-term toxic effects of cyclosporine on the kidney and the risk of renal failure has been raised. In fact, a small number of heart and other organ transplant patients receiving cyclosporine develop chronic renal failure,[87] but in most of patients, kidney function appears to be stabilized with a reduced dose of cyclosporine, even when cyclosporine is continued.[82,88] Although some progressive loss of renal function continues for up to 7 years, the rate of decline appears to be much slower after the first year.

Other Toxic Effects

Some patients treated with cyclosporine develop hepatic dysfunction, which is generally subclinical and dose dependent, especially in the first 90 days posttransplant. This hepatic toxicity is commonly characterized by mild hyperbilirubinemia and elevated serum transaminases.[89,90] In the majority of patients, these alterations in liver function are rapidly reversible by reducing the dose of cyclosporine. It is recommended that liver function tests be performed regularly for patients treated with cyclosporine.

Though not common, patients may develop mild hyperkalemia during cyclosporine therapy, partly as a result of renal dysfunction. Close monitoring of serum potassium is required, particularly in early posttransplantation.[91] If the serum potassium is less than 6 mEq/L, hyperkalemia may be managed with diuretics, but if the serum potassium is greater than 6 mEq/L, sodium polystyrene sulfonate (Kayexalate) with sorbitol should be initiated to reduce serum potassium. Potassium-sparing diuretics such as spironolactone should not be used in patients receiving cyclosporine.

Cyclosporine-induced neurotoxic effects are relatively common. In the early Canadian multicenter clinical study, 15% of patients receiving cyclosporine developed neurotoxic effects compared with 1% of the placebo group.[3] Cyclosporine-induced neurotoxicity is mild in most cases, manifesting as tremors and paresthesias. Other neurotoxic effects such as seizures and mental confusion have been uncommon. Liver transplant recipients are especially susceptible to these toxic effects of cyclosporine. De Groen et al described a syndrome of confusion, cortical blindness, quadriplegia, seizures, and coma in liver transplant recipients.[52] Hypocholesterolemia was identified as a significant risk factor for these patients. In that study, most patients who developed neurotoxic effects had extremely low total cholesterol levels (<120 mg/dL). It was explained that a high unbound fraction caused by low cholesterol, along with possible disruption of the blood–brain barrier caused by liver failure, may have contributed to these unusual neurotoxic effects.

Besides the side effects associated with cyclosporine therapy listed above, the other most common adverse reaction is hypertension.[92] Hypertension is quite common (21–100%) in the patient receiving cyclosporine.[92] Cyclosporine-associated hypertension may be related to the nephrotoxic effects of the drug as well as renal vasoconstriction. Cyclosporine-induced hypertension can usually be controlled well by various antihypertensive medications. Other minor side effects include hair overgrowth and gingival hyperplasia. Some patients tend to tolerate these adverse reactions during long-term therapy, but others need special care such as antihypertensive treatment, cosmetics, and gingivectomy.

THERAPEUTIC REGIMEN DESIGN

Therapeutic Monitoring

Table 14–5 summarizes the therapeutic ranges for the various analytic methods and blood matrices that are in clinical use.[93] Therapeutic ranges of cyclosporine are at best empirical guidelines. Because cyclosporine is generally used for prevention of rejection or graft-versus-host disease, the major limitation to defining the therapeutic ranges is the lack of standards for diagnosing toxicity or degree of immunosuppression.[94] There is no readily available marker that measures the degree of immunosuppression by cyclosporine other than acute rejection by a tissue biopsy. The only readily available test for nephrotoxicity has been serum creatinine concentration, which is insensitive to small changes in glomerular filtration rate.[95] It is difficult to establish the therapeutic ranges of cyclosporine because the clinical studies reported in the literature have often used different analytic methods, different sample matrices (serum, plasma, or whole blood), different dosing schedules, (twice daily, once daily), or different concurrent immunosuppressive agents in the various patient groups. Measuring cyclosporine concentrations, however, does help identify patients with low or high values who might benefit from dosage changes.

Whether whole blood, plasma, or serum should be used as the sample matrix has been controversial, but whole blood is recommended for several analytic reasons.[38,95] About 50% of the circulating cyclosporine in the blood is bound to erythrocytes, and concentrations depend greatly on the sample matrix chosen for analysis. Furthermore, the distribution of cyclosporine

TABLE 14–5. THERAPEUTIC RANGES OF CYCLOSPORINE

Type of Transplant	Sample Matrix	Analytic Method[a]	Target Range (ng/mL)
Kidney	Whole blood	HPLC, S-RIA, or	150–250 (<3 mo)
		S-FPIA	100–200 (>3 mo)
		NS-FPIA	400–800
	Serum/plasma	NS-FPIA	100–250
Liver	Whole blood	HPLC or S-RIA	200–300
		NS-FPIA	400–800
Heart	Whole blood	HPLC or S-RIA	150–300
Bone marrow	Serum/plasma	NS-FPIA or NS-RIA[b]	150–300

[a] HPLC, high-performance liquid chromatography; S-RIA, monoclonal radioimmunoassay specific for cyclosporine; S-FPIA, fluorescence polarization immunoassay specific for cyclosporine; NS-FPIA, nonspecific fluorescence polarization immunoassay; NS-RIA, nonspecific polyclonal radioimmunoassay.
[b] No longer available.

among plasma and blood cells is influenced by many factors such as temperature, hematocrit, drug concentrations, and incubation time. These factors may cause considerable variation in serum or plasma cyclosporine concentrations, when serum or plasma is separated from whole blood under the different conditions. Considerable efforts are involved in developing a consensus for these issues, but some issues remain unresolved.[96]

High-performance liquid chromatography (HPLC), radioimmunoassay (RIA), and fluorescence polarization immunoassay (FPIA) are the principal analytic methods available for cyclosporine monitoring.[97] HPLC is regarded as a reference standard assay; it detects cyclosporine and its metabolites separately, but requires intense labor and reliable skill for routine clinical monitoring. Specific monoclonal radioimmunoassay (S-MRIA) or specific FPIA (S-FPIA), which show good correlation to the results of HPLC, are specific for cyclosporine; however, the polyclonal radioimmunoassay (which is no longer available) and nonspecific fluorescence polarization (NS-FPIA) are nonspecific, cross-reacting with cyclosporine metabolites. There is also a nonspecific monoclonal radioimmunoassay. Results from nonspecific assay methods need to be interpreted with caution in patients with reduced hepatic function, as accumulation of metabolites occurs. Whole blood concentrations are usually much higher than serum concentrations, because cyclosporine distributes into erythrocytes. Assay accuracy is poor at concentrations of less than 50 ng/mL, which becomes important at low doses of cyclosporine.

As discussed in the previous section, the adverse reactions associated with high cyclosporine concentrations include renal dysfunction, tremor, hypertension, and hepatotoxicity. Nephrotoxicity is the most common adverse effect that is dose related; decreasing the cyclosporine dose will usually decrease the creatinine level. In renal allograft recipients, it is often difficult to differentiate between cyclosporine renal effects and acute rejection episodes. The measurement of cyclosporine concentrations may be helpful in this situation where high levels are more likely associated with cyclosporine effects and low levels with rejection.[97,98]

Clinically, 12- or 24-hour trough cyclosporine concentrations (depending on the dosing frequency) are used for monitoring therapy. There is no definite study in which cyclosporine concentrations have a better predictable value for the clinical events such as rejection or nephrotoxicity; however, because of individual variability in pharmacokinetics, the exact timing of peak concentration is not possible to predict. That is the main reason trough concentrations are used for therapeutic monitoring. Because trough concentrations may not reflect the total amount of drug exposure during the dosing interval, some transplant centers advocate that individualized oral doses be based on the area under the curve (AUC) measurement as a more useful tool to predict the clinical events.[99] So far, there is no evidence that this method has clearly better predictive value for the clinical events than trough concentration monitoring.

Dosage and Administration

Initial oral cyclosporine doses are usually about 8 to 14 mg/kg/d. For living donor kidney recipients, cyclosporine is given 1 to 2 days before transplantation to achieve therapeutic concentrations at the time of transplantation.[100] This dose is divided twice daily and adjusted to maintain the desired cyclosporine concentrations. Dosage adjustment is empiric as a result of extreme intrapatient variability in absorption and clearance. A pharmacokinetic dosing program that uses each patient's pharmacokinetic parameters will soon be available. Antilymphoblast globulin or OKT3 is often used in the early posttransplant period for cadaver kidney recipients to allow cyclosporine to be held until serum creatinine concentrations are less than 3 mg/dL, in an attempt to avoid adverse renal effects of cyclosporine.[17]

Administration of oral cyclosporine is usually preferred; however, for those patients who cannot tolerate oral therapy or whose cyclosporine absorption is poor, intravenous doses of between 3 and 6 mg/kg/d can be given. Hepatic, heart–lung, and pancreatic allograft recipients usually require intravenous cyclosporine in the first few weeks posttransplant. Loading doses are not used when beginning cyclosporine therapy as side effects would likely occur. Before use, intravenous cyclosporine solution should be diluted in 20 to 100 mL of normal saline or 5% dextrose for injection and given as a slow intravenous infusion over 2 to 6 hours. The intravenous cyclosporine dose can be given by a continuous 24-hour infusion which may reduce the renal effects of the drug. The intravenous dose is adjusted using trough levels. Blood samples for cyclosporine analysis should not be drawn from the intravenous lines used for administration, to avoid spuriously high levels. Patients being given intravenous cyclosporine can be changed to oral therapy by giving three times the intravenous dose and measuring cyclosporine concentrations.

To make the oral cyclosporine solution more palatable, patients can dilute their dose with chocolate milk or juice. A glass container should be used for mixing to avoid adsorption of the drug to wax or plastic containers.[101] To ensure cyclosporine absorption and assess the adequacy of the dose, a trough level should be taken within the first 2 or 3 days of starting therapy. Because absorption and clearance change during the first weeks of therapy, levels should be obtained at least two or three times weekly. After discharge from the hospital, levels should be obtained at least twice per week until the blood levels are stable usually within 1 or 2 months. Chronic cyclosporine dosing is guided by weekly and then monthly blood concentrations and serum creatinine levels, with most patients requiring approximately 5 to 6 mg/kg cyclosporine daily.

———————— QUESTIONS ————————————————————

1. What is the major characteristic of cyclosporine pharmacologic action and how is it related to its clinical use? (Please refer to the section Mechanism of Action.)

2. How is cyclosporine therapy initiated in solid organ transplant? (Please refer to the section Dosage and Administration.)

3. What are the issues in cyclosporine therapeutic drug monitoring regarding different sample matrices and assay methods? (Please refer to the section Therapeutic Drug Monitoring.)

4. How can cyclosporine-induced nephrotoxicity be differentiated from graft rejection in renal transplant patients?

5. What methods are used to reduce cyclosporine nephrotoxicity?

6. Cytochrome P450 enzyme-inducing agents and inhibiting agents are known to interfere with cyclosporine pharmacokinetics. What is the onset of their interactions and how long do their effects last after discontinuation of these drugs?

7. What is the role of the T-tube for cyclosporine pharmacokinetics in liver transplant patients?

REFERENCES

1. Borel IF, Feurer C, Gubler HU, Stahelin H. Biological effects of cyclosporine A: A new antilymphocytic agent. *Agents Actions.* 1976;6:468.
2. Hess AD, Colombani PM. Mechanism of action of cycloporine: Role of calmodulin, cyclophilin, and other cyclosporine-binding proteins. *Transplant Proc.* 1986;18 (suppl 5): 219.
3. Canadian Multicenter Transplant Study Group. A randomized clinical trial of cyclosporine in cadaveric renal transplantation. *N Engl J Med.* 1983;309:809.
4. Iwatsuki S, Starzl TE, Todo S, et al. Experience in 1000 liver transplants under cyclosporine–steroid therapy: A survival report. *Transplant Proc* 1988; 20(suppl 1):498.
5. Bolman RM, Olivari MT, Saffitz J, et al. Improved immunosuppression for heart transplantation. *J Heart Transplant.* 1985;4:315.
6. Sutherland DER, Gruber SA. Pancreas transplantation. *Crit Care Clin.* 1990;6(4):947.
7. Storb R, Deeg HJ, Thomas EL, et al: Preliminary results of prospective randomized trials comparing methotrexate and cyclosporine for prophylaxis of graft-versus-host disease after HLA-identical marrow transplantation. *Transplant Proc.* 1983;15:2620.
8. Nussenblatt RB, Palestine AG, Rook AH, et al. Treatment of intraocular inflammatory disease with cyclosporin A. *Lancet.* 1982;2:235.
9. Stiller C, Depre JP, Gent M, et al: Effects of cyclosporine immunosuppression in insulin-dependent diabetes of recent onset. *Science.* 1984;223:1362.

10. Tindall RFA, Rollands JA, Phillips JT, et al. Preliminary results of a double blind randomized placebo controlled trial of cyclosporine in myasthenia gravis. *N Engl J Med.* 1987;316:719.

11. Lindholm A. Factors influencing the pharmacokinetics of cyclosporine in man. *Ther Drug Monit.* 1991;13:465.

12. Kahan BD. Cyclosporine. *N Engl J Med.* 1989;321:1725.

13. Freeman DJ. Pharmacology and pharmacokinetics of cyclosporine. *Clin Biochem.* 1991;24:9.

14. Fischer G. Cyclophilin and peptidyl-prolyl *cis–trans* isomerase are probably identical proteins. *Nature.* 1989 :337:476.

15. Schumacher A, Norheim A. Progress towards a molecular understanding of cyclosporin A-mediated immunosuppression. *Clin Invest.* 1992;70:773.

16. Schreiber SL, Crabtree GR. The mechanism of action of cyclosporin A and FK 506. *Immunol Today.* 1992;13: 136.

17. Canafax DM, Min DI, Gruber SA, et al. Immunosuppression for cadaveric renal allograft recipients: A risk-factor matched comparison of the Minnesota randomized trial with an antilymphoblast globulin, azathioprine, cyclosporine and prednisone protocol. *Clin Transplant.* 1989;3:110.

18. Fahr A. Cyclosporine clinical pharmacokinetics. *Clin Pharmacokinet.* 1993;24 (6);472.

19. Drewe J, Beglinger C, Kissel T. The absorption site of cyclosporin in the human gastrointestinal tract. *Br J Clin Pharmacol.* 1992;33:39.

20. Beveridge T, Gratwohl A, Michot F, et al. Cyclosporine A: Pharmacokinetics after a single dose in man and serum levels after multiple dosing in recipients of allogeneic bone-marrow grafts. *Curr Ther Res.* 1981;30:5.

21. Ptachcinski RJ, Venkataramanan R, Burckart GJ, et al. Clinical pharmacokinetics of cyclosporine. *Clin Pharmacokinet.* 1986;11:107.

22. Lindholm A, Kahan BD. Influence of cyclosporine pharmacokinetics, trough concentrations, and AUC monitoring on outcome after kidney transplantation. *Clin Pharmacol Ther.* 1993;54:205.

23. Grevel J, Kuts K, Abish E, at al. Evidence for zero order absorption of cyclosporine. *Br J Clin Pharmacol.* 1986;22:220.

24. Reymond JP, Steimer JL, Niederberger W. On the dose dependency of cyclosporine A absorption and disposition in healthy volunteers. *J Pharmacokinet Biopharm.* 1988;16:331.

25. Lindberg A, Odlind B, Tufveson G, et al. The pharmacokinetics of cyclosporine A in uremic patients. *Transplant Proc.* 1986;18(suppl 5):144.

26. Min DL, Hwang GC, Bergstom S, et al. Bioavailability and patient acceptance of cyclosporine soft gelatin capsules in renal allograft recipients. *Ann Pharmacother.* 1992;26:175.

27. Ptachcinski RJ, Venkataramanan R, Rosenthal JT, et al. Cyclosporine kinetics in renal transplantation. *Clin Pharmacol Ther.* 1985;38:296.

28. Ptachcinski RJ, Venkataramanan R, Rosenthal JT, et al. The effect of food on cyclosporine absorption. *Transplantation.* 1985:40:174.

29. Lindholm A, Henricsson S, Dahlqvist R. The effect of food and bile acid administration on the relative bioavailability of cyclosporine. *Br J Clin Pharmacol.* 1990;29:541.

30. Gupta SK, Manfro RC, Tomlanovich SJ, et al. Effect of food on the pharmacokinetics of cyclosporine in healthy subjects following oral and intravenous administration. *J Clin Pharmacol.* 1990;30:643.

31. Odlind B, Lindberg A, Tufveson G, et al. Longitudinal study of the pharmacokinetics of cyclosporine before and after renal transplantation. *Transplant Proc.* 1986;18(suppl 5):47.

32. Atkinson K, Britton K, Paull P, et al. Detrimental effect of intestinal disease on absorption of orally administered cyclosporine. *Transplant Proc.* 1983;15:2446.

33. Burckart GJ, Starzl T, Williams L, et al. Cyclosporine monitoring and pharmacokinetics in pediatric liver transplant patients. *Transplant Proc.* 1985;17:1172.

34. Wadhwa NK, Schroeder TJ, O'Flaherty E, et al. The effect of oral metoclopramide on the absorption of cyclosporine. *Transplantation.* 1987;43:211.

35. Whitington PF, Emond JC, Whitington SH, et al. Small-bowel length and the dose of cyclosporine in children after liver transplantation. *N Engl J Med.* 1990;322:733.

36. Roberts R, Sketris IS, Abraham I, et al. Cyclosporine absorption in two patients with short-bowel syndrome. *Drug Intell Clin Pharm.* 1988;22:570.

37. Follath F, Wenk M, Vozeh S, et al. Intravenous cyclosporine kinetics in renal failure. *Clin Pharmacol Ther.* 1983;34:638.

38. Shaw LM, Bowers LD, Demers L, et al. Critical issues in cyclosporine monitoring: report of the task force on cyclosporine monitoring. *Clin Chem.* 1987;33:1269.

39. Ptachcinski R, Burckart GJ, Rosenthal JT, et al. Cyclosporine pharmacokinetics in children following cadaveric renal transplantation. *Transplant Proc.* 1985;18:766.

40. Ptachcinski R, Venkataramanan R, Burckart GJ, et al. Cycloporine kinetics in healthy volunteers. *J Clin Pharmacol.* 1987;27:243.

41. Lemaire M, Tillement JP. Role of lipoproteins and erythrocytes in the in vitro binding and distribution of cyclosporin A in the blood. *J Pharm Pharmacol.* 1982;34:715.

42. Niederberger W, et al. Distribution and binding of cyclosporine in blood and tissues. *Transplant Proc..* 1983;15:2419.

43. Rosano TG. Effect of hematocrit on cyclosporine (cyclosporin A) in whole blood and plasma of renal-transplant patients. *Clin Chem.* 1985;31:410.

44. Humbert H, Vernillet L, Cabiac MD, et al. Influence of different parameters for the monitoring of cyclosporine. *Transplant Proc.* 1990;22:1210.

45. Mraz W, Kemkes BM, Knedel M. The role of lipoproteins in exchange and transfer of cyclosporine—Results from in vitro investigations. *Transplant Proc.* 1986;18:1281.

46. Sgoutas D, Macmahon W, Love A, Jerkunica I. Interaction of cyclosporine A with human lipoproteins. *J Pharm Pharmacol.* 1986;38:583.

47. Henricsson S. A new method for measuring the free fraction of cyclosporine in plasma by equilibrium dialysis. *J Pharm Pharmacol.* 1987;39:384.

48. Legg B, Lowland M. Cyclosporine: Measurement of fraction unbound in plasma. *J Pharm Pharmcol.* 1987;39:599.

49. Lindholm A, Henricsson S. Intra- and interindividual variability in the free fraction of cyclosporine in plasma in recipients of renal transplants. *Ther Drug Monit.* 1989;11:623.

50. Atkinson K, Boland J, Britton K, Biggs J. Blood and tissue distribution of cyclosporine in humans and mice. *Transplant Proc.* 1983; 15(suppl 1):2430.

51. Flechner SM, Kolbeinsson ME, Tam J, Lum B. The impact of body weight on cyclosporine pharmacokinetics in renal transplant recipients. *Transplantation.* 1989;47:806.

52. De Groen PC, Aksamit AJ, Rakela J, et al. Central nervous system toxicity after liver transplantation: The role of cyclosporine and cholesterol. *N Engl J Med.* 1987;317:861.

53. Venkataramanan R, Koneru B, Wang C-CP, et al. Cyclosporine and its metabolites in mother and baby. *Transplantation.* 1988;46:468.

54. Kronbach T, Fischer V, Meyer UA. Cyclosporine metabolism in human liver: Identification of a cytochrome P-450III gene family as the major cyclosporine-metabolizing enzyme explains interactions of cyclosporine with other drugs. *Clin Pharmacol Ther.* 1988;43:630.

55. Colbalert J, Fabre I, Dalet I, et al. Metabolism of cyclosporine A. *Drug Metab Dispos.* 1989;17:197.

56. Maurer G, Loosli HR, Schreier E, Keller B. Disposition of cyclosporine in several animal species and man. I. Structural elucidation of its metabolites. *Drug Metab Dispos.* 1984;12:120.

57. Kolars JC, Awni WM, Merion RM, Watkins PB. First-pass metabolism of cyclosporine by the gut. *Lancet.* 1991;338:1488.

58. Yatscoff RW, Rosano TG, Bowers LD. The clinical significance of cyclosporine metabolites. *Clin Biochem.* 1991;24:23–35.

59. Ptachcinski RJ, Venkataramanan R, Burckart GJ, et al. Clinical pharmacokinetics of cyclosporine. *Clin Pharmacokinet.* 1986;11:107–132.

60. Yee GC, Kennedy MS, Storb R, Thomas ED. Effect of hepatic dysfunction on oral cyclosporine pharmacokinetics in marrow transplant patients. *Blood.* 1984;64:1277.

61. Venkataramanan R, Gray J, Ptachcinski RJ, et al. Cyclosporine kinetics in liver disease. *Clin Pharmacol Ther.* 1985;37:234.

62. Yee GC, Salomon DR. Cyclosporine. In: Evans WE, Schentag JJ, Jusko WJ, eds. *Applied Pharmacokinetics.* Vancouver: Applied Therapeutics, 1992:28.

63. Grevel J, Welsh MS, Kahan BD. Linear cyclosporine pharmacokinetics. *Clin Pharmcol Ther.* 1988;43:175.

64. Awni WM, Sawchuk RJ. The pharmacokinetics of cyclosporine. I. Single dose and constant rate infusion studies in the rabbit. *Drug Metab Dispos.* 1985;13:127.

65. Schroeder TJ, Wadhwa NK, Pesce AJ, First MR. An acute overdose of cyclosporine. *Transplantation.* 1986;41:406.

66. Krüger HU, Bross-Bach U, Proksch B, et al. Case report. A case of accidental cyclosporine overdose with pharmacokinetic analysis. *Bone Marrow Transplant.* 1988;3:167.

67. Canafax DM, Cipolle RJ, Hrushesky WJM, et al. The chronopharmacokinetics of cyclosporine and its metabolites in recipients of pancreas allografts. *Transplant Proc.* 1988;20(suppl 2): 471.

68. Venkataramanan R, Yang S, Burckart GJ, et al. Diurnal variation in cyclosporine kinetics. *Ther Drug Monit.* 1986;8:380.

69. Beveridge T, Gratwohl A, Michot F, et al. Cyclosporine A: Pharmacokinetics after a single dose in man and serum levels after multiple dosing in recipients of allogeneic bone marrow grafts. *Curr Ther Res.* 1981;30:5.

70. Buice RG, Gurley BJ, Stentz FB, et al. Cyclosporine disposition in the dog. *Transplantation.* 1985;40:483.

71. Yee GC, Mills G, Schaffer R, et al. Renal cyclosporine clearance in marrow transplant recipients: Age-related variation. *J Clin Pharmacol.* 1986;26:658.

72. Lake KD. Cyclosporine drug interactions: A review. *Cardiac Surg State Art Rev.* 1988;2:617.

73. Lake KD. Management of drug interactions with cyclosporine. *Pharmacotherapy.* 1991;11:110S.

74. Yee GC, McGuire TR. Pharmacokinetic drug interactions with cyclosporine. *Clin Pharmacokinet.* 1990;19:319,400.

75. Ferguson RM, Sutherland DER, Simmons RL, Najarian JS. Ketoconazole, cyclosporine metabolism and renal transplantation. *Lancet.* 1982;2:882.

76. Canafax DM, Graves NM, Hilligoss DM, et al. Interaction between cyclosporine and fluconazole in renal transplant recipients. *Transplantation.* 1991; 51:1014.

77. Ptachcinski RJ, Carpenter BJ, Burckart GJ, et al. Effect of erythromycin on cyclosporine levels. *N Engl J Med.* 1985:313:1416.

78. Wagner K, Philipp T, Heinemeyer G, Neumayer H. Interaction of cyclosporine and calcium antagonists. *Transplant Proc.* 1989;21:1453.

79. Normal DJ, Illingworth DR, Munson J, Hosenpud J. Myolysis and acute renal failure in a heart transplant recipient receiving lovastatin. *N Engl J Med.* 1988;318:46.

80. Dietheim AG. Clinical diagnosis and management of the renal transplant recipient with cyclosporine nephrotoxicity. *Transplant Proc..* 1986;18(2)(suppl 1):82.

81. Bennet WM. Basic mechanism and pathophysiology of cyclosporine nephrotoxicity. *Transplant Proc.* 1985;17(suppl 1):297.

82. Salomon DR. Cyclosporine nephrotoxicity and long-term renal transplantation. *Transplant Rev.* 1992;6:10.

83. Coffman TM, Carr DR, Yarger WE, et al. Evidence that renal prostaglandin and thromboxane production is stimulated in chronic cyclosporine nephrotoxicity. *Transplantation.* 1987;43:282.

84. Van Buren D, Van Buren CT, Flechner SM, et al. De novo hemolytic uremic syndrome in renal transplant recipients immunosuppressed with cyclosporine. *Surgery.* 1984;98:54.

85. Kon V, Awazu M. Endothelin and cyclosporine nephrotoxicity. *Renal Failure.* 1992;14(3):345.

86. Canafax DM, Torres A, Fryd DS, et al. The effects of delayed function on recipients of cadaveric renal allografts. *Transplantation.* 1986;41:177.

87. Myers BD, Newton L, Boshkos C, et al. Cyclosporine-associated chronic nephropathy. *N Engl J Med.* 1984;311:699.

88. Snider J, Francis DMA, Kincaid-Smith P, Walker RG. Long-term graft survival and renal function in cyclosporine-treated renal allograft recipients: Lack of evidence of nephrotoxicity. *Clin Transplant.* 1993;7:25.

89. Min DI, Monaco AP. The complications associated with transplant immunosuppression and their management. *Pharmacotherapy.* 1991;11(5):119S.

90. Rush DN. Cyclosporine toxicity to organs other than the kidney. *Clin Biochem.* 1991;24:101.

91. Sutherland DER, Strand M, Fryd DS, et al. Comparison of azathioprine–antilymphocyte globulin versus cyclosporine in renal transplantation. *Am J Kidney Dis.* 1984;3:456.

92. Weidle PJ, Vlasses PH. Systemic hypertension associated with cyclosporine: A review. *Drug Intell Clin Pharm.* 1988;22:443.

93. Lindholm A. Therapeutic monitoring of cyclosporine—An update. *Eur J Clin Pharmacol.* 1991;41:273.

94. Bowers LD. Therapeutic monitoring for cyclosporine: Difficulties in establishing a therapeutic window. *Clin Biochem.* 1991;24:81.

95. Consensus Document: Hawk's Cay meeting on therapeutic drug monitoring of cyclosporine. *Transplant Proc.* 1990;22:1357.

96. Kivistö KT. A review of assay methods for cyclosporin. *Clin Pharmacokinet.* 1992;23 (3):173.

97. Ferguson RM, Canafax DM, Sawchuk RT, Simmons RS. Cyclosporine blood level monitoring: The early posttransplant period. *Transplant Proc.* 1986;18(suppl 2):113.

98. Moyer TP, Gregory RP, Sterioff S, et al. Cyclosporine nephrotoxicity is minimized by adjusting dosage on the basis of drug concentration in blood. *Mayo Clin Proc.* 1988;63:241.

99. Grevel J, Kahan BD. Area under the curve monitoring of cyclosporine therapy: The early posttransplant period. *Ther Drug Monit.* 1991;13:-89.

100. Chan GLC, Canafax DM, Ascher NL, et al. HLA-identical renal transplantation: No rejections with a cyclosporine–azathioprine–prednisone protocol. *Clin Transplant.* 1988;2:9.

101. Ptachcinski RJ, Logue LW, Burckart GJ, Venkataramanan R. Stability and availability of cyclosporine in 5% dextrose injection or 0.9% sodium chloride injection. *Am J Hosp Pharm.* 1986;43:94.

Chapter 15

Digoxin

Alan H. Mutnick

Keep in Mind

- Identify the indication for digoxin in the patient: positive inotropic effect as in congestive heart failure, or negative chronotropic effect as in atrial fibrillation.
- Evaluate the patient for underlying processes that could alter digoxin needs.
- Assess the patient's creatinine clearance, using serum creatinine, to estimate digoxin clearance.
- Evaluate the patient's laboratory data for abnormal values that could alter normal digoxin effects.
- Evaluate the patient's status to determine if rapid loading doses are required of if slower daily maintenance dosing will suffice.
- Patients with prolonged elimination half-lives often require loading doses to achieve a rapid therapeutic benefit.
- Assess the patient's medication history to identify drugs that may alter the therapeutic response or pharmacokinetic profile of digoxin.
- Inform the patient of the frequent side effects that may herald toxicity.
- Evaluate the patient for heart rate, fluid status, pulmonary status, edema, shortness of breath, orthopnea, and dyspnea as examples for monitoring improvement or deterioration.
- Sample serum digoxin concentrations at least 4 hours and 6 to 8 hours after intravenous and oral doses, respectively. Once sampled at steady state, subsequent concentrations are generally unnecessary unless the therapeutic effect is altered, there is a change in other medications, the digoxin dosage regimen is changed, or noncompliance is suspected.
- The patient's pharmacokinetic profile may be altered as the condition improves or deteriorates.
- Do not rely on the commonly accepted therapeutic serum concentration range as a therapeutic endpoint.

CLINICAL PHARMACOLOGY AND THERAPEUTICS

Although it is now known that the primary action of digitalis is to increase the force of myocardial contraction, that mechanism of action was not determined until the drug was used in clinical practice for many years. Beginning in 1910 with Wenckebach's observations, numerous clinical studies established that digitalis glycosides were effective in heart failure, independent of cardiac rhythm, and showed that this effect was not due to a slowing of heart rate, but to a direct action in increasing the force of myocardial contraction.[1]

It is now recognized that digitalis inhibits sodium–potassium ATPase at a subcellular level.[1] The net effect of this enzyme inhibition is the intracellular accumulation of sodium ions and the loss of potassium ions from the cardiac cell. This results in a decreased rate of rise of the action potential (phase 0), a decreased conduction velocity, and increased spontaneous depolarization (phase 4). The net effect is to increase the refractory period within the atrioventricular node. This effect is also a cause for digitalis-induced reentrant tachyarrhythmias, enhanced ventricular excitability, and depression of atrioventricular conduction, all of which are common cardiac effects seen with digitalis toxicity.

Additionally, the increase in force of contraction (positive inotropic effect) has been related to the availability of rapidly exchangeable calcium, the level of which increases intracellularly with digitalis administration. Evidence to date reveals that the positive inotropic effects of digitalis glycosides result from altered excitation–contraction coupling.[2] As calcium levels are increased, there is a parallel increase in force of contraction until maximum calcium concentrations are reached.[2]

Though two mechanisms have been described that help illustrate the potential role for digitalis in the treatment of congestive heart failure and supraventricular tachyarrhythmias, additional mechanisms have been reported, and include a (1) vagal as well as extravagal mechanism that exerts a slowing effect (negative chronotropic effect) on the myocardium, (2) a parasympathetic type of effect that may be involved in the development of various toxic effects, and (3) a vasoconstrictor effect on arterial and venous smooth muscle.[2]

As discussed above, digitalis is used in situations requiring increased cardiac output or in the treatment of supraventricular arrhythmias, where digitalis exerts a negative chronotropic effect. Accepted indications for the use of digitalis are congestive heart failure, atrial fibrillation, atrial flutter, paroxysmal atrial tachycardia, and cardiogenic shock.

Though controversy exists today as when to use digitalis, the drug still plays a major role in the treatment of numerous cardiac patients. One should recognize that as additional agents become available such as inotropics, peripheral vasodilators, direct-acting antiarrhythmics, and angiotensin-converting enzyme inhibitors, there will continue to be controversy as to the appropriate place for digitalis in the treatment of congestive heart failure and supraventricular arrhythmias. This chapter deals directly with the most popular of the currently available digitalis glycosides, digoxin.

CLINICAL PHARMACOKINETICS

Absorption

Digoxin is absorbed rather passively from the duodenum and upper jejunum. The degree of absorption is dependent on dosage form as well as concomitant medications administered to patients. The oral bioavailability of digoxin, though somewhat variable, has been reported to be approximately 70% from tablets, 85% from the elixir, 95% from capsules, and approximately 80% from intramuscular administration.[3-6] In up to 10% of patients there have been reports that antibiotics (erythromycin, tetracycline) may increase the bioavailability of digoxin by preventing its metabolism by bacteria (*Eubacterium lentum*) normally located within the gastrointestinal tract prior to its absorption.[7,8] Reports in the literature describe elevations of serum digoxin concentrations on the order of 43 to 116% in patients simultaneously receiving short-term therapy with erythromycin or tetracyline and digoxin.

Coadministration of kaolin–pectin suspensions (Kaopectate) and aluminum-containing antacids (Mylanta) has been shown to reduce the degree of absorption of digoxin.[9] It has been shown that this interaction occurs because of physical adsorption; therefore, the relative time for drug administration becomes critical in determining the extent of such interactions. Ideally, administration of the kaolin–pectin suspension at least 2 hours after the digoxin has been reported to prevent such an interaction.[8] Additionally, anticholinergic substances such as propantheline, through its ability to prolong transit time, has been shown capable of increasing digoxin absorption, and metoclopramide, by increasing peristalsis, has been shown capable of reducing digoxin absorption.[10]

Distribution

The volume of distribution for digoxin is very large, and has been reported to be in the range of 7 to 8 L/kg of body weight.[5] The drug, however, shows little affinity for distribution into fat; consequently, dosing should be based on ideal body weight (IBW).[1]

Digoxin has been reported to be approximately 20 to 25% protein bound to serum albumin, and consequently, drugs such as warfarin, phenylbutazone, and clofibrate do compete for albumin binding sites, but do not result in clinically significant interactions with digoxin.[5,11] Of additional importance as it relates to target organ uptake of digoxin is the amount of digoxin taken up by myocardial tissues. Though reported to be as high as 155:1 and as low as 20:1, in adults, the usually reported myocardial/serum digoxin concentration ratios are approximately 30:1 in adults and 125:1 to 150:1 in children.[4,12] As discussed later in the chapter, this relationship becomes critical when trying to evaluate serum digoxin concentrations, where it is assumed a direct relationship exists between organ concentration and serum level if we are to appropriately monitor digoxin therapy.

Various disease processes have been shown to alter the volume of distribution for digoxin. Declining renal function has been associated with a reduction in the volume of distribution to approximately 65% of that in healthy persons, and may be due to a combination of reduced volume of extracellular fluid and reduction in the extent of binding of digoxin to important tissues such as skeletal muscle.[13]

Pregnancy has been shown to have an effect on volume of distribution of digoxin, by increasing the body space into which the drug distributes. Additionally, digoxin has been shown capable of crossing the placental barrier and has been reported to represent as much as 50% of the maternal digoxin blood concentration.[1] This poses an additional therapeutic dilemma to the pregnant patient: doses of digoxin may need to be increased because of a larger volume of distribution, but at the same time, the fetus must be protected from potentially toxic concentrations of the drug. In this situation, routine monitoring of serum digoxin concentrations may prove beneficial in monitoring digoxin to avoid subtherapeutic levels in the mother as well as the development of toxic effects in the developing fetus.

Hypothyroidism has been shown to reduce the volume of distribution, whereas hyperthyroidism has caused the opposite effect.[1] Cardiac disease, such as congestive heart failure, poses a pharmacokinetic dilemma as well as a therapeutic dilemma when administering digoxin. In this patient population, reductions in cardiac output most likely reduce the total volume of distribution for the drug and pose an increased risk of toxicity if appropriate monitoring parameters are not evaluated. As congestive heart failure worsens, and the patient begins to develop significant signs of edema, one is likely to encounter an increase in volume of distribution, necessitating closer monitoring to ensure the attainment of levels adequate to elicit a favorable therapeutic effect. Serum level digoxin determinations will prove beneficial in validating the dose, bioavailability, hemodynamic status, and elimination characteristics for this specific population.

Geriatric patients have also been reported to have altered volumes of distribution for digoxin. In this population of patients receiving digoxin, a reduced total volume of distribution can result in elevations of serum digoxin concentrations and the potential for toxicity.[11,14]

Additionally, alterations in electrolytes has been shown to alter the binding of digoxin to myocardial tissues. The binding of digoxin to the sodium–potassium adenosine triphosphatase (Na^+, K^+-ATPase) receptor is directly related to serum potassium concentrations.[15] As serum potassium levels are lowered there is an apparent increase in the binding of digoxin to the target organ myocardial tissues, and as potassium levels are increased, there is a reduction in the binding of digoxin to myocardial tissues.[16] This would help explain the reason hypokalemia potentiates digoxin toxicity. The effect of potassium-losing diuretics such as hydrochlorothiazide, chlorothiazide, and furosemide on digoxin binding to myocardial tissues as a result of reduced potassium levels must also be evaluated prior to initiating digoxin therapy.

Quinidine has been shown to displace digoxin from binding sites and reduce the volume of distribution and potentiate digoxin toxicity.[16] This is in addition to its effect on renal elimination. Quinidine has been shown to reduce renal excretion of digoxin by 25 to 40% through inhibition of active tubular secretion.[17] In general, the digoxin maintenance dose should be halved before initiation of quinidine therapy, and in patients who currently are receiving quinidine, digitalizing doses one-third normal doses should be used.[16]

Metabolism

Hepatic conversion to 3-keto- and 3-epidigoxigenin metabolites followed by conjugation describes one method for digoxin metabolism[18]; however, enterohepatic recycling of digoxin has been reported to be as high as 30% for digoxin, and the following active metabolites have been identified: digitoxigenin, bisdigitoxoside, digoxigenin monodigitoxoside, dihydrodigoxin.[1] The metabolism to these compounds is dependent primarily on gut bacterial enzymes, which act on unabsorbed drug reaching the colon, as well as on the amount of digoxin secreted into the intestine as a result of enterohepatic recycling.

Though there has been no emphasis on the metabolic pathways as a major way to remove digoxin from the body, small populations of patients may be at an added risk of digoxin toxicity if the metabolic pathways do not function properly. As mentioned previously, the broad-spectrum antibiotics erythromcyin and tetracycline have been shown capable of altering gut flora in a manner that reduces the above-mentioned metabolism of the drug, resulting in as much as a 30% increase in digoxin serum levels because of increased absorption.[8,18] Urban dwellers have been reported to be at a high risk for this interaction, as the identification of *Eubacterium lentum* among them is reported to be more common than in other populations studied.[8]

Elimination

Digoxin is excreted predominately by the renal route, where 60 to 80% of bioavailable digoxin is excreted unchanged by glomerular filtration and active tubular secretion.[5] Renal disease substantially alters the elimination half-life of digoxin. The reported half-life for digoxin in patients with normal renal function is approximately 1.6 days, whereas in anephric patients it ranges from 3.5 to 4.5 days.[5,18]

Generally, there exists controversy between creatinine clearance and steady state plasma digoxin concentrations. This becomes crucial in designing appropriate dosing regimens for patients who have some degree of renal dysfunction.[1]

The group that will be affected most by digoxin excretion is the geriatric population.[14] A gradual reduction in creatinine clearance occurs with advancing age. This requires dosage adjustments when initiating digoxin therapy. The half-life may be as low as 38 hours in young adults with normal renal function and as high as 69 hours in elderly patients.[19] Assuming that renal elimination represents approximately 75% of total body clearance of digoxin, the importance of renal function cannot be overstated. As will be discussed later, normal measures of renal function (ie, serum creatinine) do not always enable one to calculate digoxin elimination kinetics directly.

Verapamil, along with several other of the currently available calcium channel blocking agents, has been reported to reduce the renal and extrarenal elimination of digoxin.[17] Consequently, reduction of maintenance doses of digoxin with no changes in loading doses has been recommended as a way to prevent digoxin accumulation in these patients.

Pregnancy has been discussed previously as a factor that increases the volume of distribution of digoxin, and has also been associated with increases in renal elimination.[17]

A final group of patients in whom normal renal elimination is altered are those patients suffering from cardiac disease, specifically those with congestive heart failure. In this population, renal clearance of digoxin is reduced enough to allow for significant accumulation of drug if doses are not altered.

Pharmacokinetic parameters for adult and pediatric patients are summarized in Tables 15–1 and 15–2, respectively.

PHARMACODYNAMICS

Therapeutic Endpoints

Prior to developing a monitoring strategy for a drug such as digoxin, several critical assumptions are required to design effective dosing regimens. The initial assumption is that therapeutic drug monitoring reduces the variability in plasma drug concentrations. The second assumption is that a relationship exists between the plasma drug concentration and the drug's pharmacologic effect.[20]

According to the second assumption, the pharmacologic effect is proportional to the plasma drug concentration. Therefore, for therapeutic drug monitoring to be applicable to digoxin, databases must exist that substantiate a direct relationship between the concentration of

TABLE 15–1. SUMMARY OF ADULT PHARMACOKINETIC PARAMETERS

Pharmacokinetic Parameter	Normal Population	Special Populations
Intestinal absorption	70% (tablets) 85% (elixir) 95% (capsules) 80% (IM)	Reduced with concomitant use of aluminum-containing antacids and kaolin–pectin products; increased by tetracyclines
t_{max} (time to peak concentration) Volume of distribution	45–60 min 7–10 L/kg	Reduced in renal dysfunction, hypothyroidism, heart failure, geriatric patients, patients on quinidine, etc; increased in pregnancy, hyperthyroidism, severe edema
Plasma protein binding	25%	
Therapeutic plasma concentrations	0.5–2.0 ng/mL	Altered response in patients with electrolyte disturbances
$t_{1/2}$	36 h	Prolonged in renal disease, geriatric patients, and severe heart failure; reduced in pregnancy
Major routes of elimination	Renal, gastrointestinal	
Total body clearance	180 mL/min/m^2	
Renal clearance	140 mL/min/m^2	
Percentage excreted in urine as native drug		
Intravenous dose	72%	
Oral dose	54%	
Percentage excreted renally	75%	
Enterohepatic circulation	Up to 30%	
Placental transfer	Yes	
Dose adjustment with renal dysfunction	Yes	When renal function is reduced (intrinsic renal disease, aging, excessive diuretics, or severe heart failure), hepatic metabolism and fecal excretion may increase; drugs such as indomethacin, cyclosporine, quinidine and spironolactone reduce digoxin elimination by the kidney

TABLE 15–2. SUMMARY OF PEDIATRIC PHARMACOKINETIC PARAMETERS

Total body clearance
30–40 mL/min/1.73 m^2 (neonates, infants <1 mo)
130–190 mL/min/1.73 m^2 (infants, children)
Half-life, $t_{1/2}$
Preterm   60 h
Neonates 35–45 h
Infants   18–25 h
Children   36 h
Volume of distribution
Variable, but generally greater than that of adults on a L/kg basis

digoxin in the serum and the required pharmacologic effect at the designated target organ, in this case, the heart.

As discussed previously, the primary pharmacodynamic effects associated with the administration of digoxin are a dose-dependent increase in myocardial contraction (positive inotropic effect) and a dose-dependent reduction in electrical conduction at the atrioventricular (AV) node, with an associated increase in the AV node refractory period (negative chronotropic effect). The positive inotropic effect has shown to be beneficial in patients suffering from congestive heart failure. The negative chronotropic effect has been shown to be beneficial in patients suffering from supraventricular arrhythmias such as atrial fibrillation, where one goal of therapy is to slow down electrical impulses reaching the ventricles where they would have the potential to create a life-threatening arrhythmia.

The direct relationship between serum drug concentrations and digoxin pharmacodynamic effects with respect to positive inotropic effects has been more clearly defined than those involving negative chronotropic effects. Systolic time intervals have been reported to be uniquely useful to quantitate the inotropic effect of digitalis.[15] Serum digoxin concentrations ranging from 0.5 to 2.0 ng/mL have been reported successful in providing for maximal positive inotropic effects with minimal toxicity.[21]

In the case of atrial fibrillation, there are reports that increases in the serum concentration of digoxin within a therapeutic range do produce an increase in the effect of digoxin on slowing the ventricular rate.[22] This contrasts with previous reports that described lack of a direct relationship between serum digoxin concentration and reduction in ventricular rates.[23] Currently, there is good evidence that increasing the concentration of digoxin within the therapeutic range produces an increase in its ability to slow the ventricular rate in patients with atrial fibrillation.[22]

As is the case with many drugs, overlap exists between therapeutic digoxin concentrations and toxic serum drug concentrations. Numerous investigators have tried to define digoxin toxicity on the basis of serum digoxin concentrations, and the results have been mixed, with toxicity symptoms often being reported at concentrations within the therapeutic range.[24] Digoxin toxicity, however, continues to be diagnosed based on electrocardiographic, laboratory, and clinical findings in addition to the serum digoxin concentration. As evidenced by many patients receiving digoxin for its negative chronotropic effect, a serum digoxin concentration of 2.0 ng/mL may be effective in reducing the ventricular response in atrial fibrillation in one patient, whereas another patient may require a serum level of 3.0 ng/mL or more.

Aside from the pharmacodynamic differences associated with digoxin therapy, one must also identify a multitude of other clinical factors that help influence myocardial sensitivity to the actions of digoxin. Such factors as hypokalemia, hyperkalemia, hypercalcemia, hypomagnesemia, hypermagnesemia, acid–base disorders, hypoxemia, underlying heart disease, and pulmonary disease provide various levels of myocardial sensitivity that would increase/decrease responses to digoxin.[1]

The value of routine serum digoxin determinations as a means of evaluating therapeutic efficacy as well as potential toxicity is limited because of the significant overlap between nontoxic and toxic concentrations.[24] Several well-controlled studies, however, have revealed consistent results when comparing toxic concentrations with nontoxic concentrations of digoxin. The work by Smith and Haber revealed that 90% of patients without evidence of digoxin toxicity had serum digoxin levels less than 2.0 ng/mL, and 87% of patients in the toxic group had serum digoxin levels greater than 2.0 ng/mL.[25]

In our discussion of pharmacokinetics, we identified several groups of patients who had altered digoxin disposition as a result of renal impairment, thyroid disease, advanced age, and concurrent drug administration. These special groups have also revealed potential changes in drug pharmacodynamics as well.

In renal impairment, adjustments in digoxin doses to compensate for the reported reduction in the volume of distribution have shown better predictability of serum digoxin concentrations and pharmacologic response, as compared with adjustments of doses based on renal function alone.[26] This has been explained by findings that suggest a reduction in the myocardial:serum concentration ratio with diminished renal function.

Thyroid disease has also been shown to have a direct effect on the pharmacodynamics of digoxin.[1] Though the data are conflicting, hypothyroid patients seem to be more sensitive and hyperthyroid patients seem to be less sensitive to the effects of digoxin. Investigators have attempted to describe these alterations in response by describing alterations in the volume of distribution, changes in the glomerular filtration rate, malabsorption, and tissue uptake. Until agreement is obtained as to the definitive reason(s) for such pharmacodynamic changes, frequent monitoring of serum digoxin levels may prove helpful by avoiding excessive concentrations in hypothyroid patients while preventing subtherapeutic concentrations in hyperthyroid patients.

Advancing age has not been shown by itself to be a major determinant in the pharmacodynamic changes resulting from digoxin therapy. Rather, it appears to be the physiologic changes of aging that are primarily responsible for the altered pharmacokinetic parameters reported in the literature.[14] Consequently, the prolonged half-life resulting from reduced renal function and the accompanying reduction in plasma clearance of digoxin are more responsible for the increased serum digoxin concentrations than an increase or decrease in receptor sensitivity.

A final group who are at added risk when receiving digoxin are pediatric patients. The increased rates of survival of premature infants have resulted in greater use of digoxin for treatment of various anomalies that contribute to congestive heart failure.[27] Full-term infants have been shown to require more digoxin per unit of body weight and to tolerate high serum levels of digoxin better than do older children or adults[28]; however, premature infants have been shown to have longer half-lives (up to twice that of infants). Though controversy exists, it has been reported that the clinical pharmacodynamics appreciated from digoxin may occur with lower doses and subsequently lower serum digoxin concentrations than in the adult population.[27]

A recent publication addressed the issue of therapeutic drug monitoring (TDM) based on the establishment of six issued that must be considered for the application of TDM to be acceptable.[20] Such considerations for digoxin reveal the following findings:

1. There is an appropriate assay for digoxin which is accurate, precise, and reproducible, although some assays do cross-react with endogenous substances, which is of concern for older studies as well as current results.
2. Digoxin does display a substantial degree of interindividual variations with respect to absorption, distribution, and elimination and, thus, necessitates TDM.
3. An abundance of pharmacokinetic data are available for digoxin, but there is also a significant lack of studies relating such data to pharmacodynamics in patients.
4. At this time it is not totally clear whether the pharmacologic effect is proportional to the plasma digoxin concentration. As described above, when using digoxin for its negative chronotropic effects, poorly defined relationships between plasma digoxin levels and therapeutic effects would make for difficult TDM practices in some patient populations.
5. Some patient populations reveal a narrow therapeutic range for digoxin, and thus, are candidates for TDM. However, other patients may have very high serum digoxin levels and suffer no toxic effects or have seemingly therapeutic serum levels and display toxic effects.
6. Digoxin seems to elicit a constant pharmacologic effect over an extended period, consistent with TDM processes. However, despite constant plasma digoxin concentrations, changes in other variables such as potassium concentration, calcium concentration, and thyroid function can alter the pharmacologic response.
7. Many studies have been carried out that describe a "therapeutic range" and a "toxic range" for digoxin, consistent with TDM processes. However, there are also reports of patients developing toxic effects in the therapeutic range and other patients not displaying toxic effects while in the toxic range.

Though this section has attempted to address the various changes in the pharmacodynamics of digoxin, many questions still remain as to the most appropriate manner in which to monitor digoxin therapy. As can be seen by the preceding list of seven criteria, specific characteristics of digoxin make it an agent worthy of TDM and, at the same time, pose questions as to the true reliability of serum assays, therapeutic ranges, toxic ranges, and numerous other processes involved in the accurate monitoring of such therapy. Until such time when all seven criteria are fulfilled satisfactorily, the experienced clinician, capable of dealing with uncertainty, and flexible enough to adjust his or her tools to best suit the needs of each individual patient, will need to develop effective digoxin regimens by combining pharmacokinetic, pharmacodynamic, and clinical judgment to ensure the most appropriate therapeutic outcome.

Adverse Reactions

Toxic effects associated with digitalis glycosides, specifically digoxin, have been the most commonly observed drug toxic effects and potentially the most serious. The determination of effica-

TABLE 15–3. NONCARDIAC MANIFESTATIONS OF DIGITALIS INTOXICATION

Type of Symptoms	Frequency	Manifestations
Gastrointestinal	Common	Anorexia, nausea, vomiting, diarrhea, abdominal pain, constipation
Neurologic	Common	Headache, fatigue, insomnia, confusion, vertigo
	Uncommon	Delirium, psychoses, paresthesias, convulsions, neuralgia
Visual	Common	Color vision (usually green or yellow), colored halos around objects
	Uncommon	Blurring, shimmering vision
	Rare	Scotomata, micropsia, macropsia, amblyopias
Miscellaneous	Rare	Allergic (urticaria), eosinophilia, idiosyncracy, thrombocytopenia, GI hemorrhage, necrosis

Adapted from Chung EK. Digitalis intoxication. *N Eng J Med.* 1971;284:989–997.

cious as well as toxic serum digoxin concentrations has resulted in a reduction of digoxin toxicity from as high as 25% to current estimates of 2%.[15] Earlier estimates from retrospective studies of inpatients taking digitalis glycosides revealed that from 7 to 20% of patients develop toxic effects. At the same time, it had been reported that such toxicity may also be accompanied by a mortality as high as 40%.[29]

The noncardiac symptoms of digitalis toxicity are listed in Table 15–3.[30] The cardiac manifestations of the presence or absence of digitalis intoxication have been described previously, and are listed in Table 15–4.[25]

Drug–Drug Interactions

As the reader has gathered, numerous opportunities exist for additional drugs and disease processes to alter the pharmacokinetic profile of digoxin. Each pharmacokinetic parameter has been reported to be alterable through the development of drug–drug interactions. At the same time, continuous refinements in assay methods for digoxin have added to our ability to identify new drug–drug interactions as they occur. Table 15–5 provides a brief summary on some of the more commonly identified drug–drug interactions with digoxin.

THERAPEUTIC REGIMEN DESIGN

Before attempting to develop a dosage regimen for a patient about to be started on digoxin, several important issues need to be addressed prior to initiating therapy. Several key components of accurate dose calculations are listed here:

TABLE 15–4. CARDIAC CRITERIA FOR THE PRESENCE OR ABSENCE OF DIGITALIS INTOXICATION

Definite Toxicity	Possible Toxicity	No Toxicity
Sinus rhythm with second- or third-degree AV block	Marked sinus bradycardia without prior history before on digitalis	Electrocardiogram-documented stable sinus rhythm
Atrial fibrillation with high-grade AV block and PVCs, PAT with block	Atrial fibrillation with relatively slow ventricular response or occasional AV junctional escape beats	Atrial fibrillation with 70–100 beats per minute ventricle response
Supraventricular tachycardia with AV block	First-degree AV block without prior history before on digitalis or other drugs impairing conduction	Atrial flutter with AV block of 2:1 to 4:1
Frequent or multifocal ventricular premature beats or ventricular bigeminy or ventricular tachycardia	Occasional ventricular premature beats	Arrhythmia present whether patient is on or off digitalis
Arrhythmia completely resolved when digitalis is reduced or discontinued	Arrhythmia partially resolved when digitalis is reduced or stopped	

Adapted from Smith TW, Haber E. Digoxin intoxication: The relationship of clinical presentation to serum digoxin concentration. *J Clin Invest.* 1970;49:2377–2386.

1. There must exist a direct relationship between serum digoxin concentration and digoxin concentration at the target organ. In this case, the myocardium is the target organ, and a myocardial:serum concentration ratio of approximately 30:1 has been accepted.

2. Meaningful interpretation of any serum digoxin concentration requires attainment of steady state. For patients with normal renal function, this takes four to five half-lives or 6 to 8 days; in patients with renal impairment this still takes four to five half-lives, but with the half-life being as long as 4.5 days, 18 to 22 days is required for attainment of steady state.

3. Once a patient has attained steady-state serum digoxin concentrations, equilibrium must exist between the serum and target organ concentrations, in this case the myocardium and the serum. Consequently, for meaningful serum levels to be used, sampling should occur no earlier than 4 hours after an intravenous dose, 8 hours after an oral dose, and 12 hours after an intramuscular dose. Any samples drawn earlier will result in levels that *do not* reflect the direct relationship between serum concentration and myocardial concentration of digoxin.

4. Digoxin does not readily distribute into adipose tissue; consequently, lean body weight (LBW) should be used in calculating digoxin doses. It has been reported in the literature that total body stores (TBS) of 8 to 10 μg/kg digoxin are required to invoke

the positive inotropic effects of digoxin, whereas 13 to 15 μg/kg is required to invoke the negative chronotropic effects, as seen in the treatment of atrial fibrillation.

5. Though numerous methods of dosing have been described in the literature, it is crucial for the clinician involved in designing digoxin regimens to become aware of several methods and to appreciate the benefits as well as the shortcomings of each method. Of utmost importance, however, is to appreciate the fact that every method is useful to some extent, by nature of the fact that they have been designed to help remove many of the variables involved with digoxin dosing and provide a more individualized approach useful in monitoring therapy. No method can be allowed to take the place of the clinical presentation of the patient. Simply put, our goal is to identify the best way to get a therapeutic amount of digoxin into the body and, through appropriate maintenance doses, assure ourselves that this amount is allowed to remain in the body.

Determination of Serum Digoxin Concentrations

As mentioned previously, the determination by serum sampling of digoxin for efficacy as well as toxicity has improved digoxin therapy.[15] Estimation of steady-state digoxin concentrations from a single serum sample requires knowledge of both the distributive pharmacokinetic profile for a given patient and the appropriate timing of the sample for each dosing interval.[24] Additionally, an understanding of the assay technique used to assess serum digoxin concentration is required. Radioimmunoassay (RIA), enzymatic immunoassay, fluorescence polarization immunoassay, high-performance liquid chromatography, and digoxin-specific monoclonal antibodies are the various techniques that have been utilized to determine serum digoxin concentrations.

Radioimmunoassay has become more popular clinically because of its good sensitivity to levels as low as 0.2 to 0.4 ng/mL. A major point of concern regarding RIA is the low specificity and the ability for the assay to cross-react with digitalis-like substances which are present in renal failure, hepatic failure, pregnancy, some hypertensive states, and congestive heart failure.[31,32] Though the actual identity and purpose of these substances are not totally clear, they can constitute up to 50% of the total serum digoxin concentration measured by RIA.[15] It has also been reported that the major active metabolites of digoxin (eg, digoxigenin, bisdigoxiside, and monodigoxiside) react with most RIAs and, therefore, are able to be monitored, despite the appearance of digitalis-like substances.[15]

Since the identification of appropriate methods to monitor serum digoxin concentrations, much controversy has arisen as to the appropriate indications for digoxin sampling. Recommended indications for cost-effective use of digoxin serum sampling are validation of initial doses of therapy, validation of patient compliance, assessment of renal function and degree of impairment in drug elimination, validation of initial doses when interacting drugs are administered, assessment of effects of altered hemodynamics on drug distribution and elimination, assessment of nonresponse, and prevention as well as diagnosis of toxicity.[15]

It is important that the clinician use the serum digoxin concentration as a potentially valuable aid, but not depend on the assay alone for clinical decision making. It has been suggested that the use of clinical monitoring rather than clinical drug monitoring is crucial to treating a patient on digoxin effectively.

Samples taken prior to attainment of steady state do not show the true pharmacody-

TABLE 15–5. DRUGS AFFECTING THE PHARMACOKINETICS OF DIGOXIN

Agent	Alteration
Aluminum hydroxide gel	Reduced gastrointestinal absorption, which may be prevented by administering digoxin 2 h before or 2 h after these agents
Aluminum hydroxide–magnesium hydroxide compounds	
Activated charcoal	
Cholestyramine, colestipol	
Kaolin–pectin, dietary fiber	
Metoclopramide, neomycin	
Sulfasalazine	
Antibiotics (by inhibiting gut flora in select patients)	Increased absorption which may require a reduction in digoxin doses, necessitating attention to serum digoxin levels
Anticholinergics (atropine, propantheline, etc) (by reducing GI motility)	
Verapamil, diltiazem (moderate)	Reduction in renal excretion and nonrenal clearance and a reduction in volume of distribution require reduced digoxin doses and closer attention to serum digoxin levels
Spironolactone, triamterene	Reduction in renal tubular secretion of digoxin may require a reduction in digoxin doses and closer attention to serum digoxin levels
Amiodarone	Decreases renal and nonrenal clearance of digoxin, may increase digoxin bioavailability and displace digoxin from tissue stores, requiring reduction of digoxin dose and close attention to serum digoxin levels.
Quinidine	Reduced renal excretion, nonrenal clearance, volume of distribution, and tissue binding of digoxin cause a significant increase in serum digoxin levels; these effects necessitate routine monitoring of digoxin serum levels and 50% reduction in digoxin dose
Potassium-losing diuretics, (thiazides, furosemide, ethacrynic acid, etc)	Reduced potassium levels predispose patients to digoxin toxicity; serum digoxin levels *and* clinical effect must be closely monitored routinely
Amphotericin B	

Source. References 17 and 38

namic/pharmacokinetic picture for any given patient. A patient who has not received a loading dose of digoxin requires four to five half-lives to reach steady state. Even when steady state is reached, however, a major error in the use of serum digoxin assays is the failure to wait for equilibration (between serum and myocardial digoxin concentrations), which requires at least 4 hours after an intravenous dose or 8 to 12 hours after an oral dose, to allow correct interpretation of a given sample.

Consequently, a standard collection time should be established in each institution, and routine serum samples should be collected by trained individuals familiar with digoxin dosing and pharmacokinetic disposition. Many institutions have developed a morning sampling time for routine digoxin serum samples prior to administration of a patient's daily dose of digoxin. A standard collection time of 8:00 AM allows many patients to have samples drawn late enough to prevent early wakenings, but early enough to avoid interfering with morning activities, breakfast, and digoxin administration.

The digoxin assay is one of the most widely used drug assays and represents a major medical care cost, especially when used inappropriately.[15] Determination of inappropriate serum sampling practices, indications, and uses via educational programs, computer surveillance, and the like is needed to provide cost savings as well as improvement in digoxin usage.

_____ **EXAMPLE 15–1** _____

Patient A.M. is a 50-year-old white man who has currently been diagnosed with congestive heart failure (CHF). The patient stands 5 ft 6 in., weighs 180 pounds, and presents to the coronary care unit with the following laboratory values obtained while in the emergency room.

Sodium	140 mEq/L	Potassium	4.5 mEq/L
Chloride	105 mEq/L	CO_2 content	22 mEq/L
Serum creatinine	1.2 mg/100 mL	Cholesterol	190 mg/100 mL
Glucose	100 mg/100 mL	BUN	15 mg/100 mL

This patient is a rather simple case, because no mention was made of any processes that predispose him to altered pharmacodynamics or pharmacokinetics (eg, thyroid disease). One major factor for dosing digoxin centers on the renal status of the patient.

Estimation of Renal Function. The Cockcroft–Gault nomogram has been shown to be extremely helpful in the prediction of creatinine clearance from serum creatinine.[34]

$$Cl_{cr} \text{ (males)} = \frac{(140 - age) \times weight}{Cr_s \times 72}$$

$$Cl_{cr} \text{ (females)} = 0.85 \times \text{Above value}$$

where Cl_{cr} = creatinine clearance in mL/min, Cl_s = serum creatinine in mg/dL, age is in years, and weight is in kg. Therefore,

$$Cl_{cr} \text{ (A.M.)} = \frac{(140 - 50) \times 82 \text{ kg}}{1.2 \times 72}$$

$$= 85.4 \text{ mL/min.}$$

Though this does not represent the ideal renal function of 100 to 105 mL/min, it does not represent renal impairment. Consequently, no significant changes are required to account for altered volume of distribution or tissue uptake changes as discussed with renal impairment.

Estimation of Lean Body Weight (LBW). Devine has reported a method that has proven useful in converting an adult patient's height into LBW.[35] Though the method should be a helpful guide, it does require adjustments when evaluating patients with excess muscle (athletic look) as well as those with very little muscle (cachetic look)

$$LBW \text{ (males)} = 50 + 2.3 \times \text{height in in. over 5 ft}$$

$$LBW \text{ (females)} = 45 + 2.3 \times \text{height in in. over 5 ft}$$

where LBW is in kg. Therefore,

$$LBW \text{ (A.M.)} = 50 + 2.3 \times 6 = 63.8 \text{ kg} = 64 \text{ kg}$$

Estimation of Total Body Stores (TBS) Needed. In CHF one desires the positive inotropic effect for digoxin, or 8 to 10 μg/kg LBW.

$$64 \text{ kg (LBW)} \times 10 \text{ μg/kg} = 640 \text{ μg}$$

Administration of the Loading Dose. The patient is euthyroid, in normal electrolyte balance, with no other bodily abnormalities. The oral digoxin dosage will be 70% absorbed via tablets, 95% from capsules, and 100% from an intravenous dose. Depending on the acuteness of the situation, one may choose to administer a series of loading doses to obtain a therapeutic effect quickly, or administer maintenance doses over several days to appreciate a therapeutic effect. In this patient, in the hospital setting the use of a rapid load over 12 hours can be accomplished by dividing the 640 μg (0.64 mg) TBS into three doses:

IV	0.25 mg now, 0.25 mg in 6 hours, 0.125 mg in 6 hours
	Rapid load over 12 hours of 0.625 mg
Tablets	640 μg (TBS)/0.70 (absorption) = 914 μg
	or
	0.50 mg now, 0.25 mg in 6 hours, 0.125 mg in 6 hours
	Rapid load over 12 hours of 0.875 mg.
Capsules	640 μg (TBS)/0.95 (absorption) = 674 μg
	or
	0.30 mg now, 0.20 mg in 6 hours, 0.15 mg in 6 hours
	Rapid load over 12 hours of 0.65 mg

Calculation of Maintenance Dose. Previous work by Jelliffe has shown that there is a quantitative relationship between digoxin kinetics and endogenous creatinine clearance.[36] The relationship as described by Jelliffe is represented by the equation

$$D_m = \% \text{ lost/day} = \text{nonrenal losses} + \text{renal losses}$$

$$\% \text{ lost/day} = 14\% + 21\% \text{ (assuming normal renal function)}$$

As renal function changes, one is able to use Jelliffe's relationship between digoxin elimination and endogenous creatinine clearance with the following equation of a straight line.

$$\% \text{ lost/d} = 14\% + 0.20\,(\text{Cl}_{cr})$$

or

$$D_m\,(\text{mg/d}) = \frac{\text{TBS (mg)} \times \% \text{ lost/d}}{100}$$

$$\text{For patient A.M. } D_m\,(\text{mg/d}) = \frac{0.640\,(\text{mg}) \times (14\% + 0.20 \times 85)}{100}$$

$$D_m = 0.1984 \text{ mg IV}$$

$$D_m = \frac{0.1984 \text{ mg}}{0.70} = 0.28 \text{ mg tablets}$$

$$D_m = \frac{0.1984 \text{ mg}}{0.95} = 0.21 \text{ mg capsules}$$

With the available dosage forms, one would be likely to select either a 0.25-mg tablet daily or a 0.20-mg capsule daily for maintenance therapy in our patient.

Though the main goal of any dosing regimen is to reduce the variability that exists in patients due to age, weight, height, renal function, and other factors, several studies have demonstrated that very little variability in plasma digoxin levels can be accounted for by such variables. Of additional concern must also be patient compliance, concomitant drug therapy, and variations in both absorption and metabolism.

Oglivie and Ruedy used a method similar to that of Jelliffe to correct for altered renal function in patients, but chose to use BUN rather than Cr_s to calculate maintenance doses.[37] The calculation of loading doses was done by using lean body weight, in pounds, and a total dose of 7.5 μg/pound to identify a patient's required total body stores. In our case above, this would translate to the following:

Calculation of Total Body Stores

$$64 \text{ kg or } 141 \times 7.5 \text{ μg/pound} = 1058 \text{ μg or } 1.0 \text{ mg}$$

or

0.50 mg now, 0.25 mg in 6 hours, and 0.25 mg in 6 hours
for a total of 1.0 mg over 12 hours IV.

Tablets and capsules would be used in the same fashion as before, with compensation for reduced bioavailability.

Calculation of Maintenance Dose. A nomogram published by the authors revealed that our patient with a BUN of 15 would require 33.3% of his total body stores each day as maintenance, or

$$1.0 \text{ mg (TBS)} \times 33.3\% = 0.33 \text{ mg. IV}$$

or

$$\frac{0.33}{0.70} = 0.47 = 0.50 \text{ mg tablets}$$

or

$$\frac{0.33}{0.95} = 0.35 = 0.30 \text{ mg capsules}$$

Another approach to modifying digoxin dosing regimens has been described by Dettli et al as follows[38]:

Calculation of Loading Dose (LD)

$$LD = V_d \times C_pC_{max}$$
$$V_d = 4.7 + (0.028 \text{ Cl}_{cr}) \text{ L/kg} \times \text{IBW}$$
$$C_pC_{max} = 1 \text{ μg/L}$$

In our example,

$$V_d = 4.7 + (0.028 \times 85)$$
$$V_d = 7.08 \text{ L/kg} \times 64 \text{ kg.} = 453 \text{ L}$$
$$LD = 453 \text{ L} \times 1 \text{ μg/L} = 453 \text{ μg IV}$$

Calculation of Maintenance Dose (MD). Dettli et al were able to determine that the maintenance dose is a function of the patient's loading dose. However, as maintenance doses are needed to replace fractions of loading doses lost per dosing interval (τ), a simple relationship was developed:

$$MD = LD \times (1 - e^{-k_e t})$$

Dettli et al were able to describe the elimination characteristics for a drug by showing that the total fraction of the amount of drug eliminated per hour (k) is the sum of the fraction removed by nonrenal elimination (k_m) and of the fraction eliminated by the kidneys, (k_r).

$$k(\text{h}^{-1}) = k_m + k_r$$

Additionally, Dettli et al were able to show that k_r was directly related to renal elimination, that is, Cl_{cr}:[38]

$$k_e = k_m + k_r \times \text{Cl}_{cr}$$
$$= 0.00593 + 0.00013 \text{ (Cl)}_{cr}$$
$$= 0.00593 + 0.00013 \text{ (85)}$$
$$= 0.00593 + 0.01105$$
$$= 0.01698 \text{ h}^{-1}$$

At t = 24 hours

$$\text{MD IV} = 453 \text{ μg} \times (1 - 0.6653)$$

$$\text{MD IV} = 453 \times 0.33$$

$$\text{MD IV} = 150 \text{ μg daily}$$

$$\text{MD PO} = 150/F = 150/0.7 = 214 \text{ μg PO daily}$$

The assumptions are one-compartment kinetics, a fraction absorbed of 0.7, and instantaneous absorption. F is bioavailability.

In the clinical setting an alternative approach would be to select an empiric dose based on parameters like body mass, renal function, and drug interactions, and subsequently monitor serum digoxin concentrations. An initial goal of therapy would be to achieve a serum digoxin concentration of approximately 1.5 ng/mL which would correspond to a digoxin total body pool of about 10 μg/kg.

The patient in need of acute digitalization would be given a loading dose of 0.75 to 1.0 mg of digoxin administered intravenously or orally in two to three doses. Initially, the patient would receive 0.5 mg of digoxin, and then additional doses of 0.125 to 0.25 mg would be given in 8- to 12-hour intervals until an adequate response was obtained.

In the current example, our patient with a calculated lean body weight of 64 kg would receive a total dose of 11.7 to 15.6 μg/kg from the 0.75- to 1.0-mg loading dose.

After the patient had been successfully loaded with digoxin a serum digoxin concentration would allow the clinician to determine the current drug disposition in the specific patient. Once again, the serum sample is used only as a guide, and must be drawn at least 4 hours after the last intravenous dose or 8 to 12 hours after the last oral dose.

The patient would then be started on maintenance digoxin of 0.125 to 0.25 mg daily, depending on evidence of renal dysfunction, drug–drug interactions, and patient body mass.

If the patient were not in need of rapid digitalization, a daily maintenance dose of 0.125 to 0.50 mg of digoxin would have been initiated in the oral form, depending on the size of the patient, renal status, and indication for the drug, and the patient would be monitored daily for improvement in signs and symptoms. Clinical assessment parameters include slowing of heart rate, improvement in urinary output, relief of pulmonary congestion, evaluation of chest radiograph, and electrocardiogram for reduced conduction of atrial impulses into the ventricles. Additionally, assuming no alteration in renal status, a serum digoxin determination would be ordered after the patient is assumed to have attained steady state ($t_{1/2}$ = 36 hours, C_{ss} attained after 4–5 $t_{1/2}$, or 6–7 days). Note that the patient with a prolonged half-life would become a candidate for rapid loading of digoxin due to the extremely long period required to attain steady state ($t_{1/2}$ = 3–4 days, C_{ss} attained after 4–5 $t_{1/2}$, or 12–20 days).

Some situations may favor an earlier serum determination and may include addition of drugs that are known to interact with digoxin, decline in renal status, and lack of initial therapeutic response. In such situations, a serum digoxin determination may be ordered, but again, one needs to remember that the resultant level is only a rough guide for any changes in therapy. Some authors have suggested ordering baseline digoxin serum concentrations to determine the presence of digitalis-like immunoreactive substances.[15] Once again, because of the potential for excess serum determinations and resultant costs, baseline concentrations may prove beneficial in those patients predisposed to digitalis-like immunoreactive substances (eg, renal failure, pregnancy, hepatic failure)

Lewis has provided a straightforward approach to dosing digoxin in those instances where a loading dose is not required.[15] A maintenance dose of 0.25 mg is started when the creatinine clearance exceeds 20 mL/min; if the creatinine clearance is less than 20 mL/min, the maintenance dose is 0.125 mg. The serum digoxin concentration is then measured 2 days later. The 2 days reflect approximately 50% attainment in steady-state concentration for those without renal impairment. If an exceeding high or low digoxin concentration is present, the maintenance dose can be adjusted accordingly. A repeat concentration is then obtained five half-lives after a dosing change.

After receiving a serum digoxin concentration result, several important factors become important prior to any action:

1. Was the level drawn appropriately?
2. Do the levels reflect steady state, pre-steady state, and so on?
3. Is the patient predisposed to increased levels of digitalis-like immunoreactive substances?
4. Is the patient improving clinically?
5. Is the patient experiencing signs of digoxin toxicity?

For illustrative purposes for our case, a serum level drawn 23 hours after the first maintenance dose returned at 2.2 ng/mL, and the patient was complaining of nausea and blurred vision. During the rapid loading doses (a total of 1.0 mg was given), the patient's urine output increased and much of the edema had begun resolving. Lung sounds were clearing, and the patient appeared to be improving.

In the above setting, a reevaluation of the patient is needed before making any decision to reduce maintenance doses because of suspected toxicity. Serum electrolytes and creatinine need to be assessed to aid in the identification of other causes of toxicity.

In the event that no identified causes are found, one is able to use the first-order kinetics of digoxin to determine any adjustments needed in daily maintenance doses. According to first-order kinetics, a 50% reduction in daily digoxin doses from 0.25 to 0.125 mg would result in a 50% reduction in the serum digoxin concentration. A 25% reduction in daily digoxin doses from 0.25 to 0.1875 mg would result in a 25% reduction in the serum digoxin concentration. In our patient, assuming no other contributing factors, and taking into account the currently available oral preparations, our patient would have a 50% reduction in dose and an anticipated serum digoxin concentration of 1.1 ng/mL.

It is important to realize that improvement in the signs and symptoms, along with elevated serum digoxin concentration and signs of toxicity, resulted in a dose reduction. An elevated serum sample alone would not have necessitated a dosing change. If the patient was improving and had an elevated level without signs of toxicity, the clinician would not have been able to reduce the dose of digoxin as easy as in our case where the patient had signs of toxicity.

If, on the other hand, the patient experiencing digoxin toxicity with elevated levels and a good therapeutic response had coexisting factors such as hypokalemia, or was recently placed on quinidine or verapamil, or had a sudden reduction in urine output accompanied by an elevation in serum creatinine, correction of these underlying factors would have taken priority over a reduction in digoxin dose.

The physician could have supplemented with potassium or could have made a change in the digoxin dose to reflect altered pharmacokinetic disposition due to an interacting drug or reduction in digoxin elimination due to declining renal status.

I have attempted to show several examples of the earlier nomograms that had been described in the literature for dosing digoxin. At this point, no single nomogram has been shown to be perfect in its ability to predict digoxin dosing requirements for all patients evaluated; however, as has been suggested in the literature, use of any of the nomograms, along with appropriate clinical judgment, accurate determination of serum digoxin concentrations, and a total understanding of digoxin distribution kinetics, will enable the most accurate assessment of such therapy.

Digoxin Considerations in Pediatric Patients

Total Digitalizing Dose

The following doses are for intravenous administration. When oral doses are used, altered bioavailability must be compensated for, as in the adult. All doses are based on ideal body weight.

Premature newborn	20 μg/kg
Full-term newborn	30–50 μg/kg
12–24 mo	40–60 μg/kg
2–10 y	20–40 μg/kg
> 10 y	0.75–1.25 mg

Maintenance Dose

Premature infants generally require lower maintenance doses. Patients less than 10 years of age receive 20 to 30% of the total digitalizing dose in two divided doses.

Studies to date reveal that full-term infants after the first month of life up until the end of the first year of life require more digoxin per kilogram of body weight. This is due in part to a higher-than-normal volume of distribution in this patient population, as well as a higher-than-normal rate of total body clearance. The same is not the case for premature infants and full-term infants prior to the first month of life. In this situation, the literature reveals a greater sensitivity to the effects of digoxin which necessitates an alteration in prescribing.[20,21]

———— QUESTIONS ————

Patient R.A. is a 72-year-old white man admitted to the local emergency room for the treatment of acute respiratory symptoms caused by left ventricular dysfunction. On admission to the emergency room the following patient data are available:

Height:	5 ft 7 in.	Weight:	160 pounds
Na	138 mEq/L	Cl	100 mEq/L
K	4.2 mEq/L	CO_2	28 mEq/L
BUN	15 mg/100 mL	Cr_s	1.5 mg/100 mL

1. Design a treatment regimen for administering digoxin to this patient for the acute treatment of congestive heart failure?

2. Calculate an appropriate digoxin maintenance dose for chronic treatment of this patient.

3. List four subjective and four objective parameters that would aid in monitoring digoxin therapy for both therapeutic efficacy as well as digoxin toxicity.

4. Discuss the applicability of serum drug concentrations for monitoring digoxin therapy. How are serum levels used in monitoring therapy, and what conditions are required for meaningful level interpretation to exist?

5. A serum digoxin level is ordered several days after the patient has begun receiving the oral digoxin maintenance doses and returns with a reported level of 1.2 ng/mL. The patient is stated to be doing well without any complaints; however, a routine chemistry report reveals a serum potassium level of 3.6 mEq/L. What would be your recommendation to the prescriber?

6. Three days after initiating digoxin therapy, quinidine is to be given to the patient for the treatment of a supraventricular tachyarrhythmia. What are your clinical interventions prior to institution of quinidine therapy? Why?

REFERENCES

1. Davis TD, Vanderveen RL, Nienhuis M. Digoxin. In: Mungall D, ed. *Applied Clinical Pharmacokinetics.* New York: Raven Press; 1983.
2. Smith TW. Digitalis: Mechanism of action and clinical use. *N Eng J Med* 1988;318(6):358–365.
3. Keys PW. Digoxin. In: Evans WE, Jusko WJ, Schentag JJ, eds. *Applied Pharmacokinetics.* Los Angeles: Applied Therapeutics; 1982:319–349.
4. Aronson JK. Clinical pharmacokinetics of digoxin 1980. *Clin Pharmacokinet.* 1980;5:137–149.
5. Lisalo E. Clinical pharmacokinetics of digoxin. *Clin Pharmacokinet.* 1977;2:1–16.
6. Sim SK. Digoxin tablets—A review of the bioavailability problems. *Am J Hosp Pharm.* 1976; 33:44–48.
7. Aronson JK. Cardiac glycosides and drugs used in dysrhythmias. In: Dukes, ed. *Side Effects of Drugs Annual 7.* Amsterdam: Excerpta Medica; 1983: Ch 18.
8. Rodin SM, Johnson BF. Pharmacokinetic interactions with digoxin. *Clin Pharmacokinet.* 1988; 15:227–244.

9. Brown DD, Juhl RP. Decreased bioavailability of digoxin due to antacids and kaolin–pectin. *N Engl J Med.* 1976;295:1034–1037.

10. Manninen V, Melen J, Apavalahti A, et al. Altered absorption of digoxin in patients given propantheline and metoclopramide. *Lancet* 1973;1:398–400.

11. Weintraub M. Interpretation of the serum digoxin concentration. *Clin Pharmacokinet.* 1977;2:205–219.

12. Park MK, Ludden T, Arom KV, et al. Myocardial vs serum concentrations in infants and children. *Am J Dis Child.* 1982;136:418–420.

13. Reuning RH, Sans RA, Notari RF. Role of pharmacokinetics in drug dosage adjustments. I. Pharmacologic effect, kinetics and apparent volume of distribution of digoxin. *J Clin Pharmacol.* 1973;13:127–141.

14. Cusack G, Kelly J, O'Malley K, et al. Digoxin in the elderly: Pharmacokinetic consequences of old age. *Clin Pharmacol Ther.* 1979;25:772–776.

15. Lewis RP. Clinical use of serum digoxin concentrations. *Am J Cardiol.* 1992;69:97G–107G.

16. Aronson JK. Indications for the measurement of plasma digoxin concentration. *Drugs.* 1983;26:230–242.

17. Mooradian AD. Digitalis: An update of clinical pharmacokinetics, therapeutic monitoring techniques and treatment recommendations. *Clin Pharmacokinet.* 1988;15:165–179.

18. Sawyer WT. The digitalis glycosides. In: Taylor W, Diers Caviness M, eds. *A Textbook for the Clinical Application of Therapeutic Drug Monitoring.* Irving, TX: Abbott Laboratories; 1986:83–86.

19. Jelliffe RW. An improved method of digoxin therapy. *Ann Intern Med.* 1968;69:703–717.

20. Spector R, Park GD, Johnson GF, Vessell ES. Therapeutic drug monitoring. *Clin Pharmacol Ther.* 1988;43:345–353.

21. Doherty JE, de Soyza N, Kane JJ, et al. Clinical pharmacokinetics of digitalis glycosides. *Prog Cardiovasc Dis.* 1978;21:141–158.

22. Aronson JK, Hardman M. ABC of monitoring drug therapy: digoxin. *Br Med J.* 1992;305:1149–1152.

23. Redfors A. Plasma digoxin concentration—Its relation to digoxin dosage and clinical effects in patients with atrial fibrillation. *Br Heart J.* 1972;34:383–391.

24. Dobbs RJ, O'Neill CJ, Deshmikh AA, et al. Serum concentration monitoring of cardiac glycosides: How helpful is it for adjusting dosing regimens? *Clin Pharmacokinet.* 1991;20(3):175–193.

25. Smith TW, Haber E. Digoxin intoxication: The relationship of clinical presentation to serum digoxin concentration. *J Clin Invest.* 1970;49:2377–2386.

26. Koup JR, Jusko WJ, Elwood CM, et al. Digoxin pharmacokinetics: Role of renal failure in dosage regimen design. *Clin Pharmacol Ther.* 1975;18(1):9–21.

27. Pinsky WE, Jacobsen JR, Gillette PC, et al. Dosage of digoxin in premature infants. *J Pediatr.* 1979;96(4):639–642.

28. Johnson GL, Desai NS, Pauly TH, Cunningham MD. Complications associated with digoxin therapy in low-birth weight infants. *Pediatrics.* 1982;69(4):463–465.

29. Friend DG. Digitalis after two centuries. *Arch Surg.* 1976;111:14–19.

30. Chung EK. Digitalis intoxication. *N Engl J Med.* 1971;284:989–997.

31. Knoben JE, Anderson PO, eds. *Handbook of Clinical Drug Data.* Hamilton, IL: Drug Intelligence Publications; 1993:82–105.

32. Stone J, Bentur Y, Zalstein E, et al. Effect of endogenous digoxin-like substances on the interpretation of high concentration of digoxin in children. *J Pediatr.* 1990;117:321–325.

33. Dasgupta A, Saldana S, Heiman P. Monitoring free digoxin instead of total digoxin in patients with congestive heart failure and high concentrations of digoxin like immunoreactive substances. *Clin Chem.* 1990;36:2121–2123.

34. Cockcroft DW, Gault MH. Prediction of creatinine clearance from serum creatinine. *Nephron.* 1976;16:31–41.

35. Devine BJ. Gentamicin therapy. *Drug Intell Clin Pharm.* 1974;8:650–65.
36. Jelliffe RW. A mathematical analysis of digitalis kinetics in patients with normal and reduced renal function. *Math Biosci.* 1967;1:305–325.
37. Oglivie RI, Ruedy J. An educational program in digitalis therapy. *JAMA.* 1972;222(1):50–55.
38. Dettli L, Spring P, Ryler S. Multiple dose kinetics and drug dosage in patients with kidney disease. *Acta Pharmacol.* 1971;29:211–222.

Chapter 16

Lithium

Julia E. Vertrees
Larry Ereshefsky

Keep in Mind

- Lithium is a univalent cation: 1 mmol/L = 1 mEq/L.
- Administer lithium with meals or as a controlled-release product to help control adverse effects.
- Lithium can be measured in blood, saliva, red blood cells, and tears, though in general practice, only serum or plasma concentrations are measured.
- Lithium's therapeutic range is reported to be 0.4 to 1.5 mmol/L.
- The 12-hour interval has become the standard for therapeutic drug monitoring, as concentrations measured prior to 10 to 12 hours postdose may still be in the absorption and distribution phases.
- Appropriate lithium doses and serum concentrations for the maintenance phase of therapy are usually lower than the serum concentrations needed for acute symptom remission.
- Once steady-state concentrations and remission of symptoms are attained, lithium concentration checks can be performed as infrequently as every 3 months.
- Single daily dosing is possible and may help control the polyuria seen with lithium therapy.
- Response to lithium therapy is gradual: assaultive and hostile behavior usually responds within the first 1 to 3 weeks; speech and thought pattern disturbances are usually markedly reduced by the second to third week; appropriate dress and concern about previous behavior are usually noted within 2 to 4 weeks; grandiosity and delusional thinking may persist for up to 1 to 2 months.
- Mild toxic effects generally begin at lithium concentrations ≥ 1.5 mmol/L. Moderate toxicity is usually noted with serum concentrations between 1.5 and 2.5 mmol/L. Lithium concentrations greater than 2.5 mmol/L are generally associated with severe toxicity.
- Administer lithium with caution to patients concurrently receiving diuretics that act on the proximal tubule (thiazides), antipsychotics, theophylline, nonsteroidal anti-inflammatory drugs, and serotonin-specific reuptake inhibitors.

Lithium is a monovalent cation that is used primarily in the therapy of bipolar disorders (acute manic episodes and prophylaxis against recurrence). Other uses for lithium include adjunctive therapy for depression, schizophrenia, aggression, syndrome of inappropriate antidiuretic hormone (SIADH), cluster headache, and as a immunologic adjuvant.[1,2] This chapter focuses on the use of lithium in the therapy of bipolar disorder.

CLINICAL PHARMACOLOGY AND THERAPEUTICS

Lithium shares many of the physiochemical properties of the physiologic cations. It has an electrical charge similar to that of potassium and sodium and a charge density similar to that of magnesium and calcium. Because of these similarities, early theories for the mechanism of action of lithium centered around the partial substitution of lithium for these cations.[3] Difficulties with this approach arose because significant differences exist in the handling of lithium by the body. Homeostatic mechanisms maintain a large concentration gradient across cell membranes for the physiologic cations but not for lithium.[4,5] Additionally, lithium is not affected by the sodium–potassium ATPase pump to the same extent as sodium; and lithium is much more uniformly distributed intra- and extracellularly compared with the other cations.[6]

Current theories center around lithium's ability to modulate the second-messenger systems of cAMP, cGMP, and phosphatidylinositol, as well as its ability to increase the turnover rate of neurotransmitters, for example, norepinephrine and serotonin.[7–23] Lithium decouples external cell surface receptors for cAMP and cGMP from the cyclase enzyme complex located on the internal surface of cell membranes. This occurs at physiologically achievable concentrations and possibly explains the polyuria (inhibition of antidiuretic hormone-linked production of cAMP) and hypothyroidism (inhibition of thyroid stimulation hormone-linked production of cAMP) noted with lithium use.[16–18] Lithium also interferes with metabolism in the phosphatidylinositol second-messenger system, by preventing the resynthesis of phosphatidylinositol 4,5-biphosphate from inositol 1-phosphate.[19,20] As inositol does not readily cross the blood–brain barrier, the interference by lithium with phosphatidylinositol metabolism inside a cell could lead to a shortage of precursors for the resynthesis of phosphatidylinositol 4,5-biphosphate and, therefore, uncouple the agonist stimulation of a neurotransmitter (Figure 16–1). It has been further proposed that this effect may be significant only in overactive neurons, which might explain lithium's minimal effects on normal behavior.[21]

The many diverse effects of lithium make it unlikely that any one mechanism is responsible for its therapeutic effects. Complex models of dysregulation have been proposed in attempts to unify the various effects of lithium in bipolar disorders and, indeed, in all mood disorders.[24–29] Dysregulation invokes a failure of homeostatic mechanisms to regulate physiologic functions within reasonable limits. Lithium may augment homeostasis by enhancing the function of a secondary system, allowing it to take over regulatory functions.[30]

CLINICAL PHARMACOKINETICS

Table 16–1 summarizes mean pharmacokinetic data.

Dosage Forms, Absorption, and Bioavailability

Lithium ion (Li+), which is commercially available in the United States as both the carbonate and citrate salts (Table 16–2), is commonly administered by the oral route. Although a number

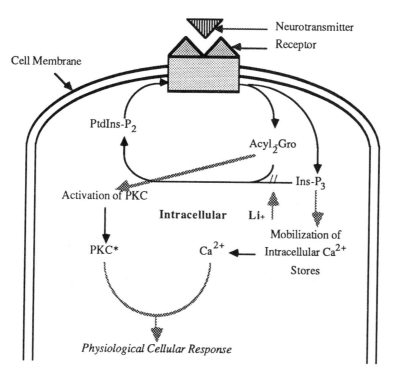

Figure 16–1. Simplified mechanism showing lithium's effects on the metabolism of the second messenger system involving phosphatidylinositol. Phosphatidylinositol 4,5-biphosphate (PtdIns-P_2) is hydrolyzed to diacylglycerol (Acyl$_2$-Gro) and inositol 1,4,5-triphosphate (Ins-P_3) by agonist neurotransmitter or drug binding the receptor on the exterior of the cell membrane. Diacylglycerol activates protein kinase C (PKC); inositol 1,4,5-triphosphate mobilizes intracellular calcium (Ca^{2+}) stores. The activated protein kinase C (PKC*) and intracellular calcium act together in stimulating the physiologic cellular response. Normally, diacylglycerol and inositol 1,4,5-triphosphate recombine to form phosphatidylinositol 4,5-biphosphate and begin the cycle again. In the presence of physiologically achieved lithium concentrations, however, the resynthesis of phosphatidylinositol 4,5-biphosphate is impaired. This leads to a less pronounced physiologic effect or uncoupling from the agonist stimulation of the neurotransmitter. (*From Weber SS, Saklad SR, Kastenholz KV. Bipolar affective disorders. In: Koda-Kimble M-A, Young LY, Kradjan WA, et al, eds. Applied Therapeutics: The Clinical Use of Drugs. Vancouver, WA: Applied Therapeutics; 1992:58-1–58-17.*)

of lithium salts are available, the carbonate is generally used because it contains more lithium by weight than other salts. Additionally carbonate products have a longer shelf-life. After oral administration, lithium is nearly completely absorbed whether given as the carbonate or citrate salt.[1,32]

Lithium absorption occurs primarily in the jejunum and ileum, with absorption decreasing

TABLE 16–1. SUMMARY OF MEAN PHARMACOKINETIC DATA[a]

Population	Half-life (h)	Volume of Distribution (L/kg)	Clearance (mL/h/kg)
Adult	α: 5.0 β: 18	0.5–1.2	Renal: 21.3–28.2[46,47,54] (10–40 mL/min[36])
Pediatric[71]	α: 6.0 β: 17.9	0.93	Renal: 21.9 Total: 40.2
Geriatric[78,79]	26.9–28.5	0.52–0.64	Renal: 13.8–15.6

[a] See also Tables 16–3 and 16–4.

along the length of the intestine. Insignificant absorption occurs in the colon.[33,34] The rate of absorption of lithium depends on the dosage form.[35,36] Following the ingestion of lithium chloride and citrate liquids, rapid absorption, with a peak concentration attained within 15 to 45 minutes, has been noted in fasting individuals. With capsule preparations, peak serum concentrations are observed within the first 1 to 3 hours and absorption is usually complete within 6 to 8 hours. Lithium's bioavailability from standard-release tablets and capsules ranges from 80 to 100%.[1,37] In a study comparing lithium citrate solution with lithium capsules, no significant differences were found between serum lithium concentrations at steady state.[38]

Administration of lithium with meals can delay its absorption significantly. Additionally, several adverse effects of lithium (tremors, polyuria, weakness, nausea, and vomiting) appear to be related to both the rate of rise in the lithium serum concentration and the absolute maximum concentration achieved. Giving lithium with meals or as a controlled-release product decreases the rate of absorption and the maximum peak concentration, and can help control these adverse effects.[39] Food's buffering effects significantly decrease the epigastric pain, burning, and anorexia noted with lithium administration.[40] Alternately, the incidence of diarrhea does not appear to be altered by product selection.

TABLE 16–2. DOSAGE FORMS AVAILABLE IN THE UNITED STATES

Product Form[a]	Brand Names	Salt Form	Dosage Unit
Tablet	Eskalith, Lithane, Lithotabs, generic	Carbonate	300 mg/8.12 mmol
Capsule	Generic	Carbonate	150 mg/4.06 mmol
	Eskalith, Lithonate, generic		300 mg/8.12 mmol
	Generic		600 mg/16.24 mmol
Extended-release tablet	Eskalith-CR	Carbonate	450 mg/12.18 mmol
Liquid	Cibalith-S	Citrate	5 mL/8 mmol (560 mg citrate salt)

[a] Lithium carbonate slow-release capsules are not commercially available in the United States.
Source. Data were taken from Reference 31.

Distribution

Lithium is distributed into total body water with an apparent steady-state volume of distribution (V_d) of 0.5 to 1.2 L/kg.[41] It is not protein bound nor metabolized, but is widely (though unevenly) distributed throughout the body.[1,36] Tissues in which lithium is found include brain, muscle, bone, and kidney. Saliva concentrations are approximately 2 times higher than serum concentrations, and thyroid concentrations are approximately 2.5 to 5 times higher. Bone seems to concentrate and retain lithium for long periods, and the effect of lithium on bone metabolism has not been fully defined. Spinal fluid lithium concentrations have been noted to be 30 to 60% of serum concentrations. Distribution of lithium in the brain shows sizable variation by region in human and animal studies.

The decline in lithium serum concentrations is best characterized by a two-compartment pharmacokinetic model. Lithium's initial apparent volume of distribution is approximately equal to the central compartment (25–40% of body weight).[1,42] The steady-state volume of distribution is approximately equal to the peripheral compartment and has been estimated to equal 50 to 100% of body weight.[42] The central and peripheral compartments together average 123% of body weight.[1] Intracellular equilibration of lithium appears to require at least 25 to 30 hours[1] and may require 3 to 10 days. A number of lithium's neurotoxic effects appear to be due to intracellular concentrations and not to serum concentrations. This long equilibration time is thought to be responsible for the lag period observed for both the therapeutic effects and some of the toxic effects of lithium.[43]

Elimination

Lithium's primary route of excretion from the body is by the kidney; other routes, including saliva, sweat, and feces, account for less than 5% of the total ingested dose.[41] Lithium clearance is directly proportional to glomerular filtration rate (GFR) and blood flow to the nephron. Renal clearance is approximately 20% of creatinine clearance, generally 10 to 40 mL/min in patients with normal renal function.[36] Sixty to eighty percent of the lithium filtered through the glomerulus is reabsorbed in the proximal tubule in competition with sodium.[1] The lithium ion is transported across biologic membranes by both active and passive mechanisms.[36]

Elimination of lithium follows a biphasic pattern, with alpha and beta half-lives of approximately 5 and 18 hours, respectively.[44] Similar to other drugs, wide interindividual variation is seen in the beta half-life. Reports have ranged from 8 to 79 hours in various studies.[42,45–49] Some literature suggests that there is a correlation between treatment duration and lithium elimination half-life. Patients on lithium therapy longer than 1 year have significantly greater half-lives than those individuals treated less than 1 year.[50] Several possible explanations exist for this observation, the most common being lithium-induced nephrotoxicity.[36] Another explanation is the observed changes in lithium transport across red blood cell (RBC) membranes as a function of time. During chronic therapy, lithium's efflux from RBCs may be reversibly decreased.[5]

Factors that influence lithium's renal clearance include a negative sodium balance or volume depletion (such as that caused by polyuria).[51] A negative sodium balance or volume depletion will lead to enhanced retention of lithium secondary to the kidney's compensatory increase in the proximal reabsorption of sodium. At the proximal tubule, lithium and sodium behave almost identically. At the distal tubule, however, reabsorptive mechanisms for sodium and potassium appear to have minimal effect on lithium clearance.

Lithium also has the ability to inhibit its own renal clearance through its inhibition of the kidney's response to antidiuretic hormone and aldosterone. At toxic plasma concentrations, lithium clearance, glomerular filtration rate, and concentrating ability are all decreased because of this reduction in the kidney's response to antidiuretic hormone and aldosterone. These alterations lead to an inhibition of the distal tubular reabsorption of sodium.[52,53] The distal tubule is especially sensitive to lithium's nephrotoxic effects because of the high nonphysiologic lithium concentrations present.[37] Although 99% of filtered water is reabsorbed, only 80% of lithium is removed from the glomerular filtrate. This yields a distal tubular concentration of 30 mmol/L at a plasma lithium concentration of 1.5 mmol/L. Compensatory stimulation of proximal tubular reabsorption of sodium, and therefore lithium, results in decreasing lithium clearance as plasma concentrations increase.[51,54]

Glomerular filtration rate, creatinine clearance, and lithium clearance all demonstrate a circadian rhythm, with increased clearances noted during the daytime. In humans, differences in mean lithium clearance between night and day of about 30% (20 mL/min versus 26 mL/min) have been reported.[55] This alteration in mean lithium clearance has been noted in addition to a significant change in lithium clearance between the upright and prone positions.[56] Postural changes appear to affect urinary lithium clearance but not salivary lithium clearance.[57] The elimination half-life of lithium also demonstrates diurnal variation along with renal clearance. The day-to-night ratio has been reported to range from 1.0 to as much as 2.5.[42,58]

Special Populations

Changes in Mood State

Alterations in lithium's volume of distribution may occur secondary to changes in mood state.[59] Biochemical theories of affective illness propose a model of abnormal concentrations of sodium, potassium, or both in the intracellular compartment.[60] Additionally, idiopathic mood swings of individual patients may be mediated by fluxes in cation transport across membranes.[44]

Renal Disease/Hemodialysis

Although contraindicated in acute renal failure, the use of lithium is possible in patients with chronic renal failure undergoing hemodialysis. A number of case reports of successful lithium maintenance therapy in such individuals now exist.[61-68] It is clear that although more complicated, lithium therapy is possible in chronic renal failure with careful patient selection and frequent laboratory monitoring.[69]

Pediatrics

Children generally have higher renal function and therefore higher lithium excretion rates are to be expected. Higher lithium excretion rates may lead to the need for higher lithium doses per kilogram of body weight to achieve similar concentrations compared with adults. This does not imply that children need higher serum lithium concentration to achieve the desired therapeutic effect.[70] Pharmacokinetic parameters have not been extensively studied in children. In a study of nine children (mean [SD] age, 10.9 [0.7]) by Vitiello and associates, the following mean pharmacokinetic parameters were observed: alpha half-life, 6.0 (1.8) hours; beta half-life, 17.9 (7.4) hours; volume of distribution, 0.93 (0.25) L/kg; renal clearance, 21.9 (9.90) mL/h/kg; total clearance, 40.2 (9.4) mL/h/kg (see Table 16–3 for comparison to adult values).[71]

It is important to note that lithium has not been approved for use in children and should therefore be used with caution. Lithium's known effects on thyroid function[72] and possible effects on bone metabolism[73] are areas of concern.[70] Children seem to be more resistant to lithium's effects on renal function, though the information is still limited[74] and proteinuria has been reported in children.[75]

Geriatrics

Elderly patients appear to have a smaller volume of distribution, about 90% of body weight versus about 120% for younger people.[76] Also, glomerular filtration rate, creatinine clearance, and lithium clearance all decrease proportionally with increasing age.[77] Several studies have explored the pharmacokinetics of the elderly (Table 16–4).[78,79] Overall, findings suggest that older individuals with normal renal function for their age may exhibit reduced lithium clearance when compared with younger adults. Additionally, the alterations in volume of distribution and clearance lead to increased half-lives and, therefore, a longer time to steady-state serum concentrations. Therefore, geriatric patients may require a smaller dosage to achieve therapeutic steady-state serum concentration and the time between dose adjustment will be longer when compared with a younger patient. Lithium doses should be reduced in direct proportion to the fraction of creatinine clearance in the patient compared with 100 mL/min/1.73 m^2.[36] These individuals tend to experience adverse effects even at lower serum concentrations.[80,81]

Pregnancy

Although lithium is generally considered teratogenic during the first trimester, the degree of risk is unclear.[82] Lithium should therefore be used in the first trimester only for women already receiving lithium, where withdrawal from lithium would endanger the mother or the pregnancy, and other less teratogenic medications, such as antipsychotics and antidepressants, cannot be used.[82,83]

Lithium is used during the second and third trimesters of pregnancy. In the later part of pregnancy, renal blood flow and glomerular filtration rate can increase by as much as 50 to 100%.[84,85] As lithium is renally cleared, lithium clearance also increases during pregnancy. After delivery, lithium clearance returns to prepregnancy values. In women who require lithium for

TABLE 16–3. COMPARISON OF PEDIATRIC AND ADULT PHARMACOKINETIC PARAMETERS

Parameter	Children[71]	Adults[46,71]	Statistic[71]
half-life (h)			
α	6.0 (1.8)		
β	17.9 (7.4)	21.39 (6.3)	Student's t 0.97, $df = 15$, NS
V_d (L/kg)	0.93 (0.25)	0.83 (0.18)	Student's t 0.90, $df = 14$, NS
Clearance (mL/h/kg)			
Renal	21.9 (9.9)		
Total	40.2 (9.4)	27.6 (4.7)	Student's t 2.99, $df = 12$, $p < .01$

TABLE 16–4. COMPARISON OF PHARMACOKINETIC VALUES IN ELDERLY VERSUS NONELDERLY ADULTS

	Hardy[79]	Chapron[78]	Adults
Gender	9 females	6 females	
Age	72.6 (5.1)[a]	80.7 (5.4)	
Weight	55.9 (10.0)	68.2 (14.4)	
V_d (L/kg)	0.64 (0.16)	0.52 (0.18)	0.75,[b] 0.85,[c] 0.7[d]
Renal clearance (mL/min/kg)	0.26 (0.08)	0.23 (0.05)	28.2,[c] 21.3,[e] 24.4[d]
Half-life (h)	26.9 (5.5)	28.5 (4.9)	19.8,[b,c] 22.6,[f] 28.9[d]
Creatinine clearance (mL/min)	69.5 (17.7)	62.3 (8.4)	
Clearance ratio (Li/creatinine)	0.20 (0.04)	0.23 (0.05)	

[a] Mean (SD).
[b] Reference 58.
[c] Reference 46.
[d] In schizophrenics.[47]
[e] Reference 54.
[f] Reference 76.

prophylaxis of manic–depressive illness during pregnancy, increased dosages are commonly needed in the last trimester to maintain constant blood concentrations. Maintenance of these higher doses after delivery may lead to lithium toxicity within 2 to 4 weeks.[84] Therefore, lithium should be discontinued several days prior to the anticipated delivery date and then restarted several days postpartum at a reduced dose.[82,86]

PHARMACODYNAMICS

Clinical Response to Lithium in Bipolar Illness

Therapeutic response to lithium is generally assessed by the evaluation of target symptoms. Hyperactivity (disturbed sleep pattern, agitation, assaultiveness, destructiveness, anxiety) is a sensitive and highly reliable indicator of the effectiveness of mania therapy. Assaultive and hostile behavior usually responds within the first 1 to 3 weeks of lithium therapy. Speech (pressured, with racing thoughts) and thought pattern disturbances (tangential associations, flight of ideas) are usually markedly reduced by the second to third week.[43] Appearance is also a useful monitoring tool. A euphoric and hypersexual patient dresses in bright colors with multiple layers of clothing and excessive makeup. An increased concern with appearance is also noted. Appropriate dress and concern about previous behavior are usually noted within 2 to 4 weeks of beginning lithium therapy.[87,88] Elevated mood, with euphoria or irritability, is typical of the classic manic patient. Euphoria is secondary to an elevated motor level, which leads to an excessive feeling of control over the environment and elevated feelings of self-esteem. These elevated feelings of self-esteem often result in grandiose delusions. Irritability usually stems from underlying grandiosity, which leads the patient to be easily provoked or excessively impatient. Grandiosity and delusional thinking may persist for up to 1 to 2 months,[89,90] though in some individuals, the grandiose delusions become fixed or encapsulated and are an integral part of the patient's life coping mechanisms. When this occurs, the delusions and grandiosity become intractable to all therapy.

Manic patients can also exhibit psychotic symptoms, similar to those seen in schizophrenia, including hallucinations, thought disorder, ideas of reference, and behavioral disorganization. Manic hyperactivity can become so severe that the flow of an individual's thoughts and motor level exceed his or her ability to control actions. Such symptoms may indicate the need for adjunctive antipsychotic therapy, at least acutely. Selected patients may require prolonged therapy with both lithium and an antipsychotic drug and may be more properly diagnosed as schizoaffective.[91,92]

Depressive symptoms include pessimism, self-reproach, anhedonia, irritability, and sadness. Thoughts generally focus on guilt, hopelessness, death, and suicide. Mood congruent psychotic features include fictitious somatic complaints and self-deprecatory hallucinations. Evaluating the clinical response of depressed patients usually includes the monitoring of motor and mental activities, mood and feeling states, sleep pattern, and psychotic features. A 2- to 4-week latency period is observed in the response of depression to lithium therapy, longer than typically seen in mania.[93] Improvement in sleep patterns is an important indicator of the onset of the clinical effect of lithium therapy. Lithium therapy corrects the diurnal rhythm disturbances responsible for disrupted sleep patterns seen in depression (difficulty in falling asleep or early-morning awakening). Vegetative signs of depression (motor and mental activity abnormalities) include psychomotor retardation, slowed thinking, poor concentration and memory, easy fatigability, decreased libido, constipation, and anorexia with weight loss.[36] The mood disturbances are among the last symptoms to respond to therapy in the depressed patient. Many individuals require up to 2 months of lithium therapy to have full symptom remission.[94]

Therapeutic Concentrations

Clinically, lithium can be measured in blood, saliva, red blood cells, and tears. In general practice, however, only serum or plasma concentrations are measured because of practical considerations and insufficient data on the correlation of saliva and RBC concentrations to response. The most common reasons for monitoring lithium concentration are to ensure that concentrations are initially within the currently accepted therapeutic range and then to monitor ongoing therapy. Additional uses include assessment of toxicity, compliance, and prediction of starting doses using pharmacokinetic techniques.

Blood (Plasma or Serum)

Either plasma or serum can be used in monitoring patients as differences in protein content of a sample have no effect on the measured lithium concentration. Flame photometry and atomic absorption spectrophotometry are the two most common methods of measuring lithium concentrations. Either may be used as they have been shown to give comparable results.[95,96] Care does need to be taken to ensure that samples for lithium determinations are not drawn in tubes containing lithium–heparin as found in some green-top tubes.[97] Additionally, a clinician should be aware that flame photometry does not give a true zero reading, even in individuals who have never been exposed to lithium.[98]

TABLE 16–5. THERAPEUTIC LITHIUM PLASMA OR SERUM CONCENTRATIONS[a]

Li⁺ (mmol/L)	Acute Use	Maintenance Use
Commonly	0.8–1.0	0.6–0.8
Occasionally	1.0–1.2	0.9–1.0
Rarely	1.2–1.5	1.0–1.2

[a] In geriatric patients or patients with an organic brain syndrome it is prudent to use a lithium serum concentration about 0.2 mmol/L lower than that shown. From Weber SS, Saklad SR, Kastenholz KV. Bipolar affective disorders. In: Koda-Kimble M-A, Young LY, Kradjan WA, et al, eds. *Applied Therapeutics: The Clinical Use of Drugs.* Vancouver, WA: Applied Therapeutics; 1992:58-1–58-17.

Lithium's therapeutic range is reported to be 0.4 to 1.5 mmol/L, depending on the stage in therapy and the patient population studied (Table 16–5). Greater than 90% of responding patients achieve good symptom remission with concentrations less than 1.2 mmol/L. The recommended ranges have crept downward over the last 10 to 15 years partly because of concerns over renal toxicity at higher lithium concentrations. The 1975 American Psychiatric Association's Task Force on Lithium Therapy[99] suggested a range of 0.7 to 1.2 mmol/L for maintenance therapy, and in 1985, the National Institutes of Health/National Institute of Mental Health Consensus Development Panel on Mood Disorders[100] suggested lithium concentrations of 0.6 to 0.8 mmol/L. Concentrations between 1.2 and 1.5 mmol/L are in a borderline toxic range but may be necessary for selected patients. Mild toxicity is not an unusual occurrence during the initial titration phase of therapy. Some patients can respond to lithium plasma concentrations of 0.4 to 0.6 mmol/L, particularly during maintenance therapy.[101]

The controversy that still exists concerning the "therapeutic range" for lithium is due, at least in part, to nonstandardized draw times for lithium blood samples used in studies assessing the therapeutic range. The currently recognized standard draw time for lithium serum concentrations (Table 16–6) is a trough measured at least 10 to 12 hours after the evening dose (based on twice-daily dosing). This 12-hour interval has become the standard for therapeutic drug monitoring, as concentrations measured prior to 10 to 12 hours postdose may still be in the absorption and distribution phases (because of variations in the dissolution times of different preparations and the differences in the absorption course among individuals). Serum concentrations determined 8 hours postdose could be 20 to 25% higher than if the same sample had been drawn 12 hours postdose. This might lead to the determination of a therapeutic range higher than necessary. Prien and Caffey,[102] while treating recurrent bipolar and unipolar depression, found that serum concentrations between 0.5 and 0.7 mmol/L were not as effective as serum concentrations of 0.8 to 1.0 mmol/L. In an additional study, concentrations of 0.9 to 1.4 mmol/L were found necessary to achieve an antimanic effect in manic patients.[103] In both studies, blood samples were collected 8 to 12 hours postdose. In contrast, samples taken later than 12 hours postdose might be as much as 15 to 20% lower when compared with 12-hour samples if drawn as late as 16 hours postdose. The effect would be to indicate a therapeutic range lower than needed for the desired effect. Such might be the case in the study by Decina and Fieve.[104] They obtained serum lithium concentrations 10 to 14 hours after the last dose in 18 recurrently depressed patients and found that serum lithium concentrations between 0.5 and 0.7 mmol/L were associ-

TABLE 16–6. STANDARDIZED LITHIUM CONCENTRATION ASSESSMENT FOR MONITORING LITHIUM THERAPY

1. The daily dose should be divided into two or more doses.
2. Blood samples should be obtained in the morning before the first lithium dose and 12 hours after the evening dose.
3. The dosage regimen should be carefully monitored at least one day before blood sampling (number of doses taken, timing of doses taken).
4. The sample should be obtained under steady-state conditions (previous therapy constant for at least 7 days).

After Amdisen A, Carson SW. Lithium. In: Evans WE, Schentag JJ, Jusko WJ, eds. *Applied Pharmacokinetics: Principles of Therapeutic Drug Monitoring.* Spokane, WA: Applied Therapeutics; 1986:978–1008.

ated with effective prophylaxis, whereas higher concentrations were no more effective in preventing relapse. Jerram and McDonald found that the relapse rate for depressed patients was equally distributed over a concentration range "just above and below 0.5–0.7 mmol/L."[105] Serum samples were drawn 12 to 16 hours after the last dose. Jann et al studied bipolar, depressed patients and found that individuals with serum lithium concentrations below 0.7 mmol/L were more susceptible to a switch into hypomania or mania when treated with tricyclic antidepressants than were those with concentrations above 0.8 mmol/L.[106] Lithium blood concentrations were sampled between 12 and 15 hours postdose.

Hence, the 12-hour postdose trough concentration determination allows greater reproducibility in the interpretation of the blood concentrations by avoiding the variation seen in serum concentrations obtained within the first 6 to 8 hours of lithium administration. When blood samples for lithium concentration determination are drawn at times other than the 12-hour standard recommendation, variations in serum concentrations can mask any correlation with response.

An additional factor in the controversy surrounding the therapeutic range for lithium concerns the "therapeutic range" being studied. There may be several different therapeutic ranges: the lithium concentration range necessary for control of an acute manic episode, to maintain remission, or for prophylaxis against new episodes. Also important is the heterogeneity of the subject population. Studies including a significant number of subjects who are treatment resistant, are rapid cyclers, and so on, could skew the observed therapeutic range for a particular effect (eg, prophylaxis).

Gelenberg et al, in an extensive review of the available literature concerning the relationship between lithium serum concentrations and successful lithium maintenance therapy, addressed a number of these points.[107] They concluded that for lithium maintenance therapy, the therapeutic range is still "obscure." Additionally, they felt that the relationship between maintenance serum lithium concentrations and adverse effects is less clear than commonly believed. This review was followed by the report of a multicenter trial comparing standard (0.8–1.0 mmol/L) and low (0.4–0.6 mmol/L) serum concentrations for maintenance therapy of bipolar disorder.[108] The study was of 94 bipolar individuals between 18 and 75 years of age. Excluded were rapid cyclers (four or more mood episodes per year) and patients who had ever carried a diagnosis of schizophrenia. Their results indicated that lithium concentrations between 0.8 and

1.0 mmol/L are more effective for maintenance therapy of bipolar illness in the population selected, although the higher concentrations are associated with a higher incidence of side effects. Therefore, although the dictum of seeking the lowest adequate dose in an attempt to decrease adverse effects is applicable to lithium, the clinician should be aware that many individuals may require long-term therapy with lithium concentrations similar to those needed for control of acute manic symptoms.

Red Blood Cells

The erythrocyte is of interest because it has been theorized that RBCs share many properties in common with neuronal cells, as RBCs possess an active transport mechanism for sodium and potassium similar to the sodium–potassium pump of nerve cells.[109] Therefore, RBCs may serve as a model for determining the distribution of lithium across neuronal membranes.[4,44] RBC and plasma lithium concentrations are commonly compared as a ratio:

$$RBC/plasma = \frac{RBC\,[Li^+]}{plasma\,[Li^+]} \times 100$$

There are four lithium transport pathways, with the Li+ – Na+ countertransport mechanism (which extrudes lithium against its electrochemical gradient) probably the single most important factor in determining intra/extracellular lithium ratios.[4,110,111] Unfortunately it is difficult to account for the multiple variables, both physiologic and treatment related, that can interfere with any of the pathways.[112] In one study, Ostrow et al found that affective illness, body mass, gender, race, and hypertension all were significantly associated with efflux rate.[113]

Several studies have found that patients responsive to lithium usually have plasma concentrations greater than 0.6 mmol/L, with RBC/plasma ratios between 30 and 40% and RBC lithium concentrations of 0.2 to 0.5 mmol/L. Early in therapy, the RBC lithium concentrations is very low, reflecting limited cellular uptake. At steady state, low RBC concentrations and low ratios are consistent with impaired cellular uptake and may be associated with poor patient response. Alternately, ratios above 50% have been associated with an increased risk of developing central nervous system toxic effects. RBC concentrations greater than 0.6 mmol/L are associated with neurotoxicity.[44,114,115] Unfortunately, others have not been able to validate the usefulness of RBC lithium concentrations in affective disorders.[116–118] Because of inter- and intrapatient variations,[118,119] routine use of RBC lithium concentrations and RBC/plasma ratios is not extensive in the clinical setting.

One possibly useful, proposed application of the RBC/plasma ratio is the monitoring of patient compliance. Patients taking lithium irregularly, or in whom the last dose was taken less than 6 hours before sampling, will have lower ratios compared with previous samples.[120–125] The key is a previous sample for comparison. Without such a sample, a RBC/plasma ratio check would be of little value.

Saliva

Shopsin et al first popularized the concept of monitoring saliva lithium concentrations after they measured lithium, sodium, and potassium in human saliva in 1969.[126] Monitoring saliva concentrations is attractive because it avoids the discomfort of venipuncture, and would be useful for patients with difficult veins or those unwilling to undergo lithium therapy because of the necessity of venipuncture.

The initial promise of saliva lithium monitoring has not been fulfilled. Although a number of studies have shown a high correlation between saliva and serum concentrations[58,126–136] significant interindividual[137–141] and intraindividual[139,142] variability has been observed. Other studies have found no significant correlation between saliva and serum concentrations.[143–145] To overcome the intraindividual variability, several authors[137,138,146] have suggested elaborate methods to control for the variability. The methods generally involve several simultaneous plasma and saliva determinations before switching to saliva determinations alone. The relationship between plasma and saliva concentrations has to be periodically reassessed to detect any changes in the ratio.

Because of the extent of the variability and the difficulty in controlling for the variability, it is unlikely that saliva concentration will ever be a viable monitoring option.

Adverse Effects

Symptomatology

The dose required to achieve therapeutic serum concentration shows wide interindividual variation. Additionally, lithium has quite a narrow therapeutic index. Over the usual therapeutic range, the plasma concentration-versus-response curve for treating manic patients with lithium is linear, and this information can be used to estimate the dose necessary to adjust a nonresponding patient's lithium concentration without exceeding the therapeutic range.[37,147] Initial serum concentrations greater than 1.5 mmol/L are associated with incipient lithium toxicity, and if dosing continues unchanged, toxic effects may occur within a few days. As lithium's nephrotoxic effect can result in a reduction of its own renal elimination, an upward spiral of the lithium serum concentration can develop when concentrations are greater than 1.2 to 1.5 mmol/L; that is, increases in lithium serum concentrations can result in further decreases in lithium clearance, which then drive the lithium serum concentration even higher.[53,77,110,148]

Mild toxic effects generally begin at lithium concentrations of 1.5 mmol/L and higher.[148] Noted effects include fine tremors of the limbs, gastrointestinal disturbances, muscle weakness, and fatigue. These symptoms may also be seen transiently at the initiation of therapy. If these effects reappear, a careful assessment should be made to determine if the patient is becoming lithium toxic. As part of the assessment, the lithium concentration should be measured and the patient should be questioned concerning recent changes in diet or physical health.[149,150]

Additionally, toxicity may appear as organicity at therapeutic serum concentrations.[151] A patient may become confused, dysarthric, and agitated, with memory impairment and cog–wheel rigidity also possible. Delirium, increased deep tendon reflexes, and seizures have also been observed during toxicity.[151,152] As equilibration of lithium into the central nervous system occurs over 3 to 7 days, symptoms of toxicity may not be apparent initially despite a toxic lithium serum concentration. Therefore, careful monitoring is necessary if lithium therapy is to continue in patients exhibiting this syndrome along with simultaneous lithium concentrations usually considered therapeutic.[152] The lithium dose ultimately should be reduced to maintain a concentration below that at which the organic symptoms appear.

The effects seen with moderate toxicity (usually noted with serum concentrations between 1.5 and 2.5 mmol/L) include sedation, lethargy, ataxia, dysarthria, headaches, increased deep tendon reflexes, hyperthermia, coarse tremors, impaired sensorium, and nystagmus. Coarse hand tremors are usually noted when serum concentration are greater than 1.5 mmol/L.[72]

Lithium concentrations greater than 2.5 mmol/L are generally associated with severe toxicity. Effects include tremors so coarse that the patient may be functionally handicapped, delirium, basal ganglia dysfunction, seizures, coma, respiratory complication, and death. Severe toxicity is generally observed only in overdose or in patients on high doses of lithium with accompanying complicating conditions (ie, diuretic therapy, infections, renal disease).[72,149]

Alterations in water and electrolyte balance are usually the cause when toxicity develops in a patient on maintenance lithium therapy. Water loss as a result of impaired renal concentrating ability appears to be a predisposing factor.[72] Reduction in the renal lithium clearance may be secondary to kidney disease or sodium deficiency.[51] Some common causes of sodium deficiency resulting in lithium toxicity include alteration in salt intake and extrarenal sodium loss, such as sweating from a fever, vomiting, and diarrhea. Drug interactions, particularly with thiazide diuretics, can also alter sodium and water balance, leading to significant toxicity (see Drug–Drug Interactions). Toxic sequelae appear to relate to both the height and duration of toxic lithium plasma concentrations.[51,153]

The onset of lithium toxicity during chronic therapy can be insidious, and the symptoms of intoxication may be more severe compared with those observed in an acutely toxic individual (eg, intentional overdose) with similar lithium serum concentrations.[154] The continual distribution of lithium into the central nervous system during chronic dosing means that the amount of lithium in the brain will be higher with chronic intoxication than the amount in the brain after acute intoxication (at least initially) for the same observed lithium plasma concentration (see Distribution). Therefore, the severity of toxicity cannot be assessed merely on the basis of lithium serum concentrations. Additional factors including nature of the toxicity (acute or chronic), length of time since reaching a toxic serum concentration, complicating medical illness, and severity of symptomology must be considered when assessing the severity of lithium toxicity. Treatment guidelines as outlined next must be considered in the light of these factors.

Treatment

Once appropriate gastrointestinal evacuation has been completed in an acute overdose, and the severity of the intoxication assessed (see discussion above), treatment of acute and chronic toxicity is the same. (A discussion of gastrointestinal decontamination is beyond the scope of this chapter.) Treatment of mild intoxication should be supportive and directed toward correction of any electrolyte or fluid imbalance. In patients with good renal function, therapy with half-normal or normal saline, at a rate sufficient to ensure a normal urine output, is the goal. Sodium should be replaced and sodium restriction avoided. Treatment with sodium chloride infusion does not appear to have an enhancing effect on lithium clearance for well-hydrated patients with normal serum sodium concentrations.[155]

Useful methods available to enhance elimination include hemodialysis, peritoneal dialysis, and arteriovenous hemodiafiltration. The use of peritoneal dialysis or forced diuresis to enhance elimination is generally reserved for situations when hemodialysis is not possible or its initiation will be delayed.[156] Additionally, the use of sodium-containing solutions in renally compromised patients is not without risks and should be done with care, if at all, in the therapy of moderate to severe lithium intoxication.[51] Individuals ill enough to require additional therapy beyond supportive care would be more appropriately treated with hemodialysis. Hemodialysis can be expected to achieve a lithium clearance of 30 to 50 mL/min, and peritoneal dialysis, 13 to 15 mL/min,[157] as compared with normal lithium clearance of 10 to 40 mL/min. Arteriovenous hemodiafiltration has been reported, in a single case, to achieve a lithium clearance of 20.5 mL/min.[158]

Though no clear-cut guidelines for patient selection exist, hemodialysis is considered the treatment of choice when the patient's clinical conditions is deteriorating or renal insufficiency is present. For all lithium-intoxicated individuals, but particularly in situations of chronic toxicity, the assessment of the severity of toxicity should not be based on lithium serum concentrations alone. Treatment recommendations are usually based both on lithium concentrations and on symptoms. Generally, patients with chronic toxicity exhibit more severe symptoms at lower concentrations than patients with acute toxicity[154] (see Symptomatology). One reasonable set of recommendations for the use of hemodialysis is that of Simard et al,[159] who recommend hemodialysis for (1) all patients with concentrations greater than 4 mmol/L, (2) symptomatic patients with concentrations greater than 2.5 mmol/L, and (3) patients in whom the lithium concentration would not be expected to fall, on its own, to 0.6 mmol/L within 36 hours, regardless of patient condition. Alternately, Amdisen suggests that hemodialysis is appropriate when the serum lithium concentration is greater than 2.5 mmol/L at 12 or more hours post-dose or when the 12-hour level is less than 2.5 mmol/L but the serum lithium concentration does not decrease by more than 10% every 3 hours.[149]

Owing to extensive intracellular stores of lithium, serum concentrations often rebound once hemodialysis is discontinued. (No rebound has been associated with peritoneal dialysis.[1]) Peak rebound concentrations are usually noted 6 to 12 hours after the end of hemodialysis. Lithium serum concentrations should be measured every 2 to 4 hours after dialysis, and hemodialysis should be repeated as necessary until the concentration remains less than 1 mmol/L.[51]

Drug–Drug Interactions

Diuretics

Sodium balance plays an important role in many of lithium's clinically significant drug–drug interactions. Alteration in the sodium balance plays a particularly important role in the modulation of lithium's renal elimination.[69,160] The reabsorption processes for lithium and sodium in the proximal tubule are nearly identical. In the distal tubules, lithium is handled differently from sodium. This difference in lithium's behavior explains why lithium's clearance can be altered by manipulation of the sodium ion. Diuretics that act on the proximal tubule can affect lithium clearance. Lithium clearance is not directly affected by distal tubule diuretic intervention.[50–52] Salt loading can increase lithium clearance by decreasing proximal tubular reabsorption of both sodium and lithium.[160]

Thiazide Diuretics. The primary site of action of thiazide-type diuretics is at the distal tubule which produces a natriuretic effect. The sodium and volume depletion caused by thiazides results in renal compensatory mechanisms that increase sodium reabsorption at the proximal tubule. This increased renal reabsorption of sodium leads to increased lithium reabsorption and, hence, an indirect decrease in lithium clearance. Himmelhock et al have shown that the decrease in lithium clearance is proportional to the thiazide dose.[161] Chlorothiazide doses of 500 mg given daily resulted in a 40% decrease in lithium clearance, whereas doses of 750 to 1000 mg chlorothiazide elevated plasma lithium concentrations by 60 to 70%. This decrease in lithium clearance occurs slowly over the first 1 to 2 weeks of therapy. In individuals who are on a low-sodium diet or who are being treated with antihypertensive agents that cause a reflex increase in sodium reabsorption in the kidney secondary to blood pressure lowering, a decrease in lithium clearance may be observed. These drug–drug interactions are highly significant and can result in clinical toxicity if the lithium dose is not adjusted based on serum concentration determinations.[69]

Alternately, this effect of thiazide-type diuretics has been used for therapeutic purposes in treating lithium-induced nephrogenic diabetes insipidus.[162] Thiazide-type diuretics are also used to enhance the efficacy of lithium therapy in refractory manic–depressive patients. Patients who cannot tolerate the gastrointestinal side effects of high doses of lithium or who otherwise require high lithium doses may benefit from combined lithium–thiazide diuretic use. The daily lithium dose can be decreased while keeping the plasma lithium concentration in the therapeutic range.[163,164]

Loop Diuretics. Several case reports of a potential interaction between loop diuretics and lithium appear in the literature.[165–168] Alternately, other reports support the safe concurrent use of loop diuretics and lithium.[169,170] Additional literature indicates that loop diuretics either have no effect on or increase lithium clearance.[54,171] Overall, the literature does not support the existence of this interaction, but as a precaution it would be prudent to assess the lithium plasma concentration when adding a loop diuretic to lithium therapy.

Antipsychotics
A significant but rare drug–drug interaction occurs between antipsychotic agents and lithium. In some patients, lithium appears to increase the severity of an individual's extrapyramidal reaction to antipsychotic agents. The higher-potency antipsychotics, especially piperazine phenothiazines, are more commonly implicated in this extrapyramidal reaction.[172] A more serious neurotoxic reaction has been reported with various antipsychotics used in combination with lithium[43,151,173–185] (including clozapine[186]), with several reports associated with irreversible brain damage.[187,188] Alternately, in multiple reports and reviews, combinations of various antipsychotics and lithium have been shown to be safe.[189–197] A review by Prakash et al summarized the interaction symptom frequency in 39 case reports: organic symptoms (82%), extrapyramidal signs (74%), cerebellar signs (26%), fever (18%), pyramidal signs (16%).[175] Although the reaction has been reported with multiple antipsychotics, there has been concern that the incidence might be increased with haloperidol.[198] Neither this issue nor the rate of occurrence of the reaction with any of the antipsychotics has been resolved. For the vast majority of patients the combination is safe. If neurotoxicity is suspected, lithium or haloperidol should be stopped promptly.

The neurotoxic reaction might illustrate pharmacologic alteration of the drug's volume of distribution. Several authors report that phenothiazines appear to increase intracellular storage of the lithium ion. In individuals in whom this increase has been noted, a lithium neurotoxic reaction appears to account for the majority of symptoms.[199,200] There is also evidence that neuroleptics (and antidepressants) may have a significant influence on lithium's distribution between plasma and tissue compartments by altering lithium transport across cell membranes.[172,201] Alterations in red blood cell lithium transport have been observed. Nemes et al found red blood cell and plasma haloperidol concentrations significantly increased after 4 weeks of combined lithium and haloperidol therapy in 17 patients with schizophrenia or schizoaffective disorder.[202] Another study also suggests that haloperidol affects red blood cell lithium transport.[203] In comparison, two other studies have found no effect of haloperidol on the lithium red blood cell/plasma ratio, but have found that phenothiazines and thioxanthenes increase the ratio.[200,204]

Theophylline

Theophylline enhances the renal elimination of lithium.[54,205–207] In one study of healthy volunteers, the lithium excretion fraction (lithium clearance/creatinine clearance) increased by 58% after the administration of a 1-g dose of oral theophylline.[54] In work by another research group,[206,207] individuals stabilized first on lithium and then titrated to therapeutic theophylline concentrations showed 11-hour lithium concentrations that were on average 21% lower than during the control period. Clinically, if the lithium dose is unaltered when theophylline is added to or subtracted from lithium therapy, the lithium concentrations would be expected to decrease or increase, respectively. This does not preclude the concurrent use of these medications; concurrent use simply requires careful lithium concentration monitoring and dose adjustment as necessary.[205]

Nonsteroidal Anti-inflammatory Drugs

Nonsteroidal anti-inflammatory drugs (NSAIDs) decrease lithium clearance by decreasing renal blood flow secondary to prostaglandin inhibition. This interaction has been reported with the following NSAIDs: diclofenac, ibuprofen, indomethacin, ketoprofen, naproxen, oxyphenylbutazone, phenylbutazone, and piroxicam.[208,209] The information to date indicates that sulindac does not interact with lithium or slightly decreases lithium concentrations.[208,210] The mechanism of the renal sparing effect may be that sulindac is metabolized in the kidney to inactive metabolites and therefore does not inhibit renal prostaglandin synthesis.[210] Aspirin also has little effect on lithium renal clearance and lithium concentrations.[208]

Serotonin-Specific Reuptake Inhibitors

Several reports exist of a possible serotonergic hyperarousal syndrome with concurrent administration of lithium with the serotonin-specific reuptake inhibitors (SSRIs) fluoxetine,[211–213] sertraline,[214] and fluvoxamine.[215,216] In one report, concurrent administration of lithium and fluoxetine led to elevated lithium concentrations (1.7 mmol/L) and neurotoxicity (stiffness of legs and arms, dizziness, ataxia, dysarthric speech) in a woman who had received 20 uneventful years of therapy with lithium alone.[212] In a second report, ataxia, coarse tremor, altered respirations, and temperature were observed to develop after addition of lithium to stable fluoxetine therapy (lithium concentrations, 0.65–1.08 mmol/L).[211] An unusual case of possible absence or complex partial seizures has been reported in a single individual (no previous seizure history) secondary to a simultaneous lithium dose increase and the addition of fluoxetine.[213] Three other medications (including two benzodiazepines at low doses) were discontinued at the same time. The seizurelike activity began approximately 1 month later and stopped after a lithium dose decrease.

In the United Kingdom, the Committee on Safety of Medicines issued a bulletin in 1989 warning of the possibility of the serotonergic hyperarousal syndrome after receiving 19 reports of adverse reactions in patients receiving fluvoxamine and lithium.[215,216] Five of the reports involved convulsions and one case involved hyperpyrexia. Alternately, Evans and Marwick reported "irresistible somnolence" several days after the addition of lithium 400 mg SR to an unspecified dose of fluvoxamine. The somnolence cleared promptly after the discontinuation of both medications and did not return once lithium alone was restarted several weeks later.[217]

Fluoxetine precipitated a switch into mania in two bipolar individuals despite apparently adequate lithium therapy.[218] Increases in lithium concentration with no toxicity were observed in this report. One of the individuals did not switch until her lithium dose was reduced secondary to the increase in the lithium concentration.

Alternately a number of reports of safe concurrent use of SSRIs and lithium appear in the literature.[219–223]

THERAPEUTIC REGIMEN DESIGN

Dosing for Acute Therapy

Approved recommendations for initial therapy in adults suggest beginning with 300 to 600 mg of lithium carbonate tablets or capsules, three times a day, or, for sustained-release products, initially 600 to 900 mg a day, with an increase on day 2 to 1200 to 1800 mg per day in three divided doses.[31] Thereafter the dosage should be individually adjusted according to serum concentrations and clinical response (target symptom response). Doses at the upper end of these recommendations may be associated with dose-limiting side effects (particularly gastrointestinal effects), which may influence patients' long-term willingness to take lithium. Therefore, beginning with a dose of 300 mg of lithium carbonate (tablets), two or three times a day for several days, before initiating the full desired starting dose, may minimize initial adverse effects and lead to increased tolerance of lithium therapy. The initial oral dose for an acute episode is in the range 24 to 48 mmol/d (900–1800 mg lithium carbonate, or 15–20 mg/kg) for an individual with normal renal function.[40] Dosage should be adjusted with serum concentrations on a biweekly or weekly basis until a serum concentration of 0.8 to 1.2 mmol/L is obtained.[31,36] In most patients, an increase of 8 mmol/d results in a 0.3 ± 0.1 mmol/L increase of Li+ in the serum.[37] Patients may occasionally require up to 80 mmol (3000 mg lithium carbonate) per day during the acute episode.[36]

An acutely manic patient may need and tolerate much higher dosages of lithium to achieve the desired therapeutic serum concentration. Once symptoms begin to remit, a decrease in the elimination rate or tolerance to the drug can occur. An alteration in the volume of distribution, a "mood-dependent compartment," may be one possible explanation for this phenomenon.[59] Individuals with poor dietary status, concurrent debilitating medical illness, and dehydration have decreased clearances when started on lithium therapy.[224,225]

Dosing for Maintenance Therapy

No clear guidelines exist for the choice of patients to receive long-term lithium therapy. Long-term therapy fits into two general types: therapy to prevent relapse after an acute episode (continuation therapy) and prophylactic therapy that follows continuation therapy or is started at some point when the patient is euthymic.[226] Factors considered in patient selection include frequency and severity of episodes, abruptness of onset of episodes, seasonality of prior episodes, prior response to medication, and possible consequences of a relapse.[226]

The appropriate lithium serum concentrations for the maintenance phase of therapy are usually lower than the serum concentrations needed for acute symptom remission [see Therapeutic Concentrations, Blood (Plasma or Serum)]. Once steady-state concentrations and symptom remission are attained, the 1985 NIH/NIMH Consensus Development Panel on Mood Disorders suggests lithium concentration checks every 1 to 3 months.[100] During times of infection, changes in diet, debilitation from any cause, or recurrence of affective symptoms or for individuals in whom control of mania is difficult to maintain, lithium serum concentrations may be more appropriately obtained monthly or more frequently as indicated by the individual circumstances. One potential cause of the recurrence of affective symptoms may be noncompliance with medication therapy. If noncompliance is suspected, a "now" lithium concentration determination might be obtained. Interpretation of such a concentration must be made carefully, as it is unlikely to be a 12-hour postdose concentration. A concentration moderately higher or lower than anticipated may simply reflect the draw time, whereas a significantly low concentration may indicate noncompliance. Alternately, an apparently toxic concentration should not trigger undue concern, unless the patient has actual symptoms of toxicity. A repeat concentration determination may be appropriate depending on the magnitude of the elevation and an interview with the patient (see Adverse Effects). Elevated concentrations may simply indicate a dose still in the absorption period, but may not necessarily indicate consistent compliance with medication therapy, as a patient might take several extra tablets just before a scheduled concentration determination in an attempt to "catch up." A more helpful therapeutic strategy to address noncompliance might be to discuss your concern with the patient and schedule a return visit with 12-hour postdose concentration determination sometime in the next few days. The interval should be short enough that steady state could not be reached if the patient immediately resumed medication therapy. Unfortunately, simple concentration determinations may be insufficient to uncover inconsistent noncompliance and do not substitute for a good relationship with both the patient and his or her family.

Polyuria and polydipsia have long been recognized as renal side effects of lithium but after a report[227] in 1977 of morphologic changes in the kidneys of patients undergoing lithium therapy, the potential nephrotoxic effects of lithium became the subject of intensive research. A discussion of lithium's nephrotoxic effects is beyond the scope of this book other than to note that although lithium can have serious renal effects, these are quite rare. The reader is referred to several studies, reviews, and texts for more extensive discussion.[228–238]

One outcome of the so-called "kidney scare"[239] has been research on different dosing strategies that might minimize lithium-induced renal effects. The impact of alterations of dose size and dose schedule on the more severe renal effects of lithium is still unclear.[228–230,232,235,238,240] Dose schedule alteration does appear to have an impact on polyuria. Some studies have noted a decreased urine volume in individuals switched from divided dosing to a single daily lithium dose.[238,241–244] Alternately, others authors have reported no alteration in urine volume with such a switch.[240,245–247] Enough data exist to suggest that in individuals bothered by polyuria, a switch to a single daily dose of lithium might be helpful in decreasing urine volume. The reader is referred to other sources for additional strategies in treating polyuria.[231]

The primary disadvantage in using a single daily dose is the confusion introduced in the use of plasma lithium concentrations to monitor lithium therapy. Data on the meaning of lithium serum concentrations in the therapy of bipolar illness have been based primarily on the 12-hour steady-state trough concentration measured during twice-daily lithium dosing.[1] Perry et al noted that when switching from twice- to once-daily dosing of lithium, the 12-hour lithium serum concentration might increase by 10% (in patients with a lithium half-life of 40 hours) to 26% (in patients with a lithium half-life of 16 hours).[241] Although changes in the 12-hour postdose concentration have not been observed in all studies evaluating a switch to once- from twice-daily dosing,[55] others have noted differences in the 12-hour postdose concentration.[42,247,248] Therefore, when choosing single daily dosing for the patient who is bothered by polyuria or who would just prefer single daily dosing, additional care must be taken to monitor the patient for the clinical indicators of relapse or toxicity, in addition to lithium serum concentrations.

Predictive Dosing Methods

As several dose adjustments may be required to find the correct dose for any given patient, pharmacokinetic models have been constructed to assist in calculating dosage requirements. The goal is to achieve a therapeutic lithium concentration with the first dosage regimen, thereby decreasing the time to response and at the same time avoiding toxicity. Requirements for such a method would be accuracy, particularly considering lithium's narrow therapeutic index, wide applicability across patient groups, and simplicity coupled with a reasonable cost. An equation that can provide a first approximation for dosing requirements is

$$D = \frac{V_d\, K_e\, \tau\, C_{av,ss}}{F} \quad or \quad D = \frac{V_d\,(0.693/t_{1/2})\, \tau\, C_{av,ss}}{F}$$

where D is dosage; V_d is volume of distribution; K_e is elimination rate constant; τ is dosing interval; $C_{av,ss}$ is average desired steady-state serum concentration; and F is fraction absorbed. All the variables in the formula are known or can be calculated. The desired steady-state serum lithium concentration and the volume of distribution ranges (0.5–1.2 L/kg) are known. The elimination rate constant can be calculated on the basis of renal clearance. The dosing interval is usually assumed to be 24 hours, and the fraction absorbed is assumed to be approximately 90%. This formula can be applied to most patients.[36]

Multiple dose prediction methods now exist based on pharmacokinetic principles. A priori methods include those of Pepin and Zetin. The Pepin method is based on population estimate of kinetic parameters.[249] It requires knowledge of the patient's age, gender, height, weight, and serum creatinine. Zetin et al developed multivariant regression models and dosing algorithms that account for dosage formulation, in- or outpatient status, presence or absence of concurrent tricyclic antidepressant administration, and patient age, gender, and weight.[250,251] The following is the second of the two dosing algorithms developed[251]:

dose = 486.8 + (746.83 × desired level) − (10.08 × age) + (5.95 × weight [kg]) + (92.01 × status) + (147.8 × sex) − (74.73 × TCA),

where status = 1 for inpatient, 0 for outpatient; sex = 1 for male, 0 for female; TCA = 1 for concurrent TCA administration, otherwise 0. The dose calculated is the daily dose of lithium carbonate.

Single-point methods include those of Cooper, Perry, and others.[252–256] Cooper et al use a lithium test dose of 600 mg and 24-hour postdose concentration determination.[257,258] A nomogram is then used to select the dosage required to achieve a serum concentration between 0.6 and 1.2 mmol/L. Note that this nomogram does not predict a specific concentration; rather, it simply indicates a dose that should place the patient's serum concentration within the range indicated by the nomogram. A simple equation also can be used instead of the nomogram:

$$Li^+ \text{ (mmol/d)} = e^{4.80 - 7.5 C_{test}}$$

Here C_{test} is the lithium plasma concentration 24 hours after 600 mg of lithium carbonate. The Perry method[259,260] uses a test dose of 1200 mg and 24-hour postdose concentration determination, with a nomogram to predict a specific steady-state serum lithium concentration.

Methods that require more than a single concentration determination include the multipoint method of Perry et al, a repeated single-point method, regression techniques, and bayesian forecasting. With the multipoint method of Perry et al, a 1200-mg test dose is given and lithium concentration is determined at 12, 24, and 36 hours.[261] Two or three of the points are then used to determine an elimination rate constant. The repeated single-point method requires that two equal-sized doses of lithium be given, separated by a time equal to the intended dosing interval, T.[262,263] A single lithium determination is made after each dose, again separated by a time equal to the intended dosing interval. The elimination rate constant is then calculated using the equation

$$k = \frac{\ln[C_1/(C_2 - C_1)]}{T} \quad or \quad \frac{0.693}{t_{1/2}} = \frac{\ln[C_1/(C_2 - C_1)]}{T}$$

All of the preceding methods can be used without the aid of a computer, though one would be useful for many of the methods. In contrast, nonlinear regression and bayesian forecasting methods require a computer. With regression techniques (linear and nonlinear),[264–266] a computer program is used to find the best-fit estimates of clearance, apparent volume of distribution, and elimination rate constant based on two or more lithium doses, and their corresponding serum concentrations. Bayesian methods begin with population estimates of pharmacokinetic parameter for clearance, apparent volume of distribution, and elimination rate constant.[267,268] Patient specific dose/concentration data are then "fit" to estimate the same parameters, and the patient-specific estimates are compared statistically with the population parameters to produce the final recommendations. Such programs generally update their population database with each patient entered and theoretically become more accurate with time for the population of patients seen at the facility using the program.

A comprehensive, comparative evaluation of the available predictive dosing methods is beyond the scope of this chapter, and the reader is referred to several reviews and studies that attempt to validate or compare the various techniques.[95,268–275] Based on the clinical experience of the authors, several comments on and recommendations for the use of predictive dosing can be made. As plasma concentration determinations are essential owing to lithium's narrow therapeutic index, empiric dosing (ie, dosing by patient response alone) is not recommended for routine clinical use.

The variability of lithium clearance relative to creatinine clearance (10–40%) and the manic patient's changing dietary and mood status all affect lithium's elimination and volume of distribution in an unpredictable fashion; hence predictive methods are still somewhat crude. Problems exist with generalizability of the predictive methods to populations other than ones similar to the population in which a method was initially developed. Blind use of any predictive method obviously should not be attempted. Additionally, although some studies have shown that several of the predictive dosing methods can safely lead to more rapid attainment of the desired serum concentration, no studies have yet been done (of which we are aware) that look at the impact of this more rapid attainment of the desired serum concentration on patient outcome. Intuitively, more rapid attainment of a presumed therapeutic serum concentration should lead to better patient outcomes, but intuition is not always borne out in controlled studies. Before we can recommend the general application of a predictive dosing technique, which may incur increased patient pain and risk, as well as increase the cost of care, controlled studies that document improved patient-driven outcomes (ie, decrease duration of symptoms, decreased need for concomitant medications, decreased length of stay, improved quality of life) need to be performed.

This notwithstanding, increasing information does support the usefulness of some type of predictive method for dosing. Based on the criteria outlined in the opening paragraph of this section (accuracy, wide applicability across patient groups, simplicity, a reasonable cost) and a current prospective study,[271] we can suggest the use of the mathematical method of Zetin and associates[67,246,247] as a reasonable choice for use in a facilities treating patients who are otherwise medically well. Its primary limitation is one shared with all current predictive methods—the problem of generalizability. For problem populations (eg, geriatric patients with cardiovascular disease or renal insufficiency, any patient whose renal function is suspect) or in those patients taking medication that may alter lithium clearance, more rigorous pharmacokinetic assessments are recommended. As we are unaware of any predictive methods that have been developed with these individuals in mind, we cannot recommend the current predictive methods for use in such patients outside a controlled study setting. It is essential to recall that use of any of the methods, in any population, does not decrease the need for frequent lithium serum concentration monitoring during therapy initiation and dose changes.

——— QUESTIONS ———

M.B. is a 36-year-old, 142-pound woman recently readmitted to the psychiatric hospital. Her husband reports that about 2 weeks ago, M.B. began sleeping less and less and that for the last few days she has not slept at all. Although employed at a rather conservative company, over the last week she has dressed for work in an increasingly colorful and provocative manner. This afternoon her husband reports that he came home to find his wife surrounded by a number of packages. She stated she had just received a big promotion and had been given the afternoon off, so she had gone on a shopping spree to celebrate (a call to her company revealed she had been sent home to change to more appropriate attire). M.B.'s husband reports that his wife has been diagnosed with bipolar disorder and had been taking lithium for several years. A pill count this afternoon revealed that she had probably not taken her lithium for about a week. On questioning, M.B. says she stopped taking her lithium late last week because she was feeling so good and wanted to feel even better.

1.   Discuss the different ways to choose a starting dose for M.B.

2. The plan is to restart her lithium with the goal of a level of 0.9 mmol/L. Calculate a starting dose using the second of the Zetin algorithms. How should this dose be given? When would it be reasonable to obtain an initial level to check your estimated dose. When would you expect the patient to be at steady state?

3. As M.B. apparently experienced an exacerbation of her mania despite reported compliance with her medication, it may be necessary to initially monitor her more closely to determine the currently appropriate therapeutic concentration for maintenance of remission (the individualized therapeutic concentration for M.B.). Discuss the usual standards for monitoring lithium therapy once the desired plasma concentration has been obtained, and how you would alter these recommendations, if at all, for M.B. Also discuss other instances where you might wish to obtain a serum concentration in addition to routine monitoring.

REFERENCES

1. Amdisen A, Carson SW. Lithium. In: Evans WE, Schentag JJ, Jusko WJ, eds. *Applied Pharmacokinetics: Principles of Therapeutic Drug Monitoring.* Spokane, WA: Applied Therapeutics; 1986:978–1008.
2. Lithium: An overview. In: Jefferson JW, Greist JH, Ackerman DL, et al, eds. *Lithium Encyclopedia for Clinical Practice.* 2nd ed. Washington, DC: American Psychiatric Press; 1987:1–31.
3. Singer I, Rotenberg D. Mechanisms of lithium action. *N Engl J Med.* 1973;289:254–260.
4. Dorus E, Pandey G, Shaughnessy R, et al. Lithium transport across red cell membrane: A cell membrane abnormality in manic–depressive illness. *Science.* 1979;205:932–934.
5. Pandey GN, Dorus E, Davis JM, et al. Lithium transport in human red blood cells: Genetic and clinical aspects. *Arch Gen Psychiatry.* 1979;36:902–908.
6. Bunney WE Jr, Pert A, Rosenblatt J, et al. Mode of action of lithium: Some biological considerations. *Arch Gen Psychiatry.* 1979;36:898–901.
7. Colburn RW, Goodwin FK, Bunney WE Jr, et al. Effect of lithium on the uptake of noradrenaline by synaptosomes. *Nature.* 1967;215:1395–1297.
8. Katz RI, Chase TN, Kopin IJ. Evoked release of norepinephrine and serotonin from brain slices: Inhibition by lithium. *Science.* 1968;162:466–467.
9. Katz RI, Kopin IJ. Release of norepinephrine-^{3}H and serotonin-^{3}H evoked from brain slices by electrical-field stimulation—Calcium dependency and the effects of lithium, ouabain, and tetrodotoxin. *Biochem Pharmacol.* 1969;18:1835–1839.
10. Corona GL, Cucchi ML, Santagostino G, et al. Blood noradrenaline and 5–HT levels in depressed women during amitriptyline or lithium treatment. *Psychopharmacology (Berl).* 1982;77:236–241.
11. Mandell AJ, Knapp S. Asymmetry and mood, emergent properties of serotonin regulation: A proposed mechanism of action of lithium. *Arch Gen Psychiatry.* 1979;36:909–916.
12. Meltzer HY, Arora RC, Goodnick P. Effect of lithium carbonate on serotonin uptake in blood platelets of patients with affective disorders. *J Affect Disord.* 1983;5:215–221.
13. Meltzer HY, Lowy M, Robertson A, et al. Effect of 5–hydroxytryptophan on serum cortisol levels in major affective disorders. III. Effect of antidepressants and lithium carbonate. *Arch Gen Psychiatry.* 1984;41:391–397.

14. Goodnick PJ, Arora RC, Jackman H, et al. Neurochemical changes during discontinuation of lithium prophylaxis. II. Alterations in platelet serotonin function. *Biol Psychiatry.* 1984;19:891–898.

15. Goodnick PH, Fieve RR. Unpublished data. Cited in: Fieve RR, Goodnick PJ. Manic depression update 1986. *Fair Oaks Hosp Psychiatry Lett.* 1986;4:29.

16. Walker JB. The effect of lithium on hormone-sensitive adenylate cyclase from various regions of the rat brain. *Biol Psychiatry.* 1974;8:245–251.

17. Belmaker RH, Kon M, Ebstein RP, et al. Partial inhibition by lithium of the epinephrine-stimulated rise in plasma cyclic-GMP in humans. *Biol Psychiatry.* 1980;15:3–8.

18. Arato M, Rihmer Z, Felszeghy K. Reduced plasma cyclic AMP level during prophylactic lithium treatment in patients with affective disorders. *Biol Psychiatry.* 1980;15:319–321.

19. Reisine T. Regulation of adrenocorticotropin release from the anterior pituitary. *Psychopharmacol Bull.* 1985;21:438–442.

20. Menkes HA, Baraban JM, Freed AN, et al. Lithium dampens neurotransmitter response in smooth muscle: Relevance to action in affective illness. *Proc Natl Acad Sci USA.* 1986;83:5727–5730.

21. Belmaker RH, Kofman O. Lithium research: State of the art. *Biol Psychiatry.* 1990;27:1279–1281. Editorial.

22. Manji HK, Hsiao JK, Risby ED, et al. The mechanisms of action of lithium. I. Effects on serotonin-ergic and noradrenergic systems in normal subjects. *Arch Gen Psychiatry.* 1991;48:505–512.

23. Risby ED, Hsiao JK, Manji HK, et al. The mechanisms of action of lithium. II. Effects on adenylate cyclase activity and β-adrenergic receptor binding in normal subjects. *Arch Gen Psychiatry.* 1991;48:513–524.

24. Kline DF. Psychotropic drugs and the regulation of behavioral activation in psychiatric illness. In: Smith WL, ed. *Drugs and Cerebral Function.* First Cerebral Function Symposium held at the Aspen Institute for Humanistic Studies, June 7–9, 1969; Aspen, CO. Springfield, IL: Charles C Thomas; 1970:69–81.

25. Goodwin FK, Bunney WE Jr. Psychobiological aspects of stress and affective illness. In: Scott JP, Senay EC, eds. *Separation and Depression: Clinical and Research Aspects.* A symposium presented at the Chicago meeting of the American Association for the Advancement of Science, 27 December 1970. Washington DC: American Association for the Advancement of Science; 1973:91–112.

26. Carroll BJ, Mendels J. Neuroendocrine regulation in affective disorders. In: Sachar EJ, ed. *Hormones, Behavior, and Psychopathology.* Papers presented at the 65th annual meeting of the American Psychopathological Association; March 1975; New York City. New York: Raven Press; 1976: 193–224.

27. Maas JW. Neurotransmitters and depression: Too much, too little, or too unstable? *Trends Neurosci.* 1979;2:306.

28. Mandell AJ, Steward KD, Knapp S, et al. Protein fluctuations and time–space asymmetries in brain. *Psychopharmacol Bull.* 1980;16:47–50.

29. Siever LJ, Davis KL. Overview: Toward a dysregulation hypothesis of depression. *Am J Psychiatry.* 1985;142:1017–1031.

30. Rosenthal J, Strauss A, Minkoff L, et al. Identifying lithium-responsive bipolar depressed patients using nuclear magnetic resonance. *Am J Psychiatry.* 1986;143:779–780.

31. Lithium (systemic). In: *USP DI, Drug Information for the Health Care Professional.* Rockville, MD: U.S. Pharmacopeial Convention; 1994;1:1770–1775.

32. Amdisen A. Variation of serum lithium concentrations during the day in relation to treatment control. Absorptive side effects and the use of slow release tablets. *Acta Psychiatr Scand.* 1969;207:55–57.

33. Amdisen A, Sjorgren J. Lithium absorption from sustained-release tablets (Duretter). *Acta Pharm Suec.* 1968;5:465–472.

34. Diamond JM, Ehrlich BE, Morawski SG, et al. Lithium absorption in tight and leaky segments of intestine. *J Membr Biol.* 1983;72:153–159.

35. Cooper TB, Simpson GM, Lee JH, et al. Evaluation of a slow-release lithium carbonate formulation. *Am J Psychiatry.* 1978;135:917–922.
36. Ereshefsky L, Jann MW. Lithium. In: Mungall D, ed. *Applied Clinical Pharmacokinetics.* New York: Raven Press; 1983:245–270.
37. Amdisen A. Serum level monitoring and clinical pharmacokinetics of lithium. *Clin Pharmacokinet.* 1977;2:73–92.
38. Heiman MF, Schwabach G, Tupin J. Liquid lithium *vs.* solid lithium: An open, cross-over, pilot study comparing oral preparations. *Dis Nerv Syst.* 1976;37:9–11.
39. Shopsin B, Gershon S. Pharmacology and toxicology of the lithium ion. In: Gershon S, Shopsin B, eds. *Lithium: Its Role in Psychiatric Research and Treatment.* London: Plenum Press, 1973:107–146.
40. Ereshefsky L, Gilderman AM, Jewett CM. Lithium therapy of manic depressive illness. Part II: Monitoring. *Drug Intell Clin Pharm.* 1979;13:492–497.
41. Jefferson JW, Greist JH. General Pharmacology. In: Jefferson JW, Greist JH, eds. *Primer of Lithium Therapy.* Baltimore: Williams and Wilkins; 1977:95–96.
42. Amdisen A. Monitoring of lithium treatment through determination of lithium concentration. *Dan Med Bull.* 1975;22:277–291.
43. Shopsin B, Gershon S, Thompson H, et al. Psychoactive drugs in mania: A controlled comparison of lithium carbonate, chlorpromazine, and haloperidol. *Arch Gen Psychiatry.* 1975;32:34–42.
44. Nelson RW, Cohen JL. Plasma and erythrocyte kinetic considerations in lithium therapy. *Am J Hosp Pharm.* 1976;33:658–664.
45. Goodnick PJ, Fieve RR, Meltzer HL. Lithium pharmacokinetics, duration of therapy, and the adenylate cyclase system. *Int Pharmacopsychiatry.* 1982;17:65–72.
46. Nielsen-Kudsk F, Amdisen A. Analysis of the pharmacokinetics of lithium in man. *Eur J Clin Pharmacol.* 1979;16:271–277.
47. Mason RW, McQueen EG, Keary PJ, et al. Pharmacokinetics of lithium: Elimination half-time, renal clearance and apparent volume of distribution in schizophrenia. *Clin Pharmacokinet.* 1978;3:241–246.
48. Poust RI, Mallinger AG, Mallinger J, et al. Pharmacokinetics of lithium in human plasma and erythrocytes. *Psychopharmacol Commun.* 1976;2:91–103.
49. Thornhill DP, Field SP. Distribution of lithium elimination rates in a selected population of psychiatric patients. *Eur J Clin Pharmacol.* 1982;21:351–354.
50. Goodnick PJ, Fieve RR, Meltzer HL, et al. Lithium elimination half-life and duration of therapy. *Clin Pharmacol Ther.* 1981;29:47–50.
51. Hansen HE, Amdisen A. Lithium intoxication. *Q J Med.* 1978;47:123–144.
52. Cox M, Singer I. Lithium and water metabolism. *Am J Med.* 1975;59:153–157.
53. Thomsen K. Renal handling of lithium at non-toxic and toxic serum lithium levels. A review. *Dan Med Bull.* 1978;25:106–115.
54. Thomsen K, Schou M. Renal lithium excretion in man. *Am J Physiol.* 1968;215:823–827.
55. Lauritsen BJ, Mellerup ET, Plenge P, et al. Serum lithium concentrations around the clock with different treatment regimens and the diurnal variation of the renal lithium clearance. *Acta Psychiatr Scand.* 1981;64:314–319.
56. Smith DF, Shimizu M. The role of plasma volume, plasma renin, and the sympathetic nervous system in the posture-induced decline in renal lithium clearance in man. *Neuropsychobiology.* 1978;4:328–332.
57. Shimizu M, Smith DF. Salivary and urinary lithium clearance while recumbent and upright. *Clin Pharmacol Ther.* 1977;21:212–215.
58. Groth U, Prellwitz W, Jahnchen E. Estimation of pharmacokinetic parameters of lithium from saliva and urine. *Clin Pharmacol Ther.* 1974;16:490–498.
59. Degkwitz R. Lithium balance studies during mania. *Int Pharmacopsychiatry.* 1979;14:199–212.

60. Tosteson DC. Lithium in mania. *Sci Am.* 1981;244:164–174.

61. Gruner JF, Dennert J, Schafer G. Lithium treatment in maintenance dialysis. Review of the literature and report of a new case on hemodialysis. *Pharmacopsychiatry.* 1991;24:13–16.

62. Lippman SB, Manshadi MS, Gultekin A. Lithium in a patient with renal failure on hemodialysis. *J Clin Psychiatry.* 1984;45:444. Letter.

63. Lippmann SB, Manshadi MS, Gultekin A. Monoamine oxidase inhibitors for depressed cardiac patients. *J Clin Psychiatry.* 1985;46:545–546. Letter.

64. Oakley WF, Clarke WF, Parsons V. The use of dialysis bath fluid as a vehicle for a drug with a narrow therapeutic index—Lithium chloride. *Postgrad Med J.* 1974;50:511–512.

65. Port FK, Kroll PD, Rosenzweig J. Lithium therapy during maintenance hemodialysis. *Psychosomatics.* 1979;20:130–131.

66. Procci WR. Mania during maintenance hemodialysis successfully treated with oral lithium carbonate. *J Nerv Ment Dis.* 1977;164:355–358.

67. Zetin M, Plon L, Vaziri N, et al. Lithium carbonate dose and serum level relationships in chronic hemodialysis patients. *Am J Psychiatry.* 1981;138:1387–1388.

68. Zuddas A, Mulas S, Del Zompo M, et al. Cluster headache: Clinical efficacy of lithium salts in a haemodialysis treated patient. *Cephalalgia.* 1985;5:95–98.

69. Lippmann S, Wagemaker H, Tucker D. A practical approach to management of lithium concurrent with hyponatremia, diuretic therapy and/or chronic renal failure. *J Clin Psychiatry.* 1981;42:304–306.

70. Children and adolescents. In: Jefferson JW, Greist JH, Ackerman DL, et al, eds. *Lithium Encyclopedia for Clinical Practice.* Washington, DC: American Psychiatric Press; 1987:180–186.

71. Vitiello B, Dehar D, Malone R, et al. Pharmacokinetics of lithium carbonate in children. *J Clin Psychopharmacol.* 1988;8:355–359.

72. Reisberg B, Gershon S. Side effects associated with lithium therapy. *Arch Gen Psychiatry.* 1979;36:879–887.

73. Birch NJ. Bone side-effects of lithium. In: Johnson FN, ed. *Handbook of Lithium Therapy.* Baltimore: University Park Press; 1980:365–371.

74. Khandelwal SW, Varma VK, Srinivasa Murthy R. Renal function in children receiving long-term lithium prophylaxis. *Am J Psychiatry.* 1984;141:278–279.

75. Lena B. Lithium therapy in hyperaggressive behavior in adolescence. In: Sandler M, ed. *Psychopharmacology of Aggression.* New York: Raven Press; 1979:197–203.

76. Lehmann K, Merten K. Die elimination von lithium in abhangigkeit vom libensalter bei gesunden und niereninsuffizienten [Elimination of lithium in dependence on age in healthy subjects and patients with renal insufficiency]. *Int J Clin Pharmacol Ther Toxicol.* 1974;10:292–298.

77. Crooks J, O'Malley K, Stevenson IH. Pharmacokinetics in the elderly. *Clin Pharmacokinet.* 1976;1:280–296.

78. Chapron DJ, Cameron IR, White LB, et al. Observations on lithium dispostition in the elderly. *J Am Geriatr Soc.* 1982;30:651–655.

79. Hardy BG, Shulman KI, MacKenzie SE., et al. Pharmacokinetics of lithium in the elderly. *J Clin Psychopharmacol.* 1987;7:153–158.

80. Foster JR, Gershell WJ, Goldfarb AI. Lithium treatment in the elderly. 1. Clinical usage. *J Gerontol.* 1977;32:299–302.

81. Hewick DS, Newbury P, Hopwood S, et al. Age as a factor affecting lithium therapy. *Br J Clin Pharmacol.* 1977;4:201–205.

82. Schou M. Lithium treatment during pregnancy, delivery, and lactation: An update. *J Clin Psychiatry.* 1990;51:410–413.

83. American Academy of Pediatrics Committee on Drugs. Psychotropic drugs in pregnancy and lactation. *Pediatrics.* 1982;69:241–244.

84. Schou M, Amdisen A, Streustrup OR. Lithium and pregnancy. II. Hazards to women given lithium during pregnancy and delivery. *Br Med J.* 1973;2:137–138.

85. Lindheimer MD, Katz AI. The renal response to pregnancy. In: Brenner BM, Rector FC, eds. *The Kidney*. Philadelphia: WB Saunders; 1981:1762–1815.

86. Shafey MH, Schou M. Lithium use and pregnancy. *J Clin Psychiatry*. 1991;52:279. Letter and Reply.

87. Ananath J, Pecknold MD. Prediction of lithium response in affective disorders. *J Clin Psychiatry*. 1978;39:95–100.

88. Ereshefsky L, Jewitt C, Gilderman A. Lithium therapy of manic depressive illness. Part I. Target symptoms, pharmacology and kinetics. *Drug Intell Clin Pharm*. 1979;13:403–408.

89. Baldessarini RJ, Lipinski JF. Lithium salts: 1970–1975. *Ann Intern Med*. 1975;83:527–533.

90. Goodwin FD, Athanasios PZ. Lithium in the treatment of mania. *Arch Gen Psychiatry*. 1979; 36:840–844.

91. Kocsis JH. Lithium in the acute treatment of mania. In: Johnson FN, ed. *Handbook of Lithium Therapy*. Baltimore: University Park Press; 1980:9–15.

92. Pope HE, Lipinski JF. Diagnosis in schizophrenia and manic–depressive illness. *Arch Gen Psychiatry*. 1978;35:811–828.

93. Carlson GA. The stages of mania. *Arch Gen Psychiatry*. 1973;28:221–228.

94. Mendels J, Ramsey TA, Dyson WL, et al. Lithium as an antidepressant. *Arch Gen Psychiatry*. 1979;36:845–846.

95. Karki S, Carson S, Holden JMC. Effect of assay methodology on the prediction of lithium maintenance dosage. *Drug Intell Clin Pharm*. 1989;23:372–375.

96. Lippmann S, Regan W, Manshadi M. Plasma lithium stability and a comparison of flame photometry and atomic absorption spectrophotometry analysis. *Am J Psychiatry*. 1981;138:1375–1377.

97. Quattrocchi FP, May B, Ackerman L. Green-top test tubes and lithium concentration. *Drug Intell Clin Pharm*. 1988;22:79.

98. Perlman BB. Limitations of laboratory methods for measuring serum levels. *J Clin Psychopharmacol*. 1988;8:442–443.

99. Cohen IM, Bunney WE Jr, Cole JO, et al. The current status of lithium therapy: Report of APA Task Force. *Am J Psychiatry*. 1975;132:997–1001.

100. NIMH/NIH Consensus Development Conference Statement: Mood disorders: pharmacological prevention of recurrences. *Am J Psychiatry*. 1985;142:469–476.

101. Hullin RP. Minimum serum lithium levels for effective prophylaxis. In: Johnson FN, ed. *Handbook of Lithium Therapy*. Baltimore: University Park Press; 1980:243–247.

102. Prien RF, Caffey EM. Relationship between dosage and response to lithium prophylaxis in recurring depression. *Am J Psychiatry*. 1976;133:567–570.

103. Prien RF, Caffey EM Jr., Klett CJ. Relationship between serum lithium level and clinical response in acute mania treated with lithium. *Br J Psychiatry*. 1972;120:409–414.

104. Decina P, Fieve RR. Prophylactic serum lithium levels in recurrent unipolar depression. *J Clin Psychopharmacol*. 1981;1:150–152.

105. Jerram TC, McDonald R. Plasma lithium control with particular reference to minimum effective levels. In: Johnson FN, Johnson S, eds. *Lithium in Medical Practice*. Proceedings of the First British Lithium Congress, University of Lancaster, England. Baltimore: University Park Press; 1978:407–415.

106. Jann MW, Bitar AH, Rao A. Lithium prophylaxis of tricyclic antidepressant-induced mania in bipolar patients. *Am J Psychiatry*. 1982;139:683–684.

107. Gelenberg AJ, Carroll JA, Baudhuin MG, et al. The meaning of serum lithium levels in maintenance therapy of mood disorders: A review of the literature. *J Clin Psychiatry*. 1989;50(suppl):17–22.

108. Gelenberg AJ, Kane JM, Keller MB, et al. Comparison of standard and low serum levels of lithium for maintenance treatment of bipolar disorder. *N Engl J Med*. 1989;321:1489–1493.

109. Mendels J, Frazer A. Alterations in cell membrane activity in depression. *Am J Psychiatry*. 1974;131:1240–1245.

110. Rafelsen O. Lithium and the kidney: Spring 1979. *Int Drug Ther Newslett*. 1979;14:25–28.

111. Ramsey TA, Frazer A, Mendels J, et al. The erythrocyte lithium–plasma lithium ratio in patients with primary affective disorder. *Arch Gen Psychiatry.* 1979;36:457–461.

112. Ostrow DG, Davis JM. Laboratory measurements in the clinical use of lithium. *Clin Neuropharmacol.* 1982;5:317–336.

113. Ostrow DG, Dorus W, Okonek A, et al. The effect of alcoholism on membrane lithium transport. *J Clin Psychiatry.* 1986;47:350–353.

114. Elizur A, Shopsin B, Gershon S, et al. Intra:extra-cellular lithium ratios and clinical course in affective states. *Clin Pharmacol Ther.* 1972;13:947–952.

115. Mendels J, Frazer A. Intra-cellular lithium concentration and clinical response: Towards a membrane theory of depression. *J Psychiatr Res.* 1973;10:9–18.

116. Flemenbaum A, Weddige R, Miller J. Lithium erythrocyte/plasma ratio as a predictor of response. *Am J Psychiatry.* 1978;135:336–338.

117. Lee CR, Hill SE, Dimitrakoudi M, et al. The relationship of plasma to erythrocyte lithium levels in patients taking lithium carbonate. *Br J Psychiatry.* 1975;127:596–598.

118. Rybakowski J, Chlopocka M, Kapelski Z, et al. Red blood cell lithium index in patients with affective disorders in the course of lithium prophylaxis. *Int Pharmacopsychiatry.* 1974;9:166–171.

119. Werstiuk ES, Rathbone MP, Grof P. Erythrocyte lithium efflux in bipolar patients and control subjects: The question of reproducibility. *Psychiatry Res.* 1984;13:175–185.

120. Frazer A, Mendels J, Brunswick D. Erythrocyte concentrations of the lithium ion: Clinical correlates in mechanisms of accumulation. *Psychopharmacol Bull.* 1978;14:14–16.

121. Carroll BJ. Prediction of treatment outcome with lithium. *Arch Gen Psychiatry.* 1979;36:870–878.

122. Brunswick DJ, Frazer A, Mendels J, et al. Red blood cell Li$^+$ to plasma Li$^+$ ratios: Are they related to plasma Li$^+$ concentrations? *Neuropsychobiology.* 1978;4:121–127.

123. Gengo F, Frazer A, Ramsey TA, et al. The lithium ratio as a guide to patient compliance. *Compr Psychiatry.* 1980;21:276–280.

124. Ayd FJ. Checking for compliance with lithium therapy. *Int Drug Ther Newslett.* 1981;16:33–34.

125. Walter-Ryan WG. Lithium index. *Hosp Community Psychiatry.* 1983;34:558–559.

126. Shopsin B, Gershon S, Pinckney L. The secretion of lithium in human mixed saliva: Effects of ingested lithium on electrolyte distribution in saliva and serum. *Int Pharmacopsychiatry.* 1969;2:148–169.

127. Neu C, DiMascio A, Williams D. Saliva lithium levels: Clinical applications. *Am J Psychiatry.* 1975;132:66–68.

128. Verghese A, Indrani N, Kuruvilla K, et al. Usefulness of saliva lithium estimation. *Br J Psychiatry.* 1977;130:149–150.

129. Honda Y, Suzuki T. Transcultural pharmacokinetic study on Li concentration in plasma and saliva. *Psychopharmacol Bull.* 1979;15:37–39.

130. Lena B, Bastable MD. The reliability of salivary lithium estimations in children. *IRCS J Med Sci.* 1978;6:280.

131. Perry R, Campbell M, Grega DM, et al. Saliva lithium levels in children: Their use in monitoring serum lithium levels and lithium side effects. *J Clin Psychopharmacol.* 1984;4:199–202.

132. Spring KR, Spirtes MA. Salivary excretion of lithium. 1. Human parotid and submaxillary secretions. *J Dent Res.* 1969;48:546–549.

133. Man PL. Correlation of saliva and serum lithium. *Psychosomatics.* 1979;20:758–759.

134. Othmer E, Powell B, Piziak VK, et al. Prospective use of saliva lithium determinations to monitor lithium therapy. *J Clin Psychiatry.* 1979;40:525–526.

135. Preskorn SH, Abernethy DR, McKnelly WV. Use of saliva lithium determinations for monitoring lithium therapy. *J Clin Psychiatry.* 1978;39:756–758.

136. Selinger D, Hailer AW, Nurnberger JI, et al. A new method for the use of salivary lithium concentration as an indicator of plasma lithium levels. *Biol Psychiatry.* 1982;17:99–102.

137. Ravenscroft P, Vozeh S, Weinstein M, et al. Saliva lithium concentrations in the management of lithium therapy. *Arch Gen Psychiatry.* 1978;35:1123–1127.

138. Rosman AW, Sczupak CA, Parkes GE. Correlation between saliva and serum lithium levels in manic–depressive patients. *Am J Hosp Pharm.* 1980;37:514–518.

139. Mathew RJ, Claghorn JL, Fenimore D, et al. Salivary lithium and lithium therapy. *Am J Psychiatry.* 1979;136:851.

140. Sims A, White AC, Garvey K. Problems associated with the analysis and interpretation of saliva lithium. *Br J Psychiatry.* 1978;132:152–154.

141. Khare CB, Sankaranarayanan A, Goel A, et al. Saliva lithium levels for monitoring lithium prophylaxis of manic–depressive psychosis. *Int J Clin Pharmacol Ther Toxicol.* 1983;21:451-453.

142. Evrard JL, Baumann P, Pera R, et al. Lithium concentrations in saliva, plasma and red blood cells of patients given lithium acetate. *Acta Psychiatr Scand.* 1978;58:67–79.

143. Prakash R, Sethi N. Lithium in saliva and serum: Some observations. *Indian J Psychiatry.* 1979; 21:256–258.

144. Sethi N, Prakash R, Sethi BB. Relationship between lithium levels of saliva and serum. *Biol Psychiatry.* 1981;16:413–414.

145. Vlaar H, Bleeker JAC, Schalken HFA. Comparison between saliva and serum lithium concentrations in patients treated with lithium carbonate. *Acta Psychiatr Scand.* 1979;60:423–426.

146. Bowden CL, Houston JP, Shulman RS, et al. Clinical utility of salivary lithium concentration. *Int Pharmacopsychiatry.* 1982;17:104–113.

147. Ereshefsky L, Stimmel GL, Hayes PE. Recognizing and treating depressive illness. *Am Pharm.* 1981;21:34–39.

148. Amdisen A. Clinical and serum level monitoring in lithium therapy and lithium intoxication. *J Anal Toxicol.* 1978;2:193–202.

149. Amdisen A. Lithium. In: Evans WE, Schentag JJ, Jusko WJ, eds. *Applied Pharmacokinetics: Principles of Therapeutic Drug Monitoring.* Spokane, WA: Applied Therapeutics; 1980: 586–617.

150. Johnson FN. The variety of models proposed for the therapeutic actions of lithium. In: Johnson FN, Johnson S, eds. *Lithium in Medical Practice.* Proceedings of the First British Lithium Congress; 15–19 July; University of Lancaster, England. Baltimore: University Park Press; 1978:305–330.

151. Rifkin A, Quitkin F, Klein DF. Organic brain syndrome during lithium carbonate treatment. *Compr Psychiatry.* 1973;14:251–254.

152. Speirs G, Hirsch SR. Severe lithium toxicity with "normal" serum concentrations. *Br Med J.* 1978;1:815–816.

153. Thomsen K, Schou M. The treatment of lithium poisoning. In: Johnson FN, ed. *Lithium Research and Therapy.* London: Academic Press; 1975:227–236.

154. Gadallah MF, Feinstein EI, Massry SG. Lithium intoxication: Clinical course and therapeutic considerations. *Mineral Electrolyte Metab.* 1988;14:146–149.

155. Jacobsen D, Aasen G, Frederichsen P, et al. Lithium intoxication: Pharmacokinetics during and after terminated hemodialysis in acute intoxications. *Clin Toxicol.* 1987;25:81–94.

156. Intoxication. In: Jefferson JW, Greist JH, Ackerman DL, et al, eds. *Lithium Encyclopedia for Clinical Practice.* Washington, DC: American Psychiatric Press; 1987:361–370.

157. Lithium. In: Rumack BH, ed. *Poisindex System, Micromedex Computerized Clinical Information System.* 79th ed. Denver: Micromedex; 1994.

158. Bellomo R, Kearly Y, Parkin G, et al. Treatment of life threatening lithium toxicity with continuous arterio-venous hemodiafiltration. *Crit Care Med.* 1991;19:836–837.

159. Simard M, Gumbiner B, Lee A, et al. Lithium carbonate: A case report and review of the literature. *Arch Intern Med.* 1989;149:36–46.

160. Demrs RG, Heninger GR. Sodium intake and lithium treatment in mania. *Am J Psychiatry.* 1971;128:132–136.

161. Himmelhock JM, Poust RI, Mallinger AG, et al. Adjustment of lithium dose during lithium–chlorothiazide therapy. *Clin Pharmacol Ther.* 1977;22:225–227.

162. Forrest JN, Cohen AD, Torretti J, et al. On the mechanism of lithium-induced diabetes insipidus in man and the rat. *J Clin Invest.* 1974;53:1115–1123.

163. Himmelhock JM, Forrest J, Neil JF, et al. Thiazide–lithium synergy in refractory mood swings. *Am J Psychiatry.* 1977;134:149–152.

164. Maletzky B. Enhancing the efficacy of lithium treatment by combined use with diuretics and low sodium diets: A preliminary report. *J Clin Psychiatry.* 1979;40:317–322.

165. Hurtig HI, Dyson WL. Lithium toxicity enhanced by diuresis. *N Engl J Med.* 1974;290:748–749.

166. Thornton WE, Pray BJ. Lithium intoxication: A report of two cases. *Can Psychiatr Assoc J.* 1975; 20:281–282.

167. Oh TE. Furosemide and lithium toxicity. *Anaesth Intensive Care.* 1977;5:60–62.

168. Huang L. Lithium intoxication with coadministration of a loop-diuretic. *J Clin Psychopharmacol.* 1990;10:228. Letter.

169. Jefferson JW, Kalin NH. Serum lithium levels and long-term diuretic use. *JAMA.* 1979;241: 1134–1136.

170. Saffer D, Coppen A. Furosemide: A safe diuretic during lithium therapy? *J Affect Disord.* 1983;5:289–292.

171. Steele TH, Manuel MA, Newton M, et al. Renal lithium reabsorption in man: Physiologic and pharmacologic determinants. *Am J Med Sci.* 1975;269:349–363.

172. Ostrow DG, Southam AS, Davis JM. Lithium–drug interactions altering the intracellular lithium level: An in vitro study. *Biol Psychiatry.* 1980;15:723–729.

173. Miller F, Menninger J, Whitcup SM. Lithium–neuroleptic neurotoxicity in the elderly bipolar patient. *J Clin Psychopharmacol.* 1986;6:176–178.

174. Smith RE, Helms PM. Adverse effects of lithium therapy in the acutely ill elderly patient. *J Clin Psychiatry.* 1982;43:94–99.

175. Prakash R, Kelwala S, Ban TA. Neurotoxicity with combined administration of lithium with a neuroleptic. *Compr Psychiatry.* 1982;23:567–571.

176. Charney DS, Kales A, Soldatos CR, et al. Somnambulistic-like episodes secondary to combined lithium–neuroleptic treatment. *Br J Psychiatry.* 1979;135:418–424.

177. Lavigne GL, Baldessarini RJ. "Equivalent" doses in medication changes. *Am J Psychiatry.* 1976; 133:851–852.

178. Addonizio G. Rapid induction of extrapyramidal side effects with combined use of lithium and neuroleptics. *J Clin Psychopharmacol.* 1985;5:296–298.

179. Slonim R, McLarty B. Sixth cranial nerve palsy—Unusual presenting symptom of lithium toxicity? *Can J Psychiatry.* 1985;30:443–444.

180. Yassa R. A case of lithium chlorpromazine interaction. *J Clin Psychiatry.* 1986;47:90–91.

181. Spring GK, Abrams R, Taylor MA. EEG observations in confirming neurotoxicity. *Am J Psychiatry.* 1979;136:1099–1100.

182. Alevizos B. Toxic reactions to lithium and neuroleptics. *Br J Psychiatry.* 1979;135:482.

183. Spring GK. Neurotoxicity with combined use of lithium and thioridazine. *J Clin Psychiatry.* 1979;40:135–138.

184. West A. Adverse effects of lithium treatment. *Br Med J.* 1977;2:642.

185. Cantor CH. Encephalopathy with lithium and thioridazine in combination. *Med J Aust.* 1986;144:164–165.

186. Blake LM, Marks RC, Luchins DJ. Reversible neurologic symptoms with clozapine and lithium. *J Clin Psychopharmacol.* 1992;12:297–299.

187. Cohen WJ, Cohen NH. Lithium carbonate, haloperidol, and irreversible brain damage. *JAMA.* 1974;230:1283–1287.

188. Singh SV. Lithium carbonate/fluphenazine decanoate producing irreversible brain damage. *Lancet.* 1982;2:278.

189. Small JG, Kellams JJ, Milstein V, et al. A placebo-controlled study of lithium compared wih neuroleptics in chronic schizophrenic patients. *Am J Psychiatry.* 1975;132:1315–1317.

190. Biederman J, Lerner Y, Belmaker RH. Combination of lithium carbonate and haloperidol in schizoaffective disorder: A controlled study. *Arch Gen Psychiatry.* 1979;36:327–333.

191. Alexander PE, van Kammen DP, Bunney WE Jr. Antipsychotic effects of lithium in schizophrenia. *Am J Psychiatry.* 1979;136:283–287.

192. Growe GA, Crayton JW, Klass DB, et al. Lithium in chronic schizophrenia. *Am J Psychiatry.* 1979;136:454–455.

193. Bigelow LB, Weinberger DR, Wyatt RJ. Synergism of combined lithium–neuroleptic therapy: A double-blind, placebo-controlled case study. *Am J Psychiatry.* 1981;138:81–83.

194. Carman JS, Bigelow LB, Wyatt RJ. Lithium combined with neuroleptics in chronic schizophrenic and schizoaffective patients. *J Clin Psychiatry.* 1981;42:124–128.

195. Baastrup PC, Hollnagel P, Sorensen R, et al. Adverse reactions in treatment with lithium carbonate and haloperidol. *JAMA.* 1976;236:2645–2646.

196. Goldney RD, Spence ND. Safety of the combination of lithium and neuroleptic drugs. *Am J Psychiatry.* 1986;143:882–884.

197. Kessel JB, Verghese C, Simpson GM. Neurotoxicity related to lithium and neuroleptic combinations? A retrospective review. *J Psychiatry Neurosci.* 1992;17:28–30.

198. Antipsychotic drugs. In: Jefferson JW, Greist JH, Ackerman DL, et al, eds. *Lithium Encyclopedia for Clinical Practice.* Washington, DC: American Psychiatric Press; 1987:105–123.

199. Jefferson JW, Geist JH. Lithium interaction with other drugs. *J Clin Psychopharmacol.* 1981;1:124–134.

200. Pandey GN, Geol I, Davis JM. Effect of neuroleptic drugs on lithium uptake by the human erythrocyte. *Clin Pharmacol Ther.* 1979;26:96–102.

201. Samoilov NN, Lyubimov BI, Sholokov VM, et al. Effect of psychotropic drugs on the pharmacokinetics of lithium [English translation]. *Bull Exp Biol Med.* 1980;89:784–785.

202. Nemes ZC, Volavka J, Cooper TB. Lithium and haloperidol. *Biol Psychiatry.* 1986;21:568–569.

203. Werstiuk ES, Grof P, Rotstein E. Effect of combined haloperidol–lithium treatment on in vitro RBC lithium uptake in patients with affective disorders. *Prog Neuropsychopharmacol Biol Psychiatry.* 1983;7:831–834.

204. Von Knorring L, Smigan L, Perris C, et al. Lithium and neuroleptic drugs in combination—Effect on lithium RBC/plasma ratio. *Int Pharmacopsychiatry.* 1982;17:287–292.

205. Sierles FS, Ossowski MG. Concurrent use of theophylline and lithium in a patient with chronic obstructive lung disease and bipolar disorder. *Am J Psychiatry.* 1982;139:117–118.

206. Perry PJ, Calloway RA, Cook BL, et al. Theophylline precipitated alterations of lithium clearance. *Acta Psychiatr Scand.* 1984;69:528–537.

207. Cook BL, Smith RE, Perry PJ, et al. Theophylline–lithium interaction. *J Clin Psychiatry.* 1985;46:278–279.

208. Anti-inflammatory drugs. In: Jefferson JW, Greist JH, Ackerman DL, et al, eds. *Lithium Encyclopedia for Clinical Practice.* Washington, DC: American Psychiatric Press; 1987:101–104.

209. Lithium–NSAIDs. In: Tatro DS, ed. *Drug Interaction Facts.* St Louis, MO: Facts and Comparisons; 1992:463.

210. Miller LG, Bowman RC, Bakht F. Sparing effect of sulindac on lithium levels. *J Fam Pract.* 1989;28:592–593.

211. Noveske FG, Hahn KR, Flynn RJ. Possible toxicity of combined fluoxetine and lithium. *Am J Psychiatry.* 1989;146:1515. Letter.

212. Salama AA, Shafey M. A case of severe lithium toxicity induced by combined fluoxetine and lithium carbonate. *Am J Psychiatry.* 1989;146:278. Letter.

213. Sacristan JA, Iglesias C, Arellano F, et al. Absence seizures induced by lithium: Possible interaction with fluoxetine. *Am J Psychiatry.* 1991;148:146–147. Letter.

214. Warrington SJ. Clinical implications of the pharmacology of sertraline. *Int Clin Psychopharmacol.* 1991;6(suppl 2):11–21.
215. Committee on Safety of Medicines. Fluvoxamine and fluoxetine—Interaction with monoamine oxidase inhibitors, lithium and tryptophan. *Curr Probl.* 1989:26.
216. Fluvoxamine maleate. In: Reynolds JEF, ed. *Martindale: The Extra Pharmacopoeia* (electronic version) (text copyright The Royal Pharmaceutical Society of Great Britain). Denver, CO: Micromedex; 1994;79.
217. Evans M, Marwick P. Fluvoxamine and lithium: An unusual interaction. *Br J Psychiatry.* 1990; 156:286. Letter.
218. Hadley A, Cason MP. Mania resulting from lithium–fluoxetine combination. *Am J Psychiatry.* 1989;146:1637–1638. Letter.
219. Burstein A. Fluoxetine–lithium treatment for kleptomania. *J Clin Psychiatry.* 1992;53:28–29. Letter.
220. Fontaine R, Ontiveros A, Elie R, et al. Lithium carbonate augmentation of desipramine and fluoxetine in refractory depression. *Biol Psychiatry.* 1991;29:946–948. Letter (published erratum appears in *Biol Psychiatry.* 1992;31:322).
221. Howland RH. Lithium augmentation of fluoxetine in the treatment of OCD and major depression: A case report. *Can J Psychiatry.* 1991;36:154–155. Letter.
222. Ontiveros A, Fontaine R, Elie R. Refractory depression: The addition of lithium to fluoxetine or desipramine. *Acta Psychiatr Scand.* 1991;83:188–192. Letter.
223. Pope HG Jr, McElroy SL, Nixon RA. Possible synergism between fluoxetine and lithium in refractory depression. *Am J Psychiatry.* 1988;145:1292–1294.
224. Mann J, Gershon S. Absolute and relative contraindications to lithium. In: Johnson FN, ed. *Handbook of Lithium Therapy.* Baltimore: University Park Press; 1980:265–278.
225. Granoff AL, Davis JM. Heat illness syndrome and lithium intoxication. *J Clin Psychiatry.* 1978;39:103–107.
226. Long-term therapy. In: Jefferson JW, Greist JH, Ackerman DL, et al, eds. *Lithium Encyclopedia for Clinical Practice.* Washington, DC: American Psychiatric Press; 1987:423–429.
227. Hestbech J, Hansen HE, Amdisen A, et al. Chronic renal lesions following long-term treatment with lithium. *Kidney Int.* 1977;12:205–213.
228. Mellerup ET, Plenge P, Rafaelsen OJ. Renal and other controversial adverse effects of lithium. In: Meltzer HY, ed. *Psychopharmacology: The Third Generation of Progress.* New York: Raven Press; 1987:1443–1448.
229. Kidney damage and renal failure. In: Jefferson JW, Greist JH, Ackerman DL, et al, eds. *Lithium Encyclopedia for Clinical Practice.* Washington, DC: American Psychiatric Press; 1987:371–379.
230. Kidney function. In: Jefferson JW, Greist JH, Ackerman DL, et al, eds. *Lithium Encyclopedia for Clinical Practice.* Washington, DC: American Psychiatric Press; 1987:386–398.
231. Polydipsia, polyuria, and diabetes insipidus. In: Jefferson JW, Greist JH, Ackerman DL, et al, eds. *Lithium Encyclopedia for Clinical Practice.* Washington, DC: American Psychiatric Press; 1987:494–501.
232. Hetmar O. The impact of long-term lithium treatment on renal function and structure. *Acta Psychiatr Scand Suppl.* 1988;345:85–89.
233. Schou M, Vestergaard P. Prospective studies on a lithium cohort. 2. Renal function. Water and electrolyte metabolism. *Acta Psychiatr Scand.* 1988;78:427–433.
234. Waller DG, Edwards JG, Papasthatis-Papayanni S. A longitudinal assessment of renal function during treatment with lithium. *Q J Med.* 1988;68:553–558.
235. Hetmar O, Brun C, Ladefoged J, et al. Long-term effects of lithium on the kidney: Functional–morphological correlations. *J Psychiatr Res.* 1989;23:285–297.
236. Schou M. Effects of long-term lithium treatment on kidney function: An overview. *J Psychiatr Res.* 1989;22:287–296.

237. Conte G, Vazzola A, Sacchetti E. Renal function in chronic lithium-treated patients. *Acta Psychiatr Scand.* 1989;79:503–504.

238. Hetmar O, Povlsen UJ, Ladefoged J, et al. Lithium: Long-term effects on the kidney. A prospective follow-up study ten years after kidney biopsy. *Br J Psychiatry.* 1991;158:53–58.

239. Schou M, Vestergaard P. Lithium and the kidney scare. *Psychosomatics.* 1981;22:92–94.

240. Muir A, Davidson R, Silverstone T, et al. Two regimens of lithium prophylaxis and renal function. *Acta Psychiatr Scand.* 1989;80:579–583.

241. Perry PJ, Dunner FL, Hahn RL. Lithium kinetics in single daily dosing. *Acta Psychiatr Scand.* 1981;64:281–294.

242. Coppen A, Bishop ME, Bailey JE, et al. Renal function in lithium and non-lithium treated patients with affective disorders. *Acta Psychiatr Scand.* 1980;62:343–355.

243. Plenge P, Mellerup ET, Bolwig TG, et al. Lithium treatment: Does the kidney prefer one daily dose instead of two? *Acta Psychiatr Scand.* 1982;66:121–128.

244. Schou M, Andisen A, Thomsen K, et al. Lithium treatment regimen and renal water handling: The significance of dosage pattern and tablet type examined through comparison of results from two clinics with different treatment regimens. *Psychopharmacology (Berl).* 1982;77:387–290.

245. Abraham G, Delva N, Waldron J, et al. Lithium treatment: A comparison of once- and twice-daily dosing. *Acta Psychiatr Scand.* 1992;85:65–69.

246. DePaulo JR, Correa EI, Sykes C, et al. Once-a-day lithium: The renal effects (paper no. 28). In: *Continuing Medical Education Syllabus and Scientific Proceedings.* Paper presented at 1984 annual meeting of the American Psychiatric Association.

247. Greil W, Bauer J, Breit J, et al. Single daily dose schedule in lithium: Long term treatment effects on pharmacokinetics and on renal and cardiac functions. *Pharmacopsychiatry.* 1985;18:106–107.

248. Vestergaard P. How does the patient prefer his lithium treatment? *Pharmacopsychiatry.* 1985;18:223–224.

249. Pepin SM, Baker DE, Nance KS, et al. Lithium dosage calculation from age, sex, height, weight, and serum creatinine. Paper presented at American Society of Hospital Pharmacists' 15th annual midyear Clinical meeting; December 9, 1980; San Francisco.

250. Zetin M, Garber D, M. C. A simple mathematical model for predicting lithium dose requirement. *J Clin Psychiatry.* 1983;44:144–145.

251. Zetin M, Garber D, De Antonio M, et al. Prediction of lithium dose: A mathematical alternative to the test dose method. *J Clin Psychiatry.* 1986;47:175–178.

252. Chang SS, Pandey GN, Dysken MW, et al. Predicting the optimal lithium dosage—A prospective study. Paper presented at 18th annual meeting of the American Society for Clinical Pharmacology and Therapeutics; March 21–23, 1979; Kansas City, MO.

253. Palladino A, Longnecker RG, Lesko LJ. Lithium-test dose methodology using flame emission photometry: Problems and alternatives. *J Clin Psychiatry.* 1983;44:7–9.

254. Slattery JT, Gibaldi M, Koup J. Prediction of maintenance dose required to attain a desired drug concentration at steady-state from a single determination after an initial dose. *Clin Pharmacokinet.* 1980;5:377–385.

255. Slattery JT. Single-point maintenance dose prediction: Role of interindividual differences in clearance and volume of distribution in choice of sampling time. *J Pharm Sci.* 1981;70:1174–1176.

256. Tyer SP, Grof P, Kalvar M, et al. Estimation of lithium dose requirement by lithium clearance, serum lithium and saliva lithium following a loading dose of lithium carbonate. *Neuropsychobiology.* 1981; 7:152–158.

257. Cooper TB, Bergner PEE, Simpson GM. 24-hour serum lithium level as a prognosticator of dosage requirements. *Am J Psychiatry.* 1973;130:601–603.

258. Cooper TB, Simpson GM. 24-hour lithium level as a prognosticator of dosage requirements: A 2-year follow-up study. *Am J Psychiatry.* 1976;4:440–443.

259. Perry PJ, Prince RA, Alexander B, et al. Prediction of lithium maintenance doses using a single-point prediction protocol. *J Clin Psychopharmacol.* 1983;3:13–17.
260. Perry PJ, Alexander B, Prince RA, et al. The utility of a single-point dosing protocol for predicting steady-state lithium levels. *Br J Psychiatry.* 1986;148:401–405.
261. Perry PJ, Alexander B, Dunner FJ, et al. Pharmacokinetic protocol for predicting serum lithium levels. *J Clin Psychopharmacol.* 1982;2:114–118.
262. Marr MA, Djuric PE, Ritschel WA, et al. Prediction of lithium carbonate dosage in psychiatric inpatients using the repeated one-point method. *Clin Pharm.* 1983;2:243–248.
263. Ritschel WA, Bananer M. Lithium dosage regimen design by the repeated one-point method. *Arzniemittelforsch Drug Res.* 1982;32:98–102.
264. Koeppe P, Hamann C. A program for nonlinear regression analysis to be used on desk-top computers. *Comput Programs Biomed.* 1980;12:121–128.
265. Swartz CM. Prediction lithium levels with a microcomputer. *Comput Psychiatry Psychol.* 1983;5: 13–17.
266. Swartz CM, Wilcox J. Characterization and prediction of lithium blood levels and clearances. *Arch Gen Psychiatry.* 1984;41:1154–1158.
267. Schumacher GE, Barr JT. Bayesian approaches in pharmacokinetic decision making. *Clin Pharm.* 1984;3:525–530.
268. Williams PJ, Browne JL, Patel RA. Bayesian forecasting of serum lithium concentrations. Comparison with traditional methods. *Clin Pharmacokinet.* 1989;17:45–52.
269. Browne JL, Patel RA, Huffman CS, et al. Comparison of pharmacokinetic procedures for dosing lithium based on analysis of prediction error. *Drug Intell Clin Pharm.* 1988;22:227–231.
270. Siemsen FK, Pasley DR. Comment: Dosing lithium. *Drug Intell Clin Pharm.* 1988;22:1005. Letter.
271. Browne JL, Huffman CS, Golden RN. A comparison of pharmacokinetic versus empirical lithium dosing techniques. *Ther Drug Monit.* 1989;11:149–154.
272. Cummings MA, Haviland MG, Cummings KL, et al. Lithium dose prediction: A prospective case series. *J Clin Psychiatry.* 1988;49:373.
273. Lobeck F, Nelson MV, Evans RL, et al. Evaluation of four methods for predicting lithium dosage. *Clin Pharm.* 1987;6:230–233.
274. Lobeck F. A review of lithium dosing methods. *Pharmacotherapy.* 1988;8:248–255.
275. Markoff RA, King M Jr. Does lithium dose prediction improve treatment efficiency? Prospective evaluation of a mathematical method. *J Clin Psychopharmacol.* 1992;12:305–308.

Chapter 17

Methotrexate

Timothy Madden
Virginia E. Eaton

Keep In Mind

- Obtain baseline assessments of renal, liver, and hematologic function with serum creatinine and creatinine clearance determinations and absolute granulocyte and platelet counts.

- Counsel the patient on the importance of good oral hygiene throughout high-dose methotrexate therapy.

- Identify risk factors for delayed methotrexate clearance: presence of a "third space" (pleural effusion, ascites) or presence of gastrointestinal obstruction.

- Maintain adequate intravenous hydration throughout high-dose methotrexate therapy using twice the patient's calculated maintenance fluid requirement. Continue until methotrexate serum concentrations are below 1 μM.

- Administer sodium bicarbonate intravenously to alkalinize the urine (maintain a pH $\geq$ 7.0). Monitor urine pH with each void and supplement with additional sodium bicarbonate until the required pH is met.

- Avoid nausea and vomiting with appropriate antiemetic therapy.

- Obtain methotrexate serum concentrations at 24, 48, and 72 hours, then daily until serum concentrations are below cytotoxic levels. Administer leucovorin based on methotrexate serum concentrations, beginning within 42 to 48 hours of the start of the methotrexate infusion.

- Continue alkalinization until methotrexate levels are 1 μM or less. Leucovorin therapy may be discontinued when methotrexate serum concentrations are below cytotoxic concentrations ($\leq 5 \times 10^{-8}$ M).

- Monitor for changes in renal function and delayed methotrexate toxicity.

- Counsel all patients on the importance of leucovorin rescue therapy and for the development of possible adverse effects.

- Avoid drugs known to alter the plasma protein binding or renal elimination of methotrexate (eg, salicylates, sulfisoxazole, nonsteroidal anti-inflammatory drugs, penicillin, probenecid).

The purpose of therapeutic drug monitoring is to ensure therapeutic efficacy while minimizing drug toxicity. A number of criteria must be fulfilled to justify the use of therapeutic drug monitoring. These requirements (Table 17–1) are used to assess the applicability of drug

TABLE 17–1. CRITERIA INDICATING THE NEED FOR THERAPEUTIC DRUG MONITORING

- Drug has a narrow therapeutic index.
- Significant pharmacokinetic variability exists within a population.
- Consequences of therapeutic failure are grave.
- Therapeutic or "target" drug concentration range must be known.
- Drug assay technology is readily available.

monitoring to the particular situation. For routine therapeutic drug monitoring to be considered for any drug, the following criteria must be met. First, the drug in question must have a narrow therapeutic index (the therapeutic drug dosage/concentration is very near that which produces toxicity); (2) within a population there must be significant variability in drug disposition; (3) the consequences of therapeutic failure must be considerable; (4) sufficient data to determine a "target" therapeutic or nontoxic concentration must exist; and (5) rapid, simple, and inexpensive assay technology must be readily available. Other variables that affect the applicability of therapeutic drug monitoring to a lesser degree are the effects of drug metabolites, route of drug administration, dosage schedule dependency, and patient's physiologic status.

Multiple clinical studies have demonstrated the value of therapeutic drug monitoring for such agents as antibiotics, anticonvulsants, and antiarrythmics. As with many of these drugs, antineoplastics typically have narrow therapeutic indices and produce severe toxic effects. These qualities coupled with the life-threatening consequences of undertreatment have led to investigations of the applicability of therapeutic drug monitoring to antineoplastic therapy. The variability in antineoplastic drug disposition is well documented, and numerous clinical trials have demonstrated a relationship between drug concentration, toxicity, and response.[1-6] Although these trials have revealed concentration–response relationships, the direct application of this information to larger populations with the purpose of defining a "therapeutic range" or target drug concentration for antineoplastic drugs has not yet been accomplished. In addition, with the exception of methotrexate, no commercial methods are currently available for rapidly quantifying antineoplastic agents in biologic fluids. The lack of simple, precise analytic methods for antineoplastic agents limits the application of routine drug monitoring in the clinical setting.

The application of these principles to antineoplastic drugs is also compounded by difficulties in relating plasma drug concentration to efficacy and toxicity. Antineoplastic agents are unlike most agents for which therapeutic drug monitoring is used in that nearly all of the important therapeutic and toxic effects of these drugs are realized after all detectable drug has been eliminated from the host. Plasma concentration–time data must therefore be retrospectively evaluated to determine the relationship between exposure and outcome.

Each of these factors has, at present, limited the routine use of therapeutic drug monitoring to a single drug, methotrexate.

CLINICAL PHARMACOLOGY AND THERAPEUTICS

Therapeutic drug monitoring principles using serum concentrations as a measure of efficacy and toxicity may be applied to high-dose methotrexate (HDMTX) therapy. HDMTX, commonly defined as 1 g/m^2 or 20 mg/kg or more of methotrexate, followed by leucovorin rescue, evolved from a desire to overcome drug resistance and to increase methotrexate penetration into pharmacologic sanctuary sites.[7-9] HDMTX, alone and in combination with other antineoplastic agents, has been successfully employed for the treatment of acute leukemias, non-Hodgkin's lymphomas, osteosarcoma, choriocarcinoma, breast cancer, and head and neck neoplasms. The initial effectiveness of HDMTX therapy was offset by a 6% incidence of drug-related deaths secondary to renal failure, severe myelosuppression, sepsis, or hemorrhage.[9] Prospective identification of risk factors for prolonged methotrexate elimination and routine monitoring of methotrexate plasma concentrations followed by appropriate leucovorin rescue provides the basis for therapeutic monitoring of methotrexate therapy.

Pharmacology

Methotrexate, 4-amino-4-deoxy-N^{10}-methylfolic acid, was first synthesized in 1949 as an analog of folic acid.[10] Chemically, methotrexate is a weak dicarboxylic acid with pK_a values of 4.8 and 5.5 and a molecular weight of 454. At physiologic pH, methotrexate is ionized and is able to cross lipid barriers, such as the blood–brain barrier, the blood–testis barrier, and the blood–eye barrier, only after high plasma concentrations are achieved.[11] Methotrexate, a weak acid, has limited solubility in an acidic environment. Solubility may be increased tenfold at pH 7.0, providing the basis for routine urinary alkalinization prior to HDMTX for the prevention of crystalluria.[12]

Mechanism of Action

Methotrexate is classified as an intracellular folate antagonist. Folates carry the one-carbon groups needed for synthesis of purine and thymidylic acid, compounds necessary for DNA synthesis and cell division. On entry into the cell, folates are reduced to tetrahydrofolates by dihydrofolate reductase (DHFR) and metabolized to polyglutamate derivatives. Both metabolites are retained in the cell and are able to perform efficiently the one-carbon transfer needed for purine synthesis.

At concentrations less than 5×10^{-6} M, methotrexate gains entry into the cell through a nonspecific energy- and temperature-dependent active transmembrane folate carrier system. This carrier system becomes saturated at 5×10^{-6} M methotrexate, and further intracellular methotrexate accumulation occurs via passive diffusion.[13,14] Intracellularly, methotrexate competes with dihydrofolates for reversible binding to DHFR[15,16] (Figure 17–1). By blocking DHFR activity, methotrexate prevents the formation of the intracellular reduced folates needed to form thymidylate and inosinic acid, which are necessary for DNA and RNA synthesis. Additionally, amino acid conversions are blocked, resulting in inhibition of protein synthesis. High free intra-

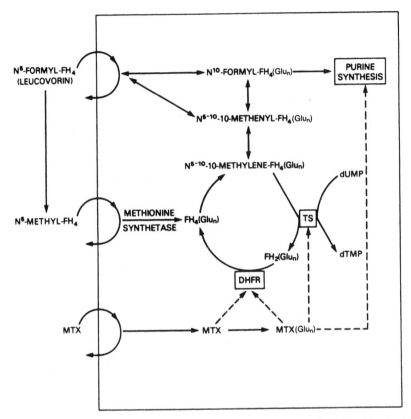

Figure 17–1. Mechanism of action of methotrexate (MTX). DHFR, dihydrofolate reductase; FH$_4$, tetrahydrofolate; Glu, glutamic acid. (*From Jolivet J, Cowan KH, Curt GA, et al. The pharmacology and clinical use of methotrexate.* N Engl J Med. *1983;309:1094–1104, with permission.*)

cellular methotrexate concentrations are required to saturate DHFR fully, as accumulated dihydrofolates resulting from methotrexate-induced metabolic blockade may continually compete for DHFR binding.[17–21] Once extracellular methotrexate concentrations fall, methotrexate dissociates from DHFR and is effluxed to maintain an intracellular:extracellular concentration equilibrium.

Methotrexate is metabolized intracellularly to polyglutamate derivatives by the enzyme folyl polyglutamate synthetase (FPGS), which forms polyglutamate derivatives of naturally occurring folates. In vitro investigations have demonstrated that methotrexate polyglutamate formation increases with increased methotrexate exposure and time, resulting in selective retention of this active methotrexate metabolite.[22–25] Methotrexate polyglutamates have been shown to bind DHFR with affinity equal to that of methotrexate, but dissociate from the enzyme more slowly and remain in the cell regardless of extracellular methotrexate concentrations. These metabolites have also been shown to prolong cytotoxicity by inhibiting thymidylate synthase and other enzymes involved in purine formation.[22,26]

Like many other antineoplastic agents, methotrexate activity has been shown to be specific for tissues undergoing rapid cell division, including bone marrow, gastrointestinal epithelium, and neoplastic tissue. Cells in S phase are primarily affected; however, at higher doses, methotrexate may arrest cellular protein synthesis commonly occurring in the G_1 phase.[27-29] In vitro studies have demonstrated that methotrexate cytotoxicity is related to both drug concentration and duration of exposure.[30,31] Studies in mice have shown that thymidylate synthesis and ultimately DNA synthesis are inhibited at extracellular methotrexate concentrations above 1×10^{-8} M, whereas purine and RNA synthesis is inhibited by methotrexate concentrations above 1×10^{-7} M. This inhibitory effect was observed to be more pronounced and of longer duration with higher methotrexate doses.[30] Normal tissues, such as the intestinal epithelium and bone marrow, displayed slower recovery, compared with tumor cells, which suggests that normal tissues may be more sensitive to the cytotoxic effects of methotrexate.[30] Methotrexate toxicity can be ameliorated by supplying cells with reduced folates, such as leucovorin, which do not require metabolic activation via the DHFR pathway.

Leucovorin (5-formyltetrahydropteroyl-L-glutamic acid, 5-formyltetrahydrofolic acid, folinic acid, or citrovorum factor) is a weak acid with high aqueous solubility. It is commercially available as a racemic mixture of *d*- and *l*- isomers, which differ in their pharmacologic and pharmacokinetic properties. The *l*-isomer is considered to be the only isomer active in the restoration of the reduced folates needed for DNA synthesis, thereby reducing the cytotoxic effects of antifolate therapy (see Figure 17–1). After administration, leucovorin is metabolized by cells of the gastrointestinal tract and the liver to tetrahydrofolate, 5-methyl tetrahydrofolate, and other reduced folates, all of which are capable of entering the folate metabolic pathway required for cellular protein synthesis.[32] In vitro studies have demonstrated that leucovorin competitively interacts at many levels to counteract methotrexate cytotoxicity.[17,33] Leucovorin and its metabolites enter the cell via the energy-dependent folate carrier system and must compete with methotrexate for cell entry. Once in the cell, some of the reduced folates undergo polyglutamation and may represent a mechanism for prolonged intracellular rescue.[32] Intracellular dihydrofolate concentrations in vitro have been observed to increase after leucovorin exposure, in a dose-dependent manner. Continued increases in intracellular dihydrofolate concentrations appear to be a function of methotrexate exposure. This observation suggests that methotrexate rescue is achieved through repletion of reduced folates with leucovorin therapy and through generation of dihydrofolates from dihydrofolate reductase inhibition.[17,33] Leucovorin repletion is not specific for methotrexate therapy, and has been shown effective in repleting reduced folates after other drug therapies known to act as folate antagonists, such as trimethoprim, trimetrexate, and pyrimethamine.

Attempts to ameliorate methotrexate cytotoxicity with leucovorin, originally investigated in cell culture and in mice, demonstrated that leucovorin effectiveness is improved when administered within 36 hours of aminopterin or methotrexate exposure.[34,35] After 42 to 44 hours, methotrexate cytotoxicity has been shown to be irreversible.[36] The amount of leucovorin needed to reverse methotrexate toxicity was related to methotrexate concentration and tumor sensitivity.[35,36] Some investigations have shown that sub- or equimolar concentrations of leucovorin were effective in reversing toxicity at methotrexate concentrations of 10^{-7} *M*, whereas others observed that much higher concentrations of leucovorin were needed to rescue cells at methotrexate concentrations ranging from 10^{-6} to 10^{-5} M.[17,35,36] Studies have shown that extracellular methotrexate concentrations exceeding 100 uM may not be effectively rescued, regardless of the leucovorin concentration.[35]

Effective leucovorin rescue originated from the desire to deliver higher doses of methotrexate, while protecting the host from substantial toxicity, in the hope of increasing the therapeutic response to methotrexate. Several early clinical trials demonstrated that leucovorin administration not only protected the host from toxic effects but achieved superior therapeutic responses.[37–39] From this preliminary work, leucovorin rescue must begin within 42 to 48 hours of the start of the methotrexate infusion or within 24 hours of the completion of methotrexate and should continue until methotrexate concentrations fall below cytotoxic levels ($<5 \times 10^{-8}$ M).[36] (*Note:* 1.0 μM = 1.0×10^{-6} M or approximately 0.5 μg/mL). Additionally, the efficacy of leucovorin rescue has been related to the route of administration. Orally administered doses above 30 to 50 mg/m^2 have demonstrated suboptimal bioavailability, as the folate-mediated carrier system in the gastrointestinal tract becomes saturated above this dose range.[40,41] It follows that parenteral leucovorin should be the preferred route when higher doses are required for adequate rescue. Intramuscular leucovorin was used in early investigations; however, this route of administration also is disadvantaged by suboptimal bioavailability.[42] The frequency of leucovorin administration should be determined by the methotrexate concentration. As leucovorin has an elimination half-life of approximately 0.7 hour, it would follow that patients with a high serum methotrexate serum concentration should initially receive leucovorin every 3 hours. If the patient demonstrates adequate methotrexate clearance, the leucovorin frequency and dose may be altered based on the methotrexate concentration.

Jaffe et al used the leucovorin rescue regimens outlined in Table 17–2 following HDMTX

TABLE 17–2. METHOTREXATE/LEUCOVORIN RESCUE TREATMENT REGIMENS PER JAFFE ET AL

Reference	Methotrexate Dosing Regimen	Leucovorin Rescue
43	1500–7500 mg/m^2 over 6 h q2wk	9–15 mg/m^2 IM q6h × 12 doses to start 2 h after completion of MTX infusion
44	1500–7500 mg/m^2 over 6 h q2wk	<0.5 m^{2a} 1.0 m^2 >1.0 m^2 5 mg 10 mg 15 mg IV q3h × 24 h followed by PO dosing q6h × 48 h
45	12.5 g/m^2 over 6 h; MTX concentrations determined 6, 24, 48, and 72 h after start of infusion	15 mg IV q3h initially; dose increased to 15–100 mg IV q3h based on toxic level criteria
46	12.5 g/m^2 over 6 h; randomized to either intravenous or intraarterial doses every 7–10 d	15 mg IV q3h initially; 100 mg q3h IV if decay abnormal; rescue to start 12 h after completion of MTX dose and to continue until level of 0.3 μM is observed

[a] Body surface area.

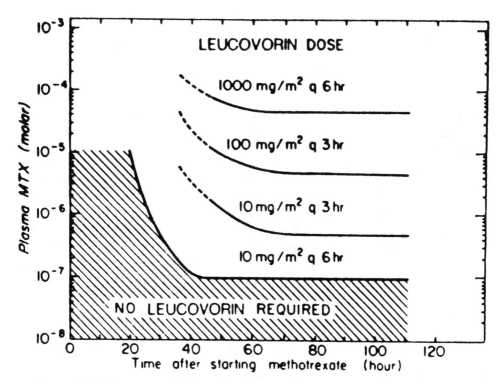

Figure 17–2. Nomogram for leucovorin rescue of high-dose methotrexate therapy. (*From Bleyer WA. New vistas for leucovorin in cancer chemotherapy. Cancer. 1989;63:995–1007, with permission.*)

for osteogenic sarcoma.[43–46] From this table, it can be seen that leucovorin rescue per the method of Jaffe et al continues until the methotrexate level drops to 0.3 μM, after which leucovorin is discontinued. This recommendation was based on the demonstration of linear, adequate methotrexate clearance, and does not address those patients with risk factors ("third spacing," bowel obstruction, renal dysfunction) for prolonged methotrexate elimination.

Bleyer proposed a nomogram approach for leucovorin dosing following methotrexate therapy (Figure 17–2). This dosing strategy was derived from leucovorin pharmacokinetic data which suggested that 100 mg/m² leucovorin resulted in a mean serum concentration of 10 μM and 1000 mg/m2 leucovorin resulted in a mean serum concentration of 100 μM.[42] From this nomogram, it is suggested that leucovorin start 36 to 42 hours after initiation of methotrexate therapy and continue until drug concentrations fall below 1.0×10^{-7} M.

Evans et al from St. Jude's Research Hospital proposed a rescue regimen for high-risk patients that is based on individual patient methotrexate pharmacokinetic data and methotrexate dosage. High risk per St. Jude's is defined as the following:

12 g/m² MTX over 6 hours   20-hour MTX level > 10 μM

<table>
<tr><td></td><td>24-hour MTX level > 5 μM</td></tr>
</table>

	24-hour MTX level > 5 μM
	44-hour MTX level > 1 μM
	Elimination $t_{1/2}$ > 3.5 hours
1.5 g/m² MTX over 24 hours	21-hour MTX level > 2.0 μM
	0.8-hour MTX level > 0.8 μM

The presence of any one of the above factors places the patient at high risk for methotrexate toxicity. Leucovorin dosage should be adjusted according to the plasma methotrexate concentrations, as shown in Table 17–3.

Methotrexate concentrations should be obtained daily in high-risk patients. For patients receiving 12 g/m², leucovorin rescue should start at 20 hours, whereas those receiving 1.5 g/m² may begin leucovorin 24 hours after completion of the methotrexate infusion.

Experimentally, other measures to reverse methotrexate toxicity have been described. One such method employs the use of carboxypeptidase G_2, a 90,000-kDa bacterial enzyme that hydrolyzes the C-terminal glutamate residue from folic acid and methotrexate, resulting in the formation of an inactive metabolite.[47,48] Preclinical investigations in mice demonstrated that the administration of methotrexate followed by carboxypeptidase G_2 protected the animal from toxic death.[48] There was, however, no difference in survival between those mice receiving leucovorin and those receiving carboxypeptidase G_2 therapy. Advantages observed in this study include

TABLE 17–3. ST. JUDE'S LEUCOVORIN RESCUE REGIMEN

Methotrexate Concentration (mM)	Leucovorin Dosage (mg/m²)
90–100	1000 q3h IV
80–90	900 q3h IV
70–80	800 q3h IV
60–70	700 q3h IV
50–60	600 q3h IV
40–50	500 q3h IV
30–40	400 q3h IV
20–30	300 q3h IV
15–20	200 q3h IV
10–15	150 q3h IV
5–10	100 q3h IV
2–5	50 q6h IV
1–2	25 q6h IV or PO
0.5–1	15 q6h IV or PO
0.1–0.5	15 q12h IV or PO
0.05–0.1	5 q12h PO or IV
<0.05	Discontinue

nonreversal of the intracellular DNA synthetic blockade, independent antitumor activity, and a short half-life compared with leucovorin. This enzyme may be additionally advantageous in the case of intrathecal methotrexate rescue, as observed in a study in rhesus monkeys.[47]

Clinical Pharmacokinetics

Pharmacokinetic data are summarized in Table 17–4.

Absorption

Absorption of methotrexate from the gastrointestinal tract is dependent on the dose administered.[49–52] Studies in animals have demonstrated that an active and passive transport system exists in the gastrointestinal tract, allowing for variable, dose-dependent absorption with methotrexate concentrations above 10^{-7} M.[53] Clinical trials have shown that bioavailability following oral administration of methotrexate is variable and incomplete.[49,50,52,54–56] Doses less than 30 mg/m^2 are completely absorbed. Higher doses have decreased bioavailability, ranging from 12 to 77%, indicating that decreased absorption is possibly due to saturable gastrointestinal transport.[49,52,57] Absorption of orally administered methotrexate is rapid, with methotrexate detectable in serum 30 minutes after oral doses and peak concentrations occurring at 1.5 hours.[52]

Factors thought to decrease the absorption of methotrexate from the gastrointestinal tract include food, particularly foods with a high fat content, and oral administration of nonabsorbable antibiotics.[58,59] There is no diurnal variation in the absorption of oral methotrexate.[60]

After subcutaneous administration, methotrexate absorption is complete and comparable to absorption after administration of low-dose oral methotrexate (7.5 mg/m^2). Peak concentrations occur 15 to 30 minutes after the administered dose.[61] At doses of 40 mg/m^2, methotrexate serum concentrations are equivalent to intravenous concentrations and exceed concentrations observed after the same oral methotrexate dose by approximately 60%.[61]

Bioavailability of methotrexate administered intramuscularly to children and adults has ranged from 75 to 100%, indicating complete absorption.[49,51,52] Intramuscular doses provide higher, more sustained serum concentrations when compared with equivalent oral doses of methotrexate.[49,51,52,62] Methotrexate concentrations can be measured 15 minutes after an intramuscular dose, with peak concentrations occurring at approximately 1 hour.[52]

Distribution

After intravenous administration methotrexate rapidly distributes to an extracellular compartment estimated to represent 18% of the total body weight.[63] At steady state the volume of distribution approximates that of total body water.[55,63] The distribution half-life ($t_{1/2,\alpha}$) ranges from 0.45 to 2.0 hours, and the $t_{1/2,\beta}$, representing primarily renal elimination, ranges from 3 to 5 hours. Triphasic elimination has been reported in many clinical investigations. The terminal-phase half-life ranges from 8 to 26 hours and represents redistribution from deep tissue sites and sanctuaries. Terminal-phase elimination has been correlated with methotrexate toxicity.

Methotrexate is approximately 40 to 50% protein bound.[55,57,64,65] Binding saturation has been observed at methotrexate concentrations greater than 5×10^{-5} M.[65] Following parenteral administration methotrexate plasma concentrations are linear with respect to dose.[55]

Distribution and retention into "third spaces," such as pleural effusions and ascitic fluid, have been demonstrated.[12,56,66] Methotrexate accumulates slowly in these fluid collections, and

TABLE 17–4. SUMMARY OF METHOTREXATE PHARMACOKINETIC DATA

Pharmacokinetic Parameter	Value		
Minimum effective concentration, intrathecal	1×10^{-6} M		
Potentially toxic concentration	5×10^{-8} M		
	1×10^{-7} M for bone marrow and GI mucosa		
Absorption			
Oral			
Doses < 30mg/m²	>80% but variable		
Doses > 30mg/m²	<25%		
Subcutaneous	100%		
Intramuscular	75–100%		
Total body clearance (mean values)			
Adults	71 mL/min/m² or 2.43 mL/min/kg		
Children	100 mL/min/m²		
Obese patients	1.6 mL/min/kg		
Elimination rate constant (mean values)			
Adults	0.306 h⁻¹		
Children	0.578 h⁻¹		
Obese patients	N/A		
Half-life (h)	α	β	γ
Adults	0.45–2.0	5.5	11–20
Children	0.03–0.13	0.9–4.0	5.3–15
Obese patients	N/A	9.3	N/A
High-risk patients		>3.5	
Intrathecal		4.5	12–18
Volume of distribution (mean values)			
Adults	0.5–1.0 L/kg		
Children	1.1 L/kg (16.4 L/m²)		
Obese patients	0.4 L/kg (total body weight)		
Protein bound	50–70%		
Clearance			
Renal	44–100%		
Nonrenal	10–40%		
Time to steady state	Not clinically relevant		
Time to peak concentration			
Oral	1–3 h		
Subcutaneous	0.25–0.5 h		
Intramuscular	0.25–1.5 h		
Major metabolites	DAMPA		
	7-OH-Methotrexate		
	7-OH-MTX Polyglutamates		
	MTX Polyglutamates		

concentrations found in these "third spaces" equal those found in plasma within 6 hours. Drug clearance from these sites is slower than from plasma, resulting in depot methotrexate concentrations that may exceed those measured in plasma during terminal elimination. Slow elimination from these loculated fluid collections results in prolongation of the terminal phase of drug elimination and continued methotrexate exposure, which may result in significant toxicity.

Methotrexate, which is ionized at physiologic pH, does not readily cross the blood–brain barrier. Penetration into the central nervous system has been shown to occur following high-dose therapy administered by either bolus or continuous infusion.[66] The steady-state plasma:CSF concentration ratio is approximately 30:1 during prolonged intravenous infusions of methotrexate.[67] Methotrexate administered intravenously in doses in excess of 1 g/m^2 have proven useful in the treatment of central nervous system leukemia.

Metabolism

Methotrexate has three principal metabolites: 4-amino-4-deoxy-N^{10}-methylpteroic acid (DAMPA),7-hydroxymethotrexate (7-OH-MTX), and methotrexate polyglutamates. DAMPA is formed by intestinal bacteria during enterohepatic circulation and has cytotoxic activity approximately 1/200th that of methotrexate, making its contribution toward methotrexate's antineoplastic action minimal.[68]

Methotrexate is oxidized in the liver to 7-OH-MTX by an aldehyde–oxidase enzyme system.[69] The aqueous solubility of this metabolite is much lower than that of the parent compound and may contribute to methotrexate renal toxicity. 7-OH-MTX enters the cell via the folate carrier system and has been shown in vitro to compete with methotrexate for intracellular transport.[70,71] This results in a decreased amount of intracellular methotrexate polyglutamation and DHFR inhibition.[69,70] 7-OH-MTX does not have the same affinity for DHFR binding as methotrexate, but has been shown in vitro to undergo polyglutamation. The polyglutamated derivative can bind DHFR, thereby augmenting methotrexate cytotoxicity.[72]

The pharmacokinetics of the 7-OH metabolite have been described in both adult and pediatric populations over a wide range of methotrexate doses.[63,66,73–75] With methotrexate doses up to 5 g/m^2, peak 7-OH-MTX concentrations ranged from 17 to 21 μM, when measured up to 24 hours after drug administration.[63,73] The concentration of 7-OH-MTX typically exceeds the concentration of the parent compound by the end of the infusion, with a peak 7-OH-MTX:MTX ratio of approximately 8:1 at 48 hours postinfusion.[63,66,73–75] 7-OH-MTX has been shown to decline biexponentially, with $t_{1/2,\alpha}$ and $t_{1/2,\beta}$ of 8 and 20 hours, respectively.[66]

The most important pharmacologic metabolite of methotrexate is the polyglutamyl derivative. This metabolite is formed intracellularly by the enzyme folyl polyglutamate synthetase (FPGS), which catalyzes the addition of up to five glutamate residues to the terminal glutamate of methotrexate. These additions increase the size of the methotrexate molecule, thereby inhibiting drug efflux from the cell. In vitro studies have demonstrated that methotrexate polyglutamate formation is a function of free intracellular methotrexate concentrations and duration of exposure.[17,22–24] Long-chain polyglutamates, desirable because they bind DHFR with affinity equal to or greater than that of methotrexate, are formed only after several hours of methotrexate exposure and may represent approximately 90% of intracellular methotrexate at 48 hours.[17,23] These metabolites are retained intracellularly regardless of methotrexate concentration, thereby contributing to sustained methotrexate cytotoxicity in susceptible cells.[22] The pharmacokinetic parameters for the polyglutamate derivatives of methotrexate have not been described.

Elimination

The primary route of methotrexate elimination is renal excretion via glomerular filtration and tubular secretion. Clinical investigations have reported that greater than 90% of the methotrexate dose may be renally eliminated within the first 24 hours.[12,55] Patients with reduced renal function are, therefore, at risk for toxic effects. Renal elimination of methotrexate and 7-OH-MTX has been shown to be enhanced when the pH of urine is maintained above 6.5.[12] Precipitation of methotrexate in the urine has been observed when the pH falls below 6.5 and may represent the mechanism for methotrexate-induced renal toxicity.[12] Maintaining adequate hydration and urinary alkalinization with oral or intravenous sodium bicarbonate or oral acetazolamide titrated to maintain a urine pH greater than 6.5 has proven effective in preventing methotrexate renal toxicity.[76]

Following high-dose therapy the elimination of methotrexate is biphasic: the beta phase represents renal elimination, and a later nonlinear gamma phase represents the liberation of drug from deep tissues. Studies have demonstrated up to tenfold variability in methotrexate clearance within a population.

Methotrexate elimination following an intrathecal dose has been described as biphasic, with half-lives of 4.5 and 12 to 18 hours. Methotrexate is eliminated from the cerebrospinal fluid by resorption and a nonspecific active transport process across the choroid plexus. Delayed clearance has been reported in patients with meningeal leukemia and in older patients, leading to toxic manifestations.[77]

Elimination from pharmacologic "third spaces," such as pleural and ascitic fluids, has been reported to be prolonged relative to methotrexate elimination from the serum. One investigator observed an elimination half-life of 27.3 hours from pleural fluid compared with 9.2 hours for plasma.[77]

Minor pathways of methotrexate elimination include bilary secretion with fecal excretion. This route accounts for less than 10% of an administered dose. Although nonrenal elimination may be considered clinically insignificant at low treatment doses, in patients receiving high-dose therapy with a reduced gastrointestinal transit time or ileus, concentrations within the gastrointestinal tract may remain cytotoxic, leading to prolonged clearance and increased risk of toxicity.[78]

The use of hemodialysis to remove methotrexate has met with limited success. In vitro investigations observed 90% removal of methotrexate from human plasma following 1 hour of hemodialysis.[79] These observations were not supported clinically, as previous attempts to hemodialyze patients with toxic methotrexate levels proved suboptimal and, in one report, inferior to enzymatic cleavage of methotrexate with carboxypeptidase G_1, a bacterial enzyme known to cleave the terminal glutamate of methotrexate, resulting in the formation of an inactive metabolite.[80-83] Peritoneal dialysis has been proven ineffective because of methotrexate's protein binding and ionization at physiologic pH.[84] The combination of hemoperfusion with charcoal filters and hemodialysis has successfully been employed in the removal of methotrexate in patients with plasma concentrations as high as 574 μM.[85-87] Patients who received the combination of hemoperfusion and hemodialysis experienced little morbidity when these procedures were combined with leucovorin and oral charcoal therapy for methotrexate removal, which demonstrates the effectiveness of combination therapy for methotrexate removal following severely toxic levels.

TABLE 17-5. SIDE EFFECTS AND ADVERSE REACTIONS

Adverse Effect	Onset/ Duration	Leucovorin Rescue Effective?	Comments
Nausea and vomiting[12,44]	1–3 d	No	Incidence may be as high as 40%; avoid with appropriate antiemetic therapy; dehydration from vomiting can potentiate MTX toxicity
Diarrhea[44]	1–3 d	Yes	Maintain adequate hydration to avoid MTX toxicity
Dermatologic toxicity[44,89,90]	1–5 d	No	Rashes reported following HDMTX: mild transient erythematous maculopapular eruptions, exacerbations of acne, vasculitis, exfoliative dermatitis, radiation recall, and reactivation of sunburn
Nephrotoxicity[12,91–94]	1–7 d	No	Manifested by increased BUN/serum creatinine, decreased MTX clearance; may be the result of MTX or metabolite precipitation in urine; avoid with alkalinization to maintain urine pH > 6.5 and vigorous hydration (3000 mL/m^2/d)
Acute hepatic toxicity[44,94]	1–10 d	No	Transient elevations in transaminases reported; may be associated with hyperbilirubinemia; return to baseline may take up to 2 wk
Mucositis[12,44,95]	3–7 d	Yes	Maintain good oral hygiene and treat with supportive measures
Conjunctivitis[96]	2–7 d	No	Burning, pruritis, "dry eyes"; may treat with topical lubricants; etiology—MTX insolubility in lacrimal fluid
Myelosuppression[44,97]	7–14 d	Yes	May support with colony-stimulating factors for prolonged myelosuppression
Transient neurologic syndrome[44,98–102]	6–20 d	unclear	Rare; may manifest as hemiplegia, speech disorder, convulsions, status epilepticus, rapidly ascending paralysis; resolves in 1–7 d; intrathecal administration may result in meningismus, tremulousness, headache, fever
Chronic leukoencephalopathy[103–107]	Months to years	Unclear	Rare, evolving toxicity; clinically manifests as lethargy, progressive dementia, seizures, spasticity; cranial irradiation, systemic and intrathecal administration of MTX, and cumulative methotrexate dose may increase risk; may be fatal

Special Populations

The pharmacokinetic parameters of methotrexate have been described in one obese patient with osteosarcoma.[88] This patient, estimated to be 184% of her ideal body weight, received an empiric methotrexate dose of 8.0 g/m^2 in combination with other antineoplastic agents on a 7-week cycle. Pharmacokinetic analysis of this patient revealed an increased steady-state volume of distribution and clearance and a terminal half-life that was similar to previously reported values. Although the authors were not able to offer specific recommendations for dosage adjustments for the obese patient, it was suggested that larger methotrexate doses may be required. This would be expected given that methotrexate distribution approximates total body water. Additionally, renal function rather than weight may help predict methotrexate pharmacokinetics in the obese patient.

PHARMACODYNAMICS

Adverse Effects

Methotrexate toxicity has been shown to correlate with plasma methotrexate concentration and duration of exposure.[27-31] The toxic effects are outlined in Table 17–5.[12,44,89–107] Risk factors include poor hydration, acidic urine pH, dehydration from vomiting or diarrhea, poor renal func-

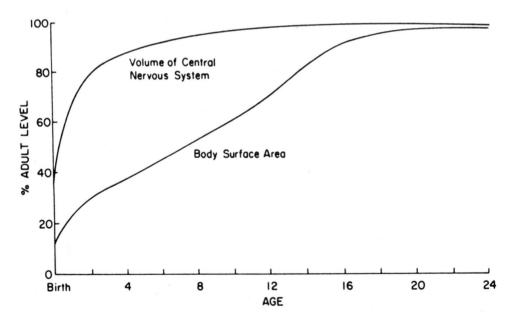

Figure 17–3. Comparison of body surface area and extracellular fluid volume of the central nervous system during childhood. (*From Bleyer WA. Clinical pharmacology of intrathecal methotrexate. II. An improved dosage regimen derived from age-related pharmacokinetics. Cancer Treat Rep. 1977;61:1419–1425, with permission.*)

tion, intestinal obstruction or decreased intestinal transit time, and presence of a third space, such as a pleural effusion or ascites.[12,108,109] It should be noted that not all toxic effects are related to folate antagonism or are reversible with leucovorin therapy.

Intrathecal Methotrexate

Dose–response correlations following intrathecal methotrexate administration have been shown to be a function of age rather than body surface area.[110] This conclusion was derived from the growth curves of the central nervous system (CNS) compared with body surface area (Figure 17–3).[111] From this curve, it can be appreciated that CNS growth does not parallel increases in body size throughout life. By 3 years of age, CNS volume has reached a plateau, whereas body surface area continues to increase until approximately 20 years of age. The volume of the CNS is thus fixed by age 3, and methotrexate doses administered intrathecally do not require adjustments for body size. This concept was demonstrated in a clinical trial comparing fixed intrathecal methotrexate doses with doses based on body surface area.[110] Adolescents who received doses based on body surface area had more toxic effects and greater morbidity related to elevated cerebrospinal fluid methotrexate concentrations, whereas younger patients had unacceptable therapeutic responses. Fixed doses based on age and cerebrospinal fluid volume produced less variability in methotrexate cerebrospinal fluid concentrations, less toxicity, and a lower relapse rate.[111] This dosing scheme is outlined in Table 17–6.

THERAPEUTIC REGIMEN DESIGN

The routine monitoring of methotrexate developed from the need to reduce the toxicity associated with high-dose methotrexate regimens. Early investigators reported a 6% mortality rate associated with the use of these regimens.[9] Since the application of pharmacokinetic monitoring, institutions such as St. Jude Children's Research Hospital have encountered no fatalities in more than 3000 courses of high-dose methotrexate therapy (Evans WE, Personal communication). These results have been obtained because of the numerous improvements in the delivery of therapy, including attention to adequate hydration, urinary alkalinization, and the use of serial plasma methotrexate concentration determinations to guide appropriate leucovorin rescue.

Numerous investigators have examined the pharmacokinetics of high-dose methotrexate administration in dosages ranging from 0.5 to 33.6 g/m^2.[66,112,113] Data from these studies have

TABLE 17–6. INTRATHECAL METHOTREXATE DOSING BASED ON PATIENT AGE

Patient Age (y)	Methotrexate Dose (mg)
<1	6
1	8
2	10
≥3	12

been used to correlate the pharmacokinetics and toxicity of methotrexate. These correlations have been used as the foundation for the development of criteria employed to identify patients at risk for developing toxic effects from methotrexate. Use of these criteria has led to the development of rational prospective monitoring of serum methotrexate concentrations in the clinical setting.

The efficacy and toxicity of methotrexate are related to both the serum *concentration* of methotrexate and the *duration* of drug exposure. Therefore, systemic clearance of methotrexate has the most profound impact on methotrexate toxicity overall. Patients with delayed methotrexate clearance are at greater risk of toxic effects, and although the criteria used to identify patients at risk vary from institution to institution, there is good agreement on the basic principles of monitoring.

The rate of systemic clearance of methotrexate varies widely, and no single predictor of methotrexate clearance (eg, creatinine clearance) other than direct monitoring of methotrexate plasma concentrations has proven useful. The rationale for prospective monitoring of methotrexate plasma concentrations after high-dose therapy is simple: (1) Delayed elimination of methotrexate results in cytotoxic drug concentrations which may persist beyond the duration of "standard" leucovorin rescue; therefore the *duration* of leucovorin rescue may not be sufficient for patients at risk. (2) As leucovorin competes with methotrexate for entry into the cell an *insufficient amount* of leucovorin may be present in the plasma, resulting in inadequate rescue. In each of these cases leucovorin administration would be tailored to the individual patient (rescue either increased, prolonged, or both) to effect successful rescue.

It is absolutely imperative that this alteration in leucovorin rescue be made promptly in these "high-risk" patients, as methotrexate toxicity may be irreversible, regardless of the administered leucovorin dose, if adequate rescue is not provided within 48 hours of methotrexate administration. Therefore, some approach to prospective identification of patients at risk for toxic effects is absolutely necessary for the safe administration of high-dose methotrexate. Because monitoring methotrexate pharmacokinetics provides the best estimate of drug clearance, plasma methotrexate concentration monitoring has been used routinely to identify patients at risk for more than a decade.

Initially, investigators used methotrexate plasma concentration at various time points, usually 24 or 48 hours after the start of the methotrexate infusion, to identify patients requiring more aggressive leucovorin rescue.[114-116] As methotrexate toxicity is related to drug exposure, a product of both concentration and time, monitoring a single methotrexate plasma concentration does not provide sufficient information for prospective identification of patients at risk. To develop an approach for the early recognition of patients at high-risk for developing methotrexate toxic effects after the administration of high-dose methotrexate, Evans et al examined methotrexate disposition and toxicity in 30 patients receiving 114 courses of high-dose methotrexate.[113] This study demonstrated that the risk factors identified (Table 17–7) enabled early recognition of patients at risk of toxic effects, allowing earlier modification of leucovorin rescue, thereby reducing or preventing toxicity. This method uses serial determination of plasma methotrexate concentration for the prospective determination of methotrexate elimination and identification of excessive plasma methotrexate concentrations.

The benefit of using such an approach is that it enables the prospective determination of patients at risk. It is this prospective assessment that permits immediate, *individualized* rescue therapy for the prevention of toxic effects.

It is clear that the institution of specific criteria for the identification of patients at risk cou-

TABLE 17–7. RISK FACTORS ASSOCIATED WITH METHOTREXATE TOXICITY

Clinical
  Renal dysfunction
  Pleural effusions
  Gastrointestinal obstruction
  Ascites
Pharmacokinetic
  24-h half-life >3.5 h
  24-h methotrexate concentration >5 μM

Adapted from Evans WE, Pratt CB, Taylor RH, et al. Pharmacokinetic monitoring of high-dose methotrexate: Early recognition of high-risk patients. *Cancer Chemother Pharmacol.* 1979;3:161–166, with permission.

pled with rational methods for determining appropriate rescue therapy has led to safer delivery of high-dose methotrexate therapy.

In the past decade our understanding of the relationship between anticancer drug pharmacokinetics and clinical effects has grown markedly. For anticancer drugs the clinical importance of these relationships was first documented in studies investigating methotrexate pharmacodynamics. Initial investigations examined the relationship between drug concentration and toxicity. Stoller, Evans, and Perez and their co-workers documented the relationship between terminal methotrexate concentration and drug toxicity.[112,113,115] Far fewer studies have successfully examined the relationship between anticancer drug concentration and efficacy. Pharmacodynamic investigations, that attempt to relate drug disposition to clinical efficacy are difficult to apply to cancer chemotherapy for a number of reasons. First, with the exception of phase I trials of new agents, most chemotherapy strategies comprise multiagent drug regimens, making it difficult to assess the impact of each agent. Second, in addition to drug treatment, multiple influences impact on successful therapy, including tumor heterogeneity, host tolerance, disease severity, drug–tumor interactions, and effects of previous treatment. Finally, a direct association between drug concentration and treatment efficacy is difficult to assess because the maximum anticancer effect (eg, tumor destruction) usually occurs after all drug has been eliminated. Nevertheless, studies have been performed that demonstrate a clear relationship between drug disposition (such as drug clearance or drug exposure) and therapeutic success. Evans et al retrospectively evaluated methotrexate disposition in 108 pediatric cancer patients with newly diagnosed acute lymphocytic leukemia (ALL). These subjects received methotrexate 1 g/m² over 24 hours for a total of 15 courses each. Those patients with a faster rate of methotrexate clearance, resulting in steady-state methotrexate concentrations less than 16 μM, were three times more likely to relapse during therapy.[3] The impact of methotrexate clearance on the outcome in childhood ALL was corroborated by Borsi and Moe, who reported higher methotrexate clearances in children with ALL who relapsed. These investigators reported that methotrexate clearance retained its prognostic significance in children with relapsed ALL who were given much higher doses of methotrexate.[40,41] These data demonstrate that knowledge of these pharmacodynamic relationships may provide for the development of individualized cancer chemotherapy regimens, which may enhance therapeutic efficacy while minimizing drug-related toxicity.

Drug–drug interactions of methotrexate are summarized in Table 17–8.[45,117–132] An algorithm for assessing and monitoring patients is provided in Figure 17–4.

TABLE 17–8. DRUG–DRUG INTERACTIONS OF PHARMACOKINETIC CONSEQUENCE

Drug	Mechanism of Interaction	Comments
Aspirin[117]	Decreased renal clearance by competition renal tubular transport	May increase the exposure to 7-OH-MTX
Probenecid[118–121]	Decreased MTX protein binding Decreased renal excretion of MTX Decreased biliary secretion	Weak organic acids compete for renal tubular transport, resulting in reabsorption of methotrexate
Nonabsorbable antibiotics[122]	Decreased MTX oral absorption by approximately 35% Decreased GI metabolism	
Sulfonamides[118,123]	Decreased MTX protein binding resulting in increased free fraction Decreased free MTX renal clearance Possible additive hematologic toxicity	Overall, results in an approximate 66% increase in systemic exposure to MTX
NSAIDs[124–126]	Decreased renal clearance by: Inhibition of prostaglandin-mediated renal perfusion rate Competition for renal tubular secretion Displacement of MTX from plasma proteins	
Penicillins[118,127]	Reduction of MTX clearance by inhibition of renal tubular secretion	
5-Fluorouracil[128,129]	Synergistic MTX cytotoxicity when administered *after* MTX	
Cisplatin[45,130]	Decreased renal elimination via cisplatin-induced renal toxicity and residual damage	Prior cisplatin therapy may be a risk factor for prolonged elimination of MTX
Cholestyramine[131]	Increased MTX biliary elimination	May have limited clinical significance, as biliary excretion is a minor pathway
Activated charcoal[132]	Acceleration of MTX elimination by interruption of enterohepatic circulation	May also be used in combination with hemodialysis/hemoperfusion

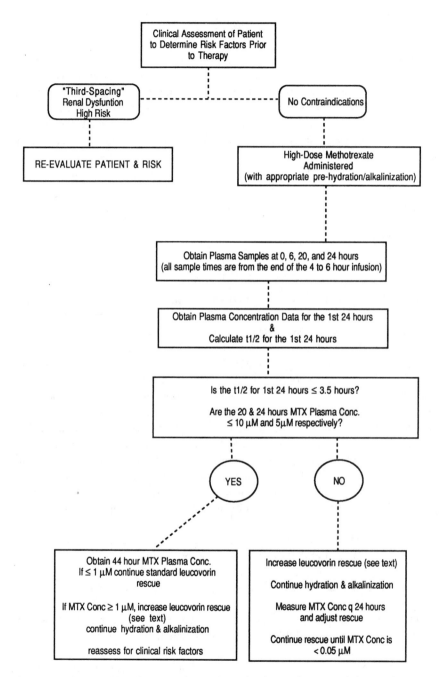

Figure 17–4. Algorithm for assessing and monitoring patients receiving methotrexate.

SUMMARY

Although anticancer drugs are among the most toxic agents administered to humans, routine therapeutic drug monitoring is currently applied only to high-dose methotrexate therapy. Several factors limit the use of antineoplastic therapeutic drug monitoring in clinical practice, including the few available methods for rapidly quantifying anticancer drugs in biologic fluids and the lack of well-established therapeutic ranges for these agents. In the future, when these limiting factors are overcome, and as disease- and population-specific pharmacodynamic data are determined for commonly used anticancer agents, therapeutic drug monitoring principles can be routinely applied to the clinical management of all patients receiving cancer chemotherapy.

———— QUESTIONS ————

T.T. is a 17-year-old black woman with osteosarcoma of the left distal femur diagnosed in 1988. Her neoadjuvant treatment consisted of 7 courses of intraarterial cisplatin 150 mg/m^2 every 2 weeks for seven courses, followed by an arthrodesis and left tarsus allo-graft. She experienced greater than 90% tumor necrosis and went on to receive doxorubicin (cumulative dose 400 mg/m^2). She developed pulmonary metastases and underwent two thoracotomies and 11 courses of ifosfamide/etoposide, resulting in a partial response. Approximately 1 year later, a right pneumonectomy was performed to decompress the right main bronchus, which had been affected by progressive disease. This resulted in a residual pleural effusion in the right chest. The chemotherapy treatment plan following the pneumonectomy consisted of 12 courses of high-dose methotrexate 12.5 g/m^2 over 6 hours followed by leucovorin rescue. Other significant medical problems include cerebral palsy and a seizure disorder treated with phenobarbital and carbamazepine, an allergy to penicillin, and an intolerance to phenytoin. Prior to the start of therapy, electrolytes and a chemistry profile were obtained and all values were within normal limits.

1. Is this patient likely to have reduced methotrexate clearance? Please list the risk factors. Is this patient at risk for methotrexate toxic effects?

2. Design an appropriate leucovorin rescue strategy for this patient.

3. In addition to adequate leucovorin rescue, what other clinical management approaches should be instituted with high-dose methotrexate therapy?

4. Are there any drug–drug interactions in the patient with seizures treated with phenobarbital and carbamazepine?

5. When may this patient be discharged from the hospital?

REFERENCES

1. Rodman JH, Abromowitch M, Sinkule JA, et al. Clinical pharmacodynamics of continuous infusion teniposide: Systemic exposure as a determinant of response in a phase I trial. *J Clin Oncol.* 1987;5:1007–1014.
2. Egorin MJ, Van Echo DA, Whitacre MY, et al. Human pharmacokinetics, excretion, and metabolism of the anthracycline antibiotic menogril and their correlation with clinical toxicities. *Cancer Res.* 1986;46:1513–1520.
3. Evans WE, Crom WR, Stewart CF, et al. Clinical pharmacodynamics of high-dose methotrexate in acute lymphocytic leukemia. *N Engl J Med.* 1986;314:471–477.
4. Milano G, Roman P, Khater R, et al. Dose versus pharmacokinetics for predicting tolerance to 5-day continuous infusion of 5-FU. *Int J Cancer.* 1988;41:537–541.
5. Egorin MJ, Van Echo DA, Olman EA, et al. Prospective validation of a pharmacologically based dosing scheme for carboplatin. *Cancer Res.* 1983;45:6502–6506.
6. Ratain MJ, Vogelzang NJ, Sinkule JA. Interpatient and intrapatient variability in vinblastine pharmacokinetics. *Clin Pharmacol Ther.* 1987;41:61–67.
7. Ackland SP, Schilsky RL. High-dose methotrexate: A critical reappraisal. *J Clin Oncol.* 1987;5:2017–2031.
8. Djerassi I. High-dose methotrexate (NSC-740) and citrovorum factor (NSC-3590) rescue: Background and rationale. *Cancer Chemother Rep.* 1975;6 (pt 3):3–6.
9. Von Hoff DD, Penta JS, Helman LJ, Slavik M. Incidence of drug-related deaths secondary to high-dose methotrexate and citrovorum factor administration. *Cancer Treat Rep.* 1977;61:745–748.
10. Seeger DR, Osulich DB, Smith JM, et al. Analogs of pteroylglutamic acid. III. 4-Amino derivatives. *J Am Chem Soc.* 1949;71:1753–1758.
11. Bleyer WA. Methotrexate: Clinical pharmacology, current status and therapeutic guidelines. *Cancer Treat Rev.* 1977;4:87–101.
12. Stoller RG, Jacobs SA, Drake JC, et al. Pharmacokinetics of high-dose methotrexate (NSC-740). *Cancer Chemother Rep.* 1975; 6:19–24.
13. Warren RD, Nichols AP, Bender RA. Membrane transport of methotrexate in human lymphoblastoid cells. *Cancer Res.* 1978;38:668–671.
14. Hill BT, Bailey BD, White JC, Goldman ID. Characteristics of transport of 4–amino antifolates and folate compounds by two lines of L5178Y lymphoblasts, one with impaired transport of methotrexate. *Cancer Res.* 1979;39:2440–2446.
15. White JC. Recent concepts on the mechanism of action of methotrexate. *Cancer Treat Rep.* 1981;65(suppl 1):3–12.
16. Waltham MC, Holland JW, Robinson SC, et al. Direct experimental evidence for competitive inhibition of dihydrofolate reductase by methotrexate. *Biochem Pharmacol.* 1988;37:535–539.
17. Boarman DM, Baram J, Allegra CJ. Mechanism of leucovorin reversal of methotrexate cytotoxicity in human MCF-7 breast cancer cells. *Biochem Pharmacol.* 1990;40:2651–2660.
18. Goldman ID, Lichenstein NS, Oliverio VT. Carrier mediated transport of the folic acid analog, methotrexate, in the L1210 leukemia cell. *J Biol Chem.* 1968;243:5007–5017.
19. Tattersall IHN, Parker LM, Pitman, Frie E. Clinical pharmacology of high-dose methotrexate (NSC-740). *Cancer Chemother Rep.* 1975;6(3):25–29.
20. White JC, Goldman ID. Mechanism of action of methotrexate: Free intracellular methotrexate required to suppress dihydrofolate reduction to tetrahydrofolate by Ehrlich ascites tumor cells in vitro. *Mol Pharmacol.* 1976;12:711–719.
21. White JC. Reversal of methotrexate binding to dihydrofolate reductase by dihydrofolate. *J Biol Chem.* 1979;254:10889–10895.
22. Jolivet J, Schilsky RL, Bailey BD, et al. Synthesis, retention, and biological activity of methotrexate polyglutamates in cultured human breast cancer cells. *J Clin Invest.* 1982;70:351–360.

23. Jolivet J, Chabner BA. Intracellular pharmacokinetics of methotrexate polyglutamates in human breast cancer cells. *J Clin Invest.* 1983;72:773–778.

24. Rosenblatt DS, Whitehead VM, Dupont MM, et al. Synthesis of methotrexate polyglutamates in cultured human cells. *Mol Pharmacol.* 1977;14:210–214.

25. Rosenblatt DS, Whitehead VM, Vera N, et al. Prolonged inhibition of DNA synthesis associated with the accumulation of methotrexate polyglutamates by cultured human cells. *Mol Pharmacol.* 1978;14:1143–1147.

26. Chabner BA. Methotrexate. In: Chabner BA, ed. *Pharmacologic Principles of Cancer Treatment.* Philadelphia: Saunders; 1982:229–255.

27. Skipper HT, Schabel FM. Quantitative and cytokinetic studies in experimental tumor models. In: Holland JF, Frei E, eds. *Cancer Medicine,* 2nd edition. Philadelphia: Lea & Febiger; 1982:663–684.

28. Ernst P, Killmann S. Perturbation of generation cycle of human leukemic myeloblasts in vivo by methotrexate. *Blood.* 1971;38:689–705.

29. Goldman ID. Effects of methotrexate on cellular metabolism: Some critical elements in the drug–cell interactions. *Cancer Treat Rep.* 1977;61:549–557.

30. Chabner BA, Young RC. Threshold methotrexate concentration for in vivo inhibition of DNA synthesis in normal and tumorous target tissues. *J Clin Invest.* 1973;52:1804–1811.

31. Pinedo HM, Chabner BA. Role of drug concentration, duration of exposure, and endogenous metabolites in determining methotrexate cytotoxicity. *Cancer Treat Rep.* 1977;61:709–715.

32. Bleyer WA. New vistas for leucovorin in cancer chemotherapy. *Cancer.* 1989;63:995–1007.

33. Allegra CJ, Boarman D. Interaction of methotrexate polyglutamates and dihydrofolate during leucovorin rescue in a human breast cancer cell line (MCF-7). *Cancer Res.* 1990;50:3574–3578.

34. Goldin A, Venditti JM, Kline I, Mantel N. Eradication of leukaemic cells (LI210) by methotrexate and methotrexate plus citrovorum factor. *Nature.* 1966;212:1548–1550.

35. Pinedo HM, Zaharko DS, Bull JM, Chabner BA. The reversal of methotrexate cytotoxicity to mouse bone marrow cells by leucovorin and nucleosides. *Cancer Res.* 1976;36:4418–4424.

36. Bernard S, Etienne MC, Fishcel JL, et al. Critical factors for the reversal of methotrexate cytotoxicity by folinic acid. *Br J Cancer.* 1991;63:303–307.

37. Levitt M, Mosher MB, DeConti RC, et al. Improved therapeutic index of methotrexate with "leucovorin rescue." *Cancer Res.* 1973;33:1729–1734.

38. Capizzi RL, Deconti RC, Marsh JC, Bertino JR. Methotrexate therapy of head and neck cancer: Improvement in therapeutic index by the use of leucovorin "rescue." *Cancer Res.* 1970;30:1782–1788.

39. Djerassi I, Rominger CJ, Kim JS, et al. Phase I study of high doses of methotrexate with citrovorum factor in patients with lung cancer. *Cancer.* 1972;30:22–30.

40. McGuire BW, Sia LL, Haynes JD, et al. Absorption kinetics of orally administered leucovorin calcium. *Natl Cancer Inst Monogr.* 1987;5:47–56.

41. Priest DG, Schmitz, JC, Bunni MA, Stuart RD. Pharmacokinetics of leucovorin metabolites in human plasma as a function of dose administered orally and intravenously. *J Natl Cancer Inst.* 1991;83:1806–1812.

42. Mehta BM, Gisolfi AL, Hutchinson DJ, et al. Serum distribution of citrovorum factor and 5-methyltetrahydrofolate following oral and IM administration of calcium leucovorin in normal adults. *Cancer Treat Rep.* 1978;62;345–350.

43. Jaffe N, Frei E, Traggis D, Bishop Y. Adjuvant methotrexate and citrovorum-factor treatment of osteogenic sarcoma. *N Engl J Med.* 1974;7:994–997.

44. Jaffee N, Traggis D. Toxicity of high-dose methotrexate (NSC-740) and citrovorum factor (NSC-3590) in osteogenic sarcoma. *Cancer Chemother Rep.* 1975;6(pt 3):31–36.

45. Jaffe N, Keifer R, Robertson R, et al. Renal toxicity with cumulative doses of *cis*-diamminedichloroplatinum-II in pediatric patients with osteosarcoma. *Cancer.* 1987;59:1577–1581.

46. Jaffe N, Raymond K, Ayala A, et al. Analysis of the efficacy of intra-arterial *cis*-diamminedichloro-platinum-II and high-dose methotrexate with citrovorum factor rescue in the treatment of primary osteosarcoma. *Reg Cancer Treat.* 1989;2:157–163.

47. Adamson PC, Balis FM, McCully CL, et al. Rescue of experimental intrathecal methotrexate overdose with carboxypeptidase-G_2. *J Clin Oncol.* 1991;9:670–674.

48. Chabner BA, Johns DG, Bertino JR. Enzymatic cleavage of methotrexate provides a method for prevention of drug toxicity. *Nature.* 1972;239:395–397.

49. Teresi ME, Crom WR, Choi KE, et al. Methotrexate bioavailability after oral and intramuscular administration in children. *J Pediatr.* 1987;110:788–792.

50. Smith DK, Omura GA, Ostroy F. Clinical pharmacology of intermediate-dose oral methotrexate. *Cancer Chemother Pharmacol.* 1980;4:117–120.

51. Freeman-Narrod M, Gerstley BJ, Engstrom PF, et al. Comparison of serum concentrations of methotrexate after various routes of administration. *Cancer.* 1975;36:1619–1624.

52. Campbell MA, Perrier DG, Dorr RT, et al. Methotrexate: Bioavailability and pharmacokinetics. *Cancer Treat Rep.* 1985;69:833–838.

53. Chungi V, Bourne D, Dittert L. Drug absorption. VIII. Kinetics of GI absorption of methotrexate. *J Pharm Sci.* 1978;67:560–562.

54. Pinkerton CR, Welshman SG, Kelly JG, et al. Pharmacokinetics of low-dose methotrexate in children receiving maintenance therapy for acute lymphoblastic leukemia. *Cancer Chemother Pharmacol.* 1982;109:36–39.

55. Henderson ES, Adamson RH, Oliverio VT. The metabolic fate of tritiated methotrexate. II. Absorption and excretion in man. *Cancer Res.* 1965;25:1018–1024.

56. Kearney PJ, Light PA, Preece A, et al. Unpredictable serum levels after oral methotrexate in children with acute lymphoblastic leukaemia. *Cancer Chemother Pharmacol.* 1979;3:117–120.

57. Wan SH, Huffman DH, Azarnoff DL, et al. Effect of route of administration and effusions on methotrexate pharmacokinetics. *Cancer Res.* 1974;34:3487–3491.

58. Cohen MH, Creaven PJ, Fossieck BH, et al. Effect of oral prophylactic broad spectrum antibiotics on the GI absorption of nutrients and methotrexate in small cell bronchogenic carcinoma patients. *Cancer.* 1976;3:1556–1559.

59. Pinkerton CR, Glasgow JFT, Welshman SG, Bridges JM. Can food influence the absorption of methotrexate in children with acute lymphoblastic leukaemia? *Lancet.* 1980;2:944–945.

60. Balis FM, Jeffries SL, Lange B, et al. Chronopharmacokinetics of oral methotrexate and 6–mercaptopurine: Is there diurnal variation in the disposition of antileukemic therapy? *Am J Pediatr Hematol/Oncol.* 1989;11:324–326.

61. Balis FM, Mirro J, Reaman GH, et al. Pharmacokinetics of subcutaneous methotrexate. *J Clin Oncol.* 1988;6:1882–1886.

62. Pinkerton CR, Welshman SG, Bridges JM. Serum profiles of methotrexate after its administration in children with acute lymphoblastic leukemia. *Br J Cancer.* 1982;45:300–303.

63. El-Yazigi A, Amer M, Al-Saleh I, Martin C. Pharmacokinetics of methotrexate and its 7-OH metabolite in cancer patients treated with different high-dose methotrexate dosage regimens. *Int J Cancer.* 1986;38:795–800.

64. Paxton J. Protein binding of methotrexate in sera from normal human beings. *J Pharmacol Methods.* 1981;3:203–213.

65. Steele WH, Lawrence JR, Stewaft JFB, et al. The protein binding of methotrexate by the serum of normal subjects. *Eur J Clin Pharmacol.* 1979;15:363–366.

66. Borsi JD, Sagen E, Romslo I, Moe PJ. Comparative study on the pharmacokinetics of 7-hydroxy-methotrexate after administration of methotrexate in the dose range of 0.5–33.6 g/m^2 to children with acute lymphoblastic leukemia. *Med Pediatr Oncol.* 1990;18:217–224.

67. Shapiro WR, Young DG, Mehta BM. Methotrexate distribution in cerebrospinal fluid after intra-

venous, ventricular, and lumbar injections. *N Engl J Med.* 1975;293:161–166.

68. Fabre G, Fabare I, Matherly LH, et al. Synthesis and properties of 7-hydroxymethotrexate polyglutamyl derivatives in Ehrlich ascites tumor cells in vitro. *J Biol Chem.* 1984;259:5066–5072.

69. Evans WE, Stewart CF, Hutson PR, et al. Disposition of intermediate-dose methotrexate in children with acute lymphocytic leukemia. *Drug Intell Clin Pharm.* 1982;16:839–842.

70. Fabre I, Fabre G, Cano JP. 7-Hydroxymethotrexate cytotoxicity and selectivity in a human Burkitt's lymphoma cell line versus human granulocytic progenitor cells: Rescue by folinic acid and nucleosides. *Eur J Cancer Clin Oncol.* 1986;22:1247–1254.

71. Allegra CJ, Chabner BA, Drake JC, et al. Enhanced inhibition of thymidylate synthase by methotrexate polyglutamates. *J Biol Chem.* 1985;260:7105–7111.

72. Fabre G, Matherly LH, Favre R, et al. In vitro formation of polyglutamyl derivatives of methotrexate and 7-hydroxymethotrexate in human lymphoblastic leukemia cells. *Cancer Res.* 1983;43:4648–4652.

73. Wolfrom C, Hepp R, Hartmann R, Breithaupt H, Henze G. Pharmacokinetic study of methotrexate, folinic acid, and their serum metabolites in children treated with high-dose methotrexate and leucovorin rescue. *Eur J Clin Pharmacol.* 1990;39:377–383.

74. Breithaupt H, Kuenzlen E. Pharmacokinetics of methotrexate and 7-hydroxymethotrexate following infusion of high-dose methotrexate. *Cancer Treat Rep.* 1982;66:1733–1735.

75. Chan KK. Metabolism of methotrexate in man after high and conventional doses. *Res Commun Chem Pathol Pharmacol.* 1980;28:551–554.

76. Shamash J, Earl H, Souhami R. Acetazolamide for alkalinisation of urine in patients receiving high-dose methotrexate. *Cancer Chemother Pharmacol.* 1991;28:150–151.

77. Bleyer WA, Drake JC, Chabner BA. Neurotoxicity and elevated cerebrospinal-fluid methotrexate concentration in meningeal leukemia. *N Engl J Med.* 1973;289:770–773.

78. Evans WE, Tsiatis A, Crom WR, et al. Pharmacokinetics of sustained serum methotrexate concentrations secondary to gastrointestinal obstruction. *J Pharm Sci.* 1981;70:1194–1198.

79. Sauer H, Fuger K, Blumenstein M. Modulation of cytotoxicity of cytostatic drugs by hemodialysis in vitro and in vivo. *Cancer Treat Rev.* 1990;17:293–300.

80. Djerassi I, Ciesielka W, Kim JS. Removal of methotrexate by filtration-adsorption using charcoal filters or by hemodialysis. *Cancer Treat Rep.* 1977;61;751–752.

81. Hande KR, Balow JE, Drake JC, et al. Methotrexate and hemodialysis. *Ann Intern Med.* 1977;87:495–496.

82. Howell SB, Blair HE, Uren J, Frei E III. Hemodialysis and enzymatic cleavage of methotrexate in man. *Eur J Cancer.* 1978;14:787–792.

83. Thierry FX, Vernier I, Dueymes JM, et al. Acute renal failure after high-dose methothrexate therapy: Role of hemodialysis and plasma exchange in methotrexate removal. *Nephron.* 1989;51:416–417.

84. Ahmad S, Shen F, Bleyer WA. Methotrexate-induced renal failure and ineffectiveness of peritoneal dialysis. *Arch Intern Med.* 1978;138:1146–1147.

85. Relling MV, Stapleton B, Ochs J, et al. Removal of methotrexate, leucovorin, and their metabolites by combined hemodialysis and hemoperfusion. *Cancer.* 1988;62:884–888.

86. Grimes DJ, Bowles MR, Buttsworth JA, et al. Survival after unexpected high serum methotrexate concentrations in a patient with osteogenic sarcoma. *Drug Saf.* 1990;5:447–454.

87. Montagne N, Milano G, Caldani C, et al. Removal of methotrexate by hemofiltration. *Cancer Chemother Pharmacol.* 1989;24:400–401. Letter to the Editor.

88. Fleming RA, Eldridge RM, Johnson CE, Stewart CF. Disposition of high-dose methotrexate in an obese cancer patient. *Cancer.* 1991;68:1247–1250.

89. Frei E III, Blum RH, Pitman SW, et al. High dose methotrexate with leucovorin rescue. *Am J Med.* 1980;68:30–36.

90. Doyle LA, Berg C, Bottino G, et al. Erythema and desquamation after high-dose methotrexate. *Cancer.* 1984;53:611–612.

91. Abelson HT, Fosburg MT, Beardsly GP, et al. Methotrexate-induced renal impairment: Clinical studies and rescue from systemic toxicity with high-dose leucovorin and thymidine. *J Clin Oncol.* 1983;1:208–216.
92. Condit PT, Chanes RE, Joel W. Renal toxicity of methotrexate. *Cancer.* 1969;23:126–131.
93. Freeman-Narrod M, Kim JS, Ohanissian H, et al. The effect of high-dose methotrexate on renal tubules as indicated by urinary lysozyme concentrations. *Cancer.* 1982;50:2775–2779.
94. Dahl MGC, Gregory MM, Scheuer PF. Liver damage due to methotrexate in patients with psoriasis. *Br Med J.* 1971;1:625–630.
95. Oliff A, Bleyer W, Poplack D. Methotrexate-induced oral mucositis and salivary methotrexate concentrations. *Cancer Chemother Pharmacol.* 1979;2:225–226.
96. Doroshow JH, Locker GYU, Gaasterland DE, et al. Ocular irritation from high-dose methotrexate therapy: Pharmacokinetics of drug in the tear film. *Cancer.* 1981;48:2158–2162.
97. Baram J, Allegra CJ, Fine RL, Chabner BA. Effect of methotrexate on intracellular folate pools in purified myeloid precursor cells from normal human bone marrow. *J Clin Invest.* 1987;79:692–697.
98. Walker RW, Allen JC, Rosen G, Caparros B. Transient cerebral dysfunction secondary to high-dose methotrexate. *J Clin Oncol.* 1986;4:1845–1850.
99. Allen JC, Rosen G. Transient cerebral dysfunction following chemotherapy for osteogenic sarcoma. *Ann Neurol.* 1978;3:441–444.
100. Packer RJ, Grossman RJ, Belasco JB. High dose systemic methotrexate-associated acute neurologic dysfunction. *Med Pediatr Oncol.* 1983;11:159–161.
101. Fritsch G, Urgan C. Transient encephalopathy during the late course of treatment with high-dose methotrexate. *Cancer.* 1984;53:1849–1851.
102. Jaffe N, Takaue Y, Anzai T, et al. Transient neurological disturbances induced by high-dose methotrexate treatment. *Cancer.* 1985;56:1356–1360.
103. Allen JC, Rosen G, Mehta BM, Horten. Leukoencephalopathy following high-dose IV methotrexate chemotherapy with leucovorin rescue. *Cancer Treat Rep.* 1980;64:1261–1273.
104. Ettinger LJ. Pharmacokinetics and biochemical effects of a fatal intrathecal methotrexate overdose. *Cancer.* 1982;50:444–450.
105. Aur RJA, Simone JV, Hustu HO, et al. Central nervous system therapy and combination chemotherapy of childhood lymphocytic leukemia. *Blood.* 1971;37:272–281.
106. Aur RJA, Hustu O, Simone J. Leukoencephalopathy (LEP) in children with acute lymphocytic leukemia (ALL) receiving preventive central nervous system (CNS) therapy. *Proc Am Assoc Cancer Res.* 1976;17:386.
107. Bleyer WA. Neurologic sequelae of methotrexate and ionizing radiation: A new classification. *Cancer Treat Rep.* 1981;65(suppl 1):89–98.
108. Chan H, Evans WE, Pratt CB. Recovery from toxicity associated with high-dose methotrexate: Prognostic factors. *Cancer Treat Rep.* 1977;61:797–804.
109. Evans WE, Pratt CB, Taylor RH, et al. Pharmacokinetic monitoring of high-dose methotrexate. *Cancer Chemother Pharmacol.* 1979;3:161–166.
110. Bleyer WA. Clinical pharmacology of intrathecal methotrexate. II. An improved dosage regimen derived from age-related pharmacokinetics. *Cancer Treat Rep.* 1977;61:1419–1425.
111. Bleyer WA, Coccia PF, Sather HN, et al. Reduction in central nervous system leukemia with a pharmacokinetically derived intrathecal methotrexate dosage regimen. *J Clin Oncol.* 1983;1:317–325.
112. Stoller RG, Hande KR, Jacobs SA, et al. Use of plasma pharmacokinetics to predict and prevent methotrexate toxicity. *N Engl J Med.* 1977;297:630–634.
113. Evans, WE, Prattt CB, Taylor RH, et al. Pharmacokinetic monitoring of high-dose methotrexate: Early recognition of high-risk patients. *Cancer Chemother Pharmacol.* 1979;3:161–166.
114. Borsi JD, Sagen E, Romslo I, Moe PJ. Rescue after intermediate and high-dose methotrexate: Background, rationale, and current practice. *Pediatr Hematol Oncol.* 1990;7:347–363.

115. Perez C, Wang YM, Sutow WW, Herson J. Significance of the 48-hour plasma level in high-dose methotrexate regimens. *Cancer Clin Trials.* 1978;1:107–111.
116. Nirenberg A, Mosende C, Mehta BM, et al. High-dose methotrexate with citrovorum factor rescue: Predictive value of serum methotrexate concentrations and corrective measures to avert toxicities. *Cancer Treat Rep.* 1977;61:1393–1396.
117. Furst DE, Herman RA, Koehnke R, et al. Effect of aspirin and sulindac on methotrexate clearance. *J Pharm Sci.* 1990;79:782–786.
118. Liegler DG, Henderson ES, Hahn MA, et al. The effect of organic acids on renal clearance of methotrexate in man. *Clin Pharmacol Ther.* 1969;10:849–857.
119. Aherne GW, Piall E, Marks V, et al. Prolongation and enhancement of serum methotrexate concentrations by probenecid. *Br Med J.* 1978;1:1097–1099.
120. Kates RE, Tozer TN. Biliary secretion of methotrexate in rats and its inhibition by probenecid. *J Pharm Sci.* 1976;65:1348–1352.
121. Bourke RS, Cheda G, Bremer A, et al. Inhibition of renal tubular transport of methotrexate by probenecid. *Cancer Res.* 1975;34:110–116.
122. Cohen MH, Creaven PJ, Fossieck BE, et al. Effect of oral prophylactic broad spectrum nonabsorbable antibiotics on the gastrointestinal absorption of nutrients and methotrexate in small cell bronchogenic carcinoma patients. *Cancer.* 1976;38:1556–1559.
123. Ferrazzini G, Klein J, Suhl H, et al. Interaction between trimethoprim–sulfamethoxazole and methotrexate in children with leukemia. *J Pediatr.* 1990;117:823–826.
124. Thyss A, Milano G, Kubar J, et al. Clinical and pharmacokinetic evidence of a life-threatening interaction between methotrexate and ketoprofen. *Lancet.* 1986;1:256–258.
125. Maiche AG. Acute renal failure to concomitant action of methotrexate and indomethacin. *Lancet.* 1986;1:1390.
126. Mandel MA. The synergistic effect of salicylates on methotrexate toxicity. *Plast Reconstr Surg.* 1976;57:733.
127. Dean R, Nachman J, Lorenzana AN. Possible methotrexate–mezlocillin interaction. *Am J Pediatr Hematol/Oncol.* 1992;14:88–92. Letter to the Editor.
128. Bertino JR, Sawicki WL, Lindquist C, et al. Schedule-dependent anti-tumor effects of methotrexate and 5–fluorouracil. *Cancer Res.* 1977;27:327–328.
129. Coates AS, Tattersall MHN, Swanson C, et al. Combination therapy with methotrexate and 5-fluorouracil: A prospective randomized clinical trial of order of administration. *J Clin Oncol.* 1984;2:756–761.
130. Crom WR, Pratt CB, Green AA, et al. The effect of prior cisplatin therapy on the pharmacokinetics of high-dose methotrexate. *J Clin Oncol.* 1984;2:655–661.
131. Erttmann R, Landbeck. Effect of oral cholestyramine on the elimination of high-dose methotrexate. *J Cancer Res Clin Oncol.* 1985;110:48–50.
132. Gadgil SD, Damle SR, Advani SH, Vaidya AB. Effect of activated charcoal on the pharmacokinetics of high-dose methotrexate. *Cancer Treat Rep.* 1982;66:1169–1171.

Chapter 18

Theophylline

Joseph S. Bertino, Jr.

Keep in Mind

- Theophylline is a methylxanthine, the mechanism of action of which is most likely adenosine antagonism, not inhibition of phosphodiesterase.

- Theophylline pharmacokinetics are very variable. Gender, age, smoking status, hepatic disease, cardiac disease, and numerous drug interactions can affect drug clearance.

- Oral absorption of theophylline, in general, is very efficient, with bioavailability averaging above 90% except for the ultraslow-release formulations.

- Theophylline is metabolized primarily by the liver, under control of the mixed-function oxidase system.

- The therapeutic range is probably 5 to 15 μg/mL, with some individuals needing higher or lower serum concentrations to attain therapeutic effect while minimizing toxic effects. In many patients with reversible airway disease, theophylline provides less than maximal bronchodilation.

- Current recommended use of theophylline in the treatment of asthma is limited based on controlled trials of other modalities such as aerosolized beta agonists in the acute treatment of asthma and cromolyn sodium in the prophylaxis of chronic reversible airway disease. Still, theophylline accounts for 1 billion dollars in drug sales in the United States yearly.

- Theophylline has a number of significant adverse effects, including tachycardia and cardiac arrhythmias, metabolic abnormalities, tremors, nausea, vomiting, behavioral disorders in children, and, rarely, seizures.

- Theophylline dosing must be individualized to reflect pharmacokinetic differences in patients. Although average loading doses (in theophylline-naive patients or in those patients with serum concentrations < 5 μg/mL) are generally about 5 mg/kg IV infused over a 20- to 30-minute period, maintenance dosing is dependent on drug clearance. Conversion of oral therapy is generally done on a 1:1 basis; however, dosage adjustments may be necessary because of reduced bioavailability of the ultraslow-release preparations.

- Theophylline is rarely a first-line therapy for reversible airway disease. Careful clinical monitoring should be coupled with the judicious use of therapeutic drug monitoring to optimize therapy.

CLINICAL PHARMACOLOGY AND THERAPEUTICS

Theophylline (1,3-dimethylxanthine) is a naturally occurring alkaloid, structurally related to caffeine and theobromine (Figure 18–1). Pharmaceutically, theophylline is poorly soluble in water (8 mg/mL at 25°C solubility). The lipophilicity of theophylline is the primary factor determining the absorption of the compound.[1]

A number of theophylline salts are available and all are synthetically prepared. Aminophylline (theophylline ethylenediamine) is a water-soluble form of theophylline that is converted to the parent compound in vivo. The theophylline content of aminophylline is approximately 85%. Oxtriphylline is a choline salt of theophylline containing approximately 64% theophylline. Theophylline calcium and theophylline sodium glycinate are two additional forms of theophylline that are commercially available.

Theophylline exhibits a number of pharmacologic actions in humans. The pharmacologic effects of theophylline have numerous explanations on a cellular basis. The first possible action is the effect of theophylline on the translocation of intracellular calcium. As theophylline concentrations well above the usually stated therapeutic range of 10 to 20 µg/mL are required to elicit this effect, this explanation is relatively unlikely.[2] The second postulated mechanism of theophylline effect is inhibition of phosphodiesterase with the resultant accumulation of the cyclic nucleotide adenosine monophosphate (cAMP). Although this had been a popular theory to explain the mechanism of action of theophylline, concentrations far exceeding the normal

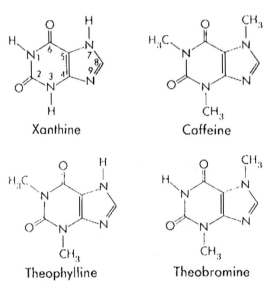

Figure 18–1. Structures of methylxanthine compounds. (*From Rall TW. Drugs used in the treatment of asthma. The methylxanthines, cromolyn sodium, and other agents. In: Goodman, Gilman A, Rall TW, eds. The Pharmacologic Basis of Therapeutics. 8th ed. New York: Pergamon Press; 1990:619, with permission.*)

range are required to elicit this effect and, thus, this theory is most likely not a valid explanation. Potentiation of prostaglandin synthesis and reduction of uptake or metabolism of catecholamines have also been postulated.[3-5] Unfortunately at this time, only limited data are available to support these mechanisms of action. A possible explanation for the cellular basis of theophylline action is blockade of adenosine receptors.[6] Theophylline acts as a competitive antagonist on both types of adenosine receptors within the therapeutic range (Figure 18–2). As adenosine receptors are found ubiquitously throughout the body, this may explain the multifactorial pharmacologic nature of theophylline.[2] It is important, however, to note that enprofylline, also a xanthine analog, does not bind to the high–affinity adenosine receptor as does theophylline, but is significantly more potent than theophylline (Figure 18–2).[7] This information may raise questions as to whether adenosine antagonism is truly the primary mechanism of theophylline's pharmacologic effects.

The pharmacologic effects of theophylline can be categorized as affecting a number of various organ systems.

Central Nervous System

Theophylline has been reported to cause a variety of central nervous system effects. In usual clinical doses, anxiety, tremors, insomnia, nervousness, headache, and nausea with or without

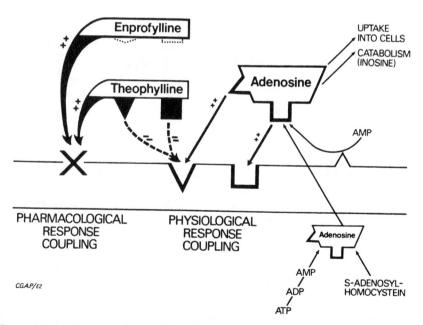

Figure 18–2. Some aspects on adenosine and xanthine are schematically depicted. (*From Persson CGA. Overview of effects of theophylline. J Allergy Clin Immunol. 1986;78:780–787, with permission.*)

vomiting have been reported.[2,7] Respiratory stimulation of the medullary centers is also seen, a pharmacologic effect that is used in treating the apnea of prematurity[8] and presumably chronic obstructive lung disease.[9,10] Another adverse central nervous system effect of theophylline is the reported association of the drug with adverse psychologic or behavioral performance.[11] Although concern for this adverse effect in children has been raised, it has been pointed out that many of the reports published on this subject have major flaws in research methodology which would negate their results.[12–14] Two additional controlled trials appear to dispute the finding that theophylline affects behavior or limits academic performance.[15,16] Finally, seizures are reported with theophylline use, with occurrences seen even in the usual stated therapeutic range.[17,18] This toxic adverse effect is covered in more detail under Adverse Effects.

Cardiovascular System

Theophylline exhibits some significant effects on the cardiovascular system which result in therapeutic and toxic effects. Ogilive et al reported increases in heart rate and contractile force with corresponding decrease in cardiac preload with theophylline concentrations in the range 10 to 20 μg/mL.[19] Although this increase in cardiac output is brief in individuals with normal cardiovascular function, this effect is more prolonged in patients with heart failure.[2] Theophylline also reduces pulmonary artery pressure and pulmonary vascular resistance, lowers right and left ventricular end-diastolic pressure, and increases right and left ventricular ejection fraction in patients with chronic obstructive pulmonary disease (COPD).[10]

Kidneys

Theophylline has long been known to increase urine production and enhance excretion of water and electrolytes in a manner similar to that of thiazide diuretics.[20] This effect, however, is transient in nature and does not seem to be secondary to increases in glomerular filtration rate or renal blood flow.[2,21] The administration of theophylline may provide additional diuretic action when combined with a loop diuretic in patients with congestive heart failure.[2]

Gastrointestinal Tract

The increase in gastric acid and pepsin secretion caused by theophylline has been well demonstrated.[22] One potential mechanism for this effect is the blockade of adenosine action (an antisecretory action) on the parietal cell.[2] In addition, theophylline has been shown to cause relaxation of the gastroesophageal sphincter.[7]

Lungs

A number of direct and indirect pulmonary effects have been attributed to theophylline. Although originally it was thought that theophylline improves mucociliary transport in patients, this effect has not been well demonstrated.[10] Theophylline enhances diaphragmatic contractility and resistance to developing fatigue of the respiratory muscles.[10] Generally, however, these pharmacologic effects occur at concentrations well above the usual stated therapeutic range; thus, in patients with chronic obstructive pulmonary disease, the improvement in ventilatory function is limited.[10] Also of note, this strengthening of diaphragmatic contractility as a result of theophylline has led to the recommendation that the drug be used to assist in weaning patients off the ventilator[23]; however, no study in adult ventilated patients has been performed to substantiate this. Theophylline also causes bronchodilation and dilation of pulmonary arterioles and increases pulmonary blood flow.

Miscellaneous Effects

A number of additional pharmacologic effects have been shown for theophylline. These include attenuation of erythropoietin production,[24] reduction in liver plasma flow,[25] small and transient increases in cortisol clearance,[26] rises in serum free fatty acids,[27,28] and potentiation of insulin release.[28] Theophylline is not known to be teratogenic.

Theophylline exhibits many pharmacologic effects in humans. Although adenosine antagonism is the proposed mechanism of action, some effects, such as its pulmonary antiasthma actions, may not be mediated by adenosine antagonism. An understanding of the pharmacologic effects of theophylline will assist the reader in better understanding the toxic side effects of the agent.

CLINICAL PHARMACOKINETICS

Despite the fact that the pharmacokinetics of theophylline have been extensively studied, numerous studies continue to be published in this area. This section attempts to summarize the major points of the published pharmacokinetic studies (Table 18–1).

TABLE 18–1. AVERAGE THEOPHYLLINE PHARMACOKINETIC PARAMETERS IN VARIOUS POPULATIONS

Population	Volume of Distribution (L/kg)	Total Body Clearance (mL/min/kg)
Neonates[a]	0.69 ± 0.95	0.29–0.8
Children		
1–9 y	0.3–0.7[b]	1.45
9–12 y	0.3–0.7[b]	1.15
Adolescents (12–16 y)	0.3–0.7[b]	0.9
Adults		
Smokers	0.3–0.7[b]	1.2
Nonsmokers	0.3–0.7[b]	0.9
Congestive heart failure, cor pulmonale	0.48–1.2	0.36
Cirrhosis	0.45–0.64	0.36

[a] Clearance depends on gestational age, degree of hepatic function maturation, and postbirth age.
[b] Average = 0.45 L/kg.

Absorption

Theophylline is currently available in a number of dosage forms. These forms include a parenteral preparation (theophylline ethylenediamine or aminophylline); oral solutions and suspensions; oral rapid-release tablets and sustained-release tablets, capsules, and granules; and rectal solutions and suppositories. This chapter does not discuss rectal administration of theophylline, as the author believes that rectal use of theophylline should be very rare. Oral theophylline solutions are considered nearly 100% bioavailable, with no significant differences being noted between the area under the curve for oral solutions and syrups versus intravenously administered doses.[29,30] This high rate of oral bioavailability suggests that no significant first-pass metabolism occurs. The average time to peak reported with the oral hydroalcoholic solution is 1.6 hours; that for the oral syrup preparation is 1.8 to 2.7 hours.[29,30] Our own data suggest a time to peak of 0.6 to 0.9 hour with theophylline hydroalcoholic solution (unpublished data). Oral theophylline tablets can be as highly bioavailable as the liquid preparations; however, great variations exist in the percentage absorbed of various solid rapid-release preparations.[30] Peak concentrations of oral non-enteric-coated tablets occur generally 1.2 to 2.0 hours after administration, reflecting the dissolution step needed for the tablets to be absorbed.[30] The concurrent ingestion of food or magnesium-containing antacids or an increase in dosage may reduce the rate but not the extent of theophylline absorption.[30–32] Other authors, however, have not found a consistent effect of magnesium- and aluminum-containing antacids on the absorption rate, lag time, time to peak concentration, or peak concentration for aminophylline tablets or the slow-release product Theo-Dur.[33]

Enteric-coated formulations of theophylline, although originally prepared to reduce the perceived direct gastrointestinal irritant effect, show reduced bioavailability and unpredictability in their absorption and should be avoided.[30,34]

Sustained-release (or controlled-release) theophylline preparations have been extensively marketed and used over the last three decades. Currently, more than a dozen preparations listed as sustained release are available in various dosage strengths. The advantages of these preparations lie in their attempt to "mimic" a constant infusion of theophylline by releasing theophylline in a slow continuous fashion for absorption from the gastrointestinal tract into the systemic circulation. This results in the ability to use less frequent dosing in certain patient populations, with the goal of increasing compliance,[35] and in the smaller peak-to-trough variations in theophylline concentrations (ie, 4–9 µg/mL over the dosing interval). The disadvantages lie in the potential for reduced bioavailability with these very slow release products,[36] as well as toxic effects due to disruption in the absorption characteristics of these slow-release products.[37] Generally, the sustained-release preparations of theophylline are bead-filled capsules or "packets" of drug embedded in a compressed tablet. The bead-filled capsules get their sustained-release characteristics by the use of varying thicknesses of coating, with the thinner coating dissolving at a faster rate than the beads with thicker coating. The drug-embedded tablets make use of an initial release of drug from the outer layer with either sustained-release beads or a slow-erosion core design.[38]

A number of issues must be considered when discussing sustained-release theophylline preparations. First, these preparations do not truly mimic a constant intravenous infusion, as drug is not released over the entire dosing interval in a zero-order fashion. Second, it is exceptionally difficult to determine the elimination rate of theophylline using a sustained-release preparation because absorption may continue for a prolonged period, making determination of the terminal portion of the elimination curve difficult to identify.[38] Third, complete bioavailability cannot be reliably obtained based on the pharmaceutical formulation and the sustained-release characteristics of the product.[38] It has become evident that the ultraslow sustained-release products such as Theo-24 and Uniphyl have significantly less bioavailability (80 and 67% bioavailability in one trial) versus products that are still sustained release but not of the ultraslow variety (Theo-Dur) or versus rapid-release products.[39] The presumed reason for this reduced bioavailability of the ultraslow-release preparations is the inability to retain the product in the gastrointestinal tract for complete absorption to take place. Fourth, the ability of the concurrent ingestion of food to affect the absorption characteristics of these sustained-release theophylline preparations is evident. In an excellent review, Jonkman noted that food had a variable effect on the rate and extent of absorption of various sustained-release theophylline products (Table 18–2).[40] The classic example of how food can affect the absorption of sustained-release theophylline was illustrated in the study of the ultraslow-release preparation Theo-24 by Hendeles et al.[41] These authors showed that administration of Theo-24 with a high-fat meal resulted in substantial increases in the 4-hour percentage of drug absorbed along with the extent of absorption. These data were confirmed by Karim et al.[42]

Another factor that has been shown to affect sustained-release theophylline absorption is circadian rhythm. Day–night differences exist in absorption, with higher peak concentrations and faster time to peak concentration being seen with morning dosing as opposed to evening dosing.[43]

TABLE 18–2. SUMMARY OF THE EFFECTS OF FOOD ON VARIOUS THEOPHYLLINE FORMULATIONS

Product	Rate of Absorption	Extent of Absorption
Solution	—[a]	—
12-h Preparations		
Sabidal	—	0
Slo-Bid Gyrocaps	− −	0
Somophyllin CRT	—	0
Theobid Duracap	0	0
Theo-Dur	− −	0
Theo-Dur Sprinkle	− − −	− − −
Theograd	—	+++
Theolair SR	− − −	—
24-h Preparations		
Dilatrane AP	—	+
Euphylong	—	—
Theo-24	+++	+++
Uniphyl	—	++

[a]0 = no effect, −/+ = slight decrease/increase (not clinically relevant); − −/++ = moderate decrease/increase; − − −/+++ = significant decrease/increase (clinically relevant).
From Jonkman JHG. Food interactions with sustained release theophylline preparations. A review. *Clin Pharmacokinet.* 1989;16:162–179, with permission.

In summary, sustained-release theophylline preparations offer dosing convenience to patients. Generally, the use of these products on a twice-daily dosing schedule will result in less peak-to-trough variations than the use of these preparations once daily, even if the product is labeled for once-daily use. Patients with rapid elimination half-lives (ie, ≤ 5 hours) or those requiring serum concentrations above 10 μg/mL may have greater therapeutic effect by dosing of these agents at least twice a day. Food effect is a real concern; thus, patients should be carefully instructed in how to take the medication and when to take it.[44] Finally, the ultraslow-release preparations such as Uniphyl and Theo-24 may show incomplete absorption because of movement of the preparation through the gastrointestinal tract before absorption is complete.

Distribution

Approximately 40% of theophylline is protein bound in humans. Following an intravenous dose, distribution is complete within 60 minutes.[45] Theophylline distributes into body water with a volume of distribution ($V_{d,ss}$) in adults ranging from 0.3 to 0.7 L/kg (average, 0.4–0.45).[45,46] In children, the volume of distribution also approaches 0.45 L/kg.[45] Larger volumes of distribution have been reported in premature newborns and in patients with hepatic cirrhosis and uncorrected acidemia.[45]

The volume of distribution of theophylline in obesity has been controversial, as it will determine whether dosing will be on the basis of ideal or total body weight. Gal et al showed that volume of distribution averaged 0.38 L/kg total body weight (TBW) for obese subjects compared with 0.48 L/kg TBW for normal-body-size subjects.[47] When comparing volumes of distribution using ideal body weight (IBW), a value of 0.77 L/kg for obese subjects versus 0.52 L/kg for normal subjects was reported. These data led the authors to suggest that loading doses of theophylline be based on TBW and maintenance doses on IBW. Two additional studies by Rohrbaugh et al[48] and Zell et al,[49] however, contradicted the findings of Gal et al, suggesting that theophylline does not distribute into adipose tissue. The data of Zell et al suggested a significant difference in volumes of distribution using TBW (0.39 L/kg) versus IBW (0.48 L/kg).[49] These authors suggested that the use of TBW for theophylline dosing may result in significant overdosing of the drug. Jewesson and Ensom suggested that neither TBW nor IBW could accurately predict volume of distribution for theophylline.[50] As the place of theophylline in therapy, along with the proposed therapeutic range, has changed since the majority of these studies were performed, it is probably judicious to use IBW for calculation of both the initial loading and maintenance doses of the drug.

Metabolism and Elimination

The major metabolic pathways for theophylline were originally discovered in the 1950s (Figure 18–3).[51,52] It has been clearly shown that three major pathways for elimination exist in adults. The first major pathway is the renal excretion of unchanged theophylline. This accounts for 5 to 15% of drug elimination.[53–55] Renal theophylline elimination is dependent on urine flow rate and is linear at rates up to 3 mL/min.[53,54]

Theophylline is metabolized primarily by the liver but exhibits nonliver blood flow-dependent characteristics. Research has shown that the enzyme P450IA2 appears to be mainly responsible for theophylline metabolism.[56] Although some data suggests that P450IA2 is responsible

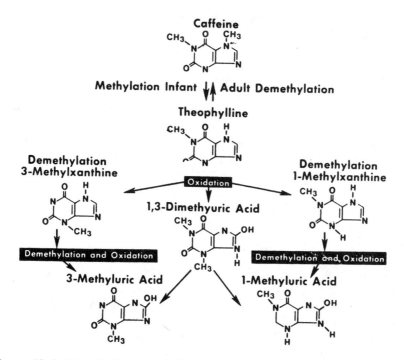

Figure 18–3. Theophylline metabolism in humans. (*From Haley TJ. Metabolism and pharmacokinetics of theophylline in human neonates, children and adults.* Drug Metab Rev. *1983;14:295–335.*)

for demethylation of theophylline, other data have shown that hydroxylation of theophylline to 1,3-dimethyluric acid (DMU) can also be mediated by this enzyme system.[57] Other in vitro data suggest that P450IA2 can both demethylate and hydroxylate theophylline, whereas P4502E1 has been shown in vitro only to hydroxylate theophylline.[58]

The second major pathway of theophylline metabolism as shown in Figure 18–3 is hydroxylation of the parent compound to DMU. This reaction proceeds by the mixed-function oxidase system (MFOS). In single-dose intravenous studies, DMU accounts for 35 to 45% of the molar dose of the drug recovered in the urine.[55,59,60] As any drug that undergoes metabolism through an enzyme-mediated system can exhibit nonlinear pharmacokinetics,[61] it is not surprising that theophylline shows dose-dependent pharmacokinetics. The data of Tang-Liu et al clearly showed that the formation pathway of DMU is saturable[54]; however, of the three major metabolic pathways involved with theophylline metabolism, the enzyme(s) responsible for DMU formation has a large capacity and a low affinity.[59] Data from other authors have substantiated this finding.[60] This suggests that elimination of theophylline by this pathway may follow a parallel zero- and first-order process. Thus, nonlinearity is not commonly seen in this pathway.

The third major pathway for theophylline metabolism is N-demethylation by the MFOS. The result of these pathways of elimination are the formation of two metabolites: 1-methylxanthine (1MX), which is further converted to 1-methyluric acid (1MU), possibly by xanthine oxidase,[62] and 3-methylxanthine (3MX). 1MU accounts for 20 to 25% of the molar quantity of theophylline excreted in the urine.[55,59,60] 3MX accounts for 13 to 17% of the molar quantity of theophylline in the urine.[55,59,60] It is unclear whether the same enzyme metabolizes theophylline to 1MX and 3MX.[63] More likely, the formation of these two different metabolites is mediated by different enzymes. These two demethylation pathways have been shown to be saturable in the therapeutic range, much more so than DMU formation.[59] In addition, the renal clearance of all of the metabolites is substantially higher than their metabolic formation and higher than the glomerular filtration rate, suggesting a renal secretory mechanism for metabolite elimination.[59]

The clinical implications of the finding of nonlinearity are important yet somewhat unclear. A number of authors have shown that total clearance of theophylline may decrease over time[64–66]; however, single-repeat-dose data from one of the same groups suggests stability of theophylline elimination rate.[67] These clinical trials generally were retrospective observations concerning nonlinear changes in presumed steady-state serum theophylline concentrations at different dosage levels.[65] This raises the question whether the zero-order kinetics that may govern some aspects of theophylline metabolism could potentially result in a substantial rise in serum concentrations with small dosage increases. It is, however, difficult to separate the results of a zero-order pharmacokinetic process from the other multitude of factors known to affect the clearance of the drug. In fact, the overall clearance process for theophylline appears to be linear, even though some of the metabolic pathways are nonlinear.[59] This difficulty in interpretation and application of the data leads to the recommendation to proceed cautiously with theophylline dosage adjustments (see Therapeutic Regimen Design).

A minor conversion pathway for theophylline in adult human beings is a methylation reaction to produce caffeine. This reaction probably occurs to a very minute extent with the resulting compound rapid metabolized to other minor metabolites.

The metabolic pathways seen for theophylline in neonates differ significantly from those in adults. Whereas in adults, conversion of theophylline to caffeine through a methylation reaction may occur with rapid conversion to caffeine metabolites to a minor extent, this reaction is an important conversion route in neonates.[68–71] Neonates excrete theophylline primarily as unchanged drug, caffeine, DMU, and 1MU. This pattern changes with increasing postconception age, however. At 28 to 32 weeks postconception, caffeine accounts for approximately 10% of the excreted dose, DMU for 20%, 1MU for 9%, 3MX for 0.5%, and unchanged theophylline for 60% (urinary metabolites).[69] By 38 to 42 weeks postconception, caffeine accounts for 10%, theobromine for 2%, DMU for 34%, 1MU for 12%, and theophylline for 43% of the urinary metabolites.[71] Thus, it appears that the oxidative metabolism system is substantially more active than the N-demethylation systems in the neonate. These drug metabolism pathways appear to mature rapidly, however, with metabolic patterns similar to those of adults by 1 year of age.[65]

Theophylline is secreted in breast milk, attaining concentrations approximately 70% of serum concentrations. No serious adverse effects have been reported in breastfed infants of mothers taking theophylline.

Elimination by Outside Pathways

Bauer et al have shown that theophylline pharmacokinetics in patients with acute and chronic renal failure are not significantly different from those in control patients.[72] An additional question relates to the effects of peritoneal and hemodialysis on theophylline elimination. Lee et al showed that intermittent peritoneal dialysis was an ineffective method of theophylline removal as compared with hemodialysis, which removed 40% of a dose.[73] As patients tend to receive hemodialysis three times weekly, the removal of this amount of theophylline during hemodialysis may decrease serum concentrations of the drug.[74] The amount of drug removed depends on the dialyzer used and the length of dialysis.[74] This author, however, believes that by dosing theophylline immediately following hemodialysis, the effect on serum concentration will be small and the postdialysis dose should raise the serum concentration adequately. The effect of continuous ambulatory peritoneal dialysis (CAPD) has been described in a limited sample of patients.[75] No substantial effect of CAPD on theophylline elimination was seen.

Normal Versus Special Populations

The pharmacokinetics of theophylline have been studied in numerous individuals with various characteristics. The author attempts to summarize these data here.

Normal Males and Females

Theophylline pharmacokinetics in normal men and women without any underlying diseases or concurrent pathophysiology differ according to smoking status and gender. Table 18–3 illustrates the average pharmacokinetic values for these groups. As is illustrated in Table 18–3, significant differences exist between smokers and nonsmokers in terms of more rapid elimination and clearance of theophylline. Significantly faster clearances and shorter half-lives exist between premenopausal women and men, regardless of smoking status for theophylline.[46,55] The reasons for these differences are not currently understood, but this has been shown in two studies with adequate numbers of subjects to detect a difference. In addition, intracycle differences in theophylline pharmacokinetics have been shown for premenopausal women at various points in the menstrual cycle.[75] These changes translate into total body clearances that are 60% faster at day 0 of the menstrual cycle compared with day 20. Unfortunately, many studies reported in the literature have not controlled for gender or menstrual cycle timing and, thus, have given the impression that no gender differences exist for theophylline pharmacokinetics. This is most likely not the case.

TABLE 18–3. CLINICAL PHARMACOKINETICS OF THEOPHYLLINE IN VARIOUS NORMAL POPULATIONS

Group	Serum Half-life (h)	Volume of Distribution	Clearance (mL/min/1.73 m²)
Nonsmokers			
Males	9.3 ± 0.9	0.41 ± 0.01	37.4 ± 4.0
Females	6.0 ± 1.8	0.34 ± 0.01	43.8 ± 6.4
Smokers			
Males	6.9 ± 1.6	0.38 ± 0.01	53.1 ± 9.4
Females	4.6 ± 0.9	0.37 ± 0.03	64.2 ± 10.6

Source. Data were taken from Reference 55.

The effect of smoking on the metabolism of theophylline has been well described.[75–81] Smokers exhibit a greater clearance as well as a shorter half-life than nonsmokers.[76] In addition, a gender-related effect is seen, with female smokers having a significantly shorter half-life and greater clearance of theophylline than male smokers.[46,55] The explanation for this increased clearance of theophylline in smokers can be explained by the increases in the clearance of the products of both demethylation and oxidation. In fact, significant differences in the clearances of DMU, 1MU, and 3MX are seen in smokers versus nonsmokers.[77–80] In addition, marijuana smoking has also been shown to increase the clearance of theophylline.[81] A partial return to non-smoking metabolic status has been shown (in men only) following 1 week of smoking abstinence.[82]

Reports of age-related metabolic differences in the metabolism of theophylline have been controversial.[83–85] Fox et al reported a faster elimination half-life and greater total body clearance in elderly subjects (> 60 years old) versus subjects younger than 60 years; however, no gender or smoking effect was noted in the elderly patients.[83] Randolph et al reported higher area under the curve (AUC) values in patients 55 to 70 years old versus younger adult subjects.[84] Jackson et al noted that theophylline clearance does not fall with increasing age until after the age of 70.[85] These studies contrast with reports in patients with pulmonary (and possibly) cardiovascular disease that note reduced clearance of theophylline in older patients.[86] The most likely explanation for the difference in theophylline pharmacokinetics between older patients with COPD and those without is the underlying disease, which results in reduction in drug clearance with dosage reduction necessary simply due to age.

On the other end of the age scale, neonates and children show remarkably different theophylline pharmacokinetics than do adults. Neonates, as discussed above, have impaired rates of theophylline metabolism and thus half-lives in the range 10 to 30 hours can be seen depending on gestational age.[68] Children over the age of 1 year can have half-lives as rapid as 2.5 to 4 hours, requiring frequent dosing.[87]

In a small trial of five women studied throughout pregnancy, Frederiksen et al noted an increase in theophylline half-life during the last trimester of pregnancy compared with the second trimester.[88] The true effect of pregnancy on theophylline pharmacokinetics in a large population is not known.

Disease States

As metabolism of theophylline is not dependent on liver blood flow, the reader could postulate that disease states that reduce liver blood flow should not significantly affect theophylline metabolism. This, however, is not the case, most likely because of the reduction in MFOS activity in states of reduced liver blood flow.

Patients with acute cardiogenic pulmonary edema (and acute congestive heart failure) show half-lives averaging 23 hours versus 6.7 hours in normal subjects.[89] Cusack et al, studying hypoxic patients with COPD, have shown that even after 48 hours of oxygen therapy, substantial reductions in theophylline clearance occur.[90]

The effect of chronic congestive heart failure on theophylline elimination has also been studied. Bauer et al noted a 50% reduction in theophylline clearance in patients with severe heart failure versus those with no heart failure.[72] This finding was also reported by Jusko et al.[91]

The effect of hepatic cirrhosis on the elimination of theophylline is a reduction in drug elimination. Piafsky et al noted a mean half-life of 25.6 hours in cirrhotic patients as compared with normal subjects, who had a mean 6.7-hour half-life.[92] Mangione et al reported similar findings.[93] In both studies, theophylline clearance was significantly reduced in cirrhotic patients.

Another disease state in which theophylline clearance is altered is cystic fibrosis. Isles et al have shown a half-life reduction of 37%, with an increase in the volume of distribution of 34% and a doubling of mean clearance, in adults with cystic fibrosis compared with normal controls.[94]

It seems clear that the administration of influenza vaccine, either as a split-virus preparation or as a whole-virus preparation, does not result in reduction in the elimination of theophylline in humans.[95,96] Acute viral illness, however, can reduce theophylline elimination, most likely as a result of the production of interferon, which inactivates the MFOS system.[97–99] More recent data, however, suggest that infection with respiratory syncytial virus, in children, does not reduce the clearance of theophylline.[100] It appears that the effect of acute viral illness is variable; thus, serum theophylline concentrations should be monitored in patients with acute viral illness.

PHARMACODYNAMICS

Drug–Drug Interactions

There is virtually an unlimited amount of information concerning drug interactions with theophylline. It is suggested that the reader consult the comprehensive review on theophylline drug interactions by Upton.[101,102] This chapter highlights significant drug–drug interactions.

Moricizine

Data concerning the antiarrhythmic agent moricizine have shown an increase in the clearance of theophylline of 20 to 40%, most likely as a result of enzyme induction.[103] It should, however, be noted that these studies were performed in normal males only. Animal studies suggest that this interaction is a result of an inhibition of conversion of theophylline to DMU and 1MU, thus indicating that both demethylation and hydroxylation are inhibited.

Rifampin

The majority of trials have suggested that rifampin acts to increase theophylline clearance and elimination in humans. The usual dosage employed in the trials was 600 mg daily. Generally, all trials have used healthy male volunteers. Straughn et al noted a mean increase in the elimination rate constant of 25% with rifampin treatment.[104] Adebayo et al reported an increase in theophylline clearance of 100% with rifampin.[105]

Oral Contraceptives

A number of trials have examined the effect of oral contraceptives on theophylline metabolism. Studies by Gardner et al[106] and Tornatore et al[107] showed theophylline clearances being reduced by approximately 30% in smoking and nonsmoking women receiving oral contraceptives.

Macrolide Antibiotics

The effect of macrolide antibiotics on the pharmacokinetics of theophylline is confusing. Generally, many of the available studies suffer from small sample size; use of varying dosages, durations of therapy, and salts of erythromycin; and inclusion of only men in the trials. In these investigations, if an effect of erythromycin on theophylline metabolism is reported, it is a reduction in clearance of 5 to 13%.[101] Erythromycin inhibits cytochrome P4503A4 but not P450IA2, which is thought to be responsible for theophylline metabolism. It is therefore difficult to surmise how this metabolic inhibition of theophylline by erythromycin may occur. One group of authors has suggested that if P4503A4 is involved with theophylline metabolism (hydroxylation to DMU), this interaction could be explained.[108] P4503A4 has been shown in vitro to hydroxylate theophylline to a small extent, but may not be the main hydroxylating enzyme.[58] These clinical trials in normal subjects contrast with reports in patients receiving theophylline and erythromycin salts for infectious diseases where theophylline toxicity has been reported to occur. As these reports are variable, patients should be monitored for theophylline toxicity when receiving erythromycin, if for no other reason than the possible reduction in theophylline clearance secondary to acute infections.

Troleandomycin (TAO), a macrolide seldom used for its antimicrobial properties, but sometimes employed because of its claimed (yet unproven in rigorous clinical studies) steroid-sparing effect, has been shown to reduce theophylline clearance on average by 50%.[109]

Clarithromycin has been shown to reduce theophylline clearance by 17% in a study of normal volunteers.[108] Midecamycin, miocamycin, and azithromycin do not appear to inhibit theophylline metabolism.[108] The data on roxithromycin show a small clearance reduction, whereas josamycin's effects are inconsistent.[108] Dirithromycin, a new macrolide derivative, has been shown to increase theophylline clearance slightly (but not statistically significantly) in healthy nonsmoking males.[110]

Calcium Channel Blockers

Verapamil, diltiazem, and nifedipine are examples of structurally dissimilar calcium channel blockers. The effects of these agents on the pharmacokinetics of theophylline are variable. Nafziger et al reported a significant decrease in theophylline clearance of 20%, an effect that was more pronounced in male smokers (whose MFOS was induced) than in male nonsmokers.[111] Sirmans et al, in 12 nonsmoking male volunteers, noted decreases in theophylline clearance of 18 and 12%, respectively, after verapamil and diltiazem.[112] These authors noted no significant changes after nifedipine treatment. Gin et al reported a decrease in theophylline clearance of 11.5% in smoking males.[113] Robson et al reported a 9% decrease in theophylline clearance with nifedipine.[114] Perhaps the most interesting trial is the one by Adebayo et al,[105] who did not observe an interaction between diltiazem and theophylline when given to nonsmoking males. Following treatment with rifampin to induce theophylline metabolism by the MFOS, the addition of diltiazem resulted in negation of the rifampin-inducing effect. This study is similar in many ways to that of Nafziger et al,[111] in which statistical differences in diltiazem effect on theophylline clearance were noted in smokers (who have induced MFOS function) but not in nonsmokers.

Calcium channel blockers may exhibit an inhibitory effect on theophylline clearance. This effect is most likely small and may be more pronounced in smokers and in patients with other reasons for induced MFOS.

Histamine Receptor Antagonists:

There is no question that cimetidine is a potent competitive inhibitor of theophylline metabolism. This effect is most likely related to dose[115] and is more significant in smokers than nonsmokers.[55,78] Cusack et al, however, found no difference in inhibition of theophylline metabolism with cimetidine in small numbers of smokers and nonsmokers.[116] Cimetidine also tends to obscure the gender differences in theophylline metabolism compared with controls, suggesting a greater effect in females versus males.[55] The effect of cimetidine occurs within 24 hours of instituting the drug. The effect generally occurs at doses of as little as 800 mg/d[115] and shows some (but not necessarily significant) increases as dosage increases.[115–118] Between 1200 and 2400 mg/d, no further reduction in theophylline clearance is noted.[119] Generally, cimetidine therapy results in a reduction in theophylline clearance of 25 to 35%.[77,115,116,119] *Cimetidine inhibits both oxidation and demethylation metabolic pathways for theophylline.*

It is clear that ranitidine and famotidine generally do not inhibit theophylline elimination and, thus, are probably the drugs of choice when theophylline and an H_2 antagonist are needed.[120,121] Similarly, roxatidine does not seem to affect the clearance of theophylline.[102]

Beta Receptor Agonists

In general, the beta adrenoceptor agonists have been shown to exhibit varying effects on elimination of theophylline. Hemstreet et al showed a 21% increase in theophylline clearance due to intravenous isoproterenol.[122] Amirav et al noted approximate doubling of theophylline clearance with the addition of intravenous albuterol.[123] Lombardi et al found no effect of oral terbutaline 5 mg every 8 hours on intravenous theophylline clearance (in healthy males),[124] whereas Garty et al reported a 25% increase in clearance in asthmatic patients.[125]

Quinolone Antibiotics

With the increasing number of quinolone antibiotics available in the marketplace, a glut of studies are available that have investigated theophylline metabolic inhibition. The oxidative and demethylation metabolic pathways of theophylline are generally affected by quinolones.[126] The presumed mechanism of quinolone inhibition is specific inhibition of the MFOS system.[126] Although data from Fuhr et al suggested that quinolones inhibited P450IA2, resulting in reduction in theophylline demethylation,[127–129] other data suggest that hydroxylation of theophylline to DMU is also inhibited by quinolones.[116,130] This finding raises a question concerning the role of P450IA2 as the only enzyme involved in the demethylation of theophylline. It appears that enoxacin is the most potent inhibitor of theophylline followed by ciprofloxacin.[126]

Enoxacin has been shown to result in a 50% reduction in theophylline clearance, an effect that appears to last 24 to 48 hours after the drug is discontinued and to be dose related.[131,132]

The effect of ciprofloxacin on the pharmacokinetics of theophylline is well described. Ciprofloxacin results in a 30% reduction in theophylline clearance.[133,134]

Norfloxacin does not produce a significant effect on theophylline metabolism.[133,135]

Other quinolones that have been investigated and not shown to exhibit significant effects on theophylline metabolism in humans include lomefloxacin,[136] ofloxacin,[137] fleroxacin,[138] and sparfloxacin.[139]

It should be noted that a number of these trials used only male subjects and excluded females. Other considerations include the use of nonsmokers in these trials. Thus, published data may not be applied to females and smokers.

Tables 18–4 to 18–6 list the major drugs that interact with theophylline. Table 18–4 notes drugs that increase theophylline clearance, Table 18–5 note drugs that decrease theophylline clearance, and Table 18–6 notes pharmacodynamic interactions with theophylline.

TABLE 18–4. DRUGS THAT INCREASE THEOPHYLLINE CLEARANCE

Albuterol	Phenobarbital
Aminoglutethimide	Phenytoin
Carbamazepine	Primidone
Isoproterenol	Rifampin
Moricizine	Sulfinpyrazone
Oral contraceptives	Terbutaline

Drug–Food Interactions

Reports in the 1970s suggested that the clearance of theophylline was substantially increased by the ingestion of beef that was broiled over charcoal (versus control subjects fed the same quantity of non-charcoal-broiled beef) compared with a phase in which no protein supplementation was given.[140] Curiously, the authors did not find an increase in theophylline clearance between the phase with no protein supplementation and the non-charcoal-broiled beef phase. Further studies, however, have noted that dietary protein supplementation (in the range of 40% of the total caloric intake as protein) results in a 25 to 50% increase in theophylline clearance.[141–144] Additionally, high carbohydrate (and low protein) intake results in a prolongation of theophylline clearance compared with a diet with 15 to 20% of the calories as carbohydrate.[139,142,144,145] Presumably, increased protein intake stimulates the MFOS to increase theophylline metabolism. It is less clear how dramatic the effect of carbohydrate intake is or what the mechanism of action is if it does reliably reduce theophylline clearance. Increased fat intake does not appear to affect theophylline pharmacokinetics (aside from the absorption of certain slow-release preparations as discussed under Absorption.[145]

There is ample evidence suggesting that the metabolic pathways of theophylline can be stimulated and inhibited by a variety of compounds.

TABLE 18–5. DRUGS THAT DECREASE THEOPHYLLINE CLEARANCE

Allopurinol	Idrocilamide
Cimetidine	Interferon Alfa
Ciprofloxacin	Isoniazid
Clarithromycin	Mexiletine
Diltiazem	Norfloxacin
Disulfiram	Ofloxacin
Enoxacin	Pefloxacin
Erythromycin	Pipemidic Acid
Etintidine	Propranolol
Felodipine	Thiabendazole
Fluvoxamine	Verapamil

TABLE 18–6. PHARMACODYNAMIC INTERACTIONS WITH THEOPHYLLINE

Acetazolamide	Increased diuretic effect
Ephedrine	Increased central system effect
Adenosine	Decreased adenosine effectiveness
Benzodiazepines	Antagonism of sedation
Lithium	Increased lithium effect as a result of increased Li concentration

Therapeutic Efficacy

Establishment of a relationship between serum theophylline concentrations and therapeutic effect is a very appealing concept. The establishment of such a relationship, given a reasonable therapeutic to toxic ratio, would result in simplification of dosage adjustment for the drug in the treatment of bronchospasm and, it is hoped, the avoidance of toxicity.

A number of investigators have attempted to establish such a pharmacokinetic–pharmacodynamic relationship for theophylline in reversible airway disease. Turner-Warwick in 1957 reported that subjective relief of symptoms of bronchospasm was noted only when the serum theophylline concentration exceeded 10 μg/mL.[146] No upper limit was established, however, and no patient in that study had a serum theophylline concentration above 18 μg/mL.

Subsequently, Jackson et al[147] and Boswell and McGinn[148] reported subjective and objective improvement at 10 and 5 to 15 μg/mL, respectively, in patients with bronchospasm. Pierson et al reported therapeutic efficacy for theophylline versus placebo in pediatric patients (less than 18 years of age) with status asthmaticus.[149] In this study, however, the authors did not examine the relationship of serum concentrations to improvements in forced expiratory volume in the first second (FEV_1) and forced vital capacity (FVC). Mitenko and Ogilvie, in a widely quoted study, noted a dose-related improvement in pulmonary function during theophylline infusions in six nonacutely ill asthmatic subjects.[150] These authors reported continuous improvement in forced FVC and FEV_1 over the theophylline concentration range 5 to 20 μg/mL, with response related to the logarithm of theophylline concentration (Figure 18–4). When examining the percentage improvement in FEV_1 versus the maximal improvement in FEV_1, $FEV_{1,max}$ (seen at 20 μg/mL), the data translate clinically into increases in FEV_1 of 50% at 5 μg/mL, 75% at 10 μg/mL, and 85% at 15 μg/mL.[151,152] This suggests that although further bronchodilation may be obtained above a serum theophylline concentration of 15 μg/mL, large increases generally are not seen above 15 μg/mL. In addition, some patients may have significant improvement in FEV_1 at 5 to 10 μg/mL. The usefulness of these data derived in six patients has been questioned.[152]

Levy and Koysooko noted an average of 80% improvement in FEV_1 at serum concentrations less than 10 μg/mL in asthmatic children.[153]

Racineux et al studied 13 patients with stable asthma examining the $FEV_1/FEV_{1,max}$.[154] A linear relationship between theophylline serum concentration and improvement in this parameter was noted. Response was 30% at 5 μg/mL, 65% at 10 μg/mL, and 85% at 15 μg/mL.[152] Given the variability in performance of pulmonary function testing (from a patient performance standpoint), and the expected variation in pharmacologic effect of theophylline based on varied severity of disease, the findings of both Mitenko and Ogilvie[150] and Racineux et al[154] may be correct.

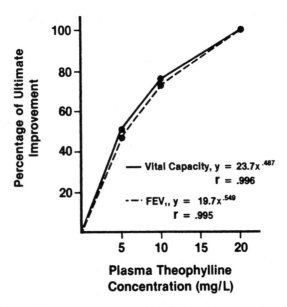

Figure 18–4. Change in vital capacity and FEV_1 in subjects with asthma studied by Mitenko and Ogilvie.[150] Plasma theophylline concentration is expressed on the abscissa. Spirometric improvement is expressed on the ordinate as a percentage of the ultimate improvement noted at a plasma theophylline concentration of 20 mg/L (the generally accepted upper limit of therapeutic values). As can be observed, most of the change occurred at plasma theophylline concentrations of 10 mg/L and less. The regressions between theophylline concentration and spirometric improvement were analyzed by use of a power function; for both power functions, exponents are < 1.0, indicating reduced response to higher concentrations of theophylline. (*From Fairshter RD, Busse WW. Theophylline—How much is enough?* J Allergy Clin Immunol. *1986;77:646–648, with permission.*)

Curiously, two studies noted positive effects of theophylline on airways at serum concentrations as low as 2 to 5 μg/mL.[155,156]

Koup and Brodsky, studying 12 hospitalized pediatric patients, noted no additional improvement in peak expiratory flow rate (PEFR), FVC, FEV_1, and midmaximal expiratory flow rate at 10.5 μg/mL versus 18.2 μg/mL theophylline.[157]

Vozeh et al noted a significant difference in FEV_1 and FVC in patients with acute bronchial obstruction (the majority of whom had COPD) with serum theophylline concentrations of 20 μg/mL versus 10 μg/mL.[158] Richer et al, using a single oral dose of theophylline, noted some correlation between PEFR and theophylline concentrations in patients with bronchial asthma but not COPD.[159] Most patients in this trial attained peak serum theophylline concentrations between 18 and 22 μg/mL; however, no significant differences in improvement in PEFR were seen in asthmatic patients with peak concentrations above 18 μg/mL. This study clearly showed that as serum concentrations (in asthmatic patients) increased above 10 μg/mL, PEFR increased. Simons et al found a good correlation between serum theophylline concentrations and FEV_1 improvements but not FVC in asthmatic children.[160]

Klein et al noted that although higher serum theophylline concentrations may be useful in acutely ill patients, in stable asthmatics, ventilatory status was not improved by serum theophylline concentrations above 12.8 μg/mL.[161] A corroborating trial was performed by Fairshter et al, who noted no differences in pulmonary function and control of asthma symptoms using sustained-release theophylline, with average theophylline concentrations of 8.8, 11.5, and 14.2 μg/mL and markedly different peak and trough concentrations.[162] Holford et al studied 174 patients, the majority with asthma (but approximately 13% with COPD), treated with theophylline during acute exacerbations.[163] The target serum concentration for half the group was 10 μg/mL, and for the other half, 20 μg/mL. Duration of hospital stay and rate and extent of improvement in peak expiratory flow rate were not significantly different between the two groups. More toxic effects were noted in the group in whom a serum concentration of 20 μg/mL was targeted.

This volume of data in many studies could be interpreted in many ways; however, given the variability in bronchospastic disease and heterogeneous response to theophylline, some conclusions can be made. It would appear that some individuals with asthma may respond significantly to theophylline at serum concentrations below 10 μg/mL. Others may not have a significant effect until serum concentrations get into the range 10 to 15 μg/mL. Still others may need up to 20 μg/mL to obtain a significant therapeutic effect. It may be prudent to set the therapeutic range for theophylline at 5 to 15 μg/mL, keeping in mind that between 5 and 10 μg/mL, some patients will not have an adequate therapeutic effect, and above 15 μg/mL, some patients may not get additional benefit.

In addition to the question of whether a relationship exists between serum concentration and effect for theophylline, studies have questioned whether clinical trials in acute asthma justify the use of theophylline. Recent data again suggest that theophylline may be a beneficial addition to the treatment of acute asthma. Wrenn et al noted that patients with asthma or COPD seen in the emergency department treated with metaproterenol and parenteral methylprednisolone had markedly decreased numbers of hospital admissions with the addition of theophylline.[164] In this trial, no objective effect on pulmonary function tests was noted; however, a measurable clinical effect was seen at 10 μg/mL. Unfortunately, the reader is unable to differentiate between the groups with asthma and COPD to see if the relationships were the same or different. Huang et al investigated the use of theophylline versus placebo in addition to parenteral corticosteroids and albuterol aerosol.[165] They found that the addition of theophylline reduced the need for beta-adrenergic nebulizer treatments and resulted in a statistically significant increase in FEV_1 versus placebo.

The data on the relationship between theophylline effect and serum concentration are exceptionally confusing. The trials have investigated patients with reversible as well as irreversible airway disease and bronchospasm, those undergoing acute as well as chronic exacerbations, and pediatric as well as adult patients. Such data raise controversies as to the usefulness of theophylline in the treatment of asthma, whether acute exacerbations or chronic therapy. Recommendations from the National Asthma Education Program have been published concerning the use of the agent[166]:

1. Theophylline is not recommended for the treatment of acute exacerbation of asthma in either children or adults in the emergency room or at home, as data have shown that no additional benefit is obtained when beta-agonist therapy is optimized for these patients. Increased adverse effects rather than increased therapeutic benefit may be seen with the use of theophylline.
2. In the hospitalized adult or pediatric patient with asthma, intravenous or oral theophylline may be used but the precise benefit that this agent adds to beta-agonist therapy is variable.
3. Theophylline is not recommended for the treatment of mild asthma in either adults or children. This agent may be useful in the treatment of moderate asthma, particularly if the patient is experiencing symptoms during the night (nocturnal asthma) and cannot get sufficient duration of action from beta agonists.[165,166] For some patients, control of nocturnal symptoms is achieved by using once daily dosing of a sustained release theophylline product. The dose is administered in the late afternoon to early evening.[167,168] The new long-acting beta agonists such as salmeterol, however, may further limit the use of theophylline.

Serum theophylline concentrations must be individualized for these patients. In any event, the therapeutic range is most likely 5 to 15 μg/mL. Some patients, however, will tolerate higher concentrations and a few will get a greater therapeutic effect. When used intravenously, theophylline is generally given as a continuous infusion in an attempt to optimize bronchodilation and minimize serum concentration fluctuations. Goldberg et al studied 11 children given theophylline by intermittent bolus and continuous infusion.[169] These authors found that FEV_1 was statistically better with the use of constant infusion. Although the use of a continuous infusion makes pharmacologic sense, no well-controlled trial in a homogeneous patient population group has conclusively shown that constant infusion is more effective than intermittent bolus. Because this is the accepted mode of therapy, and because the use of continuous infusion makes it easier to monitor serum concentrations, the use of this modality in the acute hospital situation should be promoted when oral therapy cannot be used.

As complex and confusing as the literature is on the use of theophylline in asthma, the literature on the use of theophylline in COPD is equally confusing. Eaton et al noted greater percentages of change in FEV_1 and FVC with serum theophylline concentrations of 17 to 22 μg/mL versus 9 to 12.5 μg/mL in patients with COPD[170]; however, patients could not distinguish either treatment from placebo in terms of breathlessness. Passamonte and Martinez found that serum theophylline concentrations in the range 15 to 20 μg/mL range did not result in maximal bronchodilation in COPD patients. Theophylline was found to reduce dyspnea but not improve pulmonary function tests in patients with COPD.[172] Rice et al reported that theophylline did not provide significant additional benefit to a standard treatment regimen in acute exacerbations of COPD.[173] To the contrary, Guyatt et al found that theophylline, in combination with salbutamol, provided significant benefit in COPD patients.[174] Other authors have also shown a benefit of theophylline on symptoms in COPD.[175]

The conclusion to be drawn is that theophylline may give some additional benefit (particularly subjective benefit) in the treatment of COPD.[10] No objective improvement in pulmonary function tests may be noted in COPD patients taking theophylline. The use of this agent in treating acute exacerbations of COPD is not clear.[176]

THEOPHYLLINE TOXICITY

Adverse Effects

In addition to its multitude of pharmacologic effects, theophylline can cause significant (and sometimes life-threatening) adverse effects. Two major categories of theophylline poisoning exist: the acute ingestion (often a suicide attempt) and chronic-use intoxication. Because of its complex hepatic elimination, chronic-use intoxication often occurs in the patient who can least tolerate the development of adverse effects, that is, the patient with chronic liver, pulmonary, or cardiac disease.

Acute theophylline intoxication is often a more impressive pharmacokinetic situation, but is somewhat less dangerous than chronic overdose for two main reasons. First, often the patient presenting with a single-dose acute intoxication may be a physically healthy, younger patient making a suicide gesture. These patients are less likely to have hepatic or cardiac disease, which reduce the clearance of the drug. Second, it has been shown that the 50% seizure threshold for theophylline in acute ingestions is 100 μg/mL, substantially higher than the 50% seizure level of 40 μg/mL for chronic-use intoxication.[177] Serious metabolic abnormalities have been reported with acute theophylline ingestion.[178,179] These include hypokalemia, hyperglycemia, leukocytosis (these were related to the magnitude of serum theophylline concentration), respiratory alkalosis, hypophosphatemia, and hypomagnesemia. Patients with acute intoxication present with tremors, seizures, nausea and vomiting, cardiac arrhythmias (particularly sinus tachycardia), and hypotension.[177,180] Acute overdose patients are more likely to have higher serum concentrations than chronic-use patients.[15] If a relationship exists between serum concentration and symptoms, the acute overdose situation probably lends itself more to this relationship. A 10% mortality rate along with a 27% seizure rate has been reported in acute intoxication.[15]

Chronic-use theophylline intoxication seems to be a more serious medical problem. Toxic effects in these patients may be the result of a pathophysiologic change in hepatic or cardiac function, inhibition of theophylline metabolism by drugs or acute viral illness, or medication error. Although some authors have previously tried to establish a relationship between serum theophylline concentration and symptomatology,[181,182] in chronic-use intoxication, no such relationship exists.[18] Our findings in 20 chronic-use intoxications with serum concentrations in the range 18 to 42 μg/mL included metabolic abnormalities similar to those seen in acute intoxications: gastrointestinal symptomatology in more than 50% of patients, tremors in 30%, cardiac arrhythmias in 40%, and seizures in 10%. No relationship between theophylline serum concentration and symptomatology was noted. In addition, patients did not progress from one symptom of lesser concern to seizures. Severe symptomatology was noted over the entire range of serum concentrations. Other studies have confirmed the lack of predictability of theophylline toxicity symptoms with serum concentrations in chronic-use intoxication, even in the higher serum concentration range.[183,184] Patients with a history of seizures may be prone to the development of theophylline-induced seizures. Other signs and symptoms of chronic-use theophylline intoxication include altered mental status,[184,185] hypercalcemia,[186] diarrhea,[184] rhabdomyolysis,[184] and multifocal atrial tachycardia.[187]

The management of acute versus chronic-use theophylline intoxication is somewhat varied. In both ingestions, one of the main goals is to prevent the absorption of theophylline from the gastrointestinal tract or to remove remaining drug through gastrointestinal lavage using a nasogastric hose. Activated charcoal remains the drug of choice to inhibit absorption of theophylline. As the slow and ultraslow sustained-release preparations have prolonged absorption, charcoal may be useful for up to 24 hours after ingestion. The recommended dose is 1 g/kg by mouth with 75 to 100 mL of 75% sorbitol to enhance transit through the gastrointestinal tract.[188] It is unclear whether multiple-dose activated charcoal is necessary for the continuing treatment of theophylline intoxication.[17,18] In acute intoxication, where a relationship seems to exist between serum concentration and severity of toxicity,[184] repeat-dose oral activated charcoal (which can decrease half-life by 50%) may be indicated for serum concentrations above 60 μg/mL.[17,186] In chronic-use intoxication, multiple-dose activated charcoal may not be necessary unless the patient has severe symptoms (neurologic or cardiovascular) or unless the serum concentration is above 60 μg/mL. Our findings in chronic-use intoxication suggest that discontinuing the drug and administering single-dose activated charcoal (1 g/kg with 75–100 mL of 70% sorbitol) resulted in no progression of symptoms. Multiple-dose activated charcoal did not shorten the duration of symptomatology for theophylline toxicity.[18] In theory, however, in the patient with mild symptoms but a substantially elevated serum theophylline concentration (ie, 30–60 μg/mL), the use of multiple-dose activated charcoal to reduce the serum concentration more rapidly might shorten the duration of hospitalization for the patient. If multiple-dose activated charcoal is used, doses of 10 g hourly for 12 doses or 20 g every 2 hours for 6 doses are recommended.[17] This therapy should result in significant reduction in theophylline concentrations.

The use of charcoal or resin hemoperfusion or hemodialysis for removal of theophylline from the body should be approached with extreme caution, as these modalities are associated with their own toxic effects.[17,18] In acute intoxication, these modalities should not be used unless the serum concentration is 100 μg/mL or higher or unless the patient has serious cardiac or neurologic manifestations that cannot be controlled with other interventions (such as seizures or arrhythmias).[17,177] In chronic-use intoxication, these modalities should be considered if serum theophylline concentrations are 60 μg/mL or higher and the patient has cardiac or neurologic symptoms (ie, seizures). In the face of an elevated serum concentration *without significant symptoms,* however, conservative therapy (such as oral activated charcoal) alone should be sufficient. Other authors have raised the question as to whether these invasive interventions should be used in patients older than 60 or in those with cardiac or hepatic disease and serum concentrations of 30 μg/mL or higher in chronic-use intoxications.[177,189] There is, however, little evidence that these more invasive elimination modalities reduce morbidity or mortality from theophylline intoxication.[17] In general, because of the morbidity of these invasive procedures, conservative management should be undertaken, including multiple-dose oral activated charcoal, unless the patient has significant cardiac or neurologic symptoms.

Other modalities that have been used include beta blockers and verapamil for the cardiac arrhythmias associated with theophylline intoxication. Seizures may respond to diazepam, phenytoin, or phenobarbital; however, theophylline-induced seizures generally are difficult to treat and are associated with significant mortality.[17]

THERAPEUTIC REGIMEN DESIGN

Dosing regimens for theophylline have been well worked out and approved by the Food and Drug Administration. These guidelines were established in an attempt to optimally dose theophylline while minimizing toxic effects in a majority of patients. Clinical monitoring and the judicious use of serum concentration monitoring are recommended. Tables 18–7 and 18–8 give dosage guidelines for parenteral and oral theophylline.[190,191] The dosage guidelines given differ from the FDA guidelines[192] as only one maintenance dosage level is listed rather than an initial maintenance dose for the first 12 hours followed by a lower maintenance dosage. For conversion from parenteral to oral formulations, a 1:1 ratio may be used however, it must be kept in mind that the ultra-slow release preparations may show less bioavailability than other oral preparations.

For intravenous dosing, it is recommended that the serum concentration be checked 8 hours after the initial loading dose and maintenance dose. An additional serum concentration may be checked 12 hours after the first serum concentration. Most importantly, clinical response must be assessed.

Dosage modifications for theophylline should be based on clinical response first and serum theophylline concentrations second. Although the above guidelines for oral therapy are designed to be used without checking serum theophylline concentrations, this author continues to suggest checking at least one concentration following the institution of maintenance therapy and after dosage adjustment. This recommendation is supported by experts.[191] Other schemes using graded doses increased every 3 days have been recommended and may be used.[192] These guidelines suggest maximal starting dosages of 400 mg/d in children and adults, increasing to 600 mg/d after 3 days and to 900 mg/d in another 3 days. Larger dosages may be used; however, serum concentration monitoring should be routinely performed in these instances. As noted,

TABLE 18–7. DOSAGE GUIDELINES FOR PARENTERAL THEOPHYLLINE

Patient Population	Age	Maintenance Dosage (mg/kg/h)
Neonates	0–23 d	1 mg/kg q12h[a,b]
	≥ 24 d	1.5 mg/kg q12h[a,b]
Infants	6–52 wk	(0.008)(age in wk) + 0.21[a]
Young children	1–9 y	0.8[a]
Older children and adolescent smokers	9–16 y	0.7[a]
Adult smokers	>16 y	0.7[a]
Adult nonsmokers	>16 y	0.4[a]
Adults with cardiac decompensation or hepatic disease	>16 y	0.2[a]

[a] Loading dose calculated as steady-state volume of distribution × desired concentration. Loading dose is infused over 20 to 30 minutes. In general, 1 mg/kg raises serum concentration by 2 μg/mL. For all but neonates, an average loading dose of 5 mg/kg may be used.

[b] May be given as intermittent bolus at appropriate intervals.

TABLE 18–8. DOSAGE GUIDELINES FOR ORAL THEOPHYLLINE

Patient Population	Age	Maintenance Dosage[a] (mg/kg/d)
Infants	6–52 wk	(0.3)(age in wk) + 8
Young children	1–9 y	24.0
Older children	9–12 y	20.0
Adolescents	12–16 y	18.0
Adult smokers	>16 y	13.0
Adult nonsmokers	>16 y	9.0
Adults with cardiac decompensation or hepatic disease	>16 y	4.0

[a] Median maintenance dosage. At these dosages, 20% of patients will be slightly above 20 µg/mL; the rest will be below.[169] Maintenance dosages may be given as sustained-release preparations. These can be dosed every 12 to 24 hours in adult nonsmokers and those with cardiac or hepatic disease and every 8 to 12 hours in children, adolescents, and smoking adults (children may need every 6- to 8-hour dosing).

experts do not recommend the use of theophylline as a single agent in the treatment of reversible airway disease.[166] Thus, other therapies should be optimized in addition to increasing the theophylline dose.

Increasing theophylline dose on the basis of serum concentration and clinical response is illustrated in Table 18–9.

When using the above guidelines, it is important to remember that for chronic reversible airway disease therapy, the therapeutic range is most likely 5 to 15 µg/mL; thus, these guidelines are only broad suggestions for dosage modification. Because of the variability in theophylline pharmacokinetics in humans, the multiple drug interactions, and the potential for dose-dependent kinetics, careful adjustment of theophylline doses should be undertaken. It will be a rare instance when doubling the dose will be appropriate. In the experience of this author, doubling may be performed in children with rapid clearance, but is rarely needed in other populations. In any case, the smallest daily dose that gives an adequate therapeutic response should be used. For neonates, serum concentrations below 10 µg/mL are recommended.

As with any drug therapy for which serum concentration data can be readily obtained, theophylline therapeutic drug monitoring is subject to overuse. Generally, for patients receiving parenteral continuous infusion of theophylline, a serum concentration can be obtained 8 hours after the initial loading dose and institution of maintenance dosing. This concentration can be repeated 12 hours after the first serum concentration is obtained to assess whether further accumulation is occurring. The use of repeated serum concentrations is most likely unnecessary unless the patient has significant factors that could affect clearance, the patient's bronchospasm does not improve, or his or her condition deteriorates.

For oral therapy with a sustained-release preparation, it is very difficult to predict when the peak theophylline concentration will occur. Use of serum concentrations drawn at the same time

TABLE 18–9. THEOPHYLLINE MAINTENANCE DOSE ADJUSTMENT

Measured Serum Concentration (μg/mL)	Dose Adjustment
5–7.5	Increase dose 25%; recheck serum concentration in 3 d
7.5–10	Increase dose 25% only if patient is symptomatic; recheck serum concentration in 3 d and every 6–12 mo
10–20	No change; consider decreasing dosage if >15 μg/mL
20–25	Decrease dose by 10–25%; recheck in 3 d and every 6–12 mo
25–30	Hold one dose; decrease maintenance dose by 25%; recheck in 3 d and every 6–12 mo
>30	Hold two doses; decrease maintenance dose by 50%; recheck to guide dosage adjustment; consider activated charcoal treatment for toxicity

From Hendeles L, Weinberger M, Szefler S, Ellis E. Safety and efficacy of theophylline in children with asthma. *J Pediatr.* 1992;120:177–183, with permission.

after the dose or of trough concentrations may be recommended. Dosage adjustment may proceed as indicated in Table 18–9. For rapid-release preparations, peak concentrations drawn 1 to 2.5 hours after the dose or trough concentrations may be used. In any event, dosage modification must be based on patient response and the occurrence of adverse effects.

———— QUESTIONS ————

1. J.R., a 72-year-old man with COPD, comes into the emergency room with a sinus tachycardia of 125 bpm and blood pressure of 106/70 and complains of nausea and tremors so severe that he cannot hold a pen to sign the Medicare form. He has a temperature of 38.5°C and over the last few days has developed influenza-like symptoms. At home, he has been receiving a sustained-release theophylline preparation for 12 months, 300 mg every 12 hours, with a trough serum concentration checked in his physician's office 1 month earlier of 12 μg/mL. He has no evidence of liver disease or congestive heart failure. He weighs 70 kg. The theophylline serum concentration obtained is 46.7 μg/mL. His last dose of the sustained-release theophylline preparation was 8 hours earlier. How would you treat this patient? Why has he developed theophylline toxicity?

2. Dr. Smith prescribes a sustained-release theophylline preparation, 300 mg every 12 hours, for Ms. Redmond, a 23-year-old woman with reversible airway disease. She weighs 60 kg. A trough theophylline concentration 2 weeks after institution of therapy is 10.9 μg/mL and she is asymptomatic. Ms. Redmond, while undergoing a routine chest x-ray and PPD, is diagnosed as having tuberculosis. Dr. Smith begins her on

INH 300 mg/d and rifampin 600 mg/d. After 2 weeks of TB therapy, Ms. Redmond has an acute asthmatic attack and goes to the local emergency room. Her serum theophylline concentration 6 hours after her last dose is 2.4 µg/mL. What has happened to this patient's theophylline pharmacokinetics?

3. Mr. Henry, who is receiving aminophylline tablets, 300 mg every 8 hours, has a measured theophylline trough of 4 µg/mL and is still symptomatic with his reversible airway disease. His physician tells him to double his dose to 600 mg every 8 hours and to have his theophylline concentration rechecked in 5 days. At that time Mr. Henry's trough concentration is 23 µg/mL and he has developed a tremor. What has happened to this patient to elevate his serum theophylline concentration?

4. Following the institution of theophylline therapy, Mrs. Green noted that her urine output increased dramatically, causing her to have to get up during the night to urinate two or three times. What is the explanation for this?

REFERENCES

1. Zuidema J, Merkus FWHM. Chemical and biopharmaceutical aspects of theophylline and its derivatives. *Curr Med Res Opin.* 1979;6(suppl 6):14–25.
2. Rall TW. Drugs used in the treatment of asthma. The methylxanthines, cromolyn sodium and other agents, in Goodman, Gilman A, Rall TW, eds. *The Pharmacologic Basis of Therapeutics.* 8th ed. New York: Pergamon Press; 1990:618–637.
3. Kalsner S. Mechanism of potentiation of contractor responses to catecholamines by methylxanthines and aortic strips. *Br J Pharmacol.* 1971;43:379–388.
4. Kalsner S, Frew RD, Smith GM. Mechanism of methylxanthine sensitization of norepinephrine responses in a coronary artery. *Am J Physiol.* 1975;228:1702–1707.
5. Vinegar R, Truax JF, Selph JL, et al. Potentiation of the anti-inflammatory and analgesic activities of aspirin by caffeine in the rat. *Proc Soc Exp Biol Med.* 1976;151:556–560.
6. Rall TW. Evolution of the mechanism of action of methylxanthines: From calcium mobilizers to antagonists of adenosine receptors. *Pharmacologist.* 1982;24:277–287.
7. Persson CGA. Overview of effects of theophylline. *J Allergy Clin Immunol.* 1986;78:780–787.
8. Kruter KE, Blanchard J. Management of apnea in infants. *Clin Pharm.* 1989;8:577–587.
9. Woodcock AA, Gross ER, Gellert A, et al. Effect of dihydrocodeine, ethanol and caffeine on breathlessness and exercise tolerance in patients with chronic obstructive lung disease and normal blood gases. *N Engl J Med.* 1981;305:1611–1616.
10. Hill NS. The use of theophylline in irreversible chronic obstructive pulmonary disease. *Arch Intern Med.* 1988;148:2579–2584.
11. Rachelefsky GS, Wo J, Adelson J, et al. Behavioral abnormalities in poor school performance due to oral theophylline use. *Pediatrics.* 1986;78:1133–1138.
12. Weinberger M, Lindgren S, Bender B, et al. Effects of theophylline on learning and behavior: Reason for concern or concern without reason? *J Pediatr.* 1987;111:471–473.
13. Creer TL, Kotses H, Gustafson KE, et al. A critique of studies investigating the association of theophylline through psychologic or behavioral performance. *Pediatr Asthma Allergy Immunol.* 1988; 2:169–184.
14. Creer TL, McLoughlin JA. The effects of theophylline on cognitive and behavioral performance. *J Allergy Clin Immunol.* 1989;83:1027–1029.

15. Bender B, Milgrom H. Theophylline-induced behavior change in children. *JAMA.* 1992;267: 2621–2624.

16. Lindgren S, Lokshin B, Stromquist A, et al. Does asthma or treatment with theophylline limit children's academic performance? *N Engl J Med.* 1992;327:926–930.

17. Paloucek FP, Rodvold KA. Evaluation of theophylline overdoses and toxicities. *Ann Emerg Med.* 1988;17:135–144.

18. Bertino JS Jr, Walker JW Jr. Reassessment of theophylline toxicity. Serum concentrations, clinical course, and treatment. *Arch Intern Med.* 1987;147:757–760.

19. Ogilvie RI, Fernandez PG, Winsberg F. Cardiovascular response to increasing theophylline concentrations. *Eur J Clin Pharmacol.* 1977;12:409–414.

20. Maren TH. The additive renal effect of oral aminophylline and trichlormethiazide in man. *Clin Res.* 1961;9:57.

21. Truitt EB, McKusick VA, Krantz JC. Theophylline blood levels after oral, rectal and intravenous administration in correlation with diuretic action. *J Pharmacol Exp Ther.* 1950;100:309–313.

22. Foster LJ, Treudeau WL, Goldman AL. Bronchodilator effects on gastric acid secretion. *JAMA.* 1979;241:2613–2617.

23. Sporn PHS, Morganrota ML. Discontinuation of mechanical ventilation. *Clin Chest Med.* 1988; 9:113–126.

24. Bakris GL, Souter ER, Hussey JL, et al. Effects of theophylline on erythropoietin production in normal subjects and in patients with erythrocytosis with renal transplantation. *N Engl J Med.* 1990; 323:86–90.

25. Onrot J, Shaheen O, Biaggioni I, et al. Reduction of liver plasma flow by caffeine and theophylline. *Clin Pharmacol Ther.* 1986;40:506–510.

26. Tulin-Silver J, Schteingart DE, Mathews KP. Effect of theophylline on cortisol secretion. *J Allergy Clin Immunol.* 1981;67:45–50.

27. Cathcart-Rake WF, Kyner TL, Azarnoff DL. Metabolic responses to plasma concentrations of theophylline. *Clin Pharmacol Ther.* 1979;26:89–95.

28. Ward RN, Maisels MJ. Metabolic effect of methylxanthines. *Semin Perinatol.* 1981;5:383–388.

29. Hendeles L, Weinberger M, Bighley L. Absolute bioavailability of oral theophylline. *Am J Hosp Pharm.* 1977;34:525–527.

30. Upton RA, Sansom L, Guentert TW, et al. Evaluation of the absorption from fifteen commercial theophylline products indicating deficiencies in currently available criteria. *J Pharm Biopharm.* 1980; 8:229–242.

31. Welling PG, Lions LL, Craig WA, Trochta GA. Influence of diet and fluid on bioavailability of theophylline. *Clin Pharmacol Ther.* 1975;17:475–480.

32. Arnold RA, Spurbeck GH, Shelver WH, Henderson WM. Effect of an antacid on gastrointestinal absorption of theophylline. *Am J Hosp Pharm.* 1979;36:1059–1062.

33. Reed RC, Schwartz HJ. Lack of influence of an intensive antacid regimen on theophylline bioavailability. *J Pharmacokinet Biopharm.* 1984;12:315–331.

34. Weinberger M, Hendeles L, Bighley L. The relation of product formulation to absorption of oral theophylline. *N Engl J Med.* 1978;299:852–857.

35. Stewart RB, Cluff LE. A review of medication errors in compliance in ambulant patients. *Clin Pharmacol Ther.* 1972;13:463–468.

36. Gibaldi M, Perrier D. *Pharmacokinetics.* 2nd ed. New York: Marcel Dekker; 1982:189.

37. Weinberger MW. Theophylline QID, TID, BID and now QD. A report on 24 hour dosing with slow release theophylline formulation with emphasis on analyses of data to obtain FDA approval for Theo-24. *Pharmacotherapy.* 1984;4:181–198.

38. Hendeles L, Iafrate RP, Weinberger MW. A clinical and pharmacokinetic basis for the selection and use of slow release theophylline products. *Clin Pharmacokinet.* 1984;9:95–135.

39. Hurwitz A, Karim A, Burns TS. Theophylline absorption from SR products: Comparative steady state bioavailability of once daily Theo-Dur, Theo-24 and Uniphyl. *J Clin Pharmacol.* 1987;27:855–861.

40. Jonkman JHG. Food interactions with sustained release theophylline preparations. A review. *Clin Pharmacokinet.* 1989;16:162–179.

41. Hendeles L, Weinberger MW, Milavetz G et al. Food induced "dose-dumping" from a once-a-day theophylline product as a cause of theophylline toxicity. *Chest.* 1985;87:758–765.

42. Karim A, Burns T, Janky D, Hurwitz A. Food induced changes in theophylline absorption from controlled release preparations. Part II. Importance of meal composition in dosing time relative to meal intake in assessing changes in absorption. *Clin Pharmacol Ther.* 1985;38:642–647.

43. Smolensky MH, Scott PH, Kramer WG. Clinical significance of day–night differences in serum theophylline concentrations with special reference to Theo-Dur. *J Allergy Clin Immunol.* 1986; 78:716–722.

44. Barry WH. The once daily theophylline controversy. *Pharmacotherapy.* 1984;4:167–168.

45. Hendeles L, Weinberger MW. Theophylline: A "state of the art" review. *Pharmacotherapy.* 1983; 3:2–4.

46. Nafziger AN, Bertino JS Jr. Sex related differences in theophylline pharmacokinetics. *Eur J Clin Pharmacol.* 1989;37:97–100.

47. Gal P, Jusko WJ, Yurchak AM, Franklin BA. Theophylline disposition in obesity. *Clin Pharmacol Ther.* 1978;23:438–444.

48. Rohrbaugh TM, Danish M, Ragni MC Yaffe SJ. The effect of obesity on apparent volume of distribution of theophylline. *Pediatr Pharmacol.* 1982;2:75–83.

49. Zell M, Curtis RA, Troyer WG, Fischer JH. Volume of distribution of theophylline in acute exacerbations of irreversible airway disease. *Chest.* 1985;87:212–216.

50. Jewesson PJ, Enson RJ. Difference of body fat and the volume of distribution of theophylline. *Ther Drug Monit.* 1985;7:197–201.

51. Brody BB, Axelrod J, Reichenthal J. Metabolism of theophylline "1, 3, DMX" in man. *J Biol Chem.* 1952;194:215–222.

52. Cornish HH, Christman AA. A study of the metabolism of theobromine, theophylline and caffeine in man. *J Biol Chem.* 1957;228:315–323.

53. Levy G. Koysooko R. Renal clearance of theophylline in man. *J Clin Pharmacol.* 1976;6:329–332.

54. Tang-Liu DDS, Tozer TN, Riegelman S. Urine flow dependence of theophylline renal clearance in man. *J Pharmacokinet Biopharm.* 1982;10:351–364.

55. Jennings TS, Nafziger AN, Davidson, L, Bertino JS Jr. Gender differences in hepatic induction and inhibition of theophylline pharmacokinetics and metabolism. *J Lab Clin Med.* 1993;122:208–216.

56. Campbell M, Grant DM, Inaba T, Kalow W. Biotransformation of caffeine, paraxanthine, theophylline and theobromine by polycyclic aromatic hydrocarbon-inducible cytochrome(s) P450 in human liver microsomes. *Drug Metab Dispos.* 1987;15:237–249.

57. Fuhr U, Doehmer J, Battula N, et al. Biotransformation of caffeine and theophylline in mammalian cell lines genetically engineered for expression of single cytochrome P450 isoforms. *Biochem Pharmacol.* 1992;43:225–235.

58. Gu L, Gonzalez F, Kalow W, Tang BK. Biotransformation of caffeine, paraxanthine, theobromine and theophylline by cDNA-expressed human CYP1A2 and CYP2E1. *Pharmacogenetics.* 1992;2:73–77.

59. Tang-Liu DDS, Williams RL, Riegelman S. Nonlinear theophylline elimination. *Clin Pharmacol Ther.* 1982;31:358–369.

60. Gundert-Remy U, Hildebrandt R, Hengen N, Weber E. Nonlinear elimination processes of theophylline. *Eur J Clin Pharmacol.* 1983;24:71–78.

61. Ludden TM. Nonlinear pharmacokinetics, clinical implications. *Clin Pharmacokinet.* 1991; 20:429–446.

62. Grygiel JJ, Wing LMH, Farkos J, Birkett DJ. Effects of allopurinol on theophylline metabolism and clearance. *Clin Pharmacol Ther.* 1979;26:660–667.

63. Sarkar MA, Hunt C, Guzelian PSA, Karnes HT. Characterization of human liver cytochromes P-450 involved in theophylline metabolism. *Drug Metab Dispos.* 1992;20:31–37.

64. Hendeles L, Weinberger MW, Johnson G. Monitoring serum theophylline levels. *Clin Pharmacokinet.* 1978;3:294–312.

65. Sarracin E, Hendeles L, Weinberger MW, et al. Dose dependent kinetics for theophylline: Observations among ambulatory asthmatic children. *J Pediatr.* 1980;97:825–828.

66. Weinberger MW, Ginchansky E. Dose dependent kinetics of theophylline disposition in asthmatic children. *J Pediatr.* 1977;91:820–824.

67. Milavetz G, Vaughan LM, Weinberger MW. Stability of theophylline elimination rate. *Clin Pharmacol Ther.* 1987;41:388–391.

68. Haley TJ. Metabolism and pharmacokinetics of theophylline in human neonates, children and adults. *Drug Metab Rev.* 1983;14:295–335.

69. Tserng KY, Takieddine FN, King KC. Developmental aspects of theophylline metabolism in premature infants. *Clin Pharmacol Ther.* 1983;33:522–527.

70. Tserng KY, King KC, Takieddine FN. Theophylline metabolism in premature infants. *Clin Pharmacol Ther.* 1981;29:594–600.

71. Bonati M, Latini R, Marra G, et al. Theophylline metabolism during the first month of life and development. *Pediatr Res.* 1981;15:304–308.

72. Bauer LA, Bauer SP, Blouin RA. The effect of acute and chronic renal failure on theophylline clearance. *J Clin Pharmacol.* 1982;22:65–68.

73. Lee CSC, Peterson JC, Marbury TC. Comparative pharmacokinetics of theophylline in peritoneal dialysis and hemodialysis. *J Clin Pharmacol.* 1983;23:274–280.

74. Slaughter RL, Green L, Kohli R. Hemodialysis of theophylline. *Ther Drug Monit.* 1982;4:191–193.

75. Brugerolle B, Toumi M, Faraj F, et al. Influence on the menstrual cycle on theophylline pharmacokinetics in asthmatics. *Eur J Clin Pharmacol.* 1990;39:59–61.

76. Hunt SM, Jusko WJ, Yurchak AM. Effect on smoking theophylline disposition. *Clin Pharmacol Ther.* 1976;19:546–551.

77. Grygiel JJ, Birkett DJ. Cigarette smoking and theophylline clearance and metabolism. *Clin Pharmacol Ther.* 1981;30:491–496.

78. Grygiel JJ, Miners JO, Drew R, Birkett DJ. Differential effects of cimetidine on theophylline metabolic pathways. *Eur J Clin Pharmacol.* 1984;26:335–340.

79. Dahlqvist R, Bertilsson L, Birkett DJ, et al. Theophylline metabolism in relation to antipyrine debrisoquin and sparteine metabolism. *Clin Pharmacol Ther.* 1984;35:815–821.

80. Vestal RE, Cusack BJ, Mercer GD, et al. Aging and drug interactions. 1. Effect of cimetidine and smoking on the oxidation of theophylline and cortisol in healthy men. *J Pharmacol Exp Ther.* 1987;241:488–500.

81. Jusko WJ, Schentag JJ, Clarke JH, et al. Enhanced biotransformation of theophylline in marijuana and tobacco smokers. *Clin Pharm Ther.* 1978;24:406–410.

82. Lee BL, Benowitz NL, Jacob E. Cigarette abstinence, nicotine gum and theophylline disposition. *Ann Intern Med.* 1987;106:553–555.

83. Fox RW, Sarnaan S, Bukantz SC, Lockey RF. Theophylline kinetics in a geriatric group. *Clin Pharmacol Ther.* 1983;34:60–67.

84. Randolph WC, Seaman JJ, Dickson B, et al. The effect of age on theophylline clearance in normal subjects. *Br J Clin Pharmacol.* 1986;22:603–605.

85. Jackson SHD, Johnston A, Wollard R, Turner P. The relationship between theophylline clearance and age in adult life. *Eur J Clin Pharmacol.* 1989;36:29–34.

86. Au WYW, Dutt AK, DeSoyza N. Theophylline kinetics in COPD in the elderly. *Clin Pharmacol Ther.* 1985;37:472–478.

87. Loughnan PM, Sitar DS, Ogilvie I, et al. Pharmacokinetic analysis of the disposition of intravenous theophylline in young children. *J Pediatr.* 1976;88:874–878.

88. Frederiksen MC, Ruot I, Chow MJ, Atkinson AJ Jr. Theophylline kinetics in pregnancy. *Clin Pharmacol Ther.* 1986;40:321–328.

89. Piafsky KM, Sitar DS, Rango RE, Ogilivie RI. Theophylline kinetics in acute pulmonary edema. *Clin Pharmacol Ther.* 1977;21:310–316.

90. Cusack BJ, Crowley JJ, Mercer CD, et al. Theophylline clearance in patients with severe COPD receiving supplemental oxygen in the effect of acute hypoxemia. *Am Rev Respir Dis.* 1986;133:1110.

91. Jusko WJ, Gardner MJ, Mangione A, et al. Factors affecting theophylline clearance: Age, tobacco, marijuana, cirrhosis, congestive heart failure, obesity, oral contraceptives, benzodiazepines, barbiturates and alcohol. *J Pharm Sci.* 1979;68:1358–1366.

92. Piafsky KM, Sitar DS, Rangno RE, Ogilvie RI. Theophylline disposition in patients with hepatic cirrhosis. *N Engl J Med.* 1977;296:1495–1497.

93. Mangione A, Imhoff TE, Lee RJ, et al. Pharmacokinetics of theophylline in hepatic disease. *Chest.* 1978;73:616–622.

94. Isles A, Spino M, Tachnik E, et al. Theophylline disposition in cystic fibrosis. *Am Rev Respir Dis.* 1983;127:417–421.

95. Grabowski N, May JJ, Pratt DS, et al. The effect of split virus influenza vaccination on theophylline pharmacokinetics. *Am Rev Respir Dis.* 1985;131:934–938.

96. Hannan SE, May JJ, Pratt DS, et al. The effect of whole virus influenza vaccine on theophylline pharmacokinetics. *Am Rev Respir Dis.* 1988;137:903–906.

97. Chang KC, Bauer BA, Bell TD, Choi H. Altered theophylline pharmacokinetics during acute respiratory infection. *Lancet.* 1978;1:1132–1134.

98. Mannering GJ, Renton KW, Azhary R, DeLoria LB. Effects of interferon inducing agents on hepatic cytochrome P450 drug metabolizing systems. *Ann NY Acad Sci.* 1980;350:314–321.

99. Jonkman JHG, Nicholson KG, Farrow PR, et al. Effects of alfa-interferon on theophylline pharmacokinetics on metabolism. *Br J Clin Pharmacol.* 1989;27:795–802.

100. Muslow HA, Bermard L, Brown RD, et al. Lack of effect of respiratory syncytial infection on theophylline disposition in children. *J Pediatr.* 1992;121:466–471.

101. Upton RA. Pharmacokinetic interactions between theophylline and other medication (Part 1). *Clin Pharmacokinet.* 1991;20:66–80.

102. Upton RA. Pharmacokinetic interactions between theophylline and other medications (Part 2). *Clin Pharmacokinet.* 1991;20:135–150.

103. Benedek IH, Pieniascek HJ, Davidson AF. Effect of moricizine on the pharmacokinetics of theophylline in healthy volunteers. *Pharm Res.* 1989;6:S234.

104. Straughn AB, Henderson RP, Liberman PL, Self TH. Effect of rifampin on theophylline disposition. *Ther Drug Monit.* 1984;6:153–156.

105. Adebayo GI, Akintonwa A, Mabadeje AFB. Attenuation of rifampicin-induced theophylline metabolism by diltiazem–rifampicin co-administration in healthy volunteers. *Eur J Clin Pharmacol.* 1989;37:127–131.

106. Gardner MJ, Tornatore KM, Jusko WJ, Konarkowski R. Effects of tobacco smoking and oral contraceptive use on theophylline disposition. *Br J Clin Pharmacol.* 1983;16:271–280.

107. Tornatore KM, Konarkowski R, McCarthy TL. Effect of chronic oral contraceptive steroids on theophylline disposition. *Eur J Clin Pharmacol.* 1982;23:129–134.

108. Gillum JG, Israel DS, Polk RE. Pharmacokinetic drug interactions with antimicrobial agents. *Clin Pharmacokinet.* 1993;25:450–482.

109. Weinberger MW, Hudgel D, Spector S, Chidsey C. Inhibition of theophylline clearance by TAO. *J Allergy Clin Immunol.* 1977;59:228–231.

110. Bachmann K, Nunley M, Martin M, et al. Changes of the study state pharmacokinetics of theophylline during treatment with dirithromycin. *J Clin Pharmacol.* 1990;30:1001–1005.

111. Nafziger AN, May JJ, Bertino JS Jr. Theophylline elimination by diltiazem therapy. *J Clin Pharmacol.*

1987;27:862–865.

112. Sirmans SM, Pieper JA, Lalonde RI, et al. Effect of calcium channel blockers on theophylline disposition. *Clin Pharmacol Ther.* 1988;44:29–34.

113. Gin AS, Stringer KA, Welage LS, et al. The effect of verapamil on the pharmacokinetic disposition of theophylline in cigarette smokers. *J Clin Pharmacol.* 1989;29:728–732.

114. Robson RA, Miners JO, Birkett DJ. Selective inhibitory effect of nifedipine and verapamil on oxidative metabolism colon effects on theophylline. *Br J Clin Pharmacol.* 1988;25:397–400.

115. Cohen IA, Johnson CE, Bernardi RR, et al. Cimetidine–theophylline interaction: Effects of age and cimetidine dose. *Ther Drug Monit.* 1985;37:426–434.

116. Cusack BJ, Dawson GW, Mercer GD, Vestal RE. Cigarette smoking and theophylline metabolism: Effects of cimetidine. *Clin Pharmacol Ther.* 1985;37:330–336.

117. Feely J, Pereira L, Guy E, Hockings N. Factors affecting the response to inhibition of drug metabolism by cimetidine, dose response and sensitivity of elderly and induced subjects. *Br J Clin Pharmacol.* 1984;17:77–81.

118. Cohen IH, Johnson CE, Bernard RR, et al. Cimetidine–theophylline interaction: Effects of age and cimetidine dose. *Ther Drug Monit.* 1985;7:426–434.

119. Powell JR, Rogers JF, Wargin WA, et al. Inhibition of theophylline clearance by cimetidine but not ranitidine. *Arch Intern Med.* 1984;144:484–486.

120. Kelly HW, Powell JR, Donahue JF. Ranitidine at very large doses does not inhibit theophylline elimination. *Clin Pharmacol Ther.* 1986;39:577–581.

121. Lin JH, Chremos AN, Chiou R, et al. Comparative effects of famotidine and cimetidine on pharmacokinetics of theophylline in normal volunteers. *Br J Clin Pharmacol.* 1987;24:669–672.

122. Hemstreet MP, Miles MV, Rutland RO. Effect of intravenous isoproterenol on theophylline pharmacokinetics. *J Allergy Clin Immunol.* 1982;69:360–364.

123. Amirav I, Amitai Y, Avital A, Godfray S. Enhancement of theophylline clearance by intravenous albuterol. *Chest.* 1988;94:444–445.

124. Lombardi TP, Bertino JS Jr, Goldberg A, et al. The effects of a beta-2 selective adrenergic agonist and a beta non selective antagonist on theophylline clearance. *J Clin Pharmacol.* 1987;27:523–529.

125. Garty M, Paul-Keslin L, Ilfeld DN, et al. Increased theophylline clearance in asthmatic patients due to terbutaline. *Eur J Clin Pharmacol.* 1989;36:125–128.

126. Sarkar M, Polk RE, Guzellan PS, et al. In vitro effect of fluoroquinolones on theophylline metabolism in human liver microsomes. *Antimicrob Agents Chemother.* 1990;34:594–599.

127. Fuhr U, Anders EM, Mahr G, et al. Inhibitory potency of quinolone antibacterial agents against cytochrome P4501A2 activity in vivo and in vitro. *Antimicrob Agents Chemother.* 1992;36:942–948.

128. Fuhr U, Staib AH, Kinzig M, Sorgel F. Lack of an effect of macrolides on cytochrome P4501A2 activity in human liver microsomes. Programs and Abstracts, First International Conference on the Macrolides, Azalides and Streptogramins, January 22–25, 1992; Sante Fe, NM. Abstract 206, p.47.

129. Fuhr U, Strobl G, Manaut F, et al. Quinolone antibacterial agents: Relationship between structure and in vitro inhibition of the human cytochrome P450 isoform CYP1A2. *Mol Pharmacol.* 1993;43:191–199.

130. Robson RS, Begg EJ, Atkinson HC, et al. Comparative effects of ciprofloxacin and lomefloxacin on the oxidative metabolism of theophylline. *Br J Clin Pharmacol.* 1990;29:491–493.

131. Koup JR, Toothaker RD, Tosvon E, et al. Theophylline dosage adjustment during enoxacin co-administration. *Antimicrob Agents Chemother.* 1990;34:803–807.

132. Rogge MC, Solomon WR, Sedman AJ, et al. The theophylline–enoxacin interaction: I. Effect of enoxacin dose size on theophylline disposition. *Clin Pharmacol Ther.* 1988;44:579–587.

133. Prince RA, Casabar E, Adair CG, et al. Effect of quinolone antimicrobials on theophylline pharmacokinetics. *J Clin Pharmacol.* 1989;29:650–654.

134. Schwartz J, Jauregui L, Lettieri J, Bachmann K. Impact of ciprofloxacin on theophylline clearance

and steady state concentrations in serum. *Antimicrob Agents Chemother.* 1988;32:75–77.

135. Bowles SK, Popovski Z, Rybak MJ, et al. Effect of norfloxacin on theophylline pharmacokinetics at steady state. *Antimicrob Agents Chemother.* 1988;32:510–512.

136. Nix DE, Norman A, Schentag JJ. Effect of lomefloxacin on theophylline pharmacokinetics. *Antimicrob Agents Chemother.* 1989;33:1006–1008.

137. Al-Turk WA, Shaheen OM, Othman S, et al. Effect of ofloxacin on pharmacokinetics of a single intravenous theophylline dose. *Ther Drug Monit.* 1988;10:160–163.

138. Parent M, St Laurent M, LeBelman M. Safety of fleroxacin coadministered with theophylline to young and elderly volunteers. *Antimicrob Agents Chemother.* 1990;34:1249–1253.

139. Takagi K, Yamaki K, Nadai M, et al. Effect of a new quinolone sparfloxacin on the pharmacokinetics of theophylline in asthmatic patients. *Antimicrob Agents Chemother.* 1991;35:1137–1141.

140. Kappas A, Alvares AP, Anderson KE, et al. Effect of charcoal-broiled beef on antipyrine and theophylline metabolism. *Clin Pharmacol Ther.* 1978;23:445–450.

141. Feldman CH, Hutchinson VE, Pippenger CE, et al. Effect of dietary protein in carbohydrates on theophylline metabolism in children. *Pediatrics.* 1986;66:956–962.

142. Feldman CH, Hutchinson VE, Sher TA, et al. Interaction between nutrition and theophylline metabolism in children. *Ther Drug Monit.* 1982;4:69–76.

143. Juan D, Worwag EM, Schoeller DA, et al. Effects of dietary protein on theophylline pharmacokinetics and caffeine and aminopyrine breath test. *Clin Pharmacol Ther.* 1986;40:187–194.

144. Fagan TC, Walle T, Oexmann MJ, et al. Increased clearance of propranolol in theophylline by high protein compared to high carbohydrates. *Clin Pharmacol Ther.* 1987;41:402–406.

145. Thompson PJ, Skypala I, Dawson S, et al. The effect of diet upon serum concentrations of theophylline. *Br J Clin Pharmacol.* 1983;16:267–270.

146. Turner-Warwick M. Study of theophylline plasma levels after oral administration of new theophylline compounds. *Brit Med J.* 1957;2:67–69.

147. Jackson RH, McHenry JI, Moreland FB, et al. Clinical evaluation of elixophylline with correlation of pulmonary function studies in theophylline serum levels in acute and chronic asthmatic patients. *Dis Chest.* 1964;45:75–79.

148. Boswell R, McGinn JT. Blood levels produced by three oral theophylline containing preparations. *NY J Med.* 1964;64:887–890.

149. Pierson WE, Brennan CW, Stamm SJ, VanArsdel PP. Double blind trial of aminophylline in status asthmaticus. *Pediatrics.* 1971;48:642–646.

150. Mitenko P, Ogilvie RI. Rational intravenous doses of theophylline. *N Engl J Med.* 1973;289:600–603.

151. Fairshter RD, Busse WW. Theophylline—How much is enough? *J Allergy Clin Immunol.* 1986;77:646–648.

152. Jenne JW. Reassessing the therapeutic range for theophylline on laboratory report forms, another viewpoint. *Pharmacotherapy.* 1993;13:595–597.

153. Levy G, Koysooko R. Pharmacokinetic analysis of the effect of theophylline on pulmonary function in asthmatic children. *J Pediatr.* 1975;86:789–793.

154. Racineux JL, Troussier J, Tureant A. Comparison of bronchodilator effects of salbutamol and theophylline. *Bull Eur Physiopathol Respir.* 1981;17:799–806.

155. Maselli R, Casal GL, Ellis EF. Pharmacological effect of intravenous administration of aminophylline in asthmatic children. *J Pediatr.* 1970;76:770–780.

156. Nicholson DR, Chik TW. A re-evaluation of parenteral aminophylline. *Am Rev Respir Dis.* 1973;108:241–245.

157. Koup JR, Brodsky B. Stability of pulmonary function during periodic intravenous bolus aminophylline therapy. *Ther Drug Monit.* 1979;1:85–91.

158. Vozeh S, Kewitz G, Perruchoud A, et al. Theophylline serum concentration and therapeutic effect in severe acute bronchial obstruction. The optimal use of intravenously administered aminophylline. *Am*

Rev Respir Dis. 1982;125:181–184.

159. Richer C, Mathieu M, Bah H, et al. Theophylline kinetics and ventilatory flow in bronchial asthma in chronic airflow obstruction: Influence of erythromycin. *Clin Pharmacol Ther.* 1982;31:579–586.

160. Simons FER, Luciuk GH, Simons KJ. Sustained release theophylline for treatment of asthma in preschool children. *Am J Dis Child.* 1982;136:790–793.

161. Klein JJ, Lefkowitz MS, Spector SL, Cherniack RM. Relationship between serum theophylline levels and pulmonary function before and after inhaled beta-agonist in stable asthmatics. *Am Rev Respir Dis.* 1983;127:413–416.

162. Fairshter RD, Bhola R, Thomas R, et al. Comparison of clinical effects and pharmacokinetics of once a day Uniphyl and twice a day Theo-Dur in asthmatic patients. *Am J Med.* 1985;79(6A):48–53.

163. Holford N, Black P, Couch R, et al. Theophylline target concentration in severe airways obstruction—10 or 20 mg/L? A randomized concentration controlled trial. *Clin Pharmacokinet.* 1993;25: 495–505.

164. Wrenn K, Slovis CM, Murphy F, Greengerg RS. Aminophylline therapy for acute bronchospastic disease in the emergency room. *Ann Intern Med.* 1991;115:241–247.

165. Huang D, O'Brien RG, Harman E, et al. Does aminophylline benefit adults admitted to the hospital for an acute exacerbation of asthma? *Ann Intern Med.* 1993;119:1155–1160.

166. National Asthma Education Program. *Guidelines for the Diagnosis and Management of Asthma.* Bethesda, MD: U.S. Department of Health and Human Services, Public Health Service, National Institutes of Health; June 1991.

167. Welsh PW, Reed CE, Conrad E. Timing of once-a-day theophylline dose to match peak blood level with diurnal variation in severity of asthma. *Am J Med.* 1986;80:1098–1102.

168. Arkin WW, Atkins ME, Harrison D, Stewart JH. Once-daily sustained release theophylline reduces diurnal variation in spirometry and symptomatology in adult asthmatics. *Am Rev Respir Dis.* 1987;135:316–321.

169. Goldberg P, Leffert F, Gonzalez M, et al. Intravenous aminophylline therapy for asthma. A comparison of two methods of administration in children. *Am J Dis Child.* 1980;134:596–599.

170. Eaton ML, Green BA, Church TR, et al. Effect of theophylline in irreversible air flow obstruction. *Ann Intern Med.* 1980;92:758–761.

171. Passamonte PM, Martinez AJ. Effects of inhaled atropine or metaproterenol in patients with chronic airway obstruction and therapeutic serum theophylline levels. *Chest.* 1984;85:610–615.

172. Mahler DA, Matthay RA, Schnieder PE, et al. Sustained release theophylline reduces dyspnea in nonreversible obstructive airway disease. *Am Rev Respir Dis.* 1985;131:22–25.

173. Rice KL, Leatherman JW, Dwayne PG, et al. Aminophylline for exacerbations of chronic obstructive pulmonary disease, a controlled trial. *Ann Intern Med.* 1987;107:305–309.

174. Guyatt GH, Townsend M, Pugsley SO, et al. Bronchodilators in chronic air flow limitation. Efects on airway function, exercise capacity and quality of life. *Am Rev Respir Dis.* 1987;135: 1069–1074.

175. Murciano D, Auclair MH, Pariente R, Aubier M. A randomized controlled trial of theophylline in patients with severe chronic obstructive pulmonary disease. *N Engl J Med.* 1989;320:1521–1525.

176. Lam A, Newhouse MT. Management of asthma and chronic air flow limitation. Are methylxanthines obsolete? *Chest.* 1990;98:44–52.

177. Olson KR, Benowitz NL, Woo OF, Pond SM. Theophylline overdose: Acute single ingestion versus chronic repeated overmedication. *Ann J Emerg Med.* 1985;3:386–394.

178. Hall KW, Dobsen KE, Dalton JG, et al. Metabolic abnormalities associated with intentional theophylline overdose. *Ann Intern Med.* 1984;101:457–462.

179. Shannon M, Love Joy FH Jr. Hypokalemia after theophylline intoxication. The effects of acute versus chronic poisoning. *Arch Intern Med.* 1989;149:2725–2729.

180. Amitai Y, Love Joy FH Jr. Characteristics of vomiting associated with acute sustained release the-

ophylline poisoning: Implications for management with oral activated charcoal. *Clin Toxicol.* 1987;25:539–554.

181. Zwillich CW, Sutton FD, Neff TA, et al. Theophylline induced seizures in adults: Correlation with serum concentration. *Ann Intern Med.* 1975;82:784–787.

182. Hendeles L, Bighley L, Richardson RA, et al. Frequent toxicity from intravenous aminophylline infusions in critically ill patients. *Drug Intell Clin Pharm.* 1977;12:11–18.

183. Aitken ML, Martin TR. Life threatening theophylline toxicity is not predictable by serum levels. *Chest.* 1987;91:10–14.

184. Sessler CN. Theophylline toxicity: Clinical features of 116 consecutive cases. *Am J Med.* 1990;88:567–576.

185. Wasser WG, Bronhein HE, Richardson BK. Theophylline madness. *Ann Intern Med.* 1981;95:191.

186. McPherson ML, Prince SR, Atamer ER, et al. Theophylline induced hypercalcemia. *Ann Intern Med.* 1986;105:52–54.

187. Levine JH, Michael JR, Guarnieri T. Multifocal atrial tachycardia: A toxic effect of theophylline. *Lancet.* 1985;1:12–14.

188. Goldberg MJ, Park GD, Berlinger WG. Treatment of theophylline intoxication. *J Allergy Clin Immunol.* 1986;78:811–817.

189. Shannon M. Predictors of major toxicity after theophylline overdose. *Ann Intern Med.* 1993;119:1161–1167.

190. Hendeles L, Massarari M, Weinberger M. Theophylline. In: Evans WE, Jusko WJ, Schentag JJ, eds. *Applied Pharmacokinetics.* 2nd ed. Spokane, WA: Applied Therapeutics; 1986:1105–1187.

191. Hendeles L, Weinberger M, Szefler S, Ellis E. Safety and efficacy of theophylline in children with asthma. *J Pediatr.* 1992;120:177–183.

192. McEvoy GK, ed. *American Hospital Formulary Service Drug Information.* Bethesda, MD: American Society of Hospital Pharmacists; 1991:2098–2105.

Chapter 19

Vancomycin

Keith A. Rodvold

Sharon M. Erdman

Randy D. Pryka

Keep in Mind

- Design initial doses based on total body weight and renal function; consider using one of the dosing guidelines or nomograms that represent your patient population.

- Intravenous infusions of vancomycin should be administered over a minimum of 1 hour to minimize the incidence of infusion-associated adverse reactions.

- There is a lack of correlation between serum vancomycin concentrations and efficacy.

- Data supporting a correlation between serum vancomycin concentrations and toxicity are minimal.

- Because of the multicompartment nature of the serum concentration–time profile of vancomycin, caution must be applied to the interpretation of pharmacokinetic parameters calculated with a one-compartment model.

- There exists large interpatient variation in the vancomycin pharmacokinetic parameters.

- Dosage adjustments should be based on renal function, patient population characteristics, and serum vancomycin concentrations when available.

- There is no need to monitor serum vancomycin concentrations as frequently as aminoglycoside antibiotics.

Vancomycin hydrochloride is a tricyclic glycopeptide antibiotic obtained from *Amycolatopsis orientalis* (formerly *Streptomyces orientalis* and *Nocardia orientalis*).[1,2] Vancomycin has been available since its discovery in 1956 for the systemic treatment of Gram-positive infections. During the 1960s and early 1970s, the use of vancomycin declined markedly secondary to the perception of its toxic effects and the development of antistaphylococcal penicillins and cephalosporins. There has been a resurgence in the use of vancomycin during the last 15 years because of the increasing number of patients who are immunocompromised, have indwelling foreign devices, or have methicillin-resistant staphylococcal infections.[3]

The renewed interest in vancomycin has prompted numerous studies to examine its pharmacokinetic and pharmacodynamic properties. A variety of dosing methods have emerged that are now used in clinical practice; however, skepticism exists regarding the need to monitor serum vancomycin concentrations because of the lack of conclusive evidence concerning the relationship between serum vancomycin concentrations and clinical efficacy or toxicity.[4,5]

This chapter reviews each of these issues in conjunction with the pharmacokinetic and pharmacodynamic data available for vancomycin in adult (Table 19–1) and pediatric (Table 19–2) patients. Applications of the data to the development of dosage regimens and serum concentration monitoring are also discussed.

CLINICAL PHARMACOLOGY AND THERAPEUTICS

Mechanism of Action and Spectrum of Activity

The primary mechanism of action of vancomycin is the inhibition of bacterial cell wall synthesis of multiplying microorganisms.[22] Vancomycin inhibits the second stage of peptidoglycan synthesis by binding with the essential cell wall precursor, D-alanyl-D-alanine. This mechanism differs from that of penicillins and cephalosporins, which inhibit the third stage of peptidoglycan synthesis. In addition, the antibacterial effects of vancomycin also include alteration of bacterial cell wall permeability and selective inhibition of ribonucleic acid (RNA) synthesis.[23,24]

Vancomycin is a narrow-spectrum antimicrobial agent that is bactericidal against most aerobic and anaerobic Gram-positive cocci and bacilli (Table 19–3).[25,26] Both *Staphylococcus aureus* and *Staphylococcus epidermidis,* including methicillin-resistant strains, are susceptible at minimum inhibitory concentrations (MICs) of 1 to 5 mg/L; however, the MICs of vancomycin for strains of *S. epidermidis* have occasionally been reported to be between 10 and 20 mg/L.[27] *Staphylococcus haemolyticus,* a coagulase-negative staphylococcus, has recently been reported to be resistant to both vancomycin and teicoplanin.[28]

Viridans streptococci, *Streptococcus pneumoniae,* beta-hemolytic streptococci, *Corynebacterium jeikeium,* and *Clostridia difficile* are highly susceptible to vancomycin.[25,26] *Listeria monocytogenes* is usually susceptible to vancomycin. *Lactobacillus, Actinomyces, Pediococcus, Flavobacterium meningosepticum,* and *Erysipelothrix* exhibit variable susceptibility to vancomycin.[29] Gram-negative bacteria (except occasional *Neisseria gonorrhoeae* isolates) and *Leuconostoc* species are usually resistant to vancomycin.

Vancomycin is only bacteriostatic against most strains of enterococci *(Enterococcus faecium* and *Enterococcus faecalis),* with MICs reported to be greater than 50 mg/L.[29,30] More recently, low- and high-level vancomycin resistance has been reported for *Enterococcus.* An aminoglycoside (eg, gentamicin) should be added to the vancomycin regimen for synergistic bactericidal effects against systemic enterococcal infections.

Clinical Indications

Vancomycin is used for the systemic treatment of serious Gram-positive infections (Table 19–4). Intravenous vancomycin is the drug of choice for infections caused by methicillin-resistant staphylococci.[31–33] Vancomycin is also recommended for infections caused by methicillin-

TABLE 19–1. PHARMACOKINETIC PARAMETERS (MEAN ± SD) OF VANCOMYCIN IN VARIOUS ADULT PATIENT POPULATIONS

	$V_{d,ss}$[a] (L/kg)	$t_{1/2,\alpha}$ (h)	$t_{1/2,\beta}$ (h)	Cl (mL/min)	Reference
Normal renal function	0.587 ± 0.04	0.105–0.13	7.7 ± 1.8	86.1 ± 8.9[b]	6,7
	0.49–1.25		4.7–11.2	74.3–96.2	
	0.43–1.48[c]				
Varying renal function					
Cl_{cr} >70 mL/min/1.73 m²	0.50 ± 0.20	0.40 ± 0.20	5.2 ± 2.6	98.4 ± 24.3[b]	8
Cl_{cr} 40–70 mL/min/1.73 m²	0.59 ± 0.27	0.49 ± 0.32	10.5 ± 3.6	52.6 ± 17.7[b]	
Cl_{cr} <39 mL/min/1.73 m²	0.64 ± 0.18	0.51 ± 0.21	19.9 ± 10.2	31.3 ± 14.9[b]	
Cl_{cr} >60 mL/min	0.72 ± 0.35		9.1 ± 2.8	62.7 ± 25.3	9
Cl_{cr} 10–60 mL/min	0.89 ± 0.31		32.3 ± 19.3	28.3 ± 16.0	
Cl_{cr} <10 mL/min	0.90 ± 0.21		146.7 ± 65.5	4.87 ± 2.60	
End-stage renal disease, Cl_{cr} <5 mL/min	1.00 ± 0.12	1.13 ± 0.25	121.3 ± 8.2	5.6	10
	2.92 ± 0.45[c]				
Geriatric, mean age = 68.5 y	0.76 ± 0.06	0.13 ± 0.03	12.14 ± 0.77	60 ± 3.3	11
	1.92 ± 0.30[c]				
Obese, >90% overweight	0.26 ± 0.03 TBW			187.5 ± 64.7	12
	0.68 ± 0.07 IBW				
Burn injuries, >10% BSA	0.59 ± 0.17			142.8 ± 34.5	13
Intravenous drug abuse	0.56 ± 0.12			98.0 ± 29.7	13

[a] $V_{d,ss}$, apparent volume of distribution at steady state; $t_{1/2,\alpha}$, distribution half-life; $t_{1/2,\beta}$, elimination half-life; Cl, total body clearance; Cl_{cr}, creatinine clearance; BSA, body surface area; TBW, total body weight; IBW, ideal body weight.
[b] mL/min/1.73 m².
[c] Half-life of second distribution phase for three-compartment model.

TABLE 19–2. PHARMACOKINETIC PARAMETERS OF VANCOMYCIN IN CHILDREN, INFANTS, AND NEONATES[a]

Study	PNA[a] (d)	PCA (wk)	GA (wk)	Weight (kg)	$V_{d,ss}$ (L/kg)	$t_{1/2,\alpha}$ (h)	$t_{1/2,\beta}$ (h)	Cl (mL/min)
Schaad et al[14]								
7 premature infants	3.3		32	1.23	0.736[b]	0.15	9.8	15[c]
7 premature infants	4.7		34	1.57	0.706[b]	0.05	5.9	27[c]
7 full-term infants	2.6		40	3.07	0.690[b]	0.26	6.7	30[c]
12 infants	0.26 y			4.9	0.595[b]	0.27	4.1	50[c]
4 infants	0.36 y			5.2	0.964[b]	0.49	4.1	81[c]
5 children	3.92 y			15.5	0.818[b]	0.23	2.4	163[c]
7 children	5.58 y			20.0	0.764[b]	0.50	3.0	131[c]
6 children	7.58 y			26.7	0.538[b]	0.31	2.2	134[c]
Gross et al[15]								
3 premature infants	29.0	30.0		0.83	0.970[b]		9.9	1.099[d]
6 premature infants	39.5	32.7		1.38	0.647[b]		7.1	1.053[d]
Naqvi et al[16]								
14 premature infants	8–66	<41			0.481		4.9	1.341[d]
6 premature infants	3–6.5 mo	>43			0.377		3.0	1.671[d]
Reed et al[17]								
15 premature infants (SD)	20.5	31.4	28.4	1.07	0.53		6.0	1.22
12 premature infants (SS)					0.52		6.6	1.15
Lisby-Sutch and Nahata[18]								
7 premature infants	33	32.6	27.9	1.14	0.476		7.0	0.855[d]
6 premature infants	92	44.4	32.0	3.16	0.470		2.9	2.139[d]
Kildoo et al[19]								
15 infants	29	33.2	29.0	1.30	0.48		5.6	1.37
Jarrett et al[20]								
11 premature infants	10	30.9		1.26	0.51		8.5	0.742[d]
Asbury et al[21]								
19 infants	33.9	34.2	29.3	1.78	0.52		5.6	2.38

[a] PNA, postnatal age; PCA, postconceptional age; GA, gestational age; $V_{d,ss}$, apparent volume of distribution at steady state; $t_{1/2,\alpha}$, distribution half-life; $t_{1/2,\beta}$, elimination half-life; Cl, total body clearance; SD, single-dose study; SS, steady-state study.
[b] Values represent apparent volume of distribution of beta phase. ($V_{d,\beta}$).
[c] mL/min/1.73 m².
[d] mL/min/kg.

TABLE 19–3. ANTIBACTERIAL SPECTRUM AND IN VITRO SUSCEPTIBILITY OF VANCOMYCIN

Organism	Minimum Inhibitory Concentration (mg/L)	Minimum Bactericidal Concentration (mg/L)
Staphylococcus aureus	1.56 to 3.12	1.56 to 6.25
Staphylococcus epidermidis	1.56 to 3.12	1.0 to 100
Streptococcus pyogenes	0.16 to 2.5	—
Streptococcus pneumoniae	0.29	—
Viridans streptococci	<0.1 to 1.56	<0.312 to >50
Group D streptococci		
Enterococcal	0.5 to 6.25	100 to >100
Nonenterococcal	0.1 to 1.56	0.29 to 50
Clostridium species	0.5 to 5.0	0.78 to >10
Corynebacterium species	0.5 to 5.0	0.78 to >10
Propionibacterium	0.5 to 5.0	0.78 to >10
Bacillus anthracis	0.5 to 5.0	0.78 to >10
Listeria monocytogenes	5.0	—
Lactobacilli	0.78 to >320	2.5 to >320

Adapted from Hermans PE, Wilhelm MP. Vancomycin. *Mayo Clin Proc.* 1987;62:901–905, with permission.

susceptible microorganisms in patients who are allergic to penicillins or cephalosporins. Vancomycin is also used for serious infections caused by microorganisms resistant to commonly used antimicrobial agents (eg, group JK diphtheroids, *Flavobacterium meningosepticum*) and as part of the empiric antibiotic regimen in febrile neutropenic patients.[34]

Intravenous dosages of vancomycin should be individualized and administered over a minimum of 60 minutes.[4] In treating patients with meningitis, the addition of intrathecal or intraventricular doses of vancomycin may be necessary.[35] Intraperitoneal administration of vancomycin may be a consideration in patients receiving chronic intermittent peritoneal dialysis.[36]

The in vitro synergy testing of vancomycin with gentamicin, rifampin, or both has produced conflicting results.[32,33] In penicillin-allergic patients, enterococcal infections of endocarditis and bacteremia should be treated with vancomycin plus gentamicin. The combination of vancomycin and rifampin for 6 weeks, as well as gentamicin during the first 14 days of therapy, has been suggested for the treatment of prosthetic valve endocarditis caused by methicillin-resistant coagulase-negative staphylococci.[37] The addition of gentamicin or rifampin (or both) to vancomycin therapy should be considered whenever clinical failures to vancomycin are suspected.[32]

Vancomycin is an alternative parenteral agent for endocarditis prophylaxis in dental, oral, or upper respiratory tract procedures for penicillin-allergic patients.[38] The combination of vancomycin and gentamicin can be used for endocarditis prophylaxis in patients at risk of develop-

TABLE 19–4. THERAPEUTIC AND PROPHYLACTIC USE OF VANCOMYCIN

Use	Penicillin-Allergic Patients	Non-Penicillin-Allergic Patients
Therapy		
Serious methicillin-resistant staphylococcal infections		✓
Endocarditis caused by		
Streptococcus viridans	✓	
Staphylococcus aureus (plus gentamicin)	✓	
Staphylococcus epidermidis (plus rifampin and/or gentamicin)		✓
Group D enterococci (plus gentamicin)	✓	
Group D nonenterococci (*Streptococcus bovis*)	✓	
MBC[a] <10 mg/L (vancomycin only)		
MBC ≥10 mg/L (plus gentamicin)		
Diphtheroids	✓	
Central nervous system or dialysis shunt infections caused by		
Gram-positive cocci (plus rifampin)		✓
Diphtheroids		✓
Meningitis caused by		
Gram-positive cocci	✓	
Flavobacterium		✓
Diphtheroids	✓	
Other serious infections caused by gram-positive cocci	✓	
Clostridium difficile colitis (oral vancomycin)		✓
Prophylaxis		
Endocarditis		
Oral and upper respiratory tract procedures	✓	
Gastrointestinal/genitourinary procedures (plus gentamicin)	✓	
Prosthetic implant surgery	✓	
Shunt infections in chronic hemodialysis		✓

[a] Minimum bactericidal concentration.
Adapted from Cunha BA, Ristuccia AM. Clinical usefulness of vancomycin. *Clin Pharm.* 1983;2:417–424, with permission.

ing bacteremia from various genitourinary or gastrointestinal procedures. Vancomycin is also an alternative agent for prophylaxis in patients receiving either prosthetic surgery (eg, cardiac valve or total hip replacement) or chronic hemodialysis.

Oral vancomycin is considered to be a drug of choice for serious infections of *Clostridium difficile* colitis. The usual adult dose ranges from 125 to 500 mg every 6 hours.[39] An oral vancomycin dosage of 500 mg per 1.73 m^2 every 6 hours has been recommended to treat *C. difficile* colitis in infants and children.[40] Oral vancomycin is also used for the treatment of *S. aureus* colitis and for microbial suppression in immunocompromised hosts.

CLINICAL PHARMACOKINETICS

Absorption

For the treatment of serious systemic infections, vancomycin is administered parenterally as an intravenous infusion. The recommended method is to dissolve the desired dose in 100 to 250 mL of 5% dextrose or physiologic saline and infuse the dose at a rate no faster than 15 mg per minute.[41] Administration of vancomycin by rapid or slow intravenous bolus injections is not recommended because of the possible occurrence of red-neck syndrome or hypotension. Intramuscular injections are also not recommended for the treatment of serious systemic infections, and can be very painful, causing localized erythema and swelling.

Vancomycin is administered orally for the treatment of staphylococcal ileocolitis and pseudomembranous colitis caused by *C. difficile*. When administered orally, vancomycin is not appreciably absorbed from the gastrointestinal tract in patients with normal renal function and intact bowel.[42] Geraci et al failed to detect serum vancomycin concentrations in eight normal subjects who received four 500-mg oral doses of vancomycin.[43] In addition, seven of the eight volunteers (all with normal renal function) had urine vancomycin concentrations of less than 3.8 mg/L after administration of the fourth dose, suggesting minimal absorption from the gastrointestinal tract. Oral administration of the same dose, however, did produce high enough concentrations of vancomycin in the stool (400–20,000 μg/g) of the normal volunteers to treat diarrhea caused by *S. aureus* or *C. difficile*.

Recent reports have documented serum vancomycin concentrations in the range 1.2 to 34 mg/L after the administration of oral vancomycin (125–500 mg every 6 hours) in patients with impaired renal function, or severe inflammatory bowel disease (ie, pseudomembranous colitis caused by *C. difficile*), or both.[44–47] Patients with these conditions who are to receive orally administered vancomycin should be monitored periodically for serum vancomycin concentrations, especially if high doses are anticipated to be used for prolonged periods (eg, ≥2 g/d for more than 10 days).

Distribution

The serum concentration–time profile of vancomycin is best described mathematically on the basis of a two- or three-compartment open model.[6–8,11,12,14,48] After intravenous administration, an early distribution phase is observed with a half-life of approximately 7 minutes, which is followed by a second slower distribution phase having a half-life of 30 to 90 minutes (see Table 19–1).[6,7,11]

The mean steady-state peak serum concentrations in 11 healthy volunteers immediately following 60-minute intravenous infusions of 500 mg every 6 hours and 1000 mg every 12 hours of vancomycin were 40.3 ± 6.2 and 65.7 ± 7.9 mg/L, respectively, whereas the mean steady-state trough concentrations were 11.2 ± 2.2 and 7.9 ± 1.7 mg/L, respectively.[7]

The apparent volume of distribution of vancomycin approximates or slightly exceeds total body water. Using a two-compartment model, the apparent volume of distribution ($V_{d,ss}$) of vancomycin is 0.58 ± 0.22 L/kg.[8] The mean volume of distribution appears to be significantly larger in morbidly obese patients (43 L) when compared with normal patients (28.9 L),[12] and is also larger in patients with end-stage renal disease (0.9 L/kg).[10,49,50] In addition, the volume of distribution is larger in elderly patients, possibly as a result of age-related changes in peripheral circulation and altered protein binding.[11] The volume of the central compartment (V_c) is 0.22 ± 0.12 L/kg using a two-compartment model.[8]

The penetration of vancomycin into body fluids and tissues is presented in Tables 19–5 and 19–6. After single and multiple intravenous injections, therapeutic vancomycin concentrations have been measured in ascitic, pericardial, peritoneal, pleural, and synovial fluids, with minimal amounts of vancomycin measured in bile.[43] Conflicting data exist as to whether intravenously administered vancomycin achieves appreciable concentrations in the stool.[14,43] In human tissues, vancomycin concentrates in skeletal muscle, heart valves, and bone.[43,55,56]

In patients with uninflamed meninges, vancomycin penetrates poorly into the cerebrospinal fluid (CSF).[43,62] Therapeutic vancomycin concentrations have been noted in the CSF of patients with inflamed meninges, with CSF penetration thought to be directly related to the degree of meningeal inflammation. There are, however, cases in which adequate CSF vancomycin concentrations after intravenous dosing have not been obtained, even in the presence of inflamed meninges. The combination of intravenous and intrathecal (or intraventricular) administration of vancomycin (5–20 mg every 24 hours) may be necessary in these circumstances to obtain adequate CSF concentrations in some patients.[63,64] There is currently a lack of data specifying appropriate CSF vancomycin concentrations or data confirming the safety of intraventricular vancomycin in the treatment of ventriculitis/meningitis. Peak CSF vancomycin concentrations greater than 100 mg/L have been measured following the intraventricular administration of 5 to 20 mg of vancomycin per day, and appear to have been well tolerated.[65,66] Therefore, the value of measuring CSF vancomycin concentrations is in ensuring adequate CSF concentrations against the infecting microorganism; its ability to predict the occurrence of adverse effects remains questionable.

Protein Binding

Binding of vancomycin to plasma proteins has been reported to be in the range 10 to 60%.[6,8,10,67–69] Mean values of vancomycin protein binding reported in the literature include 55% in healthy volunteers with normal renal function,[6] 30 to 40% in presumably infected patients with varying degrees of renal function (mean albumin = 2.5–2.9 g/dL),[8,68] 28.7% in burn patients (mean albumin = 2.5 g/dL),[69] and 18.5% in patients with end-stage renal disease (mean albumin = 2.78 g/dL).[10] In the concentration range 10 to 100 mg/L, vancomycin protein binding does not seem to be concentration dependent. In addition, vancomycin is bound predominantly to serum albumin rather than α_1-acid glycoprotein, as is demonstrated by a good correlation between the serum albumin concentration and the percentage of vancomycin protein bound (Figure 19–1).[69]

In a case report of a patient with immunoglobulin A myeloma who received 1 g of vancomycin every 12 hours for seven doses, unusually high serum vancomycin concentrations, a prolonged elimination half-life despite normal renal function, and a suboptimal response to vancomycin therapy were demonstrated.[70] Extensive protein binding (92–98%) of vancomycin by the immunoglobulin A protein may have accounted for these findings.

TABLE 19-5. VANCOMYCIN CONCENTRATIONS IN BODY FLUIDS AND TISSUES

Site	Intravenous Dose	N[a]	Serum Concentration (mg/L)	Site Concentration (mg/L)	Ratio of Site:Serum (%)
Body Fluids					
Aqueous humor	500 mg (S)[b]	5	13.8 (11.0–17.0)	<0.78	<5.6
Ascites	500 mg (S)	11	6.9 (6.4–8.0)	3.6 (1.5–5.2)	52
Bile	500 mg (M)	3	14.8 (9.1–20.6)	8.7 (4.8–12.5)	59
Cerebrospinal fluid	500 mg (S)	9	7.5 (5.2–10.0)	3.1 (2.0–3.6)	41
Uninflamed	500 mg (S)	9	6.3 (4.8–10.0)	0.0	0
	500 mg (M)	2	N/A	0.0	0
Meningitis					
Infants, children	10–15 mg/kg/dose (M)	3	N/A	3.1 (1.2–4.8)	
Infants, children	30–60 mg/kg/dose (M)	10	N/A	3.9 (1.0–12.3)	
Infants	10–15 mg/kg/dose (M)	2	N/A	3.1 (2.05–4.2)	
Pericardial	500 mg (S)	11	6.2 (4.4–8.7)	2.3 (0.8–5.5)	37
	500 mg (M)	3	8.6 (7.1–9.8)	6.7 (5.4–8.0)	78
Pleural	500 mg (S)	12	7.3 (2.9–10.0)	3.0 (0.0–8.1)	31
Adults	500 mg (S)	3	9.0 (8.5–9.3)	5.7 (3.3–8.1)	63
Infants.	15 mg/kg/dose (M)	1	N/A	16.0	
Synovial	500 mg (M)	6	7.0 (5.2–8.7)	5.7 (4.0–6.4)	81
Tissues					
Bone					
Cancellous	15 mg/kg/dose (S)	14	22.1 (10.5–52.9)	2.3 (0.5–16.0)[d]	13
Cortical	15 mg/kg/dose (S)	10	22.1 (10.5–52.9)	1.14 (0.0–2.58)[d]	4
Cardiac heart valve	15 mg/kg/dose (S)	33	14.2 (± 2.0 SE)	4.2 (± 1.0 SE)[d]	30
Skeletal muscle	15 mg/kg/dose (S)	33	14.2 (± 2.0 SE)	3.2 (± 0.8 SE)[d]	23

[a] N, number of subjects.
[b] S, single dose; M, multiple doses.
[c] Concentrations in mg/g.
Data are taken from References 14, 43, and 51–56.

TABLE 19–6. VANCOMYCIN CONCENTRATIONS IN PERITONEAL FLUID BY DIALYSIS METHOD

	Dosage and Route of Administration	N[a]	Time of Sampling (h)	Dialysate Concentration (mg/L)
CAPD[b] without peritonitis				
Bunke et al[57]	10 mg/kg IV (S)[c]	6	0–4	4.1 ± 0.9
			4–8	2.6 ± 0.6
			8–12	2.1 ± 0.7
			12–24	3.6 ± 0.9
	10 mg/kg IP (S)	6	0–4	106 ± 28
			4–8	9.4 ± 1.5
			8–12	1.9 ± 0.8
			12–24	1.6 ± 0.7
Morse et al[58]	15 mg/kg IV (S)	4	6	5.8 ± 2.6
		12	4.3 ± 1.8	
		48	3.0 ± 1.4	
	30 mg/kg IP (S)	4	6	610 ± 295
		12	59.2 ± 73.8	
		48	4.7 ± 2.5	
CAPD with peritonitis				
Whitby et al[59]	25 mg/kg IV (S)	6	N/A[d]	12.3 ± 0.8
Boyce et al[36]	30 mg/kg IP × 2 (given 7 d apart)	11	72	12.1 ± 4.2
			144	4.0 ± 1.5
	1 g IP followed by 30 mg/L dialysate for 5 d	8	N/A	N/A
IPD without peritonitis				
Nielsen et al[60]	1 g IV (S)	11	N/A	0–10.3
IPD with peritonitis				
Glew et al[61]	1 g IV weekly	6	N/A	0–22.5

[a] Number of subjects.
[b] CAPD, continuous ambulatory peritoneal dialysis; IPD, intermittent peritoneal dialysis.
[c] S, single dose.
[d] Not available.

Metabolism/Elimination

Vancomycin is excreted primarily through glomerular filtration, with some evidence of possible renal tubular secretion. In patients with normal renal function, 80 to 100% of an intravenously administered dose is recovered in the urine within 24 hours.[62] The total body clearance of vancomycin is linearly correlated with creatinine clearance.[9,48,71–73] Vancomycin renal clearance, however, exceeds creatinine clearance, suggesting that mechanisms other than glomerular filtration (eg, tubular secretion) play a role in vancomycin elimination.[8,11,74] The elimination half-life

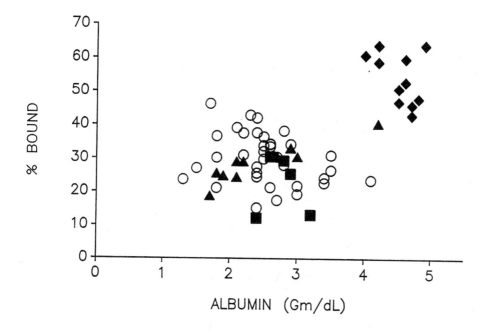

Figure 19–1. Relationship between serum albumin and percentage protein binding of vancomycin. The symbols represent individual patients from four different studies: O, Rodvold et al[8]; ■, Tan et al[10]; ▲, Zokufa et al[69]; ◆, Cutler et al.[11]

of vancomycin in patients with normal renal function is 2.9 to 13.3 hours,[6,7,9] and increases in proportion to decreases in the creatinine clearance.[8,9]

The majority of data suggest that vancomycin is excreted almost entirely by the kidneys without appreciable metabolism; however, several recent studies have suggested that some nonrenal clearance of vancomycin may occur in humans, accounting for approximately 5 to 20% of total body clearance.[8,48,74] The nonrenal clearance of vancomycin is supported by the following: renal clearance of vancomycin accounts for only 60 to 85% of the total clearance of vancomycin[8,74,75]; the y intercept is different from zero when looking at the relationship between vancomycin clearance and creatinine clearance[8,48]; and relatively high vancomycin clearances are observed in patients with impaired renal function. In contrast to a previous report,[76] dosage adjustments of vancomycin do not appear to be required in patients with hepatic impairment.[8]

Special Populations

Patients on Dialysis

The influence of dialysis procedures on the disposition of vancomycin has been studied in patients during hemodialysis, intermittent peritoneal dialysis, chronic ambulatory peritoneal dialysis, hemofiltration, and hemoperfusion. Several factors may dictate whether a drug is removed by dialysis, including the physicochemical properties of the drug, the mechanical properties of the dialysis system, the blood flow and dialysate flow during the dialysis procedure, and the pharmacokinetic characteristics of the drug.[77]

Hemodialysis has no significant effect on the elimination rate of vancomycin, so that dosage supplementation after hemodialysis is not necessary. Salem et al calculated the hemodialysis clearance of vancomycin by quantitating the amount of vancomycin removed in the dialysate.[78] Overall, less than 10% of an administered vancomycin dose is removed during routine hemodialysis, so that dosage supplementation is not required after hemodialysis. In contrast, the use of high-flux polysulfone dialyzers in two studies substantially increased the plasma clearance of vancomycin when compared with standard cuprophan dialyzers, decreasing plasma vancomycin concentrations by 49.5% during a 4-hour period[79] and 21% during a 2-hour period.[80] Because substantial amounts of vancomycin were removed during high-flux hemodialysis, dosage supplementation after the procedure was initially recommended; however, it appears as if there is a significant redistribution of vancomycin (48%), which takes approximately 12 hours after the high-flux dialysis procedure to equilibrate, so that postdialysis concentrations at 12 hours approach those observed prior to the dialysis procedure (14.5 ± 1.1 mg/L predialysis and 13.3 ± 1.0 mg/L postdialysis).[80] Therefore, recommendations for dosage supplementation following high-flux hemodialysis should be based on serum concentrations obtained at least 12 hours after the end of the procedure.

Hemoperfusion using activated charcoal or exchange resin cartridges may be useful. The clearance of vancomycin during a 4-hour hemoperfusion procedure using a Gambro charcoal cartridge was 23.6 mL/min, which increased to 85.2 mL/min during a 5-hour hemoperfusion procedure using an Amberlite resin cartridge in the same patient.[81]

Hemofiltration seems to have a significant effect on the disposition of vancomycin, by decreasing the elimination half-life and increasing the clearance of vancomycin after an intravenous dose of 18 mg/kg in patients with end-stage renal disease.[82] In addition, the mean fraction of vancomycin removed by hemofiltration was approximately 32%, so that dosage adjustment of vancomycin may be needed to maintain adequate serum vancomycin concentrations. Similar to the report regarding high-flux hemodialysis, a rebound of serum concentrations occurred following hemofiltration.

The removal of vancomycin during intermittent peritoneal dialysis remains to be elucidated. In uninfected patients, there was a 40% decline in vancomycin serum concentrations during the first 15 hours of the procedure, so that supplemental dosing may be necessary to maintain adequate concentrations.[60] Other studies have suggested minimal clearance by peritoneal dialysis. The clearance of vancomycin by intermittent peritoneal dialysis is quite variable (4–19.8 mL/min), and may have an impact on the total body clearance of vancomycin, possibly requiring some supplemental dosing.[61,83]

After the administration of intravenous vancomycin, therapeutic concentrations in peritoneal fluid are reached within 1 hour of administration, and exceed the MIC for most susceptible Gram-positive organisms for up to a 7- to 16-day period.[84,85] The serum half-life of vancomycin after intraperitoneal administration in uninfected patients undergoing continuous ambulatory peritoneal dialysis is approximately 105 hours,[58] as compared with 184 hours in patients with peritonitis.[86]

When vancomycin is administered intraperitoneally, approximately 35 to 65% of the dose is absorbed systemically in uninfected patients,[57,58,60,87] as compared with 75 to 91% in patients with peritonitis.[86] Peritoneal clearance of vancomycin is poor, representing less than 20% of the total body clearance of vancomycin.[57] The mean elimination half-life of vancomycin in the serum of patients undergoing CAPD is 66.9 hours.[87] The intraperitoneal route does not seem to be associated with any significant alterations in vancomycin pharmacokinetics.

Special Adult Patient Populations

Several patient populations have been identified in whom altered disposition of vancomycin has been observed. These include patients with impaired renal or hepatic function, morbidly obese patients, patients with burn wounds, the elderly, intravenous drug users, the critically ill, cardiac surgery patients, and pregnant patients (see Table 19–1).

Renally Impaired. Patients with renal impairment have been the most widely studied population for alterations in vancomycin disposition[8–10,48,49,88]; from these studies, many dosing methods for vancomycin have been developed. A progressive prolongation of the elimination half-life and a reduction in total body clearance of vancomycin are observed as renal function declines. In patients with a creatinine clearance of 70 mL/min or greater, the total body clearance of vancomycin is 98.4 ± 24.3 mL/min (64.4–137.9 mL/min),[8] compared with only 4.87 ± 2.60 mL/min (1.05–15.67 mL/min) in patients with end-stage renal disease on hemodialysis.[9]

As mentioned, the nonrenal clearance of vancomycin may account for approximately 5 to 20% of the total body clearance,[8,48,74] so that alterations in liver function are not likely to affect the disposition of vancomycin. It appears, however, as if the serum half-life of vancomycin may be prolonged in patients with impaired hepatic function, with no correlation between the severity of liver impairment and the degree of prolongation of the half-life or other parameters. Pachorek and Wood reported a case of a 77-year-old man with renal and hepatic dysfunction in whom the estimated and measured creatinine clearance did not solely explain the patient's vancomycin elimination half-life of 10 days.[89] Among possible explanations for this finding was that the patient may have had a greatly reduced nonrenal clearance of vancomycin secondary to hepatic dysfunction.

Geriatric Patients. The pharmacokinetics of vancomycin were assessed in older patients in a study that compared the disposition of vancomycin in six healthy elderly males (mean age, 68.5 years) as compared with 6 young healthy males (mean age, 23 years).[11] Both total clearance and renal clearance of vancomycin were decreased in the geriatric patients as compared with the young patients (60 ± 3 mL/min vs 78.3 ± 5 mL/min and 56.7 ± 3.3 mL/min vs 70 ± 5 mL/min, respectively). In addition, the geriatric patients exhibited a longer elimination half-life (12.1 hours vs 7.2 hours) and an increased apparent volume of distribution at steady state (0.76 L/kg vs 0.46 L/kg), which was attributed by the authors to enhanced tissue binding of the drug in the elderly despite similar unbound fractions. Guay et al evaluated the pharmacokinetics of vancomycin in 148 elderly (≥60 years) and 140 young (18–59 years) patients.[90] These investigators demonstrated that age is a significant predictor of total vancomycin clearance, elimination half-life, and apparent volume of distribution. These factors should be considered when dosing vancomycin in geriatric patients so that significant drug accumulation does not occur.

Obese Patients. Because obese patients undergo physiologic changes that may alter drug disposition, Blouin et al evaluated the pharmacokinetics of vancomycin in six morbidly obese (>90% overweight) patients as compared with four nonobese patients (<15% overweight).[12] The morbidly obese patients had significantly larger apparent volumes of distribution than the nonobese patients (43.0 L vs 28.9 L) and shorter elimination half-lives (3.2 hours vs 4.8 hours, respectively). Obese subjects also had significantly greater total clearances of vancomycin than nonobese patients, but not when adjusted for total body weight. Vance-Bryan et al evaluated the effect of weight on the pharmacokinetics of vancomycin in group of 107 obese (>20% above their lean body weight) and 123 nonobese adult patients.[50] These investigators demonstrated that total body weight was a significant and independent predictor of apparent volume of distribution and total body clearance of vancomycin. Therefore, larger total daily doses of vancomycin (mg/d) may be required to maintain the same concentrations in obese patients as compared with nonobese patients, and vancomycin should be dosed on a mg/kg basis using the patient's total body weight.

Burn Patients. Several studies have evaluated the pharmacokinetics of vancomycin in patients with burn injuries.[13,48,69,73,91,92] Several of these studies have shown significantly greater creatinine clearance and vancomycin clearance (up to 33%) in burn patients as compared with non-burned patients, as well as significantly shorter elimination half-lives. Burn patients required higher daily doses than nonburned patients to achieve similar serum concentrations, and they may possibly require more frequent dosing. Although the exact mechanism of the increased vancomycin clearance and dosage requirement in burn patients has not been elucidated, possible explanations for this increased clearance include increased elimination through the burn wounds, increased glomerular filtration rates, and possible altered protein binding.[13,69] Therefore, individualization of vancomycin dosing is required to avoid subtherapeutic serum concentrations in this patient population.

Intravenous Drug Abusers. One study has assessed the pharmacokinetics of vancomycin in intravenous drug abusers.[13] Intravenous drug abusers were shown to have a 31% increase in mean vancomycin clearance when compared with control subjects; however this difference did not reach statistical significance. Further study is needed in this patient population to determine if dosage adjustments are required for adequate dosing.

Critically Ill Patients. The pharmacokinetics of vancomycin have been studied in 10 critically ill patients.[93] The clearance and elimination half-life of vancomycin correlated well with underlying renal function; however, no other significant pharmacokinetic alterations were observed.

Cardiac Surgery Patients. The physiologic changes that occur during cardiopulmonary bypass include a decrease in cardiac output and organ perfusion, which may significantly alter the disposition of drugs. Several studies during cardiopulmonary bypass surgery have evaluated the pharmacokinetics of vancomycin perioperatively, as well as examined the proper dosing of vancomycin for adequate prophylactic coverage.[56,94–96] Results have shown a precipitous fall in serum vancomycin concentrations on initiation of cardiopulmonary bypass, followed by relatively constant serum concentrations maintained throughout bypass. One study has shown a rebound in vancomycin concentrations when the aorta was unclamped toward the end of bypass.[94] In addition, a dose of 15 mg/kg preoperatively provided adequate serum concentrations throughout the bypass procedures without evidence of toxicity.

Pregnant Patients. A case report in a 30-year-old intravenous drug abuser at 30 weeks of gestation demonstrated increased vancomycin dosage requirements (57 mg/kg/d) to achieve therapeutic serum concentrations.[97] Possible explanations for this increased vancomycin dosage requirement in this pregnant patient include an increase in urinary clearance of vancomycin or an increase in the volume of distribution because of pregnancy, or possibly increased vancomycin clearance secondary to intravenous drug abuse.

Children, Infants, and Neonates

Vancomycin pharmacokinetics following intravenous administration in pediatric patients have been described by either one- or two-compartment pharmacokinetic models.[14–21,98–100] As in adult patient populations, vancomycin exhibited poor absorption in two infants receiving 15 to 20 mg/kg/d oral doses with resultant serum concentrations of 0.9 and 1.5 mg/L in each infant.[14]

The majority of pharmacokinetic data for vancomycin in pediatric patient populations have been collected in preterm and low-birth-weight infants (see Table 19–2). The reported pharmacokinetic parameters of clearance and apparent volume of distribution range from 0.017 to 0.484 L/h and from 0.24 to 2.5 L, respectively, for infants with postconceptional ages of 29 to 48 weeks. A large interpatient variation in these vancomycin parameters has been observed in the neonatal and infant populations. The variation can be explained in part by inherent processes of renal maturation and changes in the ratio of intra- and extracellular fluid volume in relation to total body weight.

Pharmacokinetic parameters of vancomycin in neonates and infants have been evaluated based on the degree of maturation (Table 19–7). Several studies have shown that clearance and apparent volume of distribution directly correlate with postconceptional age and body weight.[16–19,21,98–100] Serum creatinine has also to been identified as a useful marker for correlating renal function and vancomycin clearance in infants greater than 14 days of age.[19,98–100]

The pharmacokinetic profile of vancomycin in children older than 3 years has been described in only 18 children.[14] The reported pharmacokinetic parameters of clearance and apparent volume of distribution ($V_{d,\beta}$) range from 131 to 163 mL/min/1.73 m² and from 0.538 to 0.818 L/kg, respectively. The mean elimination half-life of vancomycin in children ranges from 2.2 to 3.0 hours, compared with 4.1 to 9.8 hours in newborn and older infants.

Special Pediatric Patient Populations

Limited pharmacokinetic data are available concerning vancomycin in special pediatric patient populations. Bailie et al evaluated the peak and trough serum concentrations and dosage requirements of vancomycin in young burn patients (five of six patients between 1 and 5 years old).[92] Individualized vancomycin dosages between 52.2 and 66.8 mg/kg/d were necessary to achieve mean steady-state peak (15-minute postinfusion) and trough concentrations of 27.4 and 7.3 mg/L, respectively. This study suggests that vancomycin pharmacokinetics may be altered in pediatric burn patients.

Vancomycin pharmacokinetics have been evaluated in six infants undergoing extracorporeal membrane oxygenation (ECMO).[101] A wide interpatient variation in pharmacokinetic parameters of vancomycin was observed; however, the values were similar to those previously reported in the literature for infants not receiving ECMO. Similarly, cardiopulmonary bypass surgery has not been shown to alter the pharmacokinetics of vancomycin in children between the ages of 0.8 and 4.8 years.[102]

TABLE 19–7. SIGNIFICANT CORRELATIONS OF VANCOMYCIN PHARMACOKINETIC PARAMETERS IN INFANTS AND NEONATES

Study	Significant Correlation	Correlation Coefficient	P	Equation Describing the Correlation
Naqvi et al[16]	Cl vs PCA[a]	0.649	<.001	$V_{d,ss}$ (L) = 0.563 * Weight + 0.052
	k vs body weight	0.464	<.04	Cl (L/h) = 0.0224 * PCA − 0.639
Schaible et al[98]	$V_{d,ss}$ vs body weight[b]	0.93	<.0001	
	Cl vs PCA[b]	0.91	<.0001	
	$t_{1/2,\beta}$ vs 1/SCr[b]	0.69	<.05	
James et al[99]	Cl vs PCA	0.80	<.001	Cl (mL/min/kg) = 0.0014 * PCA$^{-1.48}$
	Cl vs body weight	0.78	<.001	Cl (mL/min/kg) = 0.00018 * weight$^{0.089}$
	Cl vs SCr	-0.74	<.005	Cl (mL/min/kg) = 2.1 * $e^{-0.00132 * SCr}$
	$t_{1/2,\beta}$ vs PCA	-0.91	<.001	$t_{1/2,\beta}$ (min) = 2.08 × 10^7 * PCA$^{-3.1}$
	$t_{1/2,\beta}$ vs body weight	-0.88	<.005	$t_{1/2,\beta}$ (min) = 4.5 × 10^5 * weight$^{-0.96}$
	$t_{1/2,\beta}$ vs SCr	0.91	<.001	$t_{1/2,\beta}$ (min) = 10.7 * SCr − 67
Reed et al[17]	$V_{d,ss}$ vs body weight[b]	0.89	<.001	
	$V_{d,ss}$ vs BSA[b]	0.89	<.001	
	$V_{d,ss}$ vs PCA[b]	0.62	<.05	
	Cl vs body weight[b]	0.89	<.001	
	Cl vs BSA[b]	0.89	<.001	
	Cl vs PCA[b]	0.62	<.05	
Lisby-Sutch and Nahata[18]	Cl vs PCA	0.863	<.0002	
	Cl vs body weight	0.867	<.0001	
	Cl vs PNA	0.873	<.0001	

Study	Correlation	r	P
Kildoo et al[19]	$V_{d,ss}$ vs GA	0.84	<.05
	$V_{d,ss}$ vs PCA	0.67	<.05
	$V_{d,ss}$ vs body weight	0.86	<.05
	Cl vs GA	0.54	<.05
	Cl vs PCA	0.88	<.05
	Cl vs body weight	0.82	<.05
	Cl vs SCr	−0.82	<.05
Leonard et al[100]	Cl vs PCA	0.724	<.005
	Cl vs SCr	−0.829	<.005
	$t_{1/2,\beta}$ vs PCA	−0.627	<.01
	$t_{1/2,\beta}$ vs SCr	0.725	<.01
Jarrett et al[20]	Cl vs SCr	−0.81	<.0027
	$t_{1/2,\beta}$ vs SCr	0.84	<.0012
Asbury et al[21]	Cl vs PCA	0.92	<.0001
	Cl vs body weight	0.85	<.0001
	Cl vs GA	0.71	<.0009
	Cl vs PNA	0.42	<.03
	$V_{d,ss}$ vs body weight	0.94	<.0001
	$V_{d,ss}$ vs BSA	0.93	<.0001
	$V_{d,ss}$ vs PCA	0.89	<.0001

[a] PCA, postconceptional age; GA, gestational age; SCr, serum creatinine; BSA, body surface area; $V_{d,ss}$, apparent volume of distribution at steady state; Cl, total body clearance; k, elimination rate constant; $t_{1/2,\beta}$, elimination half-life.

[b] Correlations represent steady-state data.

PHARMACODYNAMICS

Numerous authors have suggested various therapeutic ranges and sampling times for the appropriate monitoring of serum vancomycin concentrations.[4,5,7,9,54,103,104] These reports have led to a large disparity in the method of therapeutic drug monitoring of vancomycin. Geraci et al arbitrarily recommended peak concentrations (within 30 minutes of the end a 1-hour infusion) of 30 to 40 mg/L and trough concentrations of 5 to 10 mg/L.[43,105] This range seems acceptable and should be used in the therapeutic drug monitoring of vancomycin.[4]

Correlation of Serum Concentration With Clinical Response

Simple and conventional concepts would suggest that the recommended peak serum vancomycin concentrations of 30 to 40 mg/L are adequate for most microorganisms for which vancomycin is used clinically. In addition, serum concentrations of antibiotics are often used as surrogate markers to represent the concentration at the site of infection. For a given microorganism to be considered susceptible, the minimum inhibitory concentration (MIC) of the antibiotic must be equal to or less than achievable serum concentrations; preferably, the peak serum concentration should be four times the MIC of the infecting pathogen. The MICs and minimum bactericidal concentrations (MBCs) of most Gram-positive microorganisms for vancomycin are equal to or less than 5 mg/L (see Table 19–3). Notable exceptions are enterococci and methicillin-resistant coagulase-negative staphylococci. The recommended peak serum vancomycin concentrations of 30 to 40 mg/L are 10 to 40 times these MICs. Both serum and tissue concentrations remain above the MICs and MBCs of the infecting organism for the duration of the dosing interval when trough serum vancomycin concentrations are maintained between 5 and 10 mg/L. In addition, vancomycin demonstrates a postantibiotic effect (suppression of bacterial growth when serum concentrations are below the MIC) for several of the Gram-positive microorganisms.[106]

Serum bactericidal titers, MICs, and MBCs of vancomycin have been associated with clinical outcome in adult and pediatric patient populations.[14,18,107,108] Sorrell and colleagues demonstrated that a cure rate of 100% (eight of eight patients) was achieved when MICs for vancomycin in staphylococcal infections were less than 32 mg/L compared to only a 50% cure rate (3 of 6 patients) when MIC values were higher.[107] Louria et al demonstrated a relationship between dose, serum concentration, and bactericidal concentrations of vancomycin in only eight patients.[108] Evidence of bacteriologic eradication of staphylococci could not be demonstrated in two patients who had bactericidal concentrations of less than 1:8.

Schaad et al cured 19 of 20 pediatric patients with staphylococcal infections who demonstrated serum vancomycin concentrations greater than 12 mg/L and resultant bactericidal titers of greater than 1:8.[14] Peak serum vancomycin concentrations of 25 mg/L resulted in a median inhibitory titer of 1:32 and a median bactericidal titer of 1:16, whereas trough serum vancomycin concentrations less than 12 mg/L produced median bactericidal titers of 1:4 for isolates of *S. aureus.* When serum vancomycin concentrations were greater than 12 mg/L, all strains of *S. epidermidis* exhibited bactericidal titers of 1:8 or greater, with the exception of one strain (bactericidal titer of 1:4). In a subsequent study by this same group, 33 patients ranging in age from 1 week to 16 years demonstrated complete eradication of either *S. aureus* or *S. epidermidis* isolates in 19 of 19 patients with follow-up cultures.[108] All peak serum vancomycin concentrations (mean ± SD, 33.2 ± 9.2 mg/L) resulted in bactericidal titers ranging from 1:8 to 1:32. Finally,

Lisby-Sutch and Nahata, in a series of 30 pediatric patients, demonstrated that peak and trough vancomycin concentrations ranging from 25 to 35 mg/L and from 5 to 10 mg/L, respectively, resulted in bactericidal titers of >1:8 and 1:2.[18]

Overall, the relatively small sample size makes extrapolation of the preceding data to either adult or pediatric patients difficult; however, there appears to be a correlation between serum concentrations and serum bactericidal titers. In addition, the attainment of peak titers greater than 1:8 and of trough titers of 1:2 seems to result in improved bacteriologic and clinical outcome.

Correlation of Serum Concentrations With Toxicity

The major dose-related adverse effects associated with vancomycin are ototoxicity and nephrotoxicity. The correlations between these adverse effects and serum vancomycin concentrations are difficult to interpret because of changes in vancomycin's purity during the past 35 years, concomitant drug therapy and/or disease states, and the criteria used to define toxicity. Adverse reactions commonly associated with vancomycin therapy are summarized in Table 19–8.

Nephrotoxicity

Previous reports of vancomycin-induced nephrotoxicity could not establish a direct causal effect because many of the patients who developed nephrotoxic effects were also receiving concomitant aminoglycoside therapy, had preexisting renal disease, or had life-threatening *Staphylococcus* infections. The majority of reports implicating vancomycin as a potential nephrotoxic agent appeared in the early 1960s and may have been related, in part, to impurities in the marketed product. Data compiled recently suggest that the less purified preparations may indeed have had more nephrotoxic potential, with greater than 50% of the cases of vancomycin-induced nephrotoxicity reported during the first 6 years of clinical use.[109]

Over the last 30 years, the incidence of nephrotoxicity has not changed dramatically. The estimated incidence of vancomycin-induced nephrotoxicity is 5 to 7% when it is used as a single agent and 0 to 35% when used concurrently with an aminoglycoside.[110–116] In toxicology studies in rats and dogs, vancomycin alone had mild nephrotoxic potential[117–120]; however, the concomitant administration of vancomycin and aminoglycosides (eg, tobramycin) to rats resulted in a significant increase in nephrotoxicity compared with either agent alone.[117,119,120] A similar trend of increased nephrotoxicity in patients with the combined use of vancomycin and an aminoglycoside (eg, gentamicin and tobramycin) has been observed in some studies,[110,111,115,121,122] but not in others.[112,114,116,123]

The relationship of nephrotoxicity to vancomycin serum concentrations has been difficult to establish. In a retrospective review on the toxicity of vancomycin, two patients who developed nephrotoxic effects had trough vancomycin concentrations greater than 30 mg/L[110]; however, several other retrospective and prospective studies have associated trough vancomycin concentrations greater than 10 mg/L with the development of nephrotoxic effects.[111,112,115] Other factors that have been associated with an increased risk of nephrotoxic effects with vancomycin therapy include concomitant administration of an aminoglycoside and the length of treatment (longer than 15–21 days).[110,111,115]

In reported cases of nephrotoxicity, the renal dysfunction has been reversible, with the return of the serum creatinine to baseline following a reduction in dose or a discontinuation of therapy.

TABLE 19–8. SUMMARY OF VANCOMYCIN ADVERSE EFFECTS

Effect	Incidence	Comments
Nephrotoxicity	< 5% when used alone	Relationship of nephrotoxicity to serum concentrations is difficult to determine; tendency for troughs to be greater than 30 mg/L.
	35% when used with an aminoglycoside	Return of serum creatinine to baseline with a decrease in dose or discontinuation of vancomycin. Additive with concurrent aminoglycosides; up to 35% incidence.
Ototoxicity	1.4–5.5%	Relationship to serum concentrations is difficult to assess; most frequently associated with serum concentrations 80–100 mg/L. Pretreatment audiometric testing may be performed to monitor for high-frequency hearing loss. Use with caution in patients with renal impairment.
Red-neck syndrome	5.3–11.2%	Histamine-like reaction associated with rapid intravenous infusion; characterized by flushing, tingling, pruritus, erythema, and a macular rash. Begins 15 to 45 min after start of infusion, and abates 10 to 60 min after stopping the infusion. May be minimized by infusing at a rate of 15 mg/min or slower or by premedicating with antihistamines.
Rash	2–6%	Maculopapular or erythematous, unrelated to the red-neck syndrome. Resolves with drug discontinuation.
Thrombophlebitis, chills, fever	6%	Earlier preparations with 13% incidence. Can be minimized by diluting the drug into at least 100 mL and infusing over at least 60 min.
Neutropenia	< 2%	Reports have increased, paralleling increased use over past years. Etiology unclear, with no substantial relation to dose or serum concentrations. Returns to normal after discontinuation of vancomycin. Periodic monitoring is recommended in patients receiving vancomycin longer than 2 wk.

Ototoxicity

The first signs of ototoxicity caused by vancomycin therapy include tinnitus, dizziness, and high-frequency hearing loss occurring secondary to auditory nerve damage.[109] The majority of initial reports relating the use of vancomycin to ototoxicity are difficult to interpret because of the concurrent administration of other ototoxic medications (eg, aminoglycosides such as neomycin, streptomycin, and kanamycin), the presence of underlying renal impairment in some of the patients, and the lack of pretreatment auditory testing, making the occurrence of ototoxicity subjective. In addition, ototoxicity has not been demonstrated in guinea pigs given vancomycin alone or with ethacrynic acid,[124] but vancomycin has been shown to augment greatly the ototoxicity of gentamicin when administered concomitantly with gentamicin in guinea pigs.[125]

The incidence of vancomycin-associated ototoxicity has not changed significantly over the past few years and has been reported to be 1.4 to 5.5%.[110,113] The relationship between ototoxicity and serum concentrations is unclear because of the lack of documented timing of serum concentrations in relation to the dose in many of the reports. Ototoxicity has been most frequently associated with serum concentrations in the range 80 to 100 mg/L,[43] although it has been reported with serum concentrations between 25 and 152 mg/L.[113,126,127] The data suggest a possible causal relationship between vancomycin serum concentrations and ototoxic effects; however, it is not clear whether peak or trough vancomycin concentrations are more contributory. In addition, pretreatment audiometric testing is recommended, especially in patients with renal failure or who are receiving other ototoxic medications.

Adverse Effects Not Correlated With Serum Concentrations

Red-Neck Syndrome

Red-neck syndrome or red-man syndrome is a histamine-like reaction characterized by flushing, tingling, pruritus, tachycardia, erythema, angioedema, and a macular rash involving the face, neck, upper trunk, back, and arms.[41,128–130] It is most often associated with the rapid intravenous administration of vancomycin and the drug concentration per administration volume rather than the serum concentration of vancomycin. There have, however, been reports of red-neck syndrome following the slow infusion of vancomycin,[131] following the intraperitoneal administration of vancomycin,[132] and even following the oral administration of vancomycin for presumed pseudomembranous colitis.[133] The reaction typically begins 15 to 45 minutes after initiation of the infusion and resolves 10 to 60 minutes after its termination.

The incidence of red-man syndrome has been reported to be 5 to 47% in patients and up to 70 to 90% in healthy volunteers.[41,129,134–138] Vancomycin-induced red-man syndrome is thought to be mediated in part by histamine release. Some studies suggest that there is a relationship between the frequency and severity of the reaction and plasma histamine concentrations (as measured by the area under the plasma histamine concentration–time curve) during and after the vancomycin infusion,[129,136,138] although one study failed to show such a relationship.[41]

This reaction may be minimized or avoided by infusing vancomycin at a rate no greater than 15 mg/min.[139] Infusing a 1-g dose of vancomycin over 2 hours decreases the frequency and severity of red-man syndrome, as well as the release of histamine, as compared with a one hour infusion.[41] In addition, vancomycin desensitization (using sequential incremental doses) and the concurrent administration of antihistamines or corticosteroids have been successfully used in an attempt to decrease the severity and incidence of this reaction.[128,136,138,140]

Rashes

A maculopapular or erythematous rash may occur in 2 to 6% of patients. The rash typically resolves with discontinuation of vancomycin therapy. In addition, a recent review has reported the occurrence of exfoliative dermatitis, erythema multiforme, Stevens–Johnson syndrome, erythema bullosum, and epidermal necrolysis in patients who received vancomycin, and is typically observed between 2 and 31 days of vancomycin therapy.[141]

Thrombophlebitis, Chills, and Fever

With the earlier, less purified preparations of vancomycin, the incidence of thrombophlebitis, chills, and fever approached 50%. Since the purification of vancomycin preparations in the 1970s, the incidence of adverse effects such as thrombophlebitis, chills, and fever has been substantially reduced. Currently, the incidence of thrombophlebitis and chills ranges from 6 to 13% with the use of the more purified preparations, and may be minimized by diluting the drug into at least 100 mL of diluent and infusing the drug over at least 60 minutes. Rigors have still been reported with the use of a specific vancomycin product.[142] In addition, chemical thrombophlebitis does not appear to be directly related to serum vancomycin concentrations. Vancomycin is still a cause of drug-induced fever, despite the use of more purified products, and should be considered in any patient with prolonged fevers in whom all other etiologic causes have been eliminated.[143]

Neutropenia

The incidence of neutropenia during vancomycin therapy has increased, probably paralleling the recent increase in the use of vancomycin for serious resistant staphylococcal infections, as well as the long-term use of vancomycin for endocarditis and osteomyelitis,[144] or the sustained vancomycin concentrations in dialysis patients.[145] The exact cause of the neutropenia is unknown, although it has been postulated that vancomycin has a direct toxic effect on granulocyte production or acts possibly through an immunologically mediated pathway.[146] Vancomycin-induced neutropenia does not appear to be dose or concentration related; however, a recent report has associated the appearance of neutropenia with trough serum concentrations consistently above 10 mg/L.[147] The neutropenia generally occurs within 2 to 6 weeks of starting vancomycin therapy and returns to normal 1 to 15 days after discontinuation of the vancomycin.[144] In some cases, fever and rash may accompany the neutropenia. Periodic monitoring (eg, once weekly) is recommended if greater than 2 weeks of vancomycin therapy is to be used.

Other Adverse Effects

There have been four case reports of acute interstitial nephritis associated with vancomycin therapy,[148–151] of which only one was biopsy proven, showing diffuse interstitial, predominantly mononuclear inflammatory infiltrates.[148] The clinical picture of acute interstitial nephritis usually suggests a hypersensitivity reaction including fever, skin rash, and the acute onset of renal insufficiency. Other findings that may be present include eosinophilia and eosinophiluria. The acute interstitial nephritis associated with vancomycin therapy occurred between 7 and 28 days of vancomycin therapy and serum vancomycin concentrations were in the therapeutic range. In all cases, resolution of the symptoms and the acute renal failure were observed on discontinuation of the vancomycin therapy.

Vancomycin has also been associated with the development of thrombocytopenia in several case reports.[152–154] In all cases the patients developed severe thrombocytopenia ($<17 \times 10^9$/L); vancomycin-induced antiplatelet antibodies were demonstrated in several of the patients, suggesting an autoimmune or immune complex etiology.[152,153]

Rarely, systemic arterial hypotension and shock have been reported, most often occurring after the rapid administration of vancomycin.[139,142,155-158] Cardiac arrest has also been reported following the rapid administration of vancomycin.[157] The hypotension results from histamine release, which is most often associated with rapid infusion, and may depress cardiac function and cause peripheral vasodilation. Studies in dogs have shown the existence of dose-dependent depression of cardiac function with the administration of vancomycin, with a decrease in cardiac output and mean arterial pressure.[159] This, however, has not been demonstrated in humans.[160] Treatment of the hypotension is facilitated by the fact that these episodes are usually transient and self-limiting. Patients most often respond to repositioning, intravenous fluids, and occasionally inotropes or antihistamines.

Vancomycin has also been reported to produce an anaphylactoid reaction[161-163] characterized by dyspnea, generalized pruritus, urticaria, hypotension, and wheezing in some cases, which may respond to epinephrine. This reaction appears also to be mediated by the release of histamine and may be dose or infusion related.

Chemical peritonitis, manifested by an acute onset of abdominal pain and cloudy dialysate effluent, has been noted in several patients receiving intraperitoneal vancomycin for exit-site infections.[164,165] The peritonitis appears to be related to the route of administration, the concentration of vancomycin in the dialysate, or impurities present in the commercially available vancomycin products. The peritonitis has occurred as soon as 3 to 4 hours after the instillation of vancomycin into the peritoneal cavity and resolved without further therapy.

Other adverse reactions associated with vancomycin therapy include mononeuritis multiplex,[166] enhanced neuromuscular blockade of vecuronium,[167] and spasmodic low back pain.[168]

Drug–Drug Interactions

In contrast to the number of adverse effects associated with vancomycin therapy, there are relatively few reported interactions of vancomycin with other therapeutic agents. The most notable drug–drug interaction of vancomycin includes the increased incidence of nephrotoxicity observed with the concurrent administration of aminoglycoside antibiotics, as described earlier. Other drug interactions include the possible inactivation of vancomycin by heparin when administered through the same intravenous line.[169] This is demonstrated in a case report of an intravenous drug abuser with methicillin-resistant *S. aureus* endocarditis and deep vein thrombosis who failed to defervesce or respond bacteriologically for 7 days while heparin and vancomycin were being infused through the same line. On administration of the two agents through separate intravenous lines, the patient promptly defervesced and displayed negative blood cultures within 24 hours. In addition, in vitro studies by the same investigator demonstrated the formation of precipitates and a subsequent 50 to 60% reduction in vancomycin activity at concentrations of each agent achieved in the intravenous lines.

The concurrent administration of indomethacin and vancomycin in neonates has resulted in a markedly prolonged elimination half-life and an increased volume of distribution of vancomycin when compared with neonates who received vancomycin alone.[170] One possible explanation for this result includes a decrease in the glomerular filtration rate induced by indomethacin, impairing the renal elimination of vancomycin.

Lastly, when administered with warfarin in patients undergoing valve replacement surgery, vancomycin did not demonstrate a potentiation of the hypoprothrombinemic response when compared with cefamandole and cefazolin.[171]

Vancomycin is stable when admixed with 5% dextrose injection, with 0.9% sodium chloride injection, and in various concentrations of dextrose when stored in plastic syringes.[172,173] Vancomycin has also been shown to be stable in total parenteral nutrition (TPN) solutions containing 3% amino acids for 8 days, with and without heparin and refrigeration, and in solutions containing 1.65 and 4.25% amino acids for 4 hours at room temperature.[174,175] This allows administration of vancomycin without interruption of the TPN infusion. In addition, when administering vancomycin concomitantly with heparin in a peritoneal dialysis fluid at commonly used concentrations, there was no evidence of incompatibility for 24 hours,[176] nor were any visual precipitates observed when vancomycin was concurrently infused with methotrexate.[177]

Visual incompatibilities have been observed with the administration of vancomycin after ceftriaxone and aztreonam in the same intravenous line.[178,179] In both cases, the visual precipitate was subsequently avoided by flushing the intravenous line with 5 to 10 mL of 0.9% sodium chloride between administrations of the two agents.

Reduced vancomycin activity of up to 40% at 4 weeks has also been demonstrated in the Infusaid Drug Pump Model 100, an implantable drug pump delivery system used for osteomyelitis.[180]

THERAPEUTIC REGIMEN DESIGN

The most efficient method for providing patients with effective intravenous vancomycin therapy is for the clinician to consider the available pharmacokinetic and pharmacodynamic data to determine initial dosages, systematically monitor objective and subjective parameters, and then make appropriate dosage adjustments as indicated. Table 19–9 provides a series of monitoring parameters and questions useful in the initiation and monitoring of vancomycin therapy. This therapeutic drug monitoring process provides a standardized problem-solving approach to identifying issues associated with a patient's vancomycin therapy and individualization of dosage regimens. In addition, it is necessary for the clinician to maintain communication with physicians, nurses, laboratory technicians, and the patient to increase the effectiveness of the monitoring process.

Initial Adult Dosing Methods

The traditional approach to dosing intravenous vancomycin in adults has been the use of the original manufacturer's guidelines of 500 mg every 6 hours or 1000 mg every 12 hours. Obviously, this approach does not take into account the interpatient variability in vancomycin pharmacokinetics or simple patient characteristics such as body weight and renal function. The use of such standardized dosage regimens has also been shown to result in higher than desired steady-state serum concentrations in healthy, human volunteers with normal renal function.[7]

Several dosing guidelines, equations, and nomograms have been proposed for providing rational initial dosing regimens of vancomycin in patients with varying degrees of renal function.[127] Moellering et al constructed the first nomogram[72] (Figure 19–2), which was subsequently modified into a table for the manufacturer's package insert (Table 19–10). This nomogram is a useful source for the total daily dose of vancomycin; however, it is difficult to

Therapeutic Drug Monitoring
Gerald E. Schumacher

Table 19–18, which appears on page 622, should read as follows:

TABLE 19–18. PROPORTIONAL DOSAGE ADJUSTMENT FROM PEAK AND TROUGH SERUM VANCOMYCIN CONCENTRATIONS[a]

$$\frac{\Delta C_{ss}}{dose} = \frac{\Delta C_{ss,D}}{new\ dose}$$

$$\frac{C_{ss,peak} - C_{ss,trough}}{dose} = \frac{C_{ss,peak,D} - C_{ss,trough,D}}{new\ dose}$$

$C_{ss,peak}$ = measured peak serum vancomycin concentration (mg/L) obtained within 30 min of infusion

$C_{ss,trough}$ = measured trough serum vancomycin concentration (mg/L) obtained just before start of infusion

dose = vancomycin dose (mg) given around the measured peak and trough concentrations

$C_{ss,peak,D}$ = desired peak serum vancomycin concentration obtained within 30 min of infusion

$C_{ss,trough,D}$ = desired trough serum vancomycin concentration obtained just before start of infusion

New dose = vancomycin dose (mg) needed to achieve the desired target peak and trough concentrations

[a] Desired peak and trough serum concentrations range between 30 and 40 mg/L and between 5 and 10 mg/L, respectively.

TABLE 19–9. MONITORING OF INTRAVENOUS VANCOMYCIN THERAPY IN CLINICAL PRACTICE

I. Baseline and Follow-up Monitoring Parameters

Baseline	Follow-up
Age	
Gender	
Height	
Weight	qod
Temperature	tid
Blood urea nitrogen	q3d
Serum creatinine	q3d
Complete blood count with differential	q3d
Culture and sensitivity tests	days 2–4
Fluid status (input/output)	qd
Concomitant antibiotics	qd
Potential oto- and nephrotoxins	qd
Signs of efficacy and toxicity	qd

II. Daily Monitoring on Vancomycin Patients

1. Record monitoring parameters listed above.
2. Check current dosage regimen with nursing administration times.
3. Communicate with other health care professionals regarding patient's clinical status.
4. Determine a *plan* for each patient's treatment course.
5. Determine when the next serum vancomycin concentrations should be obtained. Ask yourself: Are serum vancomycin concentrations really needed? Will the laboratory promptly assay the samples (ie, weekends, holidays)?
6. When ordering vancomycin concentrations, communicate with the patient's nurse, ward clerk, and laboratory to ensure the proper collection of blood samples and recording of infusion and sampling times.

III. Evaluation of all Vancomycin Concentrations and Pharmacokinetic Parameters With Respect to Patient's Clinical Status

1. What is your dosage recommendation on a "mg/kg/dose" as well as "mg/kg/d"?
2. How does your final dosage recommendation compare with a similar patient population reported in the pharmacokinetic literature?
3. Have any of the following occurred that could influence your interpretation:
   a. Wrong dose administered
   b. Wrong calculation
   c. Wrong recorded information (eg, infusion time, blood sample collection)
   d. Drug not completely administered
   e. Previous dose(s) given at wrong time(s)
   f. Laboratory error in collection or assaying of samples

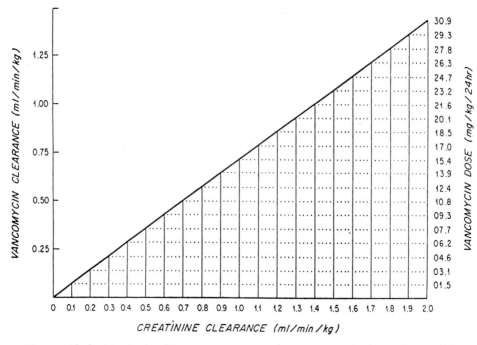

Figure 19–2. Moellering dosage nomogram for vancomycin in patients with impaired renal function. The therapeutic goal is an average steady-state concentration of 15 mg/L. The nomogram is not valid for functionally anephric patients on dialysis. Creatinine clearance should be estimated from the equations in Table 19–10. (*From Moellering RC, Krogstad DJ, Greenblatt DJ. Vancomycin therapy in patients with impaired renal function: A nomogram for dosage. Ann Intern Med. 1981;94:343–346, with permission.*)

nomogram is a useful source for the total daily dose of vancomycin; however, it is difficult to use because the calculation of creatinine clearance is in units of mL/min/kg, which can be inadvertently confused with serum creatinine. In addition, the daily maintenance dose (mg/kg/d) is without guidance in terms of a specific dose and dosing interval. A dosing chart (Table 19–11), based on a one-compartment model adaption of the Moellering nomogram, has been created to provide exact dose and dosing interval guidelines.[181]

Matzke et al have constructed a fixed-dose variable-dosing interval nomogram (Figure 19–3) based on one-compartment vancomycin pharmacokinetic parameters from 56 patients.[9] This nomogram is designed to provide a dose and dosing interval to achieve peak and trough serum vancomycin concentrations of 30 and 7.5 mg/L, respectively. Several retrospective, comparative studies suggest that the resultant serum vancomycin concentrations from this dosing method are much higher than originally predicted.[182,183] But a few investigators have shown that the Matzke nomogram performed with less bias and more precision than the Moellering nomogram.[184–186]

TABLE 19–10. VANCOMYCIN PACKAGE INSERT DOSAGE GUIDELINES FOR PATIENTS WITH RENAL IMPAIRMENT

1. The initial dose should be no less than 15 mg/kg, even in patients with mild to moderate renal insufficiency.

2. Calculate the patient's creatinine clearance (Cl_{cr}) from the following equations:

$$Cl_{cr,males} \ (mL/min) = \frac{(140 - age) * LBW^a}{72 * serum \ creatinine}$$

$$Cl_{cr,females} \ (mL/min) = \frac{(140 - age) * LBW}{72 * serum \ creatinine} * 0.85$$

3. Determine daily maintenance dose from the following table:

Creatinine Clearance (mL/min)	Vancomycin Dosage (mg/24 h)
100	1545
90	1390
80	1235
70	1080
60	925
50	770
40	620
30	465
20	310
10	155

4. **Limitations:** The table is *not* valid for functionally anephric patients. In anuria, a dose of 1000 mg (or 15 mg/kg) every 7 to 10 d has been recommended.

^{a} Lean body weight.

achieved within 24 to 48 hours by simply initiating vancomycin therapy at a dosage of 6.5 to 8 mg/kg every 6 to 12 hours.[48] Lake and Peterson designed simplified guidelines for providing dosing intervals for patients with varying degrees of renal function (Table 19–12).[104]

Rodvold et al proposed vancomycin dosing guidelines based on two-compartment pharmacokinetic parameters measured in 37 patients with varying degrees of renal function.[8] Stepwise multiple linear regression analysis revealed that creatinine clearance was the strongest predictor of vancomycin clearance, and this relationship was used to provide an equation to calculate the required daily vancomycin dose. The dosing intervals that the calculated daily dose can be divided into and administered are provided (Table 19–13). This dosing method is designed to achieve peak and trough serum vancomycin concentrations of 30 to 40 and 5 to 10 mg/L, respectively.

The choice of a particular initial dosing method should be based on comparative studies as well as experience. Perspective evaluations and comparative data assessing these dosing methods would suggest that the Moellering and Lake methods offer the least biased and most precise predictions of vancomycin dosage.[127,182,183,187,188] Experience in the authors' institutions would suggest that the Lake or Rodvold methods would provide the most reliable dosing guidelines.

TABLE 19–11. VANCOMYCIN DOSAGE CHART ADAPTED FROM FIGURE 19–2

1. Loading dose: 15 mg/kg
2. Maintenance dose: Select dose and dosing interval from the following chart based on the patient's creatinine clearance in mL/min and body weight in kg.

Creatinine Clearance[a] (mL/min)	Body weight: 40–55 kg[a] Dose: 500 mg[b]	55–75 kg 750 mg	75–100 kg 1000 mg
81–100	q8h	q12h	q18h
54–80	q12h	q18h	q24h
40–53	q18h	q24h	q36h
27–39	q24h	q36h	q48h
21–26	q36h	q48h	q72h
16–20	q48h	q60h	q84h
13–15	q60h	q84h	q108h
10–12	q72h	q108h	q144h

[a] Creatinine clearance should be estimated from the equations in Table 19–10. From Brown DL, Mauro LS. Vancomycin dosing chart for use in patients with renal impairment. *Am J Kidney Dis.* 1988;11:15–19, with permission.

Each dosing method has its limitations, and the clinician should consider monitoring serum vancomycin concentrations at least once weekly until an individualized dosage is established.

None of the preceding initial dosing methods have application to patients with severe renal impairment (creatinine clearance less than 10 mL/min and patients on dialysis). In general, initial doses of 15 mg/kg or 1000 mg every 7 to 10 days are usually recommended.[49] Monitoring of serum vancomycin concentrations, including serial collection of two or three samples separated by two to three half-lives, may be useful for determining an elimination half-life and predicting when another dose should be administered.

Initial Pediatric and Neonatal Dosing Methods

Pediatric and neonatal dosing guidelines suggested by various investigators are summarized in Table 19–14. The first dosing recommendations for both neonatal and pediatric patient populations were based on data presented by Schaad et al.[14] These dosage guidelines were based on peak serum vancomycin levels of 25 to 40 mg/L; however, a subsequent evaluation 4 years later found that the recommendation of 30 to 45 mg/kg/d for infants less than 30 days of age was associated with serum concentrations in excess of the commonly accepted therapeutic range for vancomycin.[190] Currently, dosage recommendations based on postconceptional age (PCA) and body weight seem to provide the best options for empiric dosing of infants and neonates.[16–19,98–100,191] In addition, serum creatinine may prove to be a useful guide in the empiric dosing of vancomycin in neonates and infants older than 14 days.

Selecting an empiric dosing method is difficult. Only a few of the dosing methods have been subsequently tested in patient populations other than those in which they were originally derived.[127,189–191] In addition, the highest degree of pharmacokinetic variability is seen in infants

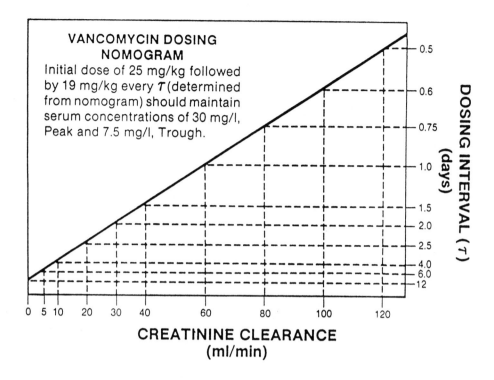

Figure 19–3. Matzke dosage nomogram for vancomycin in patients with impaired renal function. The nomogram is not valid for peritoneal dialysis patients. Creatinine clearance should be estimated from the equations in Table 19–10. Initial dose of 25 mg/kg followed by 19 mg/kg every τ (determined from nomogram) should maintain serum concentrations of 30 mg/L (peak) and 75 mg/L (trough). (*From Matzke GR, McGory RW, Halstenson CE, Keane WF. Pharmacokinetics of vancomycin in patients with various degrees of renal function. Antimicrob Agents Chemother. 1984;25:433–437, with permission.*)

derived.[127,189–191] In addition, the highest degree of pharmacokinetic variability is seen in infants less than 2 months old. Dosage individualization using a dosing method that incorporates post-conceptional age, birth weight, and/or serum creatinine, as well as measurement of steady-state vancomycin serum concentrations, seems the most prudent guide to dosing vancomycin in the pediatric and neonatal patient populations.

Serum Concentration Monitoring

The use of serum vancomycin concentrations for therapeutic drug monitoring remains contro-versial.[4,5] The large interpatient variability in pharmacokinetic parameters of vancomycin is well documented and strongly suggests the need to monitor serum vancomycin concentrations. There

TABLE 19–12. VANCOMYCIN DOSAGE GUIDELINES: "LAKE METHOD"

1. Calculate the patient's creatinine clearance (Cl_{cr}) from the following equations:

$$Cl_{cr,males} \ (mL/min) = \frac{(140 - age) * LBW^a}{72 * serum \ creatinine}$$

$$Cl_{cr,females} \ (mL/min) = \frac{(140 - age) * LBW}{72 * serum \ creatinine} * 0.85$$

   Note: Authors suggest that a value of 1.0 be used when serum creatinine is less than 1.0 mg/dL.

2. Daily maintenance dose is 8 mg/kg (LBW)^b per dose with dosing interval determined from the following table:

Creatinine Clearance (mL/min)	Dosage Interval (h)
>90	6
70–89	8
46–69	12
30–45	18
15–29	24

3. Target serum vancomycin concentrations are peaks between 20 and 30 mg/L 15 min after the end of the infusion and troughs between 5 and 10 mg/L 30 min before the next dose.

^{a} Lean body weight.
^{b} Lake and Peterson recommended LBW; we recommend using total body weight.
Source. Reference 104.

trations with clinical efficacy. Relationships between serum vancomycin concentrations and nephrotoxicity and ototoxicity have been suggested. In addition, there are several unanswered questions regarding the monitoring of serum vancomycin concentrations: (1) What ranges of peak and trough concentrations offer the greatest efficacy with minimal toxicity? (2) Do we need to monitor both peak and trough concentrations (eg, trough concentration only)? (3) When is the optimal time to monitor peak concentrations? (4) What is the most cost-effective method(s) for monitoring serum concentrations to dose vancomycin?

Table 19–15 outlines an approach to monitoring serum vancomycin concentrations. Each clinician needs to determine the importance of serum vancomycin concentrations for the individualization of drug therapy. In addition, a consensus needs to be reached with respect to the appropriate sampling times and the desired therapeutic ranges of peak and trough concentrations. Interpretation of serum vancomycin concentrations is dependent on the timing and number of serum concentrations available, as well as on the pharmacokinetic parameters derived from the results.

Serum vancomycin concentrations are currently measured by microbiologic assay, radioimmunoassay, fluorescence polarization immunoassay, enzyme multiplied immunoassay, and high-performance liquid chromatography.[192–197] A potential problem with overestimation of van-

TABLE 19–13. VANCOMYCIN DOSAGE GUIDELINES: "RODVOLD METHOD"

1. Calculate the patient's creatinine clearance (Cl_{cr}) from the following equations:

$$Cl_{cr,males} \text{ (mL/min/70 kg)} = \frac{(140 - \text{age})}{72 * \text{serum creatinine}}$$

$$Cl_{cr,females} \text{ (mL/min/70 kg)} = \frac{(140 - \text{age})}{72 * \text{serum creatinine}} * 0.85$$

2. Determine daily maintenance dose from the following equation:

$$\text{dose(mg/kg TBW}^a \text{ per 24 h)} = (0.227 * Cl_{cr}) + 5.67$$

3. The above calculated dose can be divided into and administered from the following dosing interval guidelines:

Creatinine Clearance (mL/min per 70 kg)	Dosage Interval (h)
>65	8
40–65	12
20–39	24
10–19	48

4. Target serum vancomycin concentrations are peaks between 30 and 40 mg/L immediately after the end of the infusion and troughs between 5 and 10 mg/L before the next dose.

^{a} Total body weight.
Source. Reference 8.

comycin concentrations because of the detection of vancomycin degradation products may limit the use of the fluorescence polarization immunoassay in patients on dialysis.[198–201]

Pharmacokinetics-Based Dosing Methods

Initial dosing methods provide a reasonable starting point; however, none of these methods provides for individualization of dosing regimens based on individual pharmacokinetic parameters. Several dosing methods have been suggested for dosage adjustment when serum vancomycin concentrations are available. Dosing methods that incorporate either conventional least-squares regression (Sawchuk–Zaske method[202]) or bayesian principles have tended to be less biased and more precise than the initial dosing methods.[127,185,186]

One of the most popular methods for individualizing dosages of vancomycin based on serum concentration–time data is the Sawchuk–Zaske method (Table 19–16).[185,202,203] To use this method for dosing vancomycin, several assumptions have to be made: (1) A one-compartment pharmacokinetic model is used to determine parameters and dosage regimens. (2) Peak vancomycin concentrations are obtained 1 to 3 hours after the end of the infusion to avoid the distribution phase (to meet the first assumption). (3) Serum vancomycin concentrations during the distribution phase are not important and can be ignored. (4) The therapeutic range for tar-

TABLE 19–14. SUMMARY OF DOSAGE RECOMMENDATIONS FOR NEONATES, INFANTS, AND CHILDREN

Study	PCA (wk)	Weight (g)	PNA (d)	SCr (mg/dL)	Dose and Dosing Interval
Schaade et al[14]			<7		15 mg/kg q12h
			8–30		15 mg/kg q8h
			>30		10 mg/kg q6h
					(If central nervous system infections, 15 mg/kg q6h)
Gross et al[15]	29–35	<1000	27–62		25 mg/kg loading dose, then 15 mg/kg q12h
	29–35	>1000	26–40		12.5 mg/kg loading dose, then 10 mg/kg q12h
Naqvi et al[16]	<41				15 mg/kg loading dose, then 10 mg/kg q8h
	>43				15 mg/kg loading dose, then 10 mg/kg q6h
James et al[99]	<27	<800			27 mg/kg q36h
	27–30	800–1200			24 mg/kg q24h
	31–36	1200–2000			18–27 mg/kg q12–18h
	>37	2000			22.5 mg/kg q12h
Lisby-Sutch and Nahata[18]	30–34	<1200			10 mg/kg q12h
	30–34	>1200			10 mg/kg q8h
	35–42	>1200			10 mg/kg q8h
	>42	>2000			10 mg/kg q6h
Kildoo et al[19]	>30		>14	≤0.6	10 mg/kg q8h
	>30		>14	0.7–1.2	10 mg/kg q12h
Gabriel et al[189]	<30		≤7		15 mg/kg q24h
	<30		>7	≤1.2	10 mg/kg q12h
	30–36		≤14		10 mg/kg q12h
	30–36		>14	≤0.6	10 mg/kg q8h
	30–36		>14	0.7–1.2	10 mg/kg q12h
	>36		≤7		10 mg/kg q12h
	>36		>7	≤0.6	10 mg/kg q8h
	>36		>7	0.7–1.2	10 mg/kg q12h
Leonard et al[100]	25–32	<1000			15 mg/kg q24h

[a] PCA, postconceptional age; PNA, postnatal age; SCr, serum creatinine; CNS, central nervous system.

get peak concentration may need to be lower than 30 to 40 mg/L (eg, 20 to 30 mg/L) (see Figure 19–4). (5) The period for optimal blood sampling must be adequate to determine the pharmacokinetic parameters. Although this method has been shown to offer improvement in predictive performance compared with dosing nomograms, caution must be exercised in the interpretation of the accuracy of pharmacokinetic parameter values (Table 19–17, Figure 19–5).[4,204] To obtain accurate estimates of pharmacokinetic parameters such as clearance and the apparent volume of

TABLE 19–15. APPROACH TO MONITORING SERUM VANCOMYCIN CONCENTRATIONS

I. Initial Determination of Dosage Regimen
   A. Use a method that is known to work at your institution and in the patient population to be monitored.
II. Who Should Be Monitored
   A. Monitor patients with known wide interpatient variability in renal function and vancomycin pharmacokinetic parameters; this generally includes patients who
      1. Are in intensive care units
      2. Have mild to moderate renal impairment
      3. Are in advanced renal failure
      4. Are neonates, infants, or children
      5. Are receiving concurrent aminoglycoside therapy
   B. Monitor patients with severe Gram-positive infections
III. When to Obtain Vancomycin Concentrations
   A. Obtain peak and trough concentrations at steady state.
   B. Timing of peak concentrations is dependent on the "therapeutic range you believe in." If you are using a therapeutic range of 30–40 mg/L, this means within 30 min of the completion of infusion. If you are using a one-compartment model, peak concentration should not be obtained until the distribution phase is completed (eg, greater than 1 h after the end of the infusion).
   C. Consistency is needed in obtaining "peak" concentrations for comparison with future concentrations.
   D. Obtain only trough concentrations once the dose is stabilized for the desired peak concentration.
   E. For patients in advanced renal disease, characterization of the elimination half-life may be useful for determining a dosing interval.
IV. How Often to Obtain Vancomycin Concentrations
   A. Obtain concentrations at steady state and once weekly for patients in normal renal function or mild and moderate renal impairment. Exceptions to this would include patients with changing renal function and patients who are treated concurrently with nephrotoxic agents (eg, aminoglycosides).
V. Interpretation of Vancomycin Concentrations
   A. Drug has two- and/or three-compartment characteristics.
   B. What question is trying to be answered?
   C. Different dosing approaches are dependent on sampling times:
      1. Simple percentage change using equivalent proportional changes in dose and empiric shifts of dosage interval
      2. Sawchuk–Zaske method (one-compartment model)
      3. Bayesian forecasting methods
         a. One-compartment model
         b. Two-compartment model

TABLE 19–16. EQUATIONS FOR ONE-COMPARTMENT INFUSION MODEL (SAWCHUK–ZASKE METHOD)

1. Determine the elimination half-life $(t_{1/2})$ from two or more serum vancomycin concentrations (C) from linear regression or the following equation[a]:

$$t_{1/2} = \frac{0.693}{\ln(C_1/C_2)/(t_2 - t_1)}$$

2. Determine the apparent volume of distribution $(V_{d,ss})$:

$$V_{d,ss} = (1.44 * R_0 * t_{1/2}) * \frac{1 - e^{-(0.693/t_{1/2}) * \tau}}{C_{max} - (C_{min} * e^{-(0.693/t_{1/2}) * t')}}$$

3. Choose the desired peak $(C_{max,D})$ and trough $(C_{min,D})$ serum vancomycin concentration and determine the dosing interval (τ):

$$\tau = (1.44 * t_{1/2} * \log \frac{C_{max,D}}{C_{min,D}}) + t'$$

4. Determine the infusion (R_0) and dose of vancomycin to obtain the desired peak and trough serum vancomycin concentrations:

$$R_0 = (0.693/t_{1/2}) * V_{d,ss} * C_{max,D} * \frac{1 - e^{-(0.693/t_{1/2}) * \tau}}{1 - e^{-(0.693/t_{1/2} * t')}}$$

5. Predict peak $(C_{t,max})$ concentration at time (t) after the end of the infusion and trough (C_{min}) concentration that would result from the new dosage regimen:

$$C_{t,max} = \frac{R_0 * t_{1/2} * 1.44}{V_{d,ss}} * \frac{1 - e^{-(0.693/t_{1/2}) * t'}}{C_{max} - (C_{min} * e^{-(0.693/t_{1/2}) * \tau})} * e^{-(0.693/t_{1/2}) * t}$$

$$C_{min} = C_{t,max} * e^{-(0.693/t_{1/2}) * [\tau - (t' + t)]}$$

[a] $t_{1/2}$, half-life (h); C_1 or C_2, measured serum vancomycin concentration (mg/L) obtained at specific time (h), t_1 or t_2; $V_{d,ss}$, apparent volume of distribution (L); R_0, infusion rate (mg/h); τ, dosing interval (h); C_{max}, observed maximum or peak concentration (mg/L); C_{min}, observed minimum or trough concentration (mg/L); t', length of infusion period (h); $C_{max,D}$, desired maximum or peak concentration (mg/L); $C_{min,D}$, desired minimum or trough concentration (mg/L); $C_{t,max}$, maximum or peak concentration (mg/L) at time "t"; t, time (h) after the end of the infusion.
Source: Reference 202.

distribution, up to four serum vancomycin concentrations may be needed.[205,206] Similar concerns would hold true when estimating the apparent volume of distribution with a one-compartment bayesian forecasting model.[186,206–208]

Bayesian forecasting programs that use a two-compartment model have recently been evaluated.[208–211] With the appropriate population parameter estimates and feedback steady-state serum concentrations, both initial and subsequent dosage adjustments can be accurately made.[209,211] The bayesian two-compartment model offers the advantage of using one or more serum vancomycin concentrations under either non-steady-state or steady-state conditions. The major disadvantage of this method, however, is the requirement of a computer with appropriate software.

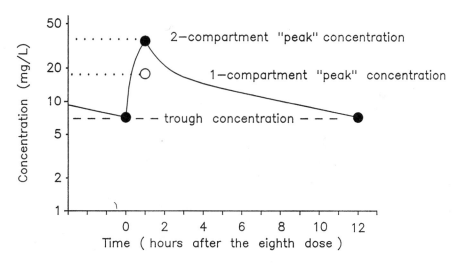

Figure 19–4. Serum concentration–time profile of vancomycin at steady state. Difference between the peak concentrations at the end of infusion for two-compartment model (●) and one-compartment model (○).

TABLE 19–17. PREDICTION ERROR FOR INDIVIDUAL ONE-COMPARTMENT PHARMACOKINETIC PARAMETERS^{a,b}

Timing of Serum Vancomycin Concentration (h after end of infusion)	C_{max} (mg/L)	$V_{d,ss}$ (L/kg)	$t_{1/2}$ (h)
0.25, 11	29.5 $(-18.0)^c$	0.44 (-37.7)	4.9 (-35.6)
0.5, 11	25.2 (-29.9)	0.54 (-23.3)	5.4 (-28.4)
1, 11	20.5 (-43.0)	0.72 (2.3)	6.4 (-16.1)
1.5, 11	18.5 (-48.6)	0.84 (19.4)	7.0 (-8.0)
3, 11	17.1 (-52.6)	0.95 (35.1)	7.5 (-0.8)

^{a} Patient characteristics: 88.5-kg male with a creatinine clearance of 117 mg/min/1.73 m^2 receiving 1-h intravenous infusion of vancomycin 1000 mg every 12 h.

^{b} Two-compartment parameters: maximum serum vancomycin concentration (C_{max}) = 36.0 mg/L, apparent volume of distribution at steady-state ($V_{d,ss}$) = 0.70 L/kg, elimination half-life ($t_{1/2}$) = 7.6 h.

^{c} Values in parentheses represent percentage prediction error associated with parameters calculated from two serum vancomycin concentrations with a one-compartment model versus two-compartment pharmacokinetic parameters for the following patient.

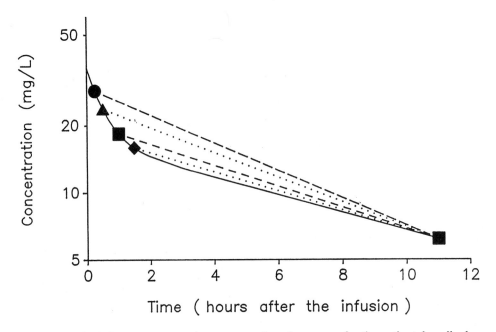

Figure 19–5. Serum vancomycin concentration–time curve for the patient described in Table 19–16. The solid line represents the actual concentrations fitted to a two-compartment pharmacokinetic model. The broken lines represent the regression line for various combinations of two serum concentrations used to determine the one-compartment pharmacokinetic parameters in Table 19–17. ●, 0.25-hour concentration; ▲, 0.5-hour concentration; ■, 1-hour concentration; ◆, 1.5-hour concentration. The 3-hour concentration was not plotted.

TABLE 19–18. PROPORTIONAL DOSAGE ADJUSTMENT FROM PEAK AND TROUGH SERUM VANCOMYCIN CONCENTRATIONS[a]

$C_{\text{ss,peak}}$	= measured peak serum vancomycin concentration (mg/L) obtained within 30 min of infusion
$C_{\text{ss,trough}}$	= measured trough serum vancomycin concentration (mg/L) obtained just before start of infusion
dose	= vancomycin dose (mg) given around the measured peak and trough concentrations
$C_{\text{ss,peak,D}}$	= desired peak serum vancomycin concentration obtained within 30 min of infusion
$C_{\text{ss,trough,D}}$	= desired trough serum vancomycin concentration obtained just before start of infusion
New dose	= vancomycin dose (mg) needed to achieve the desired target peak and trough concentrations

[a] Desired peak and trough serum concentrations range between 30 and 40 mg/L and between 5 and 10 mg/L, respectively.

Finally, a desired change in serum concentrations can be easily accomplished by using an equivalent proportional change in dose (Table 19–18). To use this approach, a set of steady-state peak and trough concentrations are needed. The peak concentration should be obtained within the first 15 to 30 minutes of completion of the intravenous infusion. Although this method does not determine individualized pharmacokinetic parameter estimates, the controversies over pharmacokinetic modeling and pharmacodynamic importance of serum vancomycin concentrations allows this oversimplified dosing technique to be useful without the need of multiple equations or a computer.

QUESTIONS

J.Z., a 22-year-old woman with a history of acute leukemia, is readmitted to the hospital on 11/21/92 with a diagnosis of Gram-negative bacteremia. Her admission laboratories include a BUN of 7 mg/dL and serum creatinine of 1.9 mg/dL. Her weight is 56 kg and her height is 67 in. She is started on piperacillin 3 g q8h and gentamicin 80 mg q8h.

On 11/26/92, J.Z. continues to have high spiking temperatures, and blood cultures from 11/24/92 report methicillin-resistant *Staphylococcus epidermidis*. Intravenous vancomycin is to be started in place of gentamicin. J.Z.'s blood chemistries have not changed since her admission.

1. Recommend a vancomycin dose (to the nearest 50 mg) and dosing interval.

Despite your recommendation, the medical team places J.Z. on intravenous vancomycin 1000 mg q12h. Three days later, a set of peak and trough serum vancomycin concentrations are obtained around the seventh vancomycin dose:

11/29/92	9:15 AM	vancomycin concentration = 19.4 mg/L
11/29/92	10:40 AM	vancomycin concentration = 64.9 mg/L

The nurse who administered the vancomycin dose recorded the infusion period as starting at 9:20 AM and finishing at 10:35 AM.

2. Recommend a vancomycin dose (to the nearest 50 mg) and dosing interval based on the serum vancomycin concentrations.

3. If this patient is going to be on vancomycin therapy for the next 2 weeks, when and how often should serum vancomycin concentrations be monitored?

REFERENCES

1. Griffith RS. Introduction of vancomycin. *Rev Infect Dis.* 1981;3(suppl):S200–S204.
2. Pfeiffer RR. Structural features of vancomycin. *Rev Infect Dis.* 1981;3(suppl):S205–S209.

3. Ena J, Dick RW, Jones RN, Wenzel RP. The epidemiology of intravenous vancomycin usage in a university hospital: A 10-year study. *JAMA.* 1993;269:598–602.

4. Rodvold KA, Zokufa H, Rotschafer JC. Routine monitoring of serum vancomycin concentrations: Can waiting be justified? *Clin Pharm.* 1987;6:655–658.

5. Edwards DJ. Therapeutic drug monitoring of aminoglycosides and vancomycin: Guidelines and controversies. *J Pharm Pract.* 1991;4:211–214.

6. Krogstad DJ, Moellering RC, Greenblatt DJ. Single-dose kinetics of intravenous vancomycin. *J Clin Pharmacol.* 1980;20:197–201.

7. Healy DP, Polk RE, Garson ML, et al. Comparison of steady-state pharmacokinetics of two dosage regimens of vancomycin in normal volunteers. *Antimicrob Agents Chemother.* 1987;31:393–397.

8. Rodvold KA, Blum RA, Fischer JH, et al. Vancomycin pharmacokinetics in patients with various degrees of renal function. *Antimicrob Agents Chemother.* 1988;32:848–852.

9. Matzke GR, McGory RW, Halstenson CE, Keane WF. Pharmacokinetics of vancomycin in patients with various degrees of renal function. *Antimicrob Agents Chemother.* 1984;25:433–437.

10. Tan CC, Lee HS, Ti TY, Lee EJC. Pharmacokinetics of intravenous vancomycin in patients with end-stage renal failure. *Ther Drug Monit.* 1990;12:29–34.

11. Cutler NR, Narang PK, Lesko LJ, et al. Vancomycin disposition: The importance of age. *Clin Pharmacol Ther.* 1984;36:803–810.

12. Blouin RA, Bauer LA, Miller DD, et al. Vancomycin pharmacokinetics in normal and morbidly obese subjects. *Antimicrob Agents Chemother.* 1982;21:575–580.

13. Rybak MJ, Albrecht LM, Berman JR, et al. Vancomycin pharmacokinetics in burn patients and intravenous drug abusers. *Antimicrob Agents Chemother.* 1990;34:792–795.

14. Schaad UB, McCracken GH, Nelson JD. Clinical pharmacology and efficacy of vancomycin in pediatric patients. *J Pediatr.* 1980;96:119–126.

15. Gross JR, Kaplan SL, Kramer WG, Mason EO. Vancomycin pharmacokinetics in premature infants. *Pediatr Pharmacol.* 1985;5:17–22.

16. Naqvi SH, Keenan WJ, Reichley RM, Fortune KP. Vancomycin pharmacokinetics in small, seriously ill infants. *Am J Dis Child.* 1986;140:107–110.

17. Reed MD, Kliegman RM, Weiner JS, et al. The clinical pharmacology of vancomycin in seriously ill preterm infants. *Pediatr Res.* 1987;22:360–363.

18. Lisby-Sutch SM, Nahata MC. Dosage guidelines for the use of vancomycin based on its pharmacokinetics in infants. *Eur J Clin Pharmacol.* 1988;35:637–642.

19. Kildoo CW, Lin ML, Gabriel MH, et al. Vancomycin pharmacokinetics in infants: Relationship to postconceptional age and serum creatinine. *Dev Pharmacol Ther.* 1990;14:77–83.

20. Jarrett RV, Marinkovich GA, Gayle E, Bass JW. Individualized pharmacokinetic profiles to compute vancomycin dosage and dosing interval in preterm infants. *Pediatr Infect Dis J.* 1993;12:156–157.

21. Asbury WH, Darsey EH, Rose WB, et al. Vancomycin pharmacokinetics in neonates and infants: A retrospective evaluation. *Ann Pharmacother.* 1993;27:490–496.

22. Nagarajan R. Antibacterial activities and modes of action of vancomycin and related glycopeptides. *Antimicrob Agents Chemother.* 1991;35:605–609.

23. Jordan DC, Mallory HDC. Site of action of vancomycin on *Staphylococcus aureus. Antimicrob Agents Chemother.* 1964;8:489–494.

24. Jordan DC, Inniss WE. Selective inhibition of ribonucleic acid synthesis in *Staphylococcus aureus* by vancomycin. *Nature.* 1959;184:1894–1895.

25. Hermans PE, Wilhelm MP. Vancomycin. *Mayo Clin Proc.* 1987;62:901–905.

26. Kucers A, Bennett NM. *The Use of Antibiotics.* 4th ed. Philadelphia: JB Lippincott; 1987:1045–1068.

27. Tuazon CU, Miller H. Clinical and microbiologic aspects of serious infections caused by *Staphylococcus epidermidis. Scand J Infect Dis.* 1983;15:347–360.

28. Schwalbe RS, Stapleton JT, Gilligan PH. Emergence of vancomycin resistance in coagulase-negative

staphylococci. *N Engl J Med.* 1987;316:927–931.

29. Johnson AP, Uttley AHC, Woodford N, George RC. Resistance to vancomycin and teicoplanin: An emerging clinical problem. *Clin Microbiol Rev.* 1990;3:280–291.

30. Courvalin P. Resistance of enterococci to glycopeptides. *Antimicrob Agents Chemother.* 1990;34: 2291–2296.

31. Brumfitt W, Hamilton-Miller J. Methicillin-resistant *Staphylococcus aureus. N Engl J Med.* 1989; 320:1188–1196.

32. Chambers HF. Methicillin-resistant staphylococci. *Clin Microbiol Rev.* 1989;1:173–186.

33. Blum RA, Rodvold KA. Recognition and importance of *Staphylococcus epidermidis* infections. *Clin Pharm.* 1987;6:464–475.

34. Hughes WT, Armstrong D, Bodey GP, et al. Guidelines for the use of antimicrobial agents in neutropenic patients with unexplained fever. *J Infect Dis.* 1990;161:381–396.

35. Luer MS, Hatton J. Vancomycin administration into the cerebrospinal fluid: A review. *Ann Pharmacother.* 1993;27:912–921.

36. Boyce NW, Wood C, Thomson NM, et al. Intraperitoneal (IP) vancomycin therapy for CAPD peritonitis: A prospective, randomized comparison of intermittent v continuous therapy. *Am J Kidney Dis.* 1988;12:304–306.

37. Karchmer AW, Archer GL, Dismukes WE. *Staphylococcus epidermidis* causing prosthetic valve endocarditis: Microbiologic and clinical observations as guides to therapy. *Ann Intern Med.* 1983;98:447–455.

38. Dajani AS, Bisno AL, Chung KJ, et al. Prevention of bacterial endocarditis: Recommendations by the American Heart Association. *JAMA.* 1990;264:2919–2922.

39. Fekety R, Silva J, Kauffman C, et al. Treatment of antibiotic-associated *Clostridium difficile* colitis with oral vancomycin: Comparison of two dosage regimens. *Am J Med.* 1989;86:15–19.

40. Batts DH, Martin D, Holmes R, et al. Treatment of antibiotic-associated *Clostridium difficile* diarrhea with oral vancomycin. *J Pediatr.* 1980;97:151–153.

41. Healy DP, Sahai JV, Fuller SH, Polk RE. Vancomycin-induced histamine release and "red man syndrome": Comparison of 1- and 2-hour infusions. *Antimicrob Agents Chemother.* 1990;34:550–554.

42. Lucas RA, Bowtle WJ, Ryden R. Disposition of vancomycin in healthy volunteers from oral solution and semi-solid matrix capsules. *J Clin Pharm Ther.* 1987;12:27–31.

43. Geraci JE, Hellman FR, Nichols DR, et al. Some laboratory and clinical experience with a new antibiotic vancomycin. *Antibiot Ann.* 1957:90–106.

44. Dudley MN, Quintiliani R, Nightingale CH, et al. Absorption of vancomycin. *Ann Intern Med.* 1984;101:144. Letter.

45. Spitzer PG, Eliopoulos GM. Systemic absorption of enteral vancomycin in a patient with pseudomembranous colitis. *Ann Intern Med.* 1984;100:533–534.

46. Thompson CM, Long SS, Gilligan PH, et al. Absorption of oral vancomycin—Possible associated toxicity. *Int J Pediatr Nephrol.* 1983;4:1–4.

47. Matzke GR, Halstenson CE, Olson PL, et al. Systemic absorption of oral vancomycin in patients with renal insufficiency and antibiotic-associated colitis. *Am J Kidney Dis.* 1987;9:422–425.

48. Rotschafer JC, Crossley K, Zaske DE, et al. Pharmacokinetics of vancomycin: Observations in 28 patients and dosage recommendations. *Antimicrob Agents Chemother.* 1982;22:391–394.

49. Cunha BA, Quintiliani R, Deglin JM, et al. Pharmacokinetics of vancomycin in anuria. *Rev Infect Dis.* 1981;3(suppl):S269–S272.

50. Vance-Bryan K, Guay DRP, Gilliland SS, et al. Effect of obesity on vancomycin pharmacokinetic parameters as determined by using a bayesian forecasting technique. *Antimicrob Agents Chemother.* 1993;37:436–440.

51. MacIlwaine WA, Sande MA, Mandell GL. Penetration of antistaphylococcal antibiotics into the human eye. *Am J Ophthalmol.* 1974;77:589–592.

52. Williams REO. L-forms of *Staphylococcus aureus*. *J Gen Microbiol*. 1963;33:325–334.
53. Congeni BL, Tan J, Salstrom SJ, Winstein L. Kinetics of vancomycin after intraventricular and intravenous administration. *Pediatr Res*. 1980;13:459. Abstract.
54. Schaad UB, Nelson JD, McCracken GH. Pharmacology and efficacy of vancomycin for staphylococcal infections in children. *Rev Infect Dis*. 1981;3(suppl):S282–S288.
55. Graziani AL, Lawson LA, Gibson GA, et al. Vancomycin concentration in infected and noninfected bone. *Antimicrob Agents Chemother*. 1988;32:1320–1322.
56. Dascher FD, Frank U, Kummel A, et al. Pharmacokinetics of vancomycin in serum and tissue of patients undergoing open-heart surgery. *J Antimicrob Chemother*. 1987;19:359–362.
57. Bunke CM, Aronoff GR, Brier ME, et al. Vancomycin kinetics during continuous ambulatory peritoneal dialysis. *Clin Pharmacol Ther*. 1983;34:631–637.
58. Morse GD, Farolino DF, Apicella MA, Walshe JJ. Comparative study of intraperitoneal and intravenous vancomycin pharmacokinetics during continuous ambulatory peritoneal dialysis. *Antimicrob Agents Chemother*. 1987;31:173–177.
59. Whitby M, Edwards R, Aston E, Finch RB. Pharmacokinetics of single dose intravenous vancomycin in CAPD peritonitis. *J Antimicrob Chemother*. 1987;19:351–357.
60. Nielsen HF, Sorensen I, Hansen HE. Peritoneal transport of vancomycin during peritoneal dialysis. *Nephron*. 1979;24:274–277.
61. Glew RH, Pavuk RA, Shuster A, Alfred HJ. Vancomycin pharmacokinetics in patients undergoing chronic intermittent peritoneal dialysis. *Int J Clin Pharmacol Ther Toxicol*. 1982;20:559–563.
62. Kirby WMM, Divelbiss CL. Vancomycin: Clinical and laboratory studies. *Antibiot Ann*. 1957:107–117.
63. Young EJ, Ratner RE, Claridge JE. Staphylococcus ventriculitis treated with vancomycin. *South Med J*. 1981;74:1014–1015.
64. Gump DW. Vancomycin for treatment of bacterial meningitis. *Rev Infect Dis*. 1981;3(suppl):S289–S292.
65. Ryan JL, Pachner A, Andriole VT, Root RK. Enterococcal meningitis: Combined vancomycin and rifampin therapy. *Am J Med*. 1980;68:449–451.
66. Bayston R, Hart CA, Barnicoat M. Intraventricular vancomycin in the treatment of ventriculitis associated with cerebrospinal fluid shunting and draining. *J Neurol Neurosurg Psychiatry*. 1987;50:1419–1423.
67. Lindholm DD, Murray JS. Persistence of vancomycin in the blood during renal failure and its treatment by hemodialysis. *N Engl J Med*. 1966;274:1047–1051.
68. Ackerman BH, Taylor EH, Olsen KM, et al. Vancomycin serum protein binding determination by ultrafiltration. *Drug Intell Clin Pharm*. 1988;22:300–303.
69. Zokufa HZ, Solem LD, Rodvold KA, et al. The influence of serum albumin and α_1-acid glycoprotein on vancomycin protein binding in patients with burn injuries. *J Burn Care Rehabil*. 1989;10:425–428.
70. Cantu TG, Dick JD, Elliott DE, et al. Protein binding of vancomycin in a patient with immunoglobulin A myeloma. *Antimicrob Agents Chemother*. 1990;34:1459–1461.
71. Nielsen HE, Hansen HE, Korsager B, Skov PE. Renal excretion of vancomycin in kidney disease. *Acta Med Scand*. 1975;197:261–264.
72. Moellering RC, Krogstad DJ, Greenblatt DJ. Vancomycin therapy in patients with impaired renal function: A nomogram for dosage. *Ann Intern Med*. 1981;94:343–346.
73. Brater DC, Bawdon RE, Anderson SA, et al. Vancomycin elimination in patients with burn injury. *Clin Pharmacol Ther*. 1986;39:631–634.
74. Golper TA, Noonan HM, Elzinga L, et al. Vancomycin pharmacokinetics, renal handling, and nonrenal clearances in normal human subjects. *Clin Pharmacol Ther*. 1988;43:565–570.
75. Munar MY, Elzinga L, Brummett R, et al. The effect of tobramycin on the renal handling of vancomycin. *J Clin Pharmacol*. 1991;31:618–623.

76. Brown N, Ho DW, Fong KL, et al. Effects of hepatic function on vancomycin clinical pharmacology. *Antimicrob Agents Chemother.* 1983;23:603–609.

77. Lee CC, Marbury TC. Drug therapy in patients undergoing haemodialysis: Clinical pharmacokinetic considerations. *Clin Pharmacokinet.* 1984;9:42–66.

78. Salem NG, Blevin RB, Matzke GR. Clearance of vancomycin by hemodialysis. In: Thirtieth Annual American Society for Artificial Internal Organs; Washington, DC; 1984;13:54. Abstract.

79. Lanese D, Alfrey PS, Molitoris BA. Markedly increased clearance of vancomycin during hemodialysis using polysulfone dialyzers. *Kidney Int.* 1989;35:1409–1412.

80. Pollard TA, Lampasona V, Akkerman S, et al. Vancomycin redistribution: Dosing recommendations following high-flux hemodialysis. *Kidney Int.* 1994;45:232–237.

81. Ahmad R, Raichura N, Kilbane V, Whitfield E. Vancomycin: A reappraisal. *Br Med J.* 1982;284:1953–1954.

82. Matzke GR, O'Connell MB, Collins AJ, Keshaviah PR. Disposition of vancomycin during hemofiltration. *Clin Pharmacol Ther.* 1986;40:425–430.

83. Magera BE, Arroyo JC, Rosansky SJ, Postic B. Vancomycin pharmacokinetics in patients with peritonitis on peritoneal dialysis. *Antimicrob Agents Chemother.* 1983;23:710–714.

84. Harford AM, Sica DA, Tartaglione T, et al. Vancomycin pharmacokinetics in continuous ambulatory peritoneal dialysis patients with peritonitis. *Nephron.* 1986;43:217–222.

85. Ayus JC, Eneas JF, Tong TG, et al. Peritoneal clearance and total body elimination of vancomycin during chronic intermittent peritoneal dialysis. *Clin Nephrol.* 1979;11:129–132.

86. Morse GD, Nairn DK, Walshe JJ. Once weekly intraperitoneal therapy for Gram-positive peritonitis. *Am J Kidney Dis.* 1987;10:300–305.

87. Pancorbo S, Comty C. Peritoneal transport of vancomycin in 4 patients undergoing continuous ambulatory peritoneal dialysis. *Nephron.* 1982;31:37–39.

88. Comstock TJ, Sica DA, Fichtl RE, Davis J. Multicompartment vancomycin kinetics in patients with end-stage renal disease. *Clin Pharmacol Ther.* 1988;44:172. Abstract.

89. Pachorek RE, Wood F. Vancomycin half-life in a patient with hepatic and renal dysfunction. *Clin Pharm.* 1991;10:297–300.

90. Guay DRP, Vance-Bryan K, Gilliland SS, et al. Comparison of vancomycin pharmacokinetics in hospitalized elderly and young patients using a bayesian forecaster. *J Clin Pharmacol.* 1993;33:918–922.

91. Garrelts JC, Peterie JD. Altered vancomycin dose vs. serum concentration relationship in burn patients. *Clin Pharmacol Ther.* 1988;44:9–13.

92. Bailie GR, Ackerman BH, Fischer JH, et al. Increased vancomycin requirements in young burn patients. *J Burn Care Rehabil.* 1984;5:376–378.

93. Garaud JJ, Regnier B, Inglebert F, et al. Vancomycin pharmacokinetics in critically ill patients. *J Antimicrob Chemother.* 1984;14(suppl D):53–57.

94. Klamerus KJ, Rodvold KA, Silverman NA, Levitsky S. Effect of cardiopulmonary bypass on vancomycin and netilmicin disposition. *Antimicrob Agents Chemother.* 1988;32:631–635.

95. Austin TW, Leake J, Coles JC, Goldbach MM. Vancomycin blood levels during cardiac bypass surgery. *Can J Surg.* 1981;24:423–425.

96. Farber BF, Karchmer AW, Buckley MJ, Moellering RC. Vancomycin prophylaxis in cardiac operations: Determination of an optimal dosage regimen. *J Thorac Cardiovasc Surg.* 1983;85:933–940.

97. Salzman C, Weingold AB, Simon GL. Increased dose requirements of vancomycin in a pregnant patient with endocarditis. *J Infect Dis.* 1987;156:409. Letter.

98. Schaible DH, Rocci ML, Alpert GA, et al. Vancomycin pharmacokinetics in infants: Relationship to indices of maturation. *Pediatr Infect Dis.* 1986;5:304–308.

99. James A, Koren G, Milliken J, et al. Vancomycin pharmacokinetics and dose recommendations for preterm infants. *Antimicrob Agents Chemother.* 1987;31:52–54.

100. Leonard MB, Koren G, Stevenson DK, Prober CG. Vancomycin pharmacokinetics in very low birth weight neonates. *Pediatr Infect Dis*. 1989;8:282–286.

101. Hoie EB, Swigart SA, Leuschen MP, et al. Vancomycin pharmacokinetics in infants undergoing extracorporeal membrane oxygenation. *Clin Pharm*. 1990;9:711–715.

102. Hatzopoulos FK, Stile-Calligaro IL, Rodvold KA, et al. Pharmacokinetics of intravenous vancomycin in pediatric cardiopulmonary bypass surgery. *Pediatr Infect Dis J*. 1993;12:300–304.

103. Fitzsimmons WE, Postelnick MJ, Tortorice PV. Survey of vancomycin monitoring guidelines in Illinois hospitals. *Drug Intell Clin Pharm*. 1988;22:598–600.

104. Lake KD, Peterson CD. A simplified dosing method for initiating vancomycin therapy. *Pharmacotherapy*. 1985;5:340–344.

105. Geraci JE. Vancomycin. *Mayo Clin Proc*. 1977;52:631–634.

106. Vogelman B, Craig WA. Kinetics of antimicrobial activity. *J Pediatr*. 1986;108:835–840.

107. Sorrell TC, Packham DR, Shanker S, et al. Vancomycin therapy for methicillin-resistant *Staphylococcus aureus*. *Ann Intern Med*. 1982;97:344–350.

108. Louria DB, Kaminski T, Buchman J. Vancomycin in severe staphylococcal infections. *Arch Intern Med*. 1961;107:225–240.

109. Bailie GR, Neal D. Vancomycin ototoxicity and nephrotoxicity. *Med Toxicol*. 1988;3:376–386.

110. Farber BF, Moellering RC. Retrospective study of the toxicity of vancomycin from 1974 to 1981. *Antimicrob Agents Chemother*. 1983;23:138–141.

111. Rybak MJ, Albrecht LM, Boike SC, Chandrasekar PH. Nephrotoxicity of vancomycin, alone and with an aminoglycoside. *J Antimicrob Chemother*. 1990;25:679–687.

112. Cimino MA, Rostein C, Slaughter RL, Emrich LJ. Relationship of serum antibiotic concentrations to nephrotoxicity in cancer patients receiving concurrent aminoglycoside and vancomycin therapy. *Am J Med*. 1987;83:1091–1097.

113. Mellor JA, Kingdom J, Cafferkey M, Keane CT. Vancomycin toxicity: A prospective study. *J Antimicrob Chemother*. 1985;15:773–780.

114. Sorrell TC, Collignon PJ. A prospective study of adverse reactions associated with vancomycin therapy. *J Antimicrob Chemother*. 1985;16:235–241.

115. Pauly DJ, Musa DM, Lestico MR, et al. Risk of nephrotoxicity with combination vancomycin–aminoglycoside antibiotic therapy. *Pharmacotherapy*. 1990;10:378–382.

116. Downs NJ, Neihart RE, Dolezal JM, Hodges GR. Mild nephrotoxicity associated with vancomycin use. *Arch Intern Med*. 1989;149:1777–1781.

117. Wold JS, Turnipseed SA. Toxicology of vancomycin in laboratory animals. *Rev Infect Dis*. 1981;3(suppl):S224–S229.

118. Appel GB, Given DB, Levine LR, Cooper GL. Vancomycin and the kidney. *Am J Kidney Dis*. 1986;8:75–80.

119. Marre R, Schulz T, Anders T, Sack K. Renal tolerance and pharmacokinetics of vancomycin in rats. *J Antimicrob Chemother*. 1984;14:253–260.

120. Wood CA, Kohlhepp SJ, Kohnen PW, et al. Vancomycin enhancement of experimental tobramycin nephrotoxicity. *Antimicrob Agents Chemother*. 1986;30:20–24.

121. Odio C, McCracken GH, Nelson JD. Nephrotoxicity associated with vancomycin–aminoglycoside therapy in four children. *J Pediatr*. 1984;105:491–493.

122. Dean RP, Wagner DJ, Tolpin MD. Vancomycin/aminoglycoside nephrotoxicity. *J Pediatr*. 1985;106:861–862.

123. Goren MP, Baker DK, Shenep JL. Vancomycin does not enhance amikacin-induced tubular nephrotoxicity in children. *Pediatr Infect Dis J*. 1989;8:278–282.

124. Brummett RE, Fox KE. Vancomycin- and erythromycin-induced hearing loss in humans. *Antimicrob Agents Chemother*. 1989;33:791–796.

125. Brummett RE, Fox KE, Jacobs F, et al. Augmented gentamicin ototoxicity induced by vancomycin in

guinea pigs. *Arch Otolaryngol Head Neck Surg.* 1990;116:61–64.

126. Traber PG, Levine DP. Vancomycin ototoxicity in a patient with normal renal function. *Ann Intern Med.* 1981;95:458–460.

127. Pryka RD, Rodvold KA, Erdman SM. An updated comparison of drug dosing methods, Part IV. Vancomycin. *Clin Pharmacokinet.* 1991;20:463–476.

128. Lin RY. Desensitization in the management of vancomycin hypersensitivity. *Arch Intern Med.* 1990;150:2197–2198.

129. Polk RE, Healy DP, Schwartz LB, et al. Vancomycin and the red-man syndrome: Pharmacodynamics of histamine release. *J Infect Dis.* 1988;157:502–507.

130. Levy M, Koren G, Dupuis L, Read SE. Vancomycin-induced red man syndrome. *Pediatrics.* 1990;86:572–580.

131. Pau AK, Khakoo R. "Red neck syndrome" with slow infusion of vancomycin. *N Engl J Med.* 1985;313:756–757. Letter.

132. Bailie GR, Kowalsky SF, Eisele G. Red-neck syndrome associated with intraperitoneal vancomycin. *Clin Pharm.* 1990;9:671–672.

133. Killian AD, Sahai JV, Memish ZA. Red man syndrome after oral vancomycin. *Ann Intern Med.* 1991;115:410–411. Letter.

134. Polk RE, Israel D, Wang J, et al. Vancomycin skin tests and prediction of "red man syndrome" in healthy volunteers. *Antimicrob Agents Chemother.* 1993;37:2139–2143.

135. Rybak MJ, Bailey EM, Warbasse LH. Absence of "red man syndrome" in patients treated with vancomycin or high-dose teicoplanin. *Antimicrob Agents Chemother.* 1992;36:1204–1207.

136. Wallace MR, Mascola JR, Oldfield EC. Red man syndrome: Incidence, etiology, and prophylaxis. *J Infect Dis.* 1991;164:1180–1185.

137. Sahai J, Healy DP, Shelton MJ, et al. Comparison of vancomycin- and teicoplanin-induced histamine release and "red man syndrome." *Antimicrob Agents Chemother.* 1990;34:765–769.

138. Sahai J, Healy DP, Garris R, et al. Influence of antihistamine pretreatment on vancomycin-induced red-man syndrome. *J Infect Dis.* 1989;160:876–881.

139. Newfield P, Roizen MF. Hazards of rapid administration of vancomycin. *Ann Intern Med.* 1979;91:581.

140. Lerner A, Dwyer JM. Desensitization to vancomycin. *Ann Intern Med.* 1984;100:157. Letter.

141. Forrence EA, Goldman MP. Vancomycin-associated exfoliative dermatitis. *Drug Intell Clin Pharm.* 1990;24:369–371.

142. Conley NS, Weiner RS, Hiemenz JW. Rigors with vancomycin. *Ann Intern Med.* 1991;115:330. Letter.

143. Clayman MD, Capaldo RA. Vancomycin allergy presenting as fever of unknown origin. *Arch Intern Med.* 1989;149:1425–1426.

144. Henry K, Steinberg I, Crossley KB. Vancomycin-induced neutropenia during treatment of osteomyelitis in an outpatient. *Drug Intell Clin Pharm.* 1986;20:783–785.

145. Milsteen S, Welik R, Heyman MR. Case report: Vancomycin-associated neutropenia in a chronic hemodialysis patient. *Am J Med Sci.* 1987;294:110–113.

146. Mackett RL, Guay DRP. Vancomycin-induced neutropenia. *Can Med Assoc J.* 1985;132:39–40.

147. Koo KB, Bachman RL, Chow AW. Vancomycin-induced neutropenia. *Drug Intell Clin Pharm.* 1986;20:780–782.

148. Codding CE, Ramseyer L, Allon M, et al. Tubulointerstitial nephritis due to vancomycin. *Am J Kidney Dis.* 1989;14:512–515.

149. Eisenberg ES, Robbins N, Lenci M. Vancomycin and interstitial nephritis. *Ann Intern Med.* 1981;95:658. Letter.

150. Ratner SJ. Vancomycin-induced interstitial nephritis. *Am J Med.* 1988;84:561–562. Letter.

151. Bergman MM, Glew RH, Ebert TH. Acute interstitial nephritis associated with vancomycin therapy. *Arch Intern Med.* 1988;148:2139–2140.

152. Walker RW, Heaton A. Thrombocytopenia due to vancomycin. *Lancet.* 1985;1:932. Letter.

153. Christie DJ, van Buren N, Lennon SS, Putnam JL. Vancomycin-dependent antibodies associated with thrombocytopenia and refractoriness to platelet transfusion in patients with leukemia. *Blood.* 1990;75:518–523.

154. Zenon GJ, Cadle RM, Hamill RJ. Vancomycin-induced thrombocytopenia. *Arch Intern Med.* 1991;151:995–996.

155. Dajee H, Laks H, Miller J, Oren R. Profound hypotension from rapid vancomycin administration during cardiac operation. *J Thor Cardiovasc Surg.* 1984;87:145–146.

156. Waters BG, Rosenberg M. Vancomycin-induced hypotension. *Oral Surg.* 1981;52:239–240.

157. Southorn PA, Plevak DJ, Wright AJ, Wilson WR. Adverse effects of vancomycin in the perioperative period. *Mayo Clin Proc.* 1986;61:721–724.

158. Glicklich D, Figura I. Vancomycin and cardiac arrest. *Ann Intern Med.* 1984;101:880. Letter.

159. Cohen LS, Wechsler AS, Mitchell JH, Glick G. Depression of cardiac function by streptomycin and other antimicrobial agents. *Am J Cardiol.* 1970;26:505–511.

160. Stier GR, McGory RW, Spotnitz WD, Schwenzer KJ. Hemodynamic effects of rapid vancomycin infusion in critically ill patients. *Anesth Analg.* 1990;71:394–399.

161. Rothenberg HJ. Anaphylactoid reaction to vancomycin. *JAMA.* 1959;171:1101–1102.

162. Symons NLP, Hobbes AFT, Leaver HK. Anaphylactoid reactions to vancomycin during anaesthesia: Two clinical reports. *Can Anaesth Soc J.* 1985;32:178–181.

163. Polk RE. Anaphylactoid reactions to glycopeptide antibiotics. *J Antimicrob Chemother.* 1991; 27(suppl B):17–29.

164. Charney DI, Gouge SF. Chemical peritonitis secondary to intraperitoneal vancomycin. *Am J Kidney Dis.* 1991;17:76–79.

165. Smith TA, Bailie GR, Eisele G. Chemical peritonitis associated with intraperitoneal vancomycin. *Drug Intell Clin Pharm.* 1991;25:602–603.

166. Leibowitz G, Golan D, Jeshurun D, Brezis M. Mononeuritis multiplex associated with prolonged vancomycin treatment. *Br Med J.* 1990;300:1344. Letter.

167. Huang KC, Heise A, Shrader AK, Tsueda K. Vancomycin enhances the neuromuscular blockade of vecuronium. *Anesth Analg.* 1990;71:194–196.

168. Gatterer G. Spasmodic low back pain in a patient receiving intravenous vancomycin during continuous ambulatory peritoneal dialysis. *Clin Pharm.* 1984;3:87–89.

169. Barg NL, Supena RB, Fekety R. Persistent staphylococcal bacteremia in an intravenous drug abuser. *Antimicrob Agents Chemother.* 1986;29:209–211.

170. Spivey JM, Gal P. Vancomycin pharmacokinetics in neonates. *Am J Dis Child.* 1986;140:859. Letter.

171. Angaran DM, Dias VC, Arom KV, et al. The comparative influence of prophylactic antibiotics on the prothrombin response to warfarin in the postoperative prosthetic cardiac valve patient. *Ann Surg.* 1987;206:155–161.

172. Gupta VD, Stewart KR, Nohria S. Stability of vancomycin hydrochloride in 5% dextrose and 0.9% sodium chloride injections. *Am J Hosp Pharm.* 1986;43:1729–1731.

173. Nahata MC, Miller MA, Durrell DE. Stability of vancomycin hydrochloride in various concentrations of dextrose injection. *Am J Hosp Pharm.* 1987;44:802–804.

174. Nahata MC. Stability of vancomycin hydrochloride in total parenteral nutrient solutions. *Am J Hosp Pharm.* 1989;46:2055–2057.

175. Schilling CG, Watson DM, McCoy HG, Uden DL. Stability and delivery of vancomycin hydrochloride when admixed in a total parenteral nutrition solution. *J Parenter Enter Nutr.* 1989;13:63–64.

176. Strong DK, Ho W, Nairn JG. Visual compatibility of vancomycin and heparin in peritoneal dialysis solutions. *Am J Hosp Pharm.* 1989;46:1832–1833.

177. Seay R, Bostrom B. Apparent compatibility of methotrexate and vancomycin. *Am J Hosp Pharm.* 1990;47:2656–2658.

178. Pritts D, Hancock D. Incompatibility of ceftriaxone with vancomycin. *Am J Hosp Pharm.* 1991;48:77.

179. Chandler SW, Folstad J, Trissel LA. Aztreonam–vancomycin incompatibility. *Am J Hosp Pharm.* 1990;47:1970.

180. Greenberg RN, Saeed AMK, Kennedy DJ, McMillian R. Instability of vancomycin in Infusaid drug pump model 100. *Antimicrob Agents Chemother.* 1987;31:610–611.

181. Brown DL, Mauro LS. Vancomycin dosing chart for use in patients with renal impairment. *Am J Kidney Dis.* 1988;11:15–19.

182. Ackerman BH. Evaluation of three methods for determining initial vancomycin doses. *Drug Intell Clin Pharm.* 1989;23:123–128.

183. Zokufa HZ, Rodvold KA, Blum RA, et al. Simulation of vancomycin peak and trough concentrations using five dosing methods in 37 patients. *Pharmacotherapy.* 1989;9:10–16.

184. Matzke GR, Kovarik JM, Rybak MJ, Boike SC. Evaluation of the vancomycin-clearance:creatinine-clearance relationship for predicting vancomycin dosage. *Clin Pharm.* 1985;4:311–315.

185. Rybak MJ, Boike SC. Individualized vancomycin dosage: Comparison with two dosage nomograms. *Drug Intell Clin Pharm.* 1986;20:64–68.

186. Garrelts JC, Godley PJ, Horton MW, Karboski JA. Accuracy of bayesian, Sawchuk–Zaske, and nomogram dosing methods for vancomycin. *Clin Pharm.* 1987;6:795–799.

187. Lake KD, Peterson CD. Evaluation of a method for initiating vancomycin therapy: Experience in 205 patients. *Pharmacotherapy.* 1988;8:284–286.

188. Musa DM, Pauly DJ. Evaluation of a new vancomycin dosing method. *Pharmacotherapy.* 6987;7:69–72.

189. Gabriel HM, Kildoo CW, Gennrich JL, et al. Prospective evaluation of vancomycin dosage guidelines for neonates. *Clin Pharm.* 1991;10:129–132.

190. Alpert G, Campos JM, Harris MC, et al. Vancomycin dosage in pediatrics reconsidered. *Am J Dis Child.* 1984;138:20–22.

191. Koren G, James A. Vancomycin dosing in preterm infants: Prospective verification of new recommendations. *J Pediatr.* 1987;110:797–798.

192. Ristuccia PA, Ristuccia AM, Bidanset JH, Cunha BA. Comparison of bioassay, high-performance liquid chromatography, and fluorescence polarization immunoassay for quantitative determination of vancomycin in serum. *Ther Drug Monit.* 1984;6:238–242.

193. Pfaller MA, Krogstad DJ, Granich GG, Murray PR. Laboratory evaluation of five assay methods for vancomycin: Bioassay, high-pressure liquid chromatography, fluorescence polarization immunoassay, radioimmunoassay, and fluorescence immunoassay. *J Clin Microbiol.* 1984;20:311–316.

194. Crossley KB, Rotschafer JC, Chern MM, et al. Comparison of a radioimmunoassay and a microbiological assay for measurement of serum vancomycin concentrations. *Antimicrob Agents Chemother.* 1980;17:654–657.

195. Ackerman BH, Berg HG, Strate RG, Rotschafer JC. Comparison of radioimmunoassay and fluorescent polarization immunoassay for quantitative determination of vancomycin concentrations in serum. *J Clin Microbiol.* 1983;18:994–995.

196. Schwenzer KS, Wang CHJ, Anhalt JP. Automated fluorescence polarization immunoassay for monitoring vancomycin. *Ther Drug Monit.* 1983;5:341–345.

197. Yeo KT, Traverse W, Horowitz GL. Clinical performance of the EMIT vancomycin assay. *Clin Chem.* 1989;35:1504–1507.

198. Morse GD, Nairn DK, Bertino JS, Walshe JJ. Overestimation of vancomycin concentrations utilizing fluorescence polarization immunoassay in patients on peritoneal dialysis. *Ther Drug Monit.* 1987;9:212–215.

199. White LO, Edwards R, Holt HA, et al. The in-vitro degradation at 37°C of vancomycin in serum, CAPD fluid and phosphate-buffered saline. *J Antimicrob Chemother.* 1988;22:739–745.

200. Anne L, Hu M, Chan K, et al. Potential problem with fluorescence polarization immunoassay cross-reactivity to vancomycin degradation product CDP-1: Its detection in sera of renally impaired patients. *Ther Drug Monit.* 1989;11:585–591.

201. Hu MW, Anne L, Forni T, Gottwald K. Measurement of vancomycin in renally impaired patient samples using a new high-performance liquid chromatography method with vitamin B_{12} internal standard: Comparison of high-performance liquid chromatography, EMIT, and fluorescence polarization immunoassay methods. *Ther Drug Monit.* 1990;12:562–569.

202. Sawchuk RJ, Zaske DE. Pharmacokinetics of dosing regimens which utilize multiple intravenous infusions: Gentamicin in burn patients. *J Pharmacokinet Biopharm.* 1976;4:183–195.

203. Birt JK, Chandler MHH. Using clinical data to determine vancomycin dosing parameters. *Ther Drug Monit.* 1990;12:206–209.

204. Ackerman BH, Olsen KM, Padilla CB. Errors in assuming a one-compartment model for vancomycin. *Ther Drug Monit.* 1990;12:304–305. Letter.

205. Albrecht LM, Rybak MJ, Boike SC, Pancorbo S. Comparison of serum sampling methods for determining vancomycin dosage regimens. *Ther Drug Monit.* 1988;10:85–90.

206. Uaamnuichai M, Day RB, Brater DC. Bayesian and least-squares methods for vancomycin dosing. *Am J Med Sci* 1987;294:100–104.

207. Pryka RD, Rodvold KA, Garrison M, Rotschafer JC. Individualizing vancomycin dosage regimens: One- versus two-compartment bayesian models. *Ther Drug Monit.* 1989;11:450–454.

208. Burton ME, Gentle DL, Vasko MR. Evaluation of a bayesian method for predicting vancomycin dosing. *Drug Intell Clin Pharm.* 1989;23:294–300.

209. Rodvold KA, Pryka RD, Garrison M, Rotschafer JC. Evaluation of a two-compartment bayesian forecasting program for predicting vancomycin concentrations. *Ther Drug Monit.* 1989;11:269–275.

210. Hurst AK, Yoshinaga MA, Mitani GH, et al. Application of a bayesian method to monitor and adjust vancomycin dosage regimens. *Antimicrob Agents Chemother.* 1990;34:1165–1171.

211. Rodvold KA, Rotschafer JC, Gilliland SS, et al. Bayesian forecasting of vancomycin concentrations with non-steady-state sampling strategies. *Ther Drug Monit.* 1994;16:37–41.

Answers

CHAPTER 1

1. One definition: The use of drug serum concentration measurements, for drugs in which there is (i) a correlation between serum concentration and response, as well as (ii) a narrow range of effective and safe concentrations, to assess patient status as an adjunct to clinical observation.

2. Most people achieve the appropriate pharmacologic effect, with minimum adverse effects, within the digoxin serum concentration range 1 to 2 ng/mL. Most patients receive a subtherapeutic effect below 1 ng/mL but a few patients require levels above 2 ng/mL. Although toxic effects occur most regularly as the level increases above 2 ng/mL, some patients demonstrate adverse reactions at concentrations below 2 ng/mL. This range applies to adult patients with normal electrolytes, thyroid status, and albumin. "Abnormals" may respond outside this range. Lastly, each patient has a patient-specific therapeutic range that may or may not correspond to the population therapeutic range of 1 to 2 ng/mL.

3. In general, it is not necessary to repeat a serum level unless there is reason to believe that the status of the patient has changed. A change in status refers to a number of different factors such as a decline in pharmacologic response, worsening illness, or alteration in pharmacokinetic parameters as a result of a change in diet, addition of new drugs to the regimen, or decline in kidney or liver function. Specifically for gentamicin, if none of the above changes is apparent, it is still usually acceptable to evaluate the serum concentration at 3-day intervals because there is a very narrow range of effective concentrations and the potential for various types of toxicity is great.

4. The most commonly monitored drugs are antibiotics like the aminoglycosides and vancomycin; antiepileptics like carbamazepine, phenytoin, and valproic acid; and the drugs digoxin, lithium, and theophylline.

5. Therapeutic drug monitoring should have a positive effect on patient outcomes if, for the drugs that are monitored using serum concentrations as part of the monitoring process, it improves the response rate to drug therapy, or decreases the time it takes to cure illness or reduce disease severity, or decreases the rate of drug-induced adverse reactions. So these factors may be studied and the data resulting from TDM patients compared with data for "control" patients not exposed to TDM. These represent patient-centered outcomes which are the primary end result desired through the use of TDM. Some sites also use system (or process)-related outcome measures to compare TDM patients with control subjects. Two such outcome measures would be the fraction of patients with drug concentrations in the therapeutic range for TDM compared with control subjects and a comparison of the fraction of patients sampled at the appropriate time.

CHAPTER 2

1. Yes. $C_{avg,ss}$ = 0.9 ng/mL. Use Equation 2–14:

$$C_{avg,ss} = \frac{(S)\,(f)\,(\text{dose}/\tau)}{Cl} = \frac{(1)\,(0.7)\,(250\ \mu g/d)}{2\ mL/kg/min} = \frac{(1)\,(0.7)\,(250/70\ \mu g/kg/d)}{2880\ mL/kg/d}$$

$$= 0.0009\ \mu g/mL = 0.9\ ng/mL$$

2. Yes. $C_{max,ss}$ = 29.4 µg/mL and $C_{min,ss}$ = 9.0 µg/mL. Use Equations 2–22 and 2–24:

$$C_{max,ss} = \frac{(S)\,(f)\,(\text{dose}/V)}{1 - 10^{-0.3(\tau/t_{1/2})}} = \frac{(1)\,(1)\,(1000\ mg/70\ kg/0.7\ L/kg)}{1 - 10^{-0.3(12h/7h)}}$$

$$= 29.4\ \mu g/mL$$

$$C_{min,ss} = (C_{max,ss})\,[10^{-0.3(\tau/t_{1/2})}] = (29.4\ \mu g/mL)\,[10^{-0.3\ (12\ h\,/\,7\ h)}]$$

$$= 9.0\ \mu g/mL$$

3. The patient's clearance is twice as fast as the population normal value: 0.08 L/kg/h. Use Equation 2–18 in rewritten form:

$$Cl = \frac{(S)\,(f)\,(\text{dose}/t_{inf})}{C_{inf,ss}} = \frac{(0.8)\,(1)\,(0.6\ mg/kg/h)}{6.0\ mg/L} = 0.08\ L/kg/h$$

4. (i) The patient needs 301 mg q4h, so use either the 250- or 375-mg dosage forms. The 250- and 375-mg doses underestimate and overestimate the revised $C_{avg,ss}$ of 5.0 µg/mL, respectively. For drugs showing linear pharmacokinetics,

$$\frac{(C_{avg,ss})_1}{(C_{avg,ss})_2} = \frac{(\text{dose rate})_1}{(\text{dose rate})_2}$$

$$\frac{(8.3\ \mu g/mL)_1}{(5.0\ \mu g/mL)_2} = \frac{(500\ mg\ q4h)_1}{(\text{dose rate})_2}$$

$$(\text{dose rate})_2 = 301\ mg\ q4h.$$

(ii) Use Equation 2–14 in rearranged form to estimate the patient's clearance:

$$Cl = \frac{(S)\,(f)\,(\text{dose}/\tau)}{C_{avg,ss}} = \frac{(0.87)\,(0.85)\,(500/70/4\ mg/kg/h)}{8.3\ mg/L}$$

$$= 0.16\ L/kg/h$$

The patient's clearance is 40% of the population value and this explains why the steady-state level is greater than expected.

5. Because $C_{max,ss}$ and $C_{min,ss}$ are commonly used as target concentration ranges for moni-

toring aminoglycosides, a logical approach is to maintain these values in the renally impaired patient similar to those expected in non-renally impaired persons. Although the nurse alone recommended a loading dose, the load will not influence the steady-state values for $C_{max,ss}$ and $C_{min,ss}$. And because the regimens have the same dosage interval, calculating one $C_{max,ss}$ and $C_{min,ss}$ set allows the other levels to be calculated by scaling up or down the nurse's levels in proportion to the variation in dosage for the other two regimens.

Use Equation 2–34 to estimate the patient's lean body weight:

ideal body weight (kg, female) = $45 + (2.3) (66 - 60) = 59$ kg (similar to her total body weight)

Use Equations 2–31 and 2–32 to estimate creatinine clearance in this female patient:

$$Cl_{cr}(males) = \frac{(140 - 30)(60)}{(3.0)(72)} = 30.6 \text{ mL/min}$$

$$Cl_{cr}(females) = 0.85 \times 30.6 = 26 \text{ mL/min}$$

Then use Equation 2–29 to estimate $(t_{1/2})_{ri}$, assuming the population mean values of $F = 0.98$, $(t_{1/2})_n = 2.5$ h, and $(Cl_{cr})_n = 120$ mL/min:

$$\frac{(t_{1/2})_n}{(t_{1/2})_{ri}} = 1 - F + F [(Cl_{cr})_{ri} / (Cl_{cr})_n]$$

$$\frac{(2.5 \text{ h})}{(t_{1/2})_{ri}} = 1 - 0.98 + 0.98 [26/120] = 0.23$$

$$(t_{1/2})_{ri} = 10.9 \text{ hours}$$

Equation 2–22 is used to estimate $C_{max,ss}$ for the nurse's regimen:

$$C_{max,ss} = \frac{(S)(f)(dose/V)}{1 - 10^{-0.3(\tau/t_{1/2})}}$$

$$C_{max,ss} = \frac{(1)(1)(0.75 \text{ mg/kg})/(0.25 \text{ L/kg})}{1 - 10^{-0.3(24 \text{ h}/10.9 \text{ h})}} = 3.8 \text{ mg/L (µg/mL)}$$

And Equation 2–24 is used to estimate $C_{min,ss}$ for the nurse's regimen:

$$C_{min,ss} = (C_{max,ss}) [10^{-0.3 (\tau/t_{1/2})}]$$

$$C_{min,ss} = (3.8) [10^{-0.3 (24 \text{ h}/10.9 \text{ h})}] = 0.8 \text{ µg/mL}$$

To estimate the $C_{max,ss}$ and $C_{min,ss}$ values for the medical resident's and pharmacy student's recommended regimens, multiply the nurse's values by two and four times, respectively:

Medical resident $C_{max,ss} = 7.6$ µg/mL and $C_{min,ss} = 1.6$ µg/mL

Pharmacy student $C_{max,ss} = 15.2$ µg/mL and $C_{min,ss} = 3.2$ µg/mL

As the tobramycin target concentration ranges for $C_{max,ss}$ and $C_{min,ss}$ are 5 to 10 and <2 µg/mL, respectively, the regimen recommended by the medical resident appears to be the most appropriate.

CHAPTER 3

1. The Total Testing Process describes all aspects of the steps of laboratory testing, beginning with a clinical question that is prompted by a patient–physician encounter and concluding with the impact of the test result on patient care. Eleven steps are included in the process. This process ensures that therapeutic drug monitoring is an orderly sequence of events and not just a numerical value for a serum drug concentration.

2. The Total Testing Process comprises preanalytical, analytical, and postanalytical components. These three components include 11 steps: preanalytic (1. clinical question, 2. test selected, 3. test ordered, 4. specimen collected); analytic (5. sample prepared, 6. analysis performed, 7. results verified); and postanalytic (8. results reported, 9. clinical answer, 10. action taken, 11. effect on patient care).

3. The pharmacist, whether acting as part of an organized TDM or clinical pharmacokinetic service or acting alone, plays a direct role in steps 2, 4, and 9, and often advises other clinicians in steps 1, 10, and 11. The test selected in step 2, the timing and method of collecting the specimen in step 4, and the interpretation of the test result in step 9 are important contributions of the pharmacist. Assisting other clinicians in defining the clinical question in step 1, monitoring the action taken in step 10, and auditing the outcome in step 11 are often ancillary but important activities of the pharmacist. In general, TDM can intervene to improve many of the steps in the Total Testing Process: providing education, drug information, and research to improve the formulation of the clinical question and interpretation of the test results; assessing the appropriateness of the TDM test order; scheduling specimen collection; developing drug dosing guidelines; and providing written and oral consultation concerning TDM results.

4. Education of clinicians, monitoring of activities, and feedback to clinicians when appropriate procedures are not met are central to improving the sample collection step. It is important to stress that samples should be obtained during the postdistribution equilibrium portion of a dosage interval once steady state has been achieved. Although waiting for postdistribution equilibrium after administering a dose is always important, some exceptions to the steady-state caveat are reasonable. If the clinician wants a serum concentration after a loading dose, that is reasonable as long as the situation and its limitations for interpretation of the test result are made clear to the practitioner. Also, it is important to stress that full information about the time of sampling, its relationship to the time of administration of the last dose, and the number of previous doses that have been given are important data for proper interpretation of the test result in step 9.

5. A number of problems may occur during the 11 steps of the Total Testing Process. The chapter stresses considerations for each of these steps. Some potential issues include inappropriate ordering of serum concentrations, poor timing of sample collection, inadequate consideration of assay selection, inconsistent follow-through on actions taken as a result of the test result, and inadequate auditing of the effect of ordering the test on patient outcome.

CHAPTER 4

1. The benefits of TDM services have been summarized in four areas:

   i. Achievement of therapeutic concentrations is associated with increased efficacy, reduced frequency of side effects, or both.

ii. Without TDM a large proportion of patients will have serum concentrations outside the therapeutic range.

iii. Making drug assays without a TDM service available to physicians does not improve the quality of treatment.

iv. Dose adjustment based on appropriate interpretation of DCMs reduces the proportion of patients with serum concentrations outside the therapeutic range.

2. Direct benefits of TDM services include improvement in survival, reduction in length of treatment, improvement in recuperation, reduction in treatment costs as a result of side effects, and improvement in patient symptoms (disease status).

3. The amount of training that will be necessary is directly related to the scope of services to be offered. Individuals who have little background in pharmacokinetics need training both in basic pharmacokinetic principles and in the application of pharmacokinetics to patient care. A number of textbooks and self-guided training manuals are available for pharmacokinetics teaching. In addition, software programs have been developed to aid in training of individuals wishing to enhance their skills in basic pharmacokinetic principles. The formation of study groups for improving pharmacokinetic skills may be useful in developing the service. It may also be advantageous to perform practice consultations on patients and scrutinize recommendations of all individuals who review the same patient for internal consistency. The practice evaluation/consultation of patients can help build the confidence of pharmacists who may have had limited experience in providing such consultation in the past.

4. Suggested steps in the development of a TDM service include the following:

    I. Instill the desire (if necessary) to provide the service in individuals who will work in and with the service

   II. Formulate a proposal and plan for service:

      A. Identify potential problems in patient care and resource utilization that might be alleviated by a clinical pharmacokinetic service (CPKS). Review the literature on the benefits of CPKSs and provide any in-house data.

      B. Determine the scope of the service.

        1. Hours of operation

        2. Number of drugs for which consultation will be provided

        3. Limitations on availability

        4. Quality assurance

      C. Evaluate the personnel available and those needed.

      D. Determine the necessity for additional training.

      E. Evaluate the equipment available and that needed.

      F. Assess the cost of the service.

      G. Develop a reimbursement plan.

  III. Recruit support for the service among other health care professionals.

  IV. Approach decision makers (administration, pharmacy and therapeutics committee, etc) with the proposal.

   V. Develop policies and procedures for the service.

  VI. Develop a promotion campaign to announce the service.

 VII. Educate ancillary personnel.

VIII. Initiate the service.

IX. Maintain a high level of visibility and promote the service.

X. Document the benefits of the service to justify its continuation.

XI. Expand the service into other areas of patient care demonstrating a need.

CHAPTER 5

1. • Understand the desired therapeutic outcome of drug therapy and a reasonable length of therapy for the individual patient.
   • Assess the potential efficacy of the drug versus other possible therapies for the specific patient.
   • Determine monitoring parameters (laboratory tests, symptom relief, etc) that will indicate optimal therapeutic outcome.
   • Determine monitoring parameters that will indicate toxic or adverse reactions caused by the drug.

2. The five important process considerations are (1) the time that the last dose was given or taken, (2) the duration of the dose infusion (if given intravenously), (3) the time that the sample was drawn, (4) the patient's relative compliance with regimen, and (5) the quality of the assay used to measure drug concentration.

3. Five factors may affect the desired target concentration: (1) alterations in protein binding that result in more or less unbound drug; (2) certain disease states and aging; (3) assay sensitivity and specificity; (4) degradation (eg, when aminoglycosides are mixed with various penicillins); (5) presence of active metabolites.

4. Drug concentration measurements drawn prior to steady state are not as useful as steady-state concentrations in determining the potential efficacy or toxicity of the current or a future regimen. Depending on whether the final concentration will be more (insufficient or no loading dose, after dose increase) or less (eg, after a loading dose that produces concentrations higher than the maintenance dose at steady state or after dose decrease), the pharmacodynamic response to the steady-state concentration may be quite different than that observed with the non-steady-state DCMs. Thus, many clinicians recommend drawing almost all DCMs at steady state.

5. Drug concentration measurements drawn prior to steadystate on an initial dosing plan can be useful aids when attempting to determine a final dose and schedule to produce desired target concentrations. Notable exceptions to the suggestion to draw DCMs at steady state would be when the patient exhibits signs and symptoms of drug toxicity prior to steady state and when compliance is in question.

CHAPTER 6

1. Intraindividual variability is concerned with the variability that occurs in drug concentrations over time in a particular patient. Patients who return to clinic on a regular basis may have

drug concentrations measured and these drug concentrations will vary from visit to visit, depending on a number of factors including drug assay variability, variability in compliance, changes in the efficiency of drug disposition within the patient over time, errors in recording times of doses and times of sampling for drug concentrations, and variability in bioavailability from visit to visit.

Interindividual variability, on the other hand, is concerned with the consistent differences in pharmacokinetic parameters across the population. Pharmacokinetic parameters of a drug may vary from individual to individual based on genetic differences, diet, exposure to environmental toxins, and so forth.

Any factor that results in consistent differences in pharmacokinetic parameters from one patient to another increases the magnitude of interindividual variability, whereas a factor that results in variability across time within an individual increases the magnitude of residual variability.

2. If the wrong pharmacokinetic structural model is selected and used to fit data, the overall tendency will be to drive up the magnitude of residual variability. This is because drug concentrations will be measured during the distribution phase of the drug for some patients and during the elimination phase for other patients. Indiscriminate pooling of these drug concentrations increases the variability in the measured drug concentrations around the typical drug concentration–time curve.

3. In the least-squares approach, the measured drug concentrations are taken to be correct and no mechanism exists to take into consideration that a drug concentration may be spurious. In the bayesian forecasting scheme, the difference between the measured and the predicted drug concentrations are weighted by the expected residual variability and there are penalties incurred for requiring clearance values that deviate from the typical values, depending on the magnitude of interindividual variability in the pharmacokinetic parameters.

Because of this distinction, bayesian estimates of pharmacokinetic parameters may not appear to fit the data very well if, for example, drug concentrations are considerably different than would be expected given the population estimates of the pharmacokinetic parameters.

4.

$$P(\text{NT}) = \frac{1}{1 + \exp^{-(-8.96 + \text{DURATION} \times 0.098 + \text{CP} \times 0.234 + \text{LIVER} \times 1.49 + \text{AGE} \times 0.051 + \text{CrCl} \times 0.02 + \text{SEX} + 0.725)}}$$

$$= \frac{1}{1 + \exp^{-(-8.96 + 10 \times 0.098 + 10 \times 0.234 + 0 \times 1.49 + 65 \times 0.051 + 40 \times 0.02 + 0 \times 0.725)}}$$

$$= \frac{1}{1 + \exp^{(-8.96 + 0.98 + 0.234 + 0 + 3.31 + 0.8 + 0)}}$$

$$= \frac{1}{1 + \exp^{-(-1.53)}}$$

$$= 17.8\%$$

Using Equation 6–16 and the patient data available, we would predict a probability of 17.8% for the patient to develop nephrotoxicity.

CHAPTER 7

1. a.

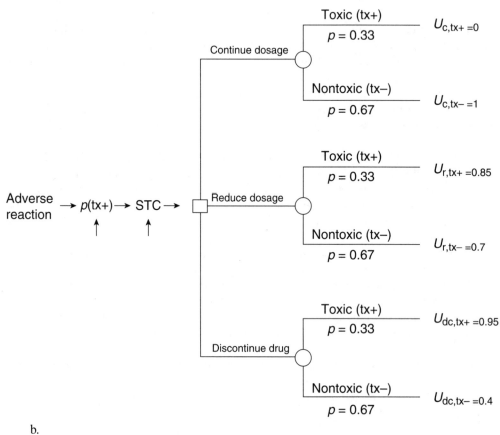

b.

$$EV_c = (0.33 \times 0) + (0.67 \times 1) = 0.67$$

$$EV_r = (0.33 \times 0.85) + (0.67 \times 0.7) = 0.75$$

$$EV_{dc} = (0.33 \times 0.95) + (0.67 \times 0.4) = 0.58$$

The best decision is to reduce the dosage regimen.

2.

a.

Test Result	Patient Status	
	Toxic (tx+)	Nontoxic (tx−)
Positive (> 22 μg/mL)	9	33
Negative (≤ 22 μg/mL)	27	131

a	b
c	d

b. True-positive rate = 0.25, true-negative rate = 0.8, positive predictive value = 0.21, negative predictive value = 0.83, and cutoff likelihood ratio positive = 1.25.

c. The test is more specific (true-negative rate of 0.8 > true-positive rate of 0.25).

d. The test is more correct in saying the patient is nontoxic when SPC is 22 µg/mL or less (negative predictive value of 0.83 > positive predictive value of 0.21).

e. The test makes more mistakes in classifying a patient as nontoxic when he or she is truly toxic (false-negative rate of 0.75 > false-positive rate of 0.20).

f. A SPC cutoff of 22 µg/mL appears to have limited usefulness in separating nontoxic from toxic patients. Test sensitivity is very low; only 25% of toxic patients show a SPC greater than 22 µg/mL. The positive predictive value is also very low; the test classifies the patient accurately for the practitioner, once a SPC is obtained, only 21% of the time. The test is much more effective at ruling toxicity out than it is at ruling toxicity in (negative predictive value of 0.83 >> positive predictive value of 0.21).

3. The following answers are true: a, d, g, and h.

4. Using the odds ratio form of Bayes' formula:

a. posttest odds = pretest odds x range likelihood ratio

$$2.7/1 = 1/2 \text{ x } 5.4$$

posttest probability = odds/1 + odds = 2.7/(1 + 2.7) = 0.73

Using the traditional form of Bayes' formula:

$$\text{Posttest probability} = \frac{p(tx+) \text{ (true-positive range rate)}}{p(tx+) \text{ (true-positive range rate)} + (1 - p(tx+)) \text{ (false-positive range rate)}}$$

$$\text{Posttest probability} = \frac{(0.33)\,(0.38)}{(0.33)\,(0.38) + (0.67)\,(0.07)} = 0.73$$

b. posttest odds = pretest odds x range likelihood ratio

$$1/4 = 1/2 \text{ x } 0.5$$

posttest probability = odds/ 1 + odds = 1/4 / (1 + 1/4) = 0.2

5.

$$T_{dc} = \frac{U_{c,tx-} - U_{dc,tx-}}{(U_{c,tx-} - U_{dc,tx-}) + (U_{dc,tx+} - U_{c,tx+})}$$

$$T_{dc} = \frac{(1.0 - 0.89)}{(1.0 - 0.89) + (0.91 - 0)} = 0.11$$

When the posttest probability of toxicity is greater than 0.11, the best decision is to discontinue the digoxin.

6. The pretest probability of 0.60 is greater than the test or discontinue threshold ($T_{t,dc}$) of 0.53, so the best decision is to discontinue theophylline without ordering a drug level.

CHAPTER 8

1. System-related outcome measures characterize various factors that contribute to the structure and process of providing an organized TDM service within the institution. These measures generally focus on the efficiency and appropriateness of delivering a TDM service and the costs associated with delivering the service (eg, percentage of drug concentration measurements that were not clinically indicated, cost of inappropriate assays). Patient-related outcome measures are more directly related to the clinical effectiveness of the TDM test or service. These measures characterize the direct outcomes of the intervention on the patient specifically or patient care in general (eg, whether the patient had a toxic effect from using the drug, percentage of patients who had toxic reactions to a drug monitored using TDM).

2. Various system-related and patient-related outcome measures are shown in Table 8–1.

3. Donabedian considered that variables used in assessing the quality of care (and thus outcomes assessment of care) could be organized in three categories called structure, process, and outcome. Figure 8–1 displays many of these variables. The structure component refers to elements like equipment and staff. The process component includes activities involved with the delivery of care including, for TDM, variables like the appropriateness of ordering samples and the timing of samples. The outcome component relates to the effect of the health care intervention on the outcome of the patient and includes, for TDM, such variables as the cure rate, toxicity rate, and cost-effectiveness of the TDM service.

4. Figure 8–1 contains many examples. One such illustration is the relationship of the use of a formal TDM service (a structure measure), and the degree of adherence to proper timing of serum concentration sampling (a process measure), to the incidence of toxicity (a patient-related outcome measure).

5. A number of studies have assessed the value of pharmacists, involved either individually or as part of an organized TDM service, in influencing important variables in the TDM process. These studies have usually been performed using an investigative design in which adherence of clinicians to the variable under study is observed pre-TDM as compared with during TDM involvement. Among many variables evaluated, three that may be identified are timing of TDM samples, as noted in Table 8–3; inappropriate responses after obtaining serum drug concentration measurements, as shown in Table 8–4; and patients with drug serum concentration measurements within the therapeutic range, as summarized in Table 8–6. The first two variables, timing and inappropriate response, are system-related administrative process variables; the third variable, dealing with levels within the therapeutic range, is an administrative outcome measure. A number of other variables have been studied.

6. A central premise of TDM is that some drugs (the TDM drugs) have a narrow range of therapeutic serum concentrations that are safe and effective. Given this, an appropriate system-related outcome measure of TDM is the fraction of patients taking TDM drugs that have serum concentrations within the generally accepted therapeutic range. Limitations from a system-related outcome viewpoint are that a serum concentration within the therapeutic range is restricted in its usefulness unless the relationship between the measurement and the time of sampling is known. If the measurement is drawn before postdistribution equilibrium or steady state is achieved, the result may be misinterpreted. From a patient-related outcome viewpoint, the fraction of patients with drug levels within the therapeutic range provides no information about the fraction of patients who responded successfully to the drug or exhibited toxic effects from using the drug.

7. Few studies to date have linked the quality of the various system-related outcome measures to patient-related measures. The assumption that the more administratively based process measures which have been the focus of TDM outcome studies (eg, measures related to the proper timing of samples, samples within the therapeutic range) actually result in more positive patient-related outcomes (eg, improved cure rate, reduced toxicity rate) is largely untested.

8. There are numerous possible answers to this question. Ried and colleagues provide one such approach. Using a meta-analysis of published studies, they compared the rate of drug-induced toxic effects for TDM drugs in patients surveilled using a TDM service as opposed to similar groups of patients monitored empirically without access to TDM. They found the odds of toxic effects were decreased for patients monitored by TDM. A related study would be the evaluation of drug effectiveness of specific TDM drugs in patients followed by a TDM service as opposed to a similar group of patients without access to TDM.

9. Quality of life encompasses a combination of the physical, psychologic, social, and economic factors that impact on the functioning of individuals. The interrelationship of these factors is shown in Figure 8–2. Quality of life is thus a multidimensional assessment of the health status of an individual. Some examples of the potential of TDM for improving quality of life include decreasing drug-induced toxic effects, increasing response to drug therapy, and decreasing the days of hospitalization.

CHAPTER 9

1a. In premature infants and neonates, dosage regimens based on postconceptional age are more appropriate than those generated using postnatal age. Postconceptional age takes into account age-related developmental physiology. In the case of renally excreted medications, kidney morphologic development is occurring up to about 34 to 36 weeks of gestation. Although nephrogenesis is essentially completed by this time, the functional capabilities of the nephrons are still evolving. A premature infant and a term infant may both have a postnatal age of 2 weeks; however, they are at different stages developmentally. Based on your review of the literature, you recommend changing empiric dosing to gentamicin 2.5 mg/kg every 18 hours. You recommend trough and peak serum concentration determinations around the third dose.

1b. On further investigation, you discover that the medication is being administered diluted in 10 mL of fluid via a Buretrol. The maintenance intravenous infusion rate is 5 mL/h and the capacity of the intravenous tubing and drip chamber is 12 mL. Given the way the drug is being administered, it is conceivable that it could take several hours for the infusion to be completed. Although the blood sampling was appropriate, the intravenous delivery system was incapable of ensuring timely and complete drug delivery at such a low infusion rate. Your interpretations of the serum concentrations are inconclusive.

To conduct a meaningful pharmacokinetic analysis and to prevent the delivery of subtherapeutic/nephrotoxic therapy, an alternative method of drug delivery is suggested. A syringe infusion pump containing the dose diluted in 2.5 mL is used to infuse the antibiotic at a rate of 5 mL/h through microbore tubing. The tubing is connected to a port close to the patient. Serum concentration determinations should be repeated around the third dose. Samples are obtained from a port different from that where the medication was infused to avoid backflow contamination.

2a. The most likely reasons for the relatively high aminoglycoside dosing commonly seen in cystic fibrosis patients include (1) the desire to achieve high peak serum concentrations, usually 8 to 12 µg/mL, to optimize pulmonary drug penetration (these levels are needed to eradicate *Pseudomonas* organisms which frequently infect the lungs in the cystic fibrosis population); and (2) the larger volume of distribution and clearance of drug in patients with severe cystic fibrosis.

2b. Several issues must be examined prior to interpretation of these results. As part of the assessment, consider the patient's prior dosing history. On his previous admission, it was determined that J.F. required a dose of 140 mg IV q8h to achieve a peak and trough pair of 8.7 and 0.5 µg/mL, respectively. Also, because of the frequency of his pulmonary exacerbations, J.F. had a permanent single-lumen injection port placed 1 year ago. All his blood work is drawn and his medication administered through this access port. The most likely causes of the observed results are contamination of blood samples by medication being infused and blood drawn from the same injection port (obtaining the samples by this route would explain the high peak concentration) and drawing of the peak level during the infusion.

2c. First, samples should never be obtained from the same port into which the medication is being infused. Second, close attention must be paid to sampling time relative to the infusion. For optimal pharmacokinetic analysis, appropriately timed serum samples should be obtained either from a separate intravenous access site (if available) or via a direct peripheral stick in the contralateral arm from which the antibiotic is being infused.

3a.. One might begin by reviewing the patient's case. How is he responding to therapy, as reflected in the white blood cell count, temperature, pulse, and overall clinical condition. You should also check his culture and sensitivity results. Next you may want to evaluate his antibiotic therapy. Let us start by determining what peak and trough concentrations we might expect from the tobramycin regimen he is receiving. We first determine his creatinine clearance. To do this we need to determine his ideal body weight using Equation 9–1. From the formula his IBW is 73 kg. His actual body weight is 101 kg (222 pounds/2.2 pounds/kg). Using Equation 9–6 we can now determine his creatinine clearance (86.2 mL/min). Plugging this value into Equation 9–9, we calculate the half-life (3.2 hours). Next we need to determine the volume of distribution. Because R.D. is overweight, we use Equations 9–3 and 9–4 to determine his dosing weight (84.2 kg). From Equation 9–5 we get a volume of distribution of 21.9 L. We now plug this information into Equations 9–14 and 9–15 to determine the expected peak and trough concentrations (assume a t' of 0.5 hour). We predict that his peak and trough concentrations will be 6.3 and 1.24 µg/mL, respectively. To verify this regimen, ask for a timed peak and trough pair to be drawn.

3b. Several possible explanations exist. The first is that the levels were obtained during the infusion. This effect could explain both the peak and trough. The high peak may result from drawing the sample from the same arm in which the dose was infused. Careful review of the timing of the infusion and serum samples ruled out these factors. The most likely cause is a lack of correlation of serum creatinine to his true kidney function. A repeat trough concentration determination revealed a similar trough and it was felt that the latter explanation was correct.

3c. If a pharmacokinetic program package is available it can be used; however, the same calculation can be managed using a scientific calculator and the following equations. First, we calculate a new half-life using the available timed samples (C_{post} = 9.4 µg/mL and C_{pre} = 5.0 µg/mL) and Equation 9–16. The dosing interval τ is equal to 8, and t_1, t_2, and t' are equal to 0.5 hour. The half-life derived from these data is 7.1 hours. Next we calculate C_{max} and C_{min} using Equations 9–17 and 9–18. These values are 9.87 and 4.76 µg/mL, respectively. Using these data, solve Equation 9–19 for V_d: $V_d = 21.95$ L. Equation 9–11 can be used to determine a new dosing interval to achieve a peak of 7.0 µg/mL and a trough of 1.5 µg/mL. Using a t' of 0.5 hour, we calculate the dosage interval to be 16.3 hours, which is rounded to 16 hours. The new dose calculated from equation 9–12 is 124.4 mg. Rounding to the nearest 10 mg results in a maintenance dose of 120 mg q16h. This regimen would yield a predicted peak and trough of 6.75 and 1.5 µg/mL, respectively (Equations 9–14 and 9–15). You would recommend a follow-up peak and trough concentration after about three to five doses.

4. Knowing that the assays for the aminoglycoside antibiotics are quite specific, you check to make sure that the samples are being run for tobramycin. You also check to make sure the patient has been receiving his doses on the correct schedule. Finally you want to check how the samples are being handled. Remember that piperacillin will inactivate tobramycin in the blood tube if allowed to sit at room temperature overnight. You recommend that peak and trough serum concentrations be drawn and that the samples be assayed quickly. If this is not possible, you suggest that the samples be spun and the serum frozen at 20 to 70°C until they can be assayed.

CHAPTER 10

1. As B.G. has congestive heart failure the initial bolus of 1 mg/kg should be halved to 0.5 mg/kg (40 mg at a rate no faster than 50 mg/min). Subsequent bolus doses should also be halved to 0.25 mg/kg or 20 mg at 5-minute intervals up to a maximum total dose of 1.5 mg/kg.

2. A total of 1 mg/kg lidocaine was administered. The usual infusion rate in a patient without heart failure would be 2 mg/min. As this patient does have heart failure the infusion rate would need to be cut by 50% to 1 mg/min.

3. Use population-based parameters:

$V_1 = 0.3$ L/kg (CHF)   0.3 L/kg $\times$ 80 kg $= 24$ L
$V_d = 0.88$ L/kg (CHF)   0.88 L/kg $\times$ 80 kg $= 70.4$ L
$Cl_{tot} = 5$ mL/min/kg (CHF with pulmonary edema $=$ class III)
$\quad = 5$ mL/min/kg $\times$ 80 kg $= 400$ mL/min
Desired serum level $= 3$ µg/mL
$C^0 (Vi) = D$ 3 µg/mL (24,000 mL) $= 72,000$ µg $= 72$ mg
$K_0 = 3$ µg/mL (400 mL/min) $= 1200$ µg/min $= 1.2$ mg/min

4. Use the Chiou equation:

V_d (population based) $= 0.88$ L/kg $\times$ 80 kg $= 70.4$ L
$K_0 = $ (initial from #3) $= 1.2$ mg/min
$K_0 = 1.2$ mg/min $\times$ 60 min/h $= 72$ mg/h
$C_1 = 3.2$ µg/mL
$C_2 = 2.8$ µg/mL
$T_1 = 1$ hour
$T_2 = 8$ hours

$$C_1 = \frac{2(72)}{3.2 + 2.8} + \frac{2(70.4)\,(3.2 - 2.8)}{(3.2 + 2.8)\,(8 - 1)} = 25.34 \text{ L/h} = 25,340 \text{ mL/h}$$

$K_0 = $ Cl (cpss)

$$K_0 = 25{,}340 \text{ mL/h } (4 \text{ μg/mL}) = 101{,}360 \text{ μg/h} = 101.36 \text{ mg/h}$$

$$\frac{101.36 \text{ mg/h}}{60 \text{ min/h}} = 1.68 \text{ mg/min} = 1.7 \text{ mg/min}$$

5. The signs and symptoms of lidocaine toxicity include confusion, agitation, vertigo, visual disturbances, tinnitus, nausea, sweating, muscle tremors, paresthesias, sinus arrest, third-degree atrioventricular block, and hypotension, and can progress to respiratory arrest, seizures, and coma. To help prevent these adverse effects careful serum level monitoring is recommended. Lidocaine levels at steady state (6–8 hours after initiation of infusion), 24 hours after initiation of infusion, and daily thereafter are recommended. In addition, because lidocaine clearance decreases during the first 24 hours every attempt should be made to decrease the infusion by 50% after 12 to 24 hours.

Amiodarone

6. Amiodarone, because of the number of potentially serious side effects, should be reserved for use when other antiarrhythmic therapies have failed. C.P. is a young individual who would probably need lifeline drug therapy. A less toxic agent would be a better first choice. If other treatments fail, amiodarone could then be tried.

7. There are two major drug interactions here that would likely occur. C.P.'s current digoxin level is 1.94 (at the upper end of normal). We could reasonably expect the level to double during the first few days of therapy. This would put the level in the toxicity range and symptoms would likely occur. The digoxin dose would need to be reduced by 50% at the onset of therapy with amiodarone to 0.125 mg daily. The prothrombin time is 19 and this could also be expected to double during the first few days of therapy and could lead to bleeding complications. The warfarin dose should also be cut in half at the onset of amiodarone therapy. Digoxin levels and prothrombin times need to be followed closely during the first few weeks of therapy. Digoxin levels every third day after the dosage reduction and every-other-day prothrombin times would be reasonable at this time.

8. The baseline laboratory monitoring parameters would include thyroid function tests (T_3, T_4, TSH), pulmonary function tests, an ophthalmologic examination, and baseline liver function tests.

9. A reasonable loading regimen would be to give 800 to 1600 mg of oral amiodarone daily for 1 to 3 weeks, then 600 mg daily for 1 month, then 200 to 400 mg daily thereafter. The doses may be divided throughout the day to decrease the incidence of gastrointestinal side effects. Intravenous amiodarone is probably not indicated in this patient and should be reserved for those patients with life-threatening, refractory arrhythmias who either need immediate treatment or are unable to take oral medications.

Procainamide

10. Calculate the intravenous loading dose for acute management:

$$\text{Weight} = 195 \text{ pounds} = 89 \text{ kg.}$$
$$V_d = \text{reduced in renal dysfunction} = 1.5 \text{ L/kg}$$
$$t_{1/2} = \text{increased with renal dysfunction} = 10 \text{ hours}$$

$$F = 0.87 \text{ for procainamide HCl}$$
$$= 0.69 \text{ for sustained-release procainamide}$$
$$C_{ss} = 4\text{–}8 \text{ mg/L (mean } 6.0 \text{ mg/L)}$$

A. $D_L = \dfrac{C_{av} \times 1.5 \text{ L/kg}}{F}$

$D_L = \dfrac{6.0 \text{ mg/L} \times 1.5 \text{ L/kg}}{0.87}$

B. $10.3 \text{ mg/kg} \times 89 \text{ kg}$

C. $D_L = 920 \text{ mg IV over 30 to 60 minutes}$

11. Calculate intravenous maintenance dose:

A. $C_{av} = \dfrac{1.44 \times R_0\, F \times t_{1/2}}{V_d}$

B. $6.00 \text{ mg/L} = \dfrac{1.44 \times R_0\, 0.87 \times 10 \text{ hours}}{1.5 \text{ L/kg}}$

C. $R_o = 0.72 \text{ mg/kg/h} = 64 \text{ mg/h} = 1.0 \text{ mg/min}$

12. Convert intravenous to oral maintenance dose:

A. $\text{Daily} = \dfrac{(C_{av} \times \text{maintenance infusion rate} \times 24 \text{ hours)} / F'}{C_{av}}$

B. $D_M = \dfrac{(6.00 \text{ mg/L} \times 64 \text{ mg/h} \times 24 \text{ hours}) / 0.69}{6.00 \text{ mg/L}}$

C. $D_M = 2.2 \text{ g in 4 doses, or } = 500 \text{ mg 6h of a sustained-release procainamide tablet}$

13. As discussed previously, controversy still exists today as to the target serum procainamide levels required for successful therapy. Of additional concern is the relationship between the active metabolite N-acetylprocainamide (NAPA) and the overall therapeutic effects of both procainamide and NAPA. Consequently, even though therapeutic procainamide levels of 4.0 to 8.0 mg/L have been described in the literature, little definitive information exists as to the levels required for both procainamide and NAPA. The clinician may find procainamide levels helpful in fine-tuning therapy, but in the long run, the electrocardiogram offers the greatest help.[142] In using the electrocardiogram, the width of the QRS complex helps the clinician determine therapeutic efficacy (reduction in arrhythmia frequency) while aiding in preventing and/or identifying toxic reactions. QRS complexes wider than 25 to 50% of the baseline widths suggest a need to adjust therapy by reducing or discontinuing procainamide therapy.

Quinidine

14. $\text{Loading dose} = \dfrac{C_{av} \times V_d}{F}$ $\qquad$ weight $= 140 \text{ pounds} = 64 \text{ kg}$

$$D_{L} = \frac{2.5 \text{ mg/L} \times 2.0 \text{ L/kg}}{0.75}$$

D_{L} = 6.7 mg/kg quinidine base or 6.70/0.83 = 8.00 mg/kg quinidine sulfate
D_{L} = 8.0 mg/kg × 64 kg = 512 mg quinidine sulfate as 100 mg every 2 hours times five or six doses

15. Maintenance Dose $= \dfrac{C_{av} \times V_{d}}{1.44 \times F \times t_{1/2}}$

   $= \dfrac{2.5 \text{ mg/L} \times 2.0 \text{ L/kg}}{1.44 \times 0.75 \times 9 \text{ hours}}$

   Maintenance Dose = 0.51 mg/kg/h = 783 mg/d quinidine base, *or* 783 mg/0.62 = 1263 mg/d of a sustained-release quinidine gluconate product, where patient could be given 648 mg (two tablets) every 12 hours to maximize patient compliance.

16. Dosing adjustments are not described in the literature for quinidine in a patient receiving digoxin; however, when quinidine is given along with digoxin, the literature does suggest a 50% reduction in digoxin doses, initially, because quinidine can significantly increase digoxin levels.

17. Quinidine is a weak base with a pK_a of 8.34, and its excretion by the kidney has been shown to be pH dependent. Though only 17% of a given quinidine dose is excreted in the urine, acidification of the urine has been shown to increase the elimination of the drug by the kidneys. As the urine pH decreases toward 6.34, a greater amount of drug is ionized, resulting in increased excretion rates.

18. Wide variations in effective quinidine blood levels, along with narrow therapeutic index, variable serum assay techniques, and altered systemic availability from various products, suggest that blood level monitoring is a useful aid in complementing the clinician's assessments. Use of serum quinidine levels in conjunction with clinical observations, such as patient complaints and electrocardiographic review, allows for prevention of quinidine toxicity and attainment of therapeutic effect.

   It should be appreciated that some of quinidine's toxic effects are not serum level dependent and may occur despite nontoxic levels.

CHAPTER 11

1. The dose of carbamazepine is started slowly in this patient and gradually increased over 4 weeks. As the dose is increased the concentration increases. When the dose is held constant, the concentration begins to decrease.

One could explain this by either poor compliance, autoinduction, or an interaction with another drug. A patient history could rule out the possibility of a drug–drug interaction. The patient history would also give an approximation of the patient's compliance. It is unlikely that the compliance would change suddenly from compliance with the initial regimen to poor compliance 1 month later with a constant dose.

The most likely explanation for this problem is autoinduction of metabolism. Carbamazepine is unique in that it induces its own metabolism. Although the dose was being increased, the autoinduction was masked. When the dose was held constant, the autoinduction was apparent.

2. In this case a maintenance dose of carbamazepine is calculated using average pharmacokinetic parameters. The patient is started on the maintenance dose as the initial dose without a titration period. She quickly achieves a concentration of 10 µg/mL and complains of central nervous system side effects.

Although the estimate of the maintenance dose is accurate, there was a lack of a titration period. With most antiepileptic drugs, there is initial central nervous system depression if initial doses are too high. This patient should have been started on a dose that was one-third to one-fourth of the estimated maintenance dose. This would have allowed time for her to develop tolerance to the central nervous system side effects.

3. This patient continued to have seizures with a phenytoin concentration of 13 µg/mL resulting from a dose of 600 mg/d. Following a 100 mg/d increase in dose, the patient developed lateral gaze nystagmus and had a serum concentration of 26 µg/mL.

Phenytoin displays Michaelis–Menten kinetics and there is a saturation point for metabolism. The nonlinear increase in concentration following the increase in dose suggests that this patient has reached the saturation point for metabolism. If the clinician feels that a new steady state has been reached, he or she can use one of the two-point nomograms to calculate a new maintenance dose. The patient may respond to a dose of 630 mg or 650 mg/d, which could be achieved with a mixture of capsules and the chewable tablet. A "rule of thumb" for phenytoin dosing is to increase the dose of phenytoin by not more than 100 mg/d if the serum concentration is less than 7 µg/mL, by not more than 50 mg/d if the concentration is between 7 and 12 µg/mL, and by not more than 30 mg/d if the serum concentration is more than 12 µg/mL.

A dosage increase of 30 mg/d would have been more appropriate in this patient.

4. A patient who has been well stabilized on phenytoin has a decrease in serum concentration in the third trimester of her pregnancy. Although one could debate the potential teratogenic potential of phenytoin versus other antiepileptic drugs in women of childbearing potential, that decision has been made. The concern is the change in serum concentration.

Compliance should be assessed. It is likely to be good given the past compliance record of this patient. Also, the times of the two serum concentrations should be compared. Assuming that extraneous factors are eliminated, the clinician is faced with a decrease in serum concentration of phenytoin in the third trimester. Several reports document that the clearance of antiepileptic drugs increases in the third trimester. The mechanism is unclear. Some have postulated an increase in free fraction, which will increase clearance and decrease total concentration. Others postulate an increase in intrinsic clearance. In this patient, the free fraction should be assessed. If this is within the usual percentage expected for phenytoin (ie, around 10% unbound), it would indicate an increase in intrinsic clearance and a need to increase the dose, especially if the patient is known to have breakthrough seizures at low concentrations. It is important to note that clearance returns to normal postpartum. Therefore, after this patient delivers, the phenytoin concentration should be checked again.

5. This patient is responding to valproic acid with a serum concentration of 60 µg/mL but complains of abdominal pain.

If the patient does not achieve total control of her seizures, the valproic acid dose could be increased. A serum concentration of 60 µg/mL is in the low "therapeutic" range; however, the size of the dose is being limited by the gastrointestinal side effects. Fewer gastrointestinal side effects are associated with the enteric-coated formulation of valproic acid (Depakote). Therefore, because this patient is responding but the dose and the continuation of therapy are limited by the side effects, a switch to the enteric-coated formulation is indicated. Also, taking the drug with food may be of some benefit. It should be remembered that taking valproic acid decreases the rate but not the extent of absorption.

6. This patient suddenly develops central nervous system side effects after successfully tolerating valproic acid for 2 years. This occurs after the addition of aspirin to her regimen. The total valproic acid concentration has decreased.

Valproic acid is highly protein bound and the binding saturates within the therapeutic range (eg, at concentrations greater than 100 µg/mL). Aspirin is also highly protein bound and has the potential to displace valproic acid from its binding site. If the free fraction of valproic acid increases, the clearance of total drug increases, which would decrease the concentration of total drug if the dose remains constant. Therefore, the free fraction of valproic acid should be measured in this patient. The aspirin should be discontinued and the patient monitored to ensure that the central nervous system side effects resolve.

7. This patient develops sudden symptoms of carbamazepine toxicity after the addition of erythromycin to his therapeutic regimen.

Erythromycin is a ubiquitous inhibitor of the cytochrome P450 enzyme system. It is well documented that erythromycin inhibits the metabolism of carbamazepine. It is therefore likely that this patient is carbamazepine toxic because of a drug–drug interaction. The dose of carbamazepine should be held and the patient should be seen to obtain a serum concentration of carbamazepine. The erythromycin should be discontinued and an alternative antibiotic should be chosen. The carbamazepine should be continued at the current dose after the central nervous system toxic effects resolve.

8. This patient is taking a relatively large dose of valproic every 8 hours but achieves a trough of only 35 µg/mL.

Therapeutic ranges are guidelines, not dogma. The first task is to determine if the patient is responding to the drug with the current serum concentrations. If she is having no seizures the concentration is "therapeutic." If the patient is having seizures, then compliance should be assessed. If this is assured, the formulation and timing of blood samples should be assessed. There is some circadian variability to the pharmacokinetics of valproic acid; however, all of this leaves the clinician with a patient with a low trough despite a large dose. There is intersubject variability in the pharmacokinetics of valproic acid. The patient should be evaluated for enzyme-inducing drugs, and the potential for a drug–drug interaction should be assessed. The possibility of malabsorption exists and the patient's stools should be observed for tablets that are absorbed. Finally, the patient may have a rapid intrinsic clearance. Therefore, a peak and a trough should be assessed. The patient may be absorbing the drug but clearing it quickly. Thus, an increase in dose is appropriate. If the patient has very high peaks and low troughs, the dosing interval could be shortened or the patient could be started on valproic acid sprinkle, which approaches a zero-order input and, thus, would minimize high peaks and low troughs.

9. Phenytoin follows Michaelis–Menten kinetics. This means that the enzymes that metab-

olize the drug may saturate and not be able to metabolize any additional substrate (ie, drug) presented to them. The equation is

$$D = \frac{V_{max} \times C_p}{K_m + C_p}$$

where D = dose (mg/d), V_{max} = maximum rate of metabolism (mg/d), K_m = a constant with a value equal to the plasma concentration at which the rate of metabolism is one-half the V_{max} (µg/mL), and C_p = plasma concentration at steady state (µg/mL). There are two unknowns in this equation: V_{max} and K_m. The clinician can use the Michaelis–Menten equation to calculate a new dose if V_{max} and K_m are known. Unfortunately these values cannot be prospectively predicted and there is significant variability in these values in the population. To approximate a dose, however, the clinician can select a value for one variable and use the equation to solve for the other variable using the concentration from a given dose. There seems to be less variability in K_m than in V_{max}. Therefore, K_m can be fixed at 4 µg/mL and the Michaelis–Menten equation used to calculate a new dose.

First, rearrange the Michaelis–Menten equation to solve for V_{max} using the known values for D and C_p and the selected value for K_m:

$$V_{max} = \frac{(K_m + C_p) * D}{C_p} = \frac{(4 \text{ µg/mL} + 8 \text{ µg/mL}) * 300 \text{ mg}}{8 \text{ µg/mL}} = 450 \text{ mg}$$

Then select a desired phenytoin concentration, for example, 15 µg/mL, and solve for a new dose using the Michaelis–Menten equation:

$$D = \frac{V_{max} * C_p}{K_m + C_p} = \frac{450 \text{ mg} * 15 \text{ µg/mL}}{4 \text{ µg/mL} + 15 \text{ µg/mL}} = 355 \text{ mg/d}$$

Phenytoin tablets contain phenytoin acid and are 100% phenytoin. Phenytoin capsules contain phenytoin sodium and are 92% phenytoin. They can, however, be used in combination to individualize the dose of phenytoin. Increase the dose in this patient to 350 mg/d and monitor the response.

An alternative method of calculating a new dose for this patient would be to use the Sheiner nomogram as described in the text.

If the patient receives two different doses and two steady-state concentrations result from those doses, V_{max} and K_m can be determined for that patient. To do this the clinician needs graph paper, where the y axis is the dose of phenytoin in mg/d and the x axis is the clearance of phenytoin expressed as dose/C_{ss} in L/d. To make this determination, the clinician first plots dose versus clearance for both dose–concentration pairs. The two points determine a straight line and the line should be extended through the y axis and the x axis. The y intercept is V_{max}, and the slope of the line is K_m. The slope is calculated as slope = $(y_1 - y_2)/(x_1 - x_2)$.

Once V_{max} and K_m have been determined for a given patient, a dose that will yield a desired serum concentration can be calculated using the Michaelis–Menten equation. Refer to Figure 2–5 for an illustration of this approach.

In all situations the clinician should remember the guideline that if the serum phenytoin is less than 7 µg/mL, the dose should not be increased by more than 100 mg/d; if the phenytoin concentration is between 7 and 12 µg/mL, the dose should not be increased by more than 50 mg/d; and if the phenytoin concentration is above 12 µg/mL, the dose should not be increased by more than 30 mg/d. The 30-mg capsule, the 50-mg tablet, and the 100-mg capsule may be used to individualize the dose of phenytoin.

10. This patient is a candidate for one of the new antiepileptic drugs. If felbamate is added to this patient's regimen, it must be remembered that felbamate will decrease the clearance of the 10, 11-diepoxide metabolite of carbamazepine. The concentration of the metabolite, which is not routinely measured, increases by 50 to 60%, whereas the concentration of the parent drug decreases by 20 to 30%. Therefore, the dose of carbamazepine should be decreased by about 30% at the time that felbamate is started.

CHAPTER 12

1. Chloramphenicol succinate, 50 mg/kg/d in four divided doses by intravenous infusion over 30 minutes, should be recommended. Hematologic function tests (ie, CBC with differential, platelet count) should be done. Peak and trough serum concentrations should be measured about 24 hours after starting therapy. If the patient's clinical status improves and the serum concentration of chloramphenicol is within the therapeutic range, there is no need to measure the chloramphenicol serum concentration again. Hematologic tests should be repeated after 7 days and every 3 days thereafter for the duration of therapy to identify potential chloramphenicol toxicity.

2. The method of infusion by gravity flow in adults has led to slower than expected delivery of drugs. Similarly, in pediatric patients the doses infused from the intravenous port of a tubing away from patient (eg, Buretrol or Volutrol) can significantly delay the delivery of drugs. The appropriateness of method of infusion, correctness of dose, and times of blood sample collection should be verified. Prolonged delivery can lead to lower than expected peak and higher than expected trough serum concentrations.

3. As many patients with cystic fibrosis are ambulatory, it would be best to give chloramphenicol base capsules. The absorption of chloramphenicol from this product does not depend on pancreatic enzymes, as is the case with oral chloramphenicol palmitate. Cystic fibrosis patients with lower than normal levels of pancreatic lipase may not fully convert chloramphenicol palmitate to active chloramphenicol.

4. Phenobarbital has been shown to induce the metabolism of chloramphenicol. Thus, serum chloramphenicol concentration is likely to decrease during concurrent therapy. This may require an increase in chloramphenicol dose. Chloramphenicol does not influence the disposition of phenobarbital. If phenobarbital therapy is to be continued, chloramphenicol should be remeasured to ensure its therapeutic concentration. Similarly, if phenobarbital is discontinued, the concentration of chloramphenicol should be remeasured to avoid toxic concentrations.

CHAPTER 13

1a. Perphenazine is a competitive inhibitor of NT metabolism resulting in an increase in plasma NT concentration. Her antidepressant response has deteriorated because her plasma NT concentration is outside the therapeutic window of 50 to 150 ng/mL. If her auditory hallucinations have resolved, the perphenazine could be discontinued with no change in her NT dose. A return to the previous plasma NT concentration would be expected along with a return of her antidepressant response. Alternatively, if the perphenazine is continued, the NT dose could be reduced to bring the plasma NT concentration back into the therapeutic window.

1b. Phenytoin (Dilantin) is an enzyme-inducing agent and has increased the metabolic clearance of NT. The NT dose should be increased to bring the plasma NT concentration back into the therapeutic window of 50 to 150 ng/mL. If Dilantin is discontinued while M.S. is still on NT, then reduce the NT dose back to 100 mg/d.

2. G.R. is a rapid hydroxylator of DMI. Approximately one third of rapid hydroxylators may show nonlinear DMI kinetics. G.R.'s hydroxylation enzymes may have become saturated, resulting in a nonlinear increase in the plasma DMI concentration. G.R's problem urinating and dizziness are adverse effects to his high plasma DMI concentration. You should recommend decreasing the DMI dose to 100 mg/d and monitoring G.R.'s antidepressant response, resolution of adverse effects, and plasma DMI concentration. If the DMI dose needs to be increased from 100 mg/d, doses should be made in small increments, such as 25 mg and monitored closely to avoid excessive increases in the plasma DMI concentration.

3. The new antihypertensive agent may competitively inhibit the metabolism of NT, causing T.P.'s plasma NT concentration to increase. You would want to alert the clinic psychiatrist about this possible drug interaction so that T.P.'s plasma NT concentration could be monitored for any significant changes. Learning whether T.P. is a rapid or slow hydroxylator gives you more information about the likelihood of a significant drug–drug interaction. Rapid hydroxylators are more likely to have significant alterations in NT clearance when P450IID6 inhibitors are introduced compared with slow hydroxylators. Also, approximately one third of rapid hydroxylators can exhibit nonlinear pharmacokinetics, which could occur with the introduction of a P450IID6 inhibitor. Both of these factors increase the need for TDM in this patient.

CHAPTER 14

1. Cyclosporine selectively inhibits production of soluble proliferative factors, interleukin-2 (IL-2) and other cytokines. This mechanism is similar to that of the new immunosuppressive agent tacrolimus (FK-506).[102] IL-2 and other cytokines are necessary for helper and cytotoxic T-cell activation, proliferation, and maturation. A lack of cytokine disrupts the activation and proliferation of the helper and cytotoxic T cells that are essential for the rejection process. Once IL-2 gene has been expressed on T cells, however, cyclosporine is unable to inhibit IL-2-dependent activation, because it does not block IL-2 receptor expression or binding of IL-2 on its receptor. In addition, suppressor T cells are relatively spared by cyclosporine therapy, which is important for halting the progress of autoimmune diseases. Cyclosporine is used mainly for prevention of rejection and it is not as effective as corticosteroids or OKT3 in reversing the acute rejection

process once the rejection develops. It does not suppress bone marrow function, which differentiates it from other immunosuppressive agents such as azathioprine.

2. Initial oral cyclosporine doses are usually about 8 to 14 mg/kg/d. For living donor kidney recipients, cyclosporine is given 1 to 2 days before transplantation to achieve therapeutic concentrations at the time of transplantation. This dose is divided twice daily and adjusted to maintain the desired cyclosporine concentrations. Dosage adjustment is empiric as a result of extreme intrapatient variability in absorption and clearance. Administration of oral cyclosporine is usually preferred; however, for those patients who cannot tolerate oral therapy in which cyclosporine absorption is poor, intravenous doses between 3 and 6 mg/kg/d can be given. Hepatic, heart–lung, and pancreatic allograft recipients usually require intravenous cyclosporine in the first few weeks posttransplant. Loading doses are not used when beginning cyclosporine therapy, as side effects would likely occur. The intravenous cyclosporine dose can be given by a continuous 24-hour infusion, which may reduce the renal effects of the drug. To ensure cyclosporine absorption and assess the adequacy of the dose, a trough level should be taken within the first 2 or 3 days of starting therapy. Because absorption and clearance change during the first weeks of therapy, levels should be obtained at least two or three times weekly. After discharge from the hospital, levels should be obtained at least twice per week until the blood levels are stable; usually within 1 or 2 months. Chronic cyclosporine dosing is guided by weekly and then monthly blood concentrations and serum creatinine levels, with most patients requiring approximately 5 to 6 mg/kg cyclosporine daily.

3. Because of the potential variability of the temperature-dependent distribution of cyclosporine between whole blood and plasma, whole blood was recommended as the sample matrix for analysis of cyclosporine. Currently, most transplant centers use whole blood as the sample matrix of choice. High-performance liquid chromatography (HPLC), radioimmunoassay (RIA), and fluorescence polarization immunoassay (FPIA) are the principal analytic methods available for cyclosporine monitoring.

HPLC: HPLC is the reference analytic method and has specificity to detect parent drug and metabolites separately; however, it requires intense labor and technical support for routine reliable monitoring.

RIA: There are three types of radioimmunoassay: nonspecific, specific, and polyclonal. Polyclonal radioimmunoassay, which has cross-reactivity with the parent drug and other metabolites, was first used for routine serum cyclosporine monitoring, and early therapeutic drug monitoring studies showed the clinical utility of this analytic method. Polyclonal RIA is no longer available, and at present, nonspecific RIA using monoclonal antibodies is commercially available. With whole blood as sample matrix, results averaging three to five times higher than those obtained with HPLC have been reported. Specific RIAs employ either a ^{3}H or a ^{125}I tracer and specific monoclonal antibody. These methods still have some cross-reactivity and tend to overestimate actual cyclosporine concentrations compared with HPLC, though RIAs show relatively small variability.

FPIA: There are two types of FPIA, a nonspecific polyclonal FPIA, which generally gives similar results to those of polyclonal RIAs, and specific monoclonal FPIA. Both procedures were developed by the Abbott Company and require the TDx instruments. The FPIA with specific monoclonal antibodies still has some cross-reactivity, and FPIA values were, on average, 24% higher than those obtained by HPLC.

4. There is no definite method to differentiate cyclosporine-induced nephrotoxicity from

graft rejection except for renal tissue biopsy. In both cases, renal dysfunction occurs, which manifests as rising serum creatinine and BUN with reduced urine output; however, it is important to diagnose correctly because the treatments are opposite. Clinically, graft rejection generally manifests as rapidly rising serum creatinine, BUN, graft tenderness, fever, chills, and malaise as well as low cyclosporine trough concentration. On the other hand, cyclosporine-induced nephrotoxicity causes more insidious increases in serum creatinine and BUN over several days with high cyclosporine trough levels. But individual sensitivity to cyclosporine nephrotoxic effects are widely variable and some patients may develop renal toxic effects with low cyclosporine concentrations.

5. Various attempts have been made to manage cyclosporine-induced nephrotoxicity. The most widely accepted method, therapeutic monitoring of blood (or serum) cyclosporine concentrations, has met with modest success. Most transplant clinicians agree that cyclosporine concentrations should be monitored to reduce the toxicity while achieving the optimal effect. Unfortunately, the relationship between cyclosporine concentrations and toxicity (or efficacy) and the therapeutic levels have not been well established. Some patients develop nephrotoxic effects at subtherapeutic levels, whereas others experience graft rejection at relatively high trough concentrations of cyclosporine. Despite its limitations, monitoring of blood concentrations gives a reasonable guideline for managing cyclosporine-induced toxic effects. If toxic levels or upper therapeutic levels occur with a slow rising creatinine but without the obvious signs of graft rejection, such as fever and graft tenderness, then cyclosporine dose should be reduced by 50 mg/d and the creatinine and cyclosporine levels rechecked. If the serum creatinine continues to rise with a low cyclosporine level, graft rejection is likely. Biopsy should be performed to differentiate nephrotoxicity from graft rejection.

Second, various protocol modifications have been made to reduce the nephrotoxic effects of cyclosporine while maintaining its efficacy. In the case of kidney transplantation, the initial delayed renal allograft function appears to be accentuated in the presence of graft ischemia, as often occurs in cadaveric kidneys. Many transplant centers have tried sequential initiation of cyclosporine with other agents to avoid cyclosporine use until the period of acute tubular necrosis has been resolved. During the initial period of acute tubular necrosis, antilymphocyte globulin (or OKT3) with azathioprine and prednisone are used in place of cyclosporine, with a subsequent switch to cyclosporine when diuresis has ensued and the serum creatinine level has fallen below approximately 3 mg/dL. This sequential initiation of cyclosporine appears to shorten the oliguric period and the duration of dialysis among patients having delayed graft function. Some transplant centers have attempted to replace cyclosporine with conventional protocols (azathioprine and prednisone) after a certain period to avoid the chronic toxicity of cyclosporine. These attempts produced mixed results: some demonstrated reasonable success, whereas others showed unacceptably high rejection rates. Most transplant centers in this country remain reluctant to accept this method because of its high risk of rejection and graft failure.

Third, various drugs have been used to prevent cyclosporine nephrotoxicity. Calcium channel blockers, such as verapamil and diltiazem, seem to reduce the nephrotoxic effects of cyclosporine as well as the incidence of delayed graft function. Before and immediately after surgery, diltiazem and verapamil have been used to reduce nephrotoxicity and delayed graft function. These approaches have some advantages, because most patients have mild hypertension after transplantation, which can be treated by these drugs. Both drugs can increase cyclosporine blood concentrations by delaying cyclosporine clearance, which requires lower overall cyclosporine doses to maintain the same trough level. Close monitoring of cyclosporine concentration is required while these drugs are used with cyclosporine to maintain the therapeutic cyclosporine levels. Thromboxane synthetase inhibitors are still undergoing clinical trials to evaluate their efficacy in preventing cyclosporine-induced nephrotoxicity.

6. Anticonvulsants such as phenytoin, phenobarbital, and carbamazepine and the antitubercular drug rifampicin are well known cytochrome P450 enzyme inducers. When these drugs are added to the regimen of a patient receiving cyclosporine, cyclosporine concentrations are decreased significantly, and generally two to five times the normal dose is required to maintain therapeutic trough concentrations. The ratio of cyclosporine concentration to dose decreases within 48 hours and remains low as long as the enzyme-inducing drug therapy is used. After these drugs are discontinued, this effect lasts at least 2 weeks. Among anticonvulsants, valproic acid does not induce this effect and can be used as an alternative.

Macrolide antibiotics such as erythromycin; azole antifungal agents such as ketoconazole, fluconazole, and itraconazole; and calcium channel blockers such as diltiazem and verapamil inhibit the cytochrome P450 enzymes and increase cyclosporine trough concentrations when added to the regimen of a patient receiving cyclosporine. The potency of each drug in inhibiting cytochrome P450 varies, but ketoconazole appears to be the most potent inhibitor; it reduces cyclosporine dosage by 88% while maintaining the same therapeutic concentrations. The increase in cyclosporine trough concentrations begins within 2 days and gradually returns to normal over several weeks after discontinuation of these drugs. During this period, more frequent monitoring is necessary.

7. Bile acids act as an emulsifying agent for lipophilic substances in the gastrointestinal tract, such as cyclosporine. Bile acids are necessary for adequate absorption of cyclosporine in the gastrointestinal tract. During the initial period after liver transplant, a T-tube is placed for monitoring bile acid production and bile acid will be drained externally. Insufficient bile acid in the gastrointestinal tract is one of the major causes of poor bioavailability, and it generally requires much higher doses of oral cyclosporine in the liver transplant patient compared with other transplant patients before T-tube clamping. After 1 to 2 weeks when total bilirubin approaches less than 3 mg/dL, the T-tube will be clamped and bile acids will be directed to the duodenum. After the T-tube is clamped, cyclosporine absorption significantly improves and cyclosporine toxicity may develop if the cyclosporine dose is not reduced.

CHAPTER 15

1. 5 ft 7 in. = 50 kg + (2.3 kg × 7 in.) = 66 kg IBW.
    a. Desired total body stores = 10–13 µg/kg = 660–858 µg. This patient requires 0.75–1.0 mg of digoxin.
    b. The acuteness of the patient's symptoms necessitates the use of a rapid parenteral loading dose rather than a slow load with intermittent daily maintenance doses. Therefore, rapid digitalization would occur intravenously at 6-hour intervals as follows:
       • 0.50 mg IV stat
       • 0.25 mg IV in 6 hours (if inadequate response)
       • 0.125 mg IV in 6 hours (if inadequate response)
       • 0.125 mg IV in 6 hours (if inadequate response)

The total loading dose is 0.75–1.0 mg IV over 12–18 hours (depending on individual response). Prior to administration of each dose, the patient's clinical status is checked for improvement and deterioration.

2. The percentage of drug lost per dosing interval represents the maintenance dose needed by the patient.

A. % loss per day = $14\% + Cl_{cr} \times 0.20$

$$Cl_{cr} = \frac{(140 - age) \times IBW}{70 \times Cr_s}$$

$$= \frac{(140 - 72) \times 66\ kg}{70 \times 1.5}$$

$$= 42.7\ mL/min$$

% loss per day = $14\% + (42.7 \times 0.20)$

$$= 22.5\% \text{ loss every 24 hours}$$

B. 22.5% of 750 μg (total body stores) = $0.225 \times 750 = 168.75$ mg IV

C. $\dfrac{168.75\ mg\ IV}{\%\ absorption}$ = oral dose of tablets, capsules, elixirs

$$\frac{168.75}{0.70} = 240\ \mu g = 0.24\ mg$$

or one 0.25-mg tablet orally every day

In the clinical setting this patient would probably be given 0.25 mg orally of a tablet or 0.2 mg orally of a capsule.

3. It is of primary importance in monitoring our patient receiving digoxin to assess those parameters, subjective and objective, that show improvement in disease symptoms without the development of symptoms of digoxin toxicity:

	Subjective	Objective
Therapeutic efficacy	Easier breathing	Improved paroxysmal nocturnal dyspnea (PND)
	Less fatigue	Diminished pulmonary rales
	Less shortness of breath	Reduced jugular venous distension
	Reduction in use of pillows to sleep	Decreased organomegaly
	Reduction in peripheral edema	Decrease in heart size on chest x-ray
		Loss of weight
		Loss of fluids (input/output)
Toxicity	Gastrointestinal upset	Potassium levels
	Visual disturbances	Serum digoxin concentration
	Dizziness	Serum creatinine for digoxin elimination alterations
	Flip–flop feelings in the chest	Electrocardiogram for digoxin-associated arrythmias

4. Though still somewhat controversial, the literature reports a direct relationship between therapeutic effects and serum levels of 0.5 to 2.0 µg/mL. Additionally, as serum levels approach 2.0 µg/mL, there is reportedly an associated increase in toxic effects. For serum digoxin levels to have clinical applicability, two conditions must be met after initiating therapy.

- Serum levels must be determined after the patient has attained steady-state digoxin concentrations.
- Serum levels must be drawn during the postabsorptive phase of any given dosing interval when the drug has reached equilibrium between the myocardium and the serum.

Levels that are not drawn under appropriate conditions lead to clinically misleading information.

5. As had been discussed on several occasions, it is crucial to review the serum sample along with the overall clinical status of the patient prior to making any recommendations. Of interest in this case is the low potassium level in this patient, which would predispose the patient to digoxin toxicity, even if serum digoxin levels are within the reported therapeutic range. Our patient has no complaints at this time, but it is recommended that a potassium supplement be administered to the patient and the clinical status reevaluated after such supplementation. It would be premature to alter digoxin doses at this time, but as long as the potassium level is low, close monitoring of this patient is required to identify potential signs of digoxin toxicity.

6. As a result of the documented drug–drug interactions described between digoxin and quinidine, closer attention to serum digoxin concentrations prior to quinidine therapy is needed. Quinidine has been shown to reduce digoxin's renal clearance while additionally altering its volume of distribution with a resultant increase in serum digoxin concentrations. A serum level obtained prior to quinidine therapy will enable the clinician to reduce the digoxin dose as needed prior to a potential doubling in serum levels after initiating quinidine therapy. It has been suggested in the literature that the digoxin dose be reduced by 50% when initiating quinidine therapy, to avoid inducing digoxin toxicity.

CHAPTER 16

As M.B. has been on lithium therapy for several years, apparently successfully until this current episode, it may be reasonable to use her previous dose and corresponding lithium serum concentration as a starting point. The important point to consider here is exactly what lithium concentration she was maintained on for the last few years: Was it higher or lower than 0.8 mmol/L. M.B. apparently relapsed while taking her lithium and stopped it only after the manic episode was underway. Also recall that patients experiencing an acute manic episode often require higher lithium plasma concentrations during the initial part of therapy versus maintenance therapy.

If M.B. is maintained at a concentration below 0.8 mmol/L, then the usually linear relationship of lithium dose to plasma concentration, in the therapeutic range, can be used to adjust the dose to achieve a lithium concentration greater than 0.8 mmol/L. In most patients, an increase of 8 mmol/d will result in an increase of 0.3 ± 0.1 mmol/L in the lithium plasma concentration. Even if she had been maintained at a lithium concentration of 0.8 mmol/L or higher prior to relapse, the concentration still may need to be adjusted upward. In this case the same proportionality can be used to adjust her lithium dose, but extra care needs to be taken in monitoring her therapy because she may need lithium concentrations in the range 1.0 to 1.5 mmol/L for control of this acute episode.

If no information concerning M.B.'s previous dose was available, she could simply be started at an initial dose of 300 mg of lithium carbonate three times a day for several days, and then the dose could be adjusted to achieve the desired plasma concentration as discussed in the section Dosing for Acute Therapy.

Monitoring of the lithium level acutely would be as described in the following question, except that an interim level prior to steady state would be of increased importance if the target lithium concentration is greater than 1.0 mmol/L. It is essential that the following be kept in mind before starting lithium therapy in any patient who might have been on lithium in the recent past, particularly when the history of the last ingested dose is unclear. As M.B. is reported to have taken no lithium for about a week and, therefore, her lithium plasma concentration would be expected to be zero, this kind of a history should never be taken as fact. A lithium concentration should always be measured to confirm the history prior to the initiation of therapy.

Alternately, one of the predictive dosing methods discussed could be used to estimate a reasonable starting dose for M.B..

2. The Zetin equation is:

$$dose = 486.8 + (746.83 \times desired\ level) - (10.08 \times age) + (5.95 \times weight\ [kg]) + (92.01 \times status) + (147.8 \times sex) - (74.73 \times TCA)$$

where status = 1 for inpatient, 0 for outpatient; sex = 1 for male, 0 for female; TCA = 1 for concurrent TCA administration, otherwise 0. The dose calculated is the daily dose of lithium carbonate.

As M.B. is to be treated as an inpatient, status = 1, she is female so sex = 0, and no TCA will be used so that factor = 0 in the algorithm. This gives the following when the appropriate substitutions are made:

$$dose = 486.8 + (746.83 \times 0.9\ mmol/L) - (10.08 \times 36\ years) + (5.95 \times [142/2.2]\ kg) + (92.01 \times 1) + (147.8 \times 0) - (74.73 \times 0)$$
$$= 1272\ mg\ lithium\ carbonate$$

Rounding to the nearest 300 mg gives a reasonable starting dose of 1200 mg per day of lithium carbonate. To use the 12-hour lithium serum concentration to monitor the progress of therapy, the dose will need to be divided into two doses of 600 mg each of lithium carbonate.

Using an average adult half-life of 18 hours, M.B. would be expected to be at steady state in about 5 days (18 hours × 7 half-lives to steady state = 5.25 days). Therefore, a level should be checked at this time point. Additionally, to ensure that the dose has not been overestimated, it would be reasonable to check a level after several days of therapy. Between 75 and 87.5% of the steady-state concentration should be achieved in 36 to 54 hours (two to three half-lives) based on an 18-hour half-life. The need for this interim level is unclear; simple clinical monitoring for toxicity is sufficient in many cases. But because the toxic symptoms of lithium can display a lag period, an interim level is not an unreasonable precaution. A basic requirement for the use of any of the prospective dosing methods is familiarity with the tendency of the method to over- or underestimate the dose in a given patient population. Therefore, when beginning to use a method for a certain patient population, the clinician would be wise to check interim levels until an understanding of the limitations of the method is achieved.

3. There are no specific standards for lithium concentration determination. Generally a weekly concentration is determined until symptom stability is obtained and then for 1 to 2 weeks afterward to ensure stability of the lithium concentration. Weekly monitoring would be reinstituted at later points in therapy if a dose adjustment is required. Once control of the mood disor-

der is gained and the patient enters maintenance therapy, it is typical to obtain a level every 3 months. Situations where increased frequency of concentration determination would be appropriated include intercurrent infection, changes in diet, debilitation from any cause, and recurrence of affective symptoms. Additionally, it may be desirable to monitor the lithium concentration monthly for individuals in whom control of mania is difficult to maintain. Increased frequency of monitoring must be balanced by the invasiveness of the blood collection, which may be poorly tolerated by many individuals and cannot substitute for good clinical observation. For these individuals, patient and family education on the importance of monitoring for prodromal indications of relapse for the specific patient, along with prompt reporting of such symptoms, may be a more effective strategy than increased frequency of concentration monitoring.

"Now" lithium concentration determination may be considered if toxicity or noncompliance is suspected. Unfortunately, such determinations are difficult to interpret as they are rarely taken at the 12-hour postdose time point. A concentration moderately higher or lower than anticipated may simply be due to the draw time, whereas a significantly low concentration may indicate noncompliance. Alternately, an apparently toxic concentration should not trigger undue concern in an individual with no symptoms of toxicity. A repeat concentration determination may be appropriate depending on the magnitude of the elevation and an interview with the patient. Elevated concentrations may simply indicate a dose still in the absorption period, but may not necessarily indicate consistent compliance with medication therapy, as a patient might take several extra tablets just before a scheduled concentration determination in an attempt to "catch up." A more helpful therapeutic strategy to address noncompliance might be to discuss your concern with the patient and schedule a return visit with 12-hour postdose concentration determination sometime in the next few days. The interval should be short enough that steady state could not be reached if the patient immediately resumed medication therapy. Unfortunately, simple concentration determinations may be insufficient to uncover inconsistent noncompliance and do not substitute for a good relationship with both the patient and his or her family.

CHAPTER 17

1. This patient has the following risk factors:
   - Prior cisplatin therapy: Although this patient experienced greater than 90% tumor necrosis from intraarterial cisplatin therapy, she was left with residual renal failure. Prior to starting methotrexate therapy, a 12-hour urine collection was obtained, and a creatinine clearance of 30 mL/min/1.73 m^2 was estimated. As methotrexate is eliminated primarily by renal mechanisms, patients with renal dysfunction would be placed at high risk for delayed elimination.
   - Pleural effusion: Pleural effusions, ascites, and other pharmacologic "third spaces" may sequester methotrexate for extended periods, leading to prolonged systemic exposure. If prolonged elimination is documented by serial methotrexate plasma concentrations, clinical management includes thoracentesis, to drain the pleural cavity of pleural fluid harboring methotrexate, and adequate leucovorin rescue, to protect normal host tissue from methotrexate toxicity. This patient experienced delayed elimination after receiving the first course of high-dose methotrexate. A log concentration versus time plot (see Figure A–1) revealed prolonged elimination after approximately

72 hours. The elimination half-life for the first 24 hours may be calculated with the following formulas:

$$t_{1/2} = 0.693 / K_{el}$$

$$K_{el} = \ln (C_1/C_2) / \Delta T$$

From the data presented on the graph, the following may be calculated:

$$K_{el} = \ln(1149/13.5) / 18 \text{ hours}$$

$$= 0.25 \text{ hour}^{-1}$$

$$t_{1/2} = 0.693/0.25 \text{ hour}^{-1}$$

$$= 2.77 \text{ hours}$$

This calculated half-life reflects the renal elimination of methotrexate, and because it is under 3.5 hours, the patient would not be considered high risk for methotrexate toxicity within the first 24 hours. It would appear that the renal dysfunction present in this patient is not clinically affecting the renal excretion of methotrexate during the first 24 hours. Concentrations after 24 hours reflect tissue redistribution, which is a nonlinear process. Calculating the half-life beyond the initial 24-hour elimination, therefore, would not be adequate for monitoring patients at risk. One would require serial methotrexate concentrations every 12 to 24 hours to make an appropriate leucovorin dosage recommendation.

2. The leucovorin rescue strategy proposed by Evans et al for high-risk patients would be an appropriate approach, based on the following table:

MTX Concentration (mM)	LCV Dosage (mg/m^2)
90–100	1000 q3h IV
80–90	900 q3h IV
70–80	800 q3h IV
60–70	700 q3h IV
50–60	600 q3h IV
40–50	500 q3h IV
30–40	400 q3h IV
20–30	300 q3h IV
15–20	200 q3h IV
10–15	150 q3h IV
5–10	100 q3h IV
2–5	50 q6h IV
1–2	25 q6h IV or PO
0.5–1	15 q6h IV or PO
0.1–0.5	15 q12h IV or PO
0.05–0.1	5 q12h PO or IV
<0.05	Discontinue

A leucovorin dose of at least 150 mg/m^2 IV q3h should be instituted at 48 hours so that the patient is protected against excessive gastrointestinal toxic effects or profound neutropenia. Serial methotrexate concentrations should be obtained every 24 hours to ensure appropriate leucovorin dosage and methotrexate metabolic clearance. Leucovorin rescue should continue until methotrexate concentrations are below cytotoxic levels (0.05 μM). In addition to adequate leucovorin, thoracentesis may be attempted to remove the methotrexate depot. Other interventions, such as oral cholestyramine, have not been successful in the clinical setting and should be reserved for cases of methotrexate overdose in combination with charcoal dialysis.

3. Adequate hydration and alkalinization should begin 12 to 24 hours prior to methotrexate administration and continue until methotrexate concentrations are below 1 μM. This patient should be given IV fluid at the rate of 3000 mL/m^2/24 hours with adequate bicarbonate to maintain the urine pH above 6.5 to 7.0. As high-dose methotrexate may be moderately emetogenic, antiemetic therapy should be in place. Many antiemetic regimens exist, and the appropriate regimen should be tailored to meet the needs of the individual patient. Because this patient has a history of seizure disorders, butyrophenones and phenothiazines should be avoided. Serotonin antagonists, metoclopramide, or ondansetron would be acceptable in this case.

If this patient's BSA is 1.35 m^2, appropriate orders for hydration and antiemetics would state:

- IV fluid—D5W with sodium bicarbonate 50 mEq/L to run at 170 mL/h (3 L/m^2/24 hour).
- Please check urine pH with each void. If pH is below 6.5, increase bicarbonate in IV fluid to 100 mEq/L.
- Strict I/O and daily weight, vital signs every shift.
- Ondansetron 10 mg IVPB 30 minutes prior to methotrexate administration and q8h around the clock. For breakthrough nausea, may give an additional ondansetron 10 mg IVPB.

(*Note:* In clinical trials, ondansetron has been administered as a continuous infusion. An alternate approach employed at the M. D. Anderson Cancer Center is to supply ondansetron in the IV hydration. To avoid physical incompatibility, sodium acetate rather than sodium bicarbonate should be used for alkalinization. The new order might read: D5W with sodium acetate 70 mEq, ondansetron 6 mg, to run at 170 mL/h. For breakthrough nausea or vomiting, ondansetron 5 to 10 mg may be administered IVPB prn.)

4. This patient may be at risk for seizure activity during high-dose methotrexate therapy because of increased renal elimination of phenobarbital. The percentage of phenobarbital excreted in the urine as parent drug ranges from 20 to 40%. Because phenobarbital is a weak acid and therefore ionized at an alkaline pH, the alkalinization required to facilitate methotrexate clearance would also enhance phenobarbital clearance by decreasing renal reabsorption.

It would be reasonable to obtain phenobarbital serum concentrations prior to high-dose methotrexate therapy and serially during routine alkalinization. The patient should be observed for seizures, and prn orders for lorazepam for breakthrough seizures should be obtained. To reestablish an adequate phenobarbital concentration, the patient may be dosed based on the following equation:

$$\text{incremental loading dose} = (C_{p,\text{desired}} - C_{p,\text{observed}}) \times \text{volume of distribution}$$

As phenobarbital has a long half-life, it should be recognized that several days to weeks is needed to reestablish a steady-state situation.

5. The patient with no nausea or vomiting demonstrating adequate oral intake may be discharged on oral leucovorin with appropriate clinic follow-up. Compliance with clinic visits should be stressed, as inadequate leucovorin rescue may result in mucositis, diarrhea, and profound neutropenia. The patient with prolonged methotrexate elimination should remain hospitalized with hydration until the methotrexate concentration falls below 1 μM. Once this concentration is achieved, oral leucovorin therapy may be started and the patient discharged with daily clinic appointments for methotrexate serum concentrations and leucovorin adjustments.

CHAPTER 18

1. Treatment for J.R. consists of the following:
- Intravenous hydration
- Activated charcoal 1 g/kg with 100 mL of 70% sorbitol (Do not administer multiple-dose activated charcoal.)
- Admission to hospital for observation

The patient is most likely in a toxic condition (assuming that his compliance has not changed), secondary to the acute viral infection reducing the clearance of theophylline.

2. The patient, assuming she has been compliant, most likely has had a significant mixed-function oxidase induction from rifampin which has increased her theophylline clearance.

3. Theophylline can have dose-dependent pharmacokinetics. The most likely explanation is that the dose of 1800 mg/d exceed the V_{max} of theophylline and Mr. Henry accumulated drug.

4. Theophylline exerts a diuretic action on the kidney, hence the increased water loss.

CHAPTER 19

1. Any of the initial adult dosing methods could be used. The following recommendations would result depending on the method chosen:

Moellering's Nomogram: $Cl_{cr,female}$ = 0.73 mL/min/kg
   Loading Dose: 15 mg/kg = 840 mg
   Dose: 10.8 mg/kg/24 hrs = 604.8 mg/24 hours
   Thus: 850 mg initially and then 600 mg q24h or 300 mg q12h

Brown's Table: $Cl_{cr,female}$ = 41 mL/min
   Loading Dose: 15 mg/kg = 840 mg
   Dose: 750 mg/dose
   Interval: q24h
   Thus: 850 mg initially and then 750 mg q24h

Matzke's Nomogram: $Cl_{cr,female}$ = 41 mL/min
   Loading Dose: 25 mg/kg = 1400 mg
   Dose: 19 mg/kg/dose = 1064 mg/dose
   Interval: q36h
   Thus: 1400 mg initially and then 1050 mg q36h

Lake's Guidelines: $Cl_{cr,female}$ = 41 mL/min
Dose: 8 mg/kg/dose = 448 mg/dose
Interval: q18h
Thus: 450 mg q18h

Rodvold's Guidelines: $Cl_{cr,female}$ = 53 mL/min/70 kg
Dose: 17.7 mg/kg/24 hours = 991 mg/24 hours
Interval: q12h
Thus: 500 mg q12h

2. You could use the proportional dosing method, Sawchuk–Zaske one-compartment model, or bayesian one- or two-compartment model if you had the computer software.

Proportional Dosing Method

- 1000 mg produces a change in peak to trough concentrations of 64.9 mg/L − 19.4 mg/L = 45.5 mg/L. So, every 100 mg of vancomycin produces a concentration change of 4.6 mg/L.
- As the trough concentration is greater then 10 mg/L with an q12h interval, you would empirically change the interval to q24h to lower the trough toward 5 to 10 mg/L.
- A change in concentration of about 25 mg/L is needed to achieve peaks of 30 to 40 mg/L from 5 to 10 mg/L. Thus, 550 mg should be infused over 60 minutes q24h.

Sawchuk–Zaske Method

- Calculated parameters: C_{max} = 65.5 mg/L; $V_{d,ss}$ = 0.34 L/kg; $t_{1/2}$ = 6.1 hours.
- Recommended dose (infused over 60 minutes) and predicted serum vancomycin concentrations for this dosage: 500 mg q12h, resulting in C_{max} = 33.2 mg/L and C_{min} = 9.5 mg/L.

Bayesian One-Compartment Model[207]

- Calculated parameters: $V_{d,ss}$ = 0.61 L/kg; $t_{1/2}$ = 10.7 hours; Cl = 37 mL/min.
- Recommended dose (infused over 60 minutes) and predicted serum vancomycin concentration for this dosage: 1000 mg q24h, resulting in C_{max} = 35.5 mg/L and C_{min} = 8.1 mg/L.

Bayesian Two-Compartment Model[207, 209, 211]

- Calculated parameters: $V_{d,ss}$ = 0.64 L/kg; $t_{1/2}$ = 10.8 hours; Cl = 42 mL/min.
- Recommended dose (infused over 60 minutes) and predicted serum vancomycin concentration for this dosage: 750 mg q24h, resulting in C_{max} = 36.2 mg/L and C_{min} = 4.9 mg/L.

3. A set of peak and trough serum concentrations collected once weekly should be more than adequate. Some clinicians may use only a trough concentration to monitor therapy after the first set of peak and trough concentrations have been obtained. More aggressive monitoring may be needed if the patient's renal function changes or other nephrotoxic agents are concurrently being administered (eg, aminoglycosides). The timing of peak concentrations (eg, 15, 30, or 60 minutes after the end of the infusion) depends on how the clinician will use the concentrations in further calculations as well as the therapeutic range used for the interpretation. Trough concentrations should be obtained just before the next dose is administered.

Index